The Respiratory Tract in Pediatric Critical Illness and Injury

Derek S. Wheeler, Hector R. Wong, and Thomas P. Shanley (Eds.)

The Respiratory Tract in Pediatric Critical Illness and Injury

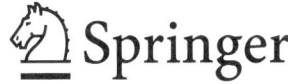

Editors
Derek S. Wheeler, MD
Assistant Professor of Clinical Pediatrics
University of Cincinnati College of Medicine
Division of Critical Care Medicine
Cincinnati Children's Hospital Medical Center
Cincinnati, OH, USA

Hector R. Wong, MD
Professor of Pediatrics
University of Cincinnati College of Medicine
Director, Division of Critical Care Medicine
Cincinnati Children's Hospital Medical Center
Cincinnati, OH, USA

Thomas P. Shanley, MD
Ferrantino Professor of Pediatrics and
    Communicable Diseases
University of Michigan Medical Center
Director, Division of Critical Care Medicine
C.S. Mott Children's Hospital
Ann Arbor, MI, USA

ISBN 978-1-84800-924-0   e-ISBN 978-1-84800-925-7
DOI 10.1007/978-1-84800-925-7

British Library Cataloguing in Publication Data
A catalogue record for this book is available from the British Library

Library of Congress Control Number: 2008940131

Springer Science+Business Media
springer.com

Preface

The principal role of the respiratory system is to permit efficient exchange of respiratory gases (O_2 and CO_2) with the environment. The respiratory system is unique in that it is constantly exposed to a barrage of foreign substances from both the internal environment (at any one point in time, approximately one-half of the cardiac output is received by the lungs) and the external environment (with each breath, the respiratory tract is exposed to pollens, viruses, bacteria, smoke, etc). According to the Centers for Disease Control and Prevention, diseases of the respiratory system were the seventh and eighth leading causes of deaths in children aged 1 to 19 years in 2003 [1]. Dr. George A. Gregory, one of the founding fathers of pediatric critical care medicine, once estimated that acute respiratory failure accounts for nearly 50% of all admissions to the pediatric intensive care unit (PICU) [2]. Just as important are the many diseases that affect the respiratory system that are not associated with acute respiratory failure, but nevertheless constitute a major portion of the practice of pediatric critical care medicine, some of which account for significant morbidity and mortality [3]. Once again, we would like to dedicate this textbook to our families and to the physicians and nurses who provide steadfast care every day in pediatric intensive care units across the globe.

Derek S. Wheeler
Hector R. Wong
Thomas P. Shanley

References

1. Martin JA, Kochanek KD, Strobino DM, Guyer B, MacDorman MF. Annual summary of vital statistics—2003. Pediatrics 2005;115:619–34.
2. Gregory GA. Respiratory Failure in the Child. New York: Churchill Livingstone, 1981.
3. Vidyasagar D. Clinical Diagnosis of Respiratory Failure in Infants and Children. New York: Churchill Livingstone, 1981.

Preface to *Pediatric Critical Care Medicine: Basic Science and Clinical Evidence*

The field of critical care medicine is growing at a tremendous pace, and tremendous advances in the understanding of critical illness have been realized in the last decade. My family has directly benefited from some of the technological and scientific advances made in the care of critically ill children. My son Ryan was born during my third year of medical school. By some peculiar happenstance, I was nearing completion of a 4-week rotation in the newborn intensive care unit (NICU). The head of the pediatrics clerkship was kind enough to let me have a few days off around the time of the delivery—my wife, Cathy, was 2 weeks past her due date and had been scheduled for elective induction. Ryan was delivered through thick meconium-stained amniotic fluid and developed breathing difficulty shortly after delivery. His breathing worsened over the next few hours, so he was placed on the ventilator. I will never forget the feelings of utter helplessness my wife and I felt as the NICU transport team wheeled Ryan away in the transport isolette. The transport physician, one of my supervising third-year pediatrics residents during my rotation the past month, told me that Ryan was more than likely going to require extracorporeal membrane oxygenation (ECMO). I knew enough about ECMO at that time to know that I should be scared! The next 4 days were some of the most difficult moments I have ever experienced as a parent, watching the blood being pumped out of my tiny son's body through the membrane oxygenator and roller pump, slowly back into his body (Figures 1 and 2). I remember the fear of each day when we would be told of the results of his daily head ultrasound, looking for evidence of intracranial hemorrhage, and then the relief when we were told that there was no bleeding. I remember the hope and excitement on the day Ryan came off ECMO, as well as the concern when he had to be sent home on supplemental oxygen. Today, Ryan is

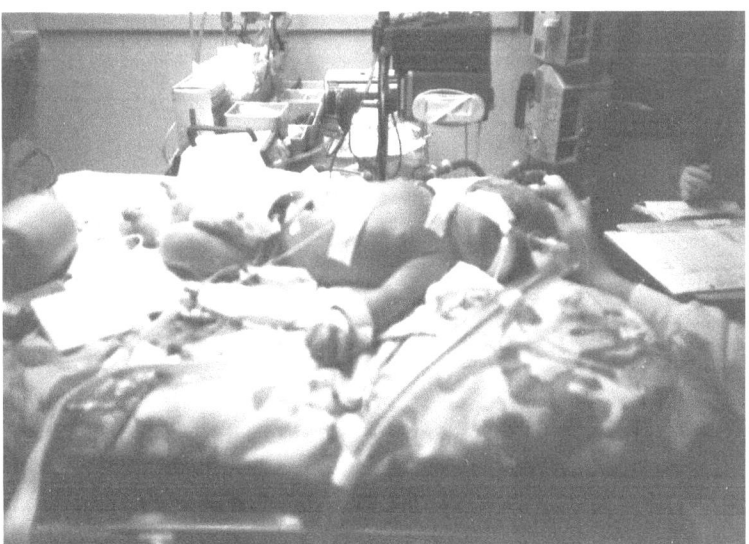

FIGURE 1

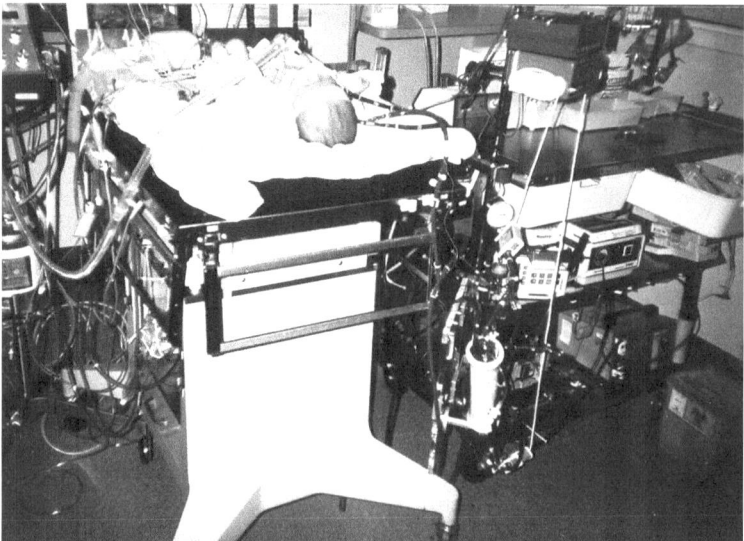

FIGURE 2

happy, healthy, and strong. We are thankful to all the doctors, nurses, respiratory therapists, and ECMO specialists who cared for Ryan and made him well. We still keep in touch with many of them. Without the technological advances and medical breakthroughs made in the fields of neonatal intensive care and pediatric critical care medicine, things very well could have been much different. I made a promise to myself long ago that I would dedicate the rest of my professional career to advancing the field of pediatric critical care medicine as payment for the gifts with which we, my wife and I, have been truly blessed. It is my sincere hope that this textbook, which has truly been a labor of joy, will educate a whole new generation of critical care professionals and in so doing help make that first step toward keeping my promise.

Derek S. Wheeler

Contents

Contributors

John H. Arnold, MD
Associate Professor of Anesthesia
Harvard Medical School
Senior Associate in Anesthesiology,
    Critical Care
Medical Director, Respiratory Care
Children's Hospital Boston
Boston, MA, USA

Margaret A. Chase, MD
Division of Critical Care Medicine
Cincinnati Children's Hospital
    Medical Center
Cincinnati, OH, USA

Patricia R. Chess, MD
Associate Professor of Pediatrics and
    Biomedical Engineering
University of Rochester Medical Center
Division of Neonatology
Golisano Children's Hospital at Strong
    Rochester
Rochester, NY, USA

David N. Cornfield, MD
Professor of Pediatrics
Stanford University School of Medicine
Divisions of Pediatric Pulmonology and
    Critical Care Medicine
Lucille Packard Children's Hospital
Palo Alto, CA, USA

Peter N. Cox, MBChB, DCH, FFARCS, FRCP
Associate Professor of Anaesthesia and
    Critical Care Medicine
University of Toronto School of Medicine
Departments of Critical Care Medicine and
    Lung Biology
The Hospital for Sick Children, Toronto
Toronto, Ontario, Canada

Martha A.Q. Curley, RN, PhD, FAAN
Assistant Professor of Anesthesiology

Harvard Medical School
Director Critical Care and Cardiovascular
    Nursing Research
Children's Hospital Boston
Boston, MA, USA

Heidi J. Dalton, MD, FCCM
Professor of Pediatrics
George Washington University
Department of Critical Care Medicine and
    Anesthesiology
Director, PICU and Pediatric ECMO
Children's National Medical Center
Washington, DC, USA

Emily L. Dobyns, MD
Associate Professor of Pediatrics
University of Colorado Health
    Sciences Center
Division of Critical Care Medicine
The Children's Hospital Denver
Denver, CO, USA

Jeffrey R. Fineman, MD
Professor of Pediatrics
Medical Director, Cardiac Intensive Care Unit
University of California, San Francisco
San Francisco, CA, USA

Eva N. Grayck, MD
Associate Professor of Pediatrics
University of Colorado Health
    Sciences Center
Division of Critical Care Medicine
The Children's Hospital Denver
Denver, CO, USA

Margaret F. Guill, MD
Professor of Pediatrics
Medical College of Georgia
Chief, Section of Pulmonary Medicine
MCG Children's Medical Center
Augusta, GA, USA

Imad Y. Haddad, MD
Department of Pediatrics
Banner Medical Center
Phoenix, AZ, USA

Suriyanarayana P. Hariprakash, MBBS,
    DCH, MRCP, MRCPCH
University of Toronto School of Medicine
Departments of Critical Care Medicine
The Hospital for Sick Children, Toronto
Toronto, Ontario, Canada

Howard E. Jeffries, MD, MPH, MBA
Clinical Assistant Professor of Pediatrics
University of Washington School
    of Medicine
Children's Hospital and Regional
    Medical Center
Seattle, WA, USA

Brian P. Kavanagh, MB, BSc, MRCP, FRCP
Associate Professor of Anesthesia and
    Medicine
University of Toronto
Director of Research
Department of Critical Care Medicine
The Hospital for Sick Children
Toronto, Ontario, Canada

Alik Kornecki, MD
Department of Paediatrics
London Health Sciences Center
University of Western Ontario
London, Ontario, Canada

Ann Marie LeVine, MD
Assistant Professor of Pediatrics
University of Florida College of Medicine
Division of Critical Care Medicine
Shands Hospital for Children
Gainesville, FL, USA

John Marcum, MD
Division of Critical Care Medicine
Children's Hospital of Los Angeles
Los Angeles, CA, USA

Lynn D. Martin, MD
Professor of Anesthesiology and Pediatrics
    (adjunct)
University of Washington School of
    Medicine
Director, Department of Anesthesiology and
    Pain Medicine
Children's Hospital and Regional Medical
    Center
Seattle, WA, USA

Nilesh M. Mehta, MD, MRCPCH
Children's Hospital Boston
Boston, MA, USA

Renuka Mehta, MBBS
Assistant Professor of Pediatrics
Medical College of Georgia
Section of Critical Care Medicine
MCG Children's Medical Center
Augusta, GA, USA

Christopher J.L. Newth, MB, FRCPC
Professor of Pediatrics
University of Southern California Keck
    School of Medicine
Division of Critical Care Medicine
Children's Hospital Los Angeles
Los Angeles, CA, USA

Robert H. Notter, MD, PhD
Professor of Pediatrics and Environmental
    Medicine
University of Rochester Medical Center
Golisano Children's Hospital at Strong
    Rochester
Rochester, NY, USA

Peter Oishi, MD
Instructor
Department of Pediatrics
University of California, San Francisco
Division of Critical Care Medicine
UCSF Children's Hospital
San Francisco, CA, USA

Kristen Page, PhD
Research Assistant Professor of Pediatrics
University of Cincinnati College of Medicine
Division of Critical Care Medicine
Cincinnati Children's Hospital Medical
    Center
Cincinnati, OH, USA

Michael J. Rutter, FRACS
Associate Professor of Surgery
University of Cincinnati College of Medicine
Director of Clinical Research
Division of Pediatric Otolarnygology/Head
    and Neck Surgery
Cincinnati Children's Hospital Medical
    Center
Cincinnati, OH, USA

Thomas P. Shanley, MD
Associate Professor of Pediatrics and
    Communicable Diseases
University of Michigan Medical Center
Director, Division of Critical Care Medicine
C.S. Mott Children's Hospital
Ann Arbor, MI, USA

Shinya Tsuchida, MD
Departments of Critical Care Medicine and
    Anesthesia
Program in Lung Biology

The Hospital for Sick Children
University of Toronto
Toronto, Ontario, Canada

Kathleen M. Ventre, MD
Assistant Professor of Pediatrics
University of Utah School School
  of Medicine
Division of Critical Care Medicine
Primary Children's Medical Center
Salt Lake City, UT, USA

Michael Vish, MD
Division of Critical Care Medicine
Cincinnati Children's Hospital Medical Center
Cincinnati, OH, USA

Zhengdong Wang
Department of Pediatrics
University of Rochester Medical Centre
Rochester, NY, USA

Derek S. Wheeler, MD
Assistant Professor of Clinical Pediatrics
University of Cincinnati College of Medicine
Division of Critical Care Medicine

Cincinnati Children's Hospital Medical Center
Cincinnati, OH, USA

Douglas F. Willson, MD
Associate Professor of Pediatrics
University of Virginia Health
  Sciences Center
Director, Division of Pediatric Critical Care
University of Virginia Children's Medical
  Center
Charlottesville, VA, USA

Robert E. Wood, MD, PhD
Professor of Pediatrics
University of Cincinnati College of Medicine
Division of Pulmonary Medicine
Cincinnati Children's Hospital Medical Center
Cincinnati, OH, USA

Angela T. Wratney, MD, MHSc
Associate Professor of Pediatrics
The George Washington University School of
  Medicine
Division of Pediatric Critical Care Medicine
Children's National Medical Center
Washington, DC, USA

1
Respiratory Physiology

Howard E. Jeffries and Lynn D. Martin

Introduction

Understanding and managing respiratory failure remains a cornerstone of critical care practice, as over half of all admissions to pediatric critical care units are related to respiratory issues. The unique aspects of a developing pulmonary system demand an in-depth knowledge of these changes and their impact on diagnostics and therapeutics. Only by understanding the normal function of the respiratory system is the critical care physician able to begin to formulate mechanisms for supporting a failing physiology. This chapter introduces the developmental aspects of anatomy and physiology as they relate to the respiratory system and discusses pulmonary circulation and ventilation perfusion inequality and the physiologic effects of mechanical ventilation.

Developmental Anatomy

During the embryonic period, the airways first appear as a ventral outpouching of the primitive foregut. The lung develops through five stages (Figure 1.1), beginning with the embryonic stage in the fourth week during which the two main bronchi are formed. By the end of the pseudoglandular stage (week 16) all major conducting airways have formed, including the terminal bronchioles [1]. The canalicular stage is characterized by the development of respiratory bronchioles and the initiation of surfactant production [2]. During the saccular and alveolar stages the respiratory system continues to mature, with decreased interstitial tissue, thinning distal airway walls, the formation of alveoli, and increasing surfactant production. The pulmonary vasculature develops in tandem with the airways, eventually resulting in the completion of the extensive pulmonary capillary network by the alveolar stage.

At birth, the lung must make a dramatic transformation from a liquid-containing structure to one capable of supporting complete gas exchange requirements. The lung contains approximately 30 mL/kg of fetal lung liquid just before birth [3], and the lung becomes a net absorber of fluid rather than a secretor of fluid. The exact mechanisms for this transformation are unknown, although chloride ion transport opening sodium channels in the presence of catecholamines has been implicated [4]. Over the remainder of childhood, the lung will continue to grow and mature, and the 20 million alveolar saccules present at birth [5] will increase to 300 million alveoli by 8 years of age [6]. The increase in alveoli parallels the increase in alveolar surface area from $2.8\,m^2$ at birth, to $32\,m^2$ at 8 years of age, and $75\,m^2$ by adulthood [6]. Alveolar multiplication appears to be the major mechanism for lung growth, although some growth has also been attributed to the growth of individual alveoli.

The adult lung contains anatomic channels that permit ventilation distal to an area of obstruction (Figure 1.2). Two channels have been identified in normal human lungs, interalveolar (pores of Kohn) and bronchoalveolar (Lambert's channel). Interbronchiolar channels are not found in healthy lungs but develop during disease processes. Pores of Kohn appear as holes in alveolar walls in the first and second years of life [7]. Lambert's channels are found after 6 years of age [8]. The absence of these collateral pathways places infants and children at risk for the development of atelectasis and resulting ventilation/perfusion inequality [9].

Developmental Mechanics of Breathing

Elastic Properties of the Lung and Chest Wall

The lung is an elastic structure and will decrease its size whenever possible. However, the presence of the chest wall, which, in contrast to the lung, pulls outward at low volumes and inward at high volumes, retards this tendency [10]. Lung recoil has been shown to increase with age in children over 6 years of age [11] and may relate to elastin deposition [12]. The presence of an air–liquid interface increases the elastic recoil of the lung because of surface tension forces. Surface tension is the force that acts across the surface of a liquid, as the attractive forces between liquid molecules are stronger than the forces between liquid and gas molecules [13]. Saline-filled lung units, in which the surface tension forces have been abolished, was demonstrated by Von Neergaard in early surface tension experiments in the 1920s to be far more compliant (Figure 1.3). The decrease in surface tension forces likely resulted in a

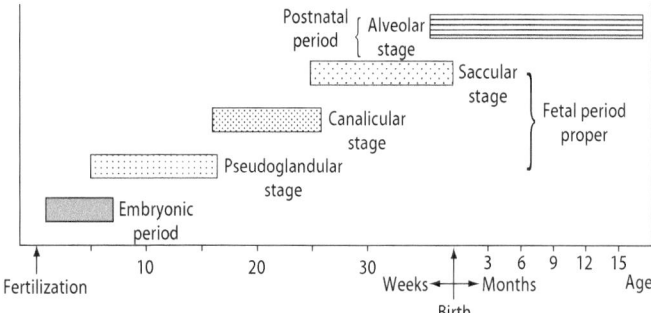

FIGURE 1.1. Stages of lung development. (From Burri PH. Annu Rev Physiol 1984;46: 612–628, with permission.)

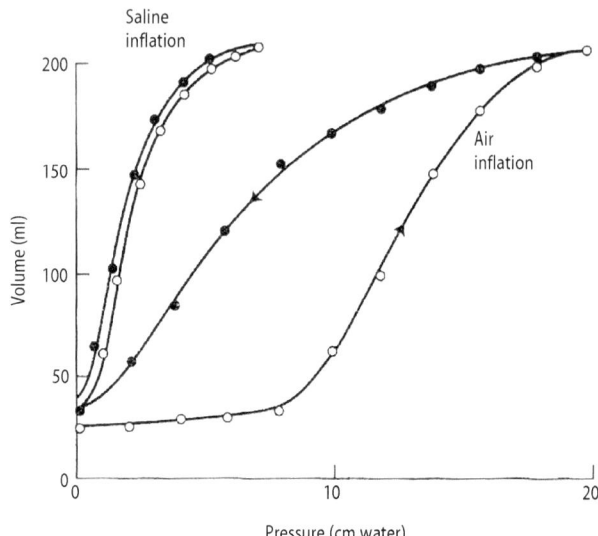

FIGURE 1.3. Pressure–volume curves of air and saline. Open circles represent inflation, and closed circles represent deflation. The compliance of the saline-filled lung is greater than the air-filled lung. (From West JB. Respiratory Physiology—The Essentials. Philadelphia: Lippincott Williams & Wilkins; 2000:84, with permission.)

reduction in lung elastic recoil [13]. Surfactant, a phospholipid–protein complex, has been shown to profoundly lower surface tension. The intermolecular repulsive forces oppose the normal attractive forces, and this effect is amplified at lower lung volumes, with compression of the surfactant complex. Traditional understanding of surface tension notes the significant role that surfactant plays in lung stabilization in accordance with the law of Laplace, stating that the pressure across a surface (P) is equal to 2 times the surface tension (T) divided the radius (r):

$$P = 2T/r$$

However, this is likely inefficient to explain lung stabilization in its entirety. The interdependence model of the lung, in which lung units share planar rather than spherical walls, gives credence to tissue forces playing a role (Figure 1.4). In all likelihood, lung stability results from a combination of these two forces.

Compliance of the Lung and Chest Wall

The pressure–volume curve of the air-filled lung is depicted in Figure 1.3. The slope of the curve, volume change per unit pressure,

is equal to the compliance of the lung (C = $\Delta V/\Delta P$). Normally, the lung is quite compliant; however, at the extremes of lung inflation and deflation, as seen from the graph, that compliance is reduced. Lung compliance depends on both the elasticity of the tissue and the original lung volume before inflation, as much larger pressures are needed to inflate lungs from lower lung volumes. Compliance, defined as the change in volume per change in pressure, when measured at zero airflow is termed the *static compliance*. However, lung compliance may also be measured during slow breathing; this value is termed *dynamic compliance*. Dynamic compliance also reflects the intrinsic elastic properties of the lung, although it is influenced by the respiratory rate and level of airway resistance [14].

$$C_{static} = \frac{\text{Tidal volume (corrected)}}{\text{Plateau pressure} - \text{Positive end-expiratory pressure}}$$

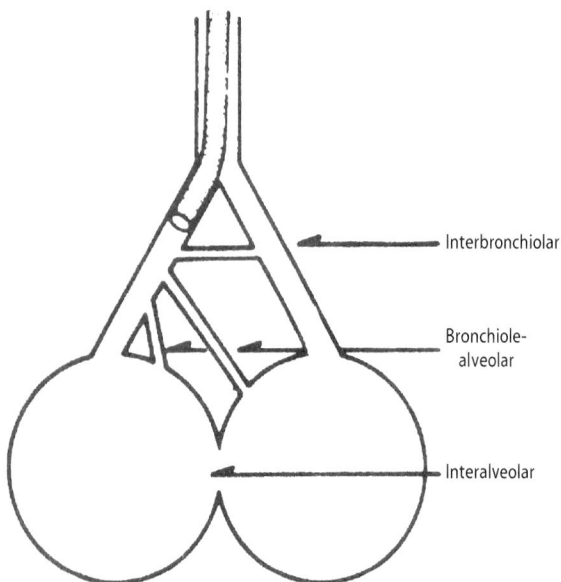

FIGURE 1.2. The various pathways for collateral ventilation. (From Menkes HA, Traystman RJ. Collateral ventilation. Am Rev Respir Dis 1977;116:287, with permission.)

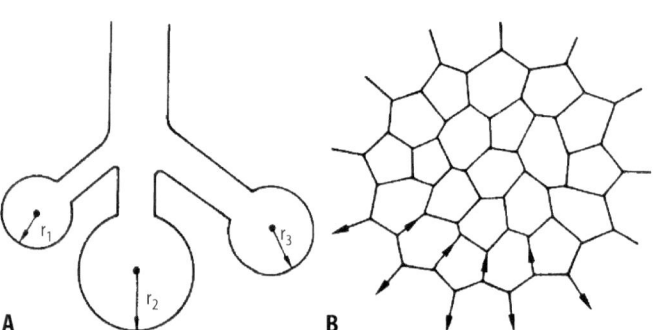

FIGURE 1.4. **(A)** Classic model of the distal lung in which individual alveoli are controlled by Laplace's law. Small alveoli would empty into large alveoli. **(B)** Interdependence model of the lung in which alveoli share common planar and not spherical walls. Any decrease in the size of one alveolus would be stabilized by the adjacent alveoli. (From Weibel ER, Bachofen H. News Physiol Sci 1987;2:72–75, with permission.)

$$C_{dynamic} = \frac{\text{Tidal volume (corrected)}}{\text{Peak inspiratory pressure} - \text{Positive end-expiratory pressure}}$$

During the first year of life, the compliance of the respiratory system (C_T) increases by as much as 150% [15]. The increase in lung compliance is responsible for the majority of the gain, outstripping the increase in chest wall compliance. The compliance of the chest wall (C_{CW}) is measured by examining the difference between the esophageal/pleural pressure (P_{PL}) and the atmosphere (P_A) per change in volume ($C_{CW} = V/([P_A - P_{PL}])$). The infant chest wall is remarkably compliant (Figure 1.5), and compliance decreases with increasing age. The elastic recoil of an infant's chest wall is close to zero and with age increases because of the progressive ossification of the rib cage and increased intercostal muscle tone [16]. In addition, the moving of the abdominal compartment caudally with the attainment of an upright posture has also been theorized to play a role in increasing outward recoil of the adult chest.

The functional significance of the decreased recoil of the infant chest wall increases the possibility of lung collapse in the setting of lung disease. The excessive compliance of the infant chest wall requires the infant to perform more work than an adult chest to move a similar tidal volume. During an episode of respiratory distress, an infant will develop severe retractions in order to maintain

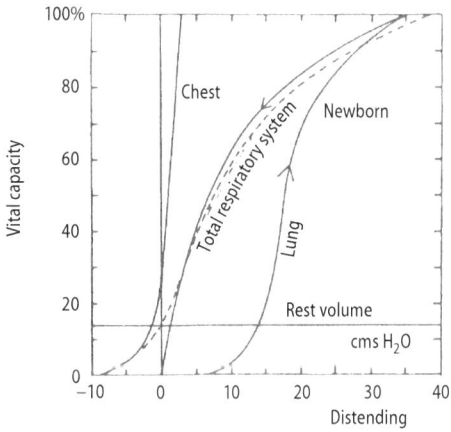

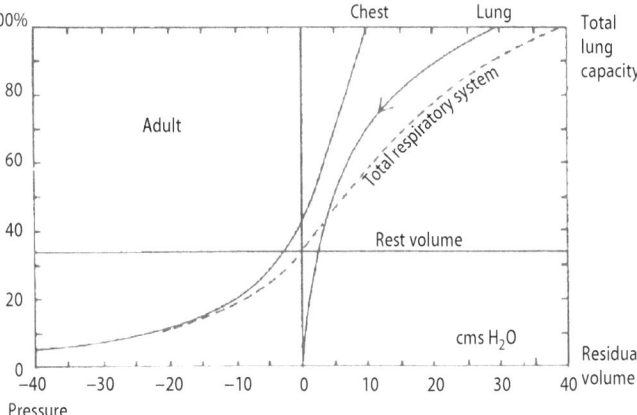

FIGURE 1.5. Static pressure–volume curves in the newborn and in the adult. (From Smith CA, Nelson NM. The Physiology of the Newborn Infant. Springfield, IL: Charles C. Thomas; 1976;205, with permission.)

ventilation and oxygenation. However, a significant portion of the energy generated is wasted through the distortion of the highly compliant rib cage during negative pressure generation from diaphragmatic contraction [17]. It has been observed that some infants will stop breathing from fatigue when faced with excessive respiratory demands. This impression of diaphragmatic fatigue and failure has been confirmed through electromyographic measurements of the diaphragms of fatiguing infants who become apneic in the face of increased work of breathing [18].

Airway Resistance

In order for air to move in and out of the lungs, gas must flow from an area of higher pressure to one of lower pressure. According to Ohm's law, the pressure gradient that faces a substance (gas or liquid) is equal to the product of the flow rate times the resistance to flow (pressure gradient [P] = flow rate [V] × resistance [R]). The components of pulmonary resistance to gas flow include (1) the inertia of the respiratory system (effectively negligible), (2) the frictional resistance of the chest wall tissue (negligible), (3) the frictional resistance of the lung tissue (20% of pulmonary resistance), and (4) the frictional resistance of the airways to the flow of air (majority of pulmonary resistance) [19].

The extent of the pressure drop and its relationship to the airflow rate depend on the pattern of flow, either laminar or turbulent. In laminar flow, air travels down a tube in parallel to the side of the tube; however, when variation in the flow rate develops because of a sudden rise in gas flow rate, a narrowing of the tube or the encountering of an acute angle, the flow becomes turbulent. Laminar flow of air is governed by the Hagen-Poiseuille law (also known as Poiseuille's law), where $P = (V)(8l\eta/\pi r^4)$; in this equation, l is the length of the tube, r is the radius of the tube, and η is the viscosity of the gas. Through rearranging the terms, it can be noted that resistance is mostly determined by the radius of the tube, in that $R = P/V = 8l\eta/\pi r^4$. Turbulent flow has different properties from laminar flow, as it is proportional to the square of the flow rate: $P = KV^2$ and becomes more dependent on the gas density instead of the viscosity [20]. Clinical attempts to exploit the properties of turbulent gas flow have been made in the patients with both upper and lower airway obstruction (i.e., croup and asthma). In both of these settings, the introduction of helium-oxygen admixtures is an attempt to introduce helium, a gas with a lower density than oxygen, in order to promote airflow in turbulent airways.

The main site of airway resistance in the adult is the upper airway; however, it has been shown that peripheral airway resistance in children younger than 5 years of age is four times higher than adults [21]. This may explain the high incidence of lower airway obstructive disease in infants and young children, especially when considering Poiseuille's law and the dramatic increase in resistance that is seen with only a small amount of airway obstruction. Within the bronchial tree, direct measurements of the pressure drop have found that the major site of resistance is the medium-sized bronchi and that little of the total resistance to air flow is determined by the smaller airways. The resistance of these bronchi is determined by the presence of exogenous materials, autonomic regulation of bronchial smooth muscle, and lung volume. As lung volume increases, a radial traction is imparted to the surrounding lung tissue, which increases the intraluminal caliber of these bronchi and reduces their resistance (Figure 1.6) [22].

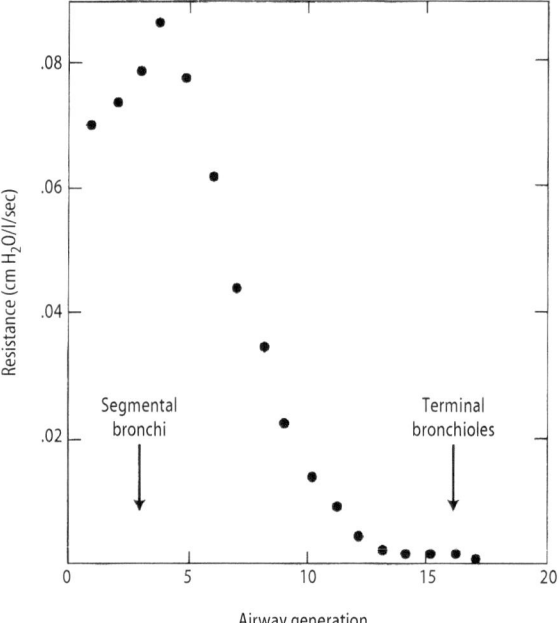

FIGURE 1.6. The relationship between airway resistance and lung volume. Conductance, the reciprocal of airway resistance, is a straight line. (From West JB. Respiratory Physiology—The Essentials. Philadelphia: Lippincott Williams & Wilkins; 2000:95, with permission.)

During illness airway resistance can be increased from either intraluminal obstruction or extrinsic compression. Extrinsic compression can occur from a variety of etiologies, including the finding of airway collapse during forced expiration secondary to dynamic compression of the airway. During normal exhalation, there is a pressure drop from the alveolus to the mouth, which allows for air flow; however, there continues to be a favorable transmural pressure gradient and cartilaginous support, which maintains airway patency (transmural pressure gradient = intraluminal pressure – pleural pressure). On the contrary, during a forced expiration maneuver, the pleural pressure raises significantly, decreasing the transmural pressure gradient, causing the airway caliber to narrow. At some location along the airway during the forced expiration maneuver, the intraluminal pressure will equal the intrapleural pressure. This is termed the *equal pressure point* (EPP). Beyond this point, forces favoring airway collapse exceed those favoring patency (tethering action of lung tissue and rigid cartilage), resulting in airway collapse [23]. In the presence of bronchopulmonary dysplasia, bronchomalacia, and tracheomalacia, these mechanisms are amplified, leading to earlier symptoms of airway collapse [24].

Lung Volumes

An understanding of static lung volumes and the developmental impacts are critical to evaluating and subsequently treating infants and children with respiratory disease. Volumes and capacities of the lungs are affected by several factors, specifically muscle strength, the static–elastic characteristics of the chest wall and lungs, and patient age [25]. The traditional spirometric tracing in Figure 1.7 depicts tidal breathing followed by maximal inspiratory and expiratory efforts. Five lung volumes are shown. Tidal volume

is defined as the amount of gas moved during normal breathing, and residual volume is defined as the amount of gas that remains in the lung after a maximal expiration. Four capacities, which are composed of multiple volumes, are also shown. Vital capacity is defined as the volume of gas that may be exhaled from the lung following a maximal inspiration. Functional residual capacity (FRC) is defined as the gas that remains in the lung at the end of a tidal breath. This gas serves as a reservoir of oxygen during expiration and accordingly is a very important construct in the understanding of respiratory pathophysiology. It is now discussed at length.

Functional residual capacity in a normal lung is the same as the end-expiratory lung volume (EELV); however, in diseased or injured lung, EELV may be greater or less than FRC. Functional residual capacity is determined by the static balance between the outward recoil of the chest wall and the inward recoil of the lung. However, in infants, the outward recoil is quite small, and the inward recoil is only slightly less than that in adults [26]. Accordingly, the static balance of forces results in a low ratio of FRC to total lung capacity (TLC) of approximately 10%–15%, limiting gas exchange. However, when measured in the dynamic state, that ratio of FRC/TLC in infants approximates the adult value of 40% [27]. Therefore, the dynamic EELV of infants is much greater than that predicted by the static balance of forces.

The mechanism for this difference in static versus dynamic FRC/TLC ratio in infants relates to the mechanism of breath termination. Adults cease expiration at low flow rates, whereas infants will abruptly terminate expiration [28] at high flow rates (Figure 1.8). Infants utilize two mechanisms to end expiration: the postinspiratory activity of the diaphragm and expiratory laryngeal braking [29,30]. The expiratory braking mechanism is an active process in which the resistance in the upper airway is increased by laryngeal narrowing during expiration. This generates positive end-expiratory pressure, resulting in an EELV that is above FRC. These mechanisms are both arousal and gestational age dependent. During REM sleep in premature infants, both postinspiratory activity of the diaphragm and laryngeal braking are reduced, although braking appears preserved during non-REM sleep [31,32]. This may exacerbate the loss of oxygen stores during apnea, leading to the clinical finding of significant desaturation and bradycardia in premature infants.

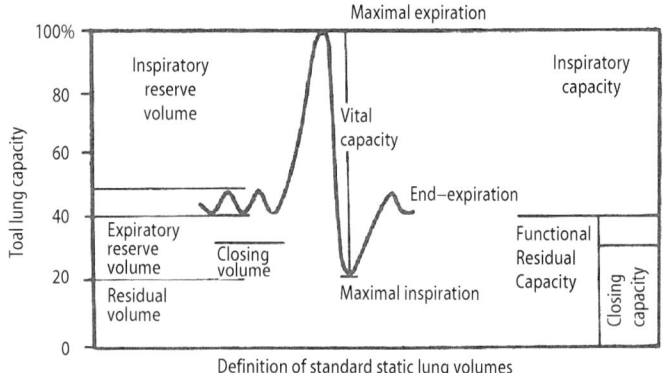

FIGURE 1.7. Typical spirometric tracing that depicts tidal breathing followed by a maximal inspiration and then a maximal expiration. Five volumes and five capacities are shown. (From Smith CA, Nelson NM. The Physiology of the Newborn Infant. Springfield, IL: Charles C. Thomas; 1976;206, with permission.)

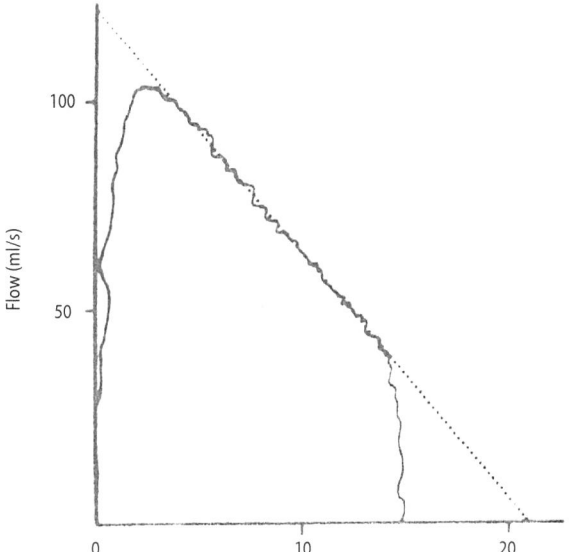

FIGURE 1.8. Passive flow-volume curve that demonstrates the abrupt onset of inspiration in an infant much above passive functional residual capacity. (From Le Souef PN, et al. Am Rev Respir Dis 1984;129:552–556, with permission.)

The final volume and capacity not fully considered to this point are closing volume and closing capacity. The closing capacity is composed of residual volume and closing volume and is defined as the volume of gas that remains in the lung when small alveoli and airways in dependent regions of the lung are collapsed or considered closed. When closing capacity exceeds FRC, by definition, some lung units are closed during a portion of tidal breathing. If closing capacity ever exceeds the tidal volume, then these lung units will be closed during all phases of tidal breathing. These concepts are important in pediatrics, as children younger than 6 years of age have a closing capacity greater than FRC in the supine position [33]. This finding has been attributed to reduce inward recoil of the lung. This concept becomes clinically important in critically ill infants and children, in whom elevated closing capacity leading to areas of collapse results in ventilation and perfusion inequality, resulting in pathophysiologic intrapulmonary shunting. Ventilation–perfusion matching is discussed at length later in this chapter.

Physiologic Effects of Mechanical Ventilation

Since the introduction of mechanical ventilation into the intensive care unit, there has been an explosion of new ventilators and ventilatory techniques to treat patients with respiratory failure. Physicians contemplating the use of mechanical ventilation must be familiar with these therapeutic options and their potential benefits and associated risks. A detailed understanding of the physiologic and pathophysiologic effects of mechanical ventilation is crucial to improve the outcomes of patients with respiratory failure.

Maintenance of Oxygenation

The partial pressure of oxygen in the alveolus (PAO_2) is one of the primary determinants of arterial oxygen tension and is the chief target of alterations in mechanical ventilation. The PAO_2 is deter-

mined by the alveolar gas equation: $PAO_2 = PiO_2 - PACO_2$, where PiO_2 is the partial pressure of inspired oxygen and $PACO_2$ is the partial pressure of alveolar carbon dioxide. The PiO_2 is determined by the fraction of inspired oxygen, the barometric pressure ($P_B = 760\,mm\,Hg$ at sea level), and the partial pressure of water vapor ($P_{H2O} = 47\,mm\,Hg$). Thus the $PiO_2 = FiO_2 \cdot (P_B - P_{H2O}) = 150\,mm\,Hg$ in room air at sea level. For clinical purposes, $PACO_2$ is assumed to equal the partial pressure of arterial carbon dioxide ($PaCO_2 = 40\,mm\,Hg$) divided by the respiratory quotient (RQ; determined by the mix of metabolic substrates and usually estimated to be approximately 0.8), resulting in $50\,mm\,Hg$. Substituting these values for PiO_2 and $PACO_2$, respectively, into the previous equation yields the classic alveolar gas equation: $PAO_2 = FiO_2 \cdot (P_B - P_{H2O}) - PaCO_2/RQ$. The latter equation yields a PAO_2 of 100 to 120 mm Hg in room air at sea level.

The alveolar gas equation reveals three etiologies for hypoxemia (Table 1.1): (1) low FiO_2 (i.e., hypoxic gas mixture); (2) low barometric pressure (i.e., high altitude); and (3) hypoventilation. The first two are rarely causes of hypoxemia, and an important principle of the alveolar gas equation can be gleaned by examining the last situation. A decrease in alveolar ventilation by 50% in room air at sea level will yield a PAO_2 of 50 mm Hg, a clinically significant level of hypoxemia. However, with the administration of 25% inspired oxygen, the PAO_2 increases to 78 mm Hg, a nonhypoxemic concentration. Thus, a very small increase in inspired oxygen tension will easily overcome hypoxemia caused solely by hypoventilation.

The difference between the partial pressure of oxygen in the alveolus (PAO_2) and that in the pulmonary capillary (PaO_2), approximately 10 mm Hg under normal conditions, is caused by the diffusion barrier of alveolar–capillary membrane and the overall ventilation–perfusion (V/Q) ratio of the lung. While the former is easily overcome by increase inspired oxygen concentration and rarely is a cause for clinically significant hypoxemia, the same cannot be said for the latter. The principal etiology for clinically significant hypoxemia is pulmonary pathology associated with decreased lung volumes, reduced lung compliance, and an increased proportion of low V/Q compartments of the lung [34]. Under severe conditions, areas of the lung may become completely atelectatic and lead to right-to-left intrapulmonary shunting. One of the primary objectives of mechanical ventilation is to restore normal lung volumes and mechanics through the application of continuous positive airway pressure (CPAP). A useful clinical index of the effect of changes of ventilation variables is mean airway pressure (P_{aw}) [35]. Mean airway pressure is defined by the following equation:

$$P_{aw} = (\text{Peak inspiratory pressure [PIP]} - \text{Positive end-expiratory pressure [PEEP]}) \cdot (T_i/T_i + T_e) + PEEP$$

TABLE 1.1. Alveolar partial pressures of oxygen under various conditions.

Condition	$FiO_2 (P_B - P_{H2O}) - PaCO_2/RQ$	$= PAO_2$ (mmHg)
Normal	0.21 (760 − 47) − 40/0.8	100
Hypoxic gas mixture at sea level	0.15 (760 − 47) − 40/0.8	57
Normoxic, hypobaric pressure	0.21 (560 − 47) − 40/0.8	58
Normoxic, hypoventilation at sea level	0.21 (760 − 47) − 80/0.8	50
Hypoventilation with supplemental O_2	0.25 (760 − 47) − 80/0.8	78

Source: Adapted from Martin L. Mechanical ventilation, respiratory monitoring and the basics of pulmonary physiology. In: Tobias JD, ed. Pediatric Critical Care: The Essentials. Armonk, NY: Futura; 1999:58.

Accordingly, alterations in peak inspiratory and end-expiratory pressures, ventilator rate, and inspiratory to expiratory (I:E) ratio can increase P_{aw}, which can recruit atelectatic or poorly ventilated alveolar units, thereby restoring normal V/Q matching and decreasing intrapulmonary shunt [36]. The restoration of lung volumes frequently allows a dramatic reduction in the inspired oxygen concentration as well as improving respiratory mechanics and decreasing the work of breathing. These improvements may allow for the partial or complete restoration of spontaneous ventilation, which is associated with several possible advantages (improved V/Q matching, decreased risk of barotraumas, diminished adverse effects of continuous positive pressure ventilation) [37].

From the previous discussion, the major etiologic factors producing hypoxemia can be listed as (1) hypoxic gas mixture, (2) hypoventilation, (3) ventilation–perfusion mismatch, (4) diffusion abnormalities of the alveolar–capillary membrane, (5) high altitude, and (6) true shunt related to cyanotic, congenital heart disease.

Maintenance of Alveolar Ventilation

A second goal of mechanical ventilation is to augment or control alveolar ventilation. Respiratory failure is frequently defined in terms of $PaCO_2$, which is inversely related to alveolar ventilation (V_A): $PaCO_2 \propto V_{CO2}/V_A$, where V_{CO2} is carbon dioxide production. Alveolar ventilation is also defined (at normal ventilator frequencies) as $V_A = f(V_T - V_D)$, where V_T is tidal volume, V_D is dead space volume, and f is the respiratory frequency. Alterations in V_T and/or f, which are the components of minute ventilation (V_E), will result in changes in $PaCO_2$. Clinicians may fail to account for the third component in these equations, namely, V_D. The relationship between V_E and $PaCO_2$ can be described by the following: $PaCO_2 = 0.863\ V_{CO2}/[V_E(1 - V_D/V_T)]$, where V_{CO2} is the metabolically produced carbon dioxide at standard temperature and pressure.

Most of V_D in normal individuals is the result of the volume of the conducting airways (anatomic V_D). Because the anatomic dead space is relatively constant, with an increasing V_T, V_D/V_T tends to decrease and rarely exceeds 0.3. In patients with intrinsic lung disease undergoing mechanical ventilation, V_D/V_T has been found to exceed 0.6 and is primarily caused by continued ventilation of poorly perfused regions of the lungs (alveolar V_D). In this setting, increases in V_T may not decrease V_D/V_T because higher alveolar pressures as a result of increases in V_T on V_D/V_T can be facilitated by measurement of V_D/V_T using capnography: $V_D/V_T = (PaCO_2 - P_{ET}CO_2)/ PaCO_2$, where $P_{ET}CO_2$ is the partial pressure of carbon dioxide in exhaled gas, commonly referred to as *end-tidal carbon dioxide*. In summary, three factors must be considered when changes in $PaCO_2$ occur: (1) changes in metabolic V_{CO2}, (2) alterations in V_E as a result of increases or decreases in V_T and f, and (3) modifications of V_D.

Mechanics of Ventilation

A simplified single-compartment model of the lungs composed of a single, cylindrical flow-conducting tube (i.e., conducting airways) connected to a single, spherical elastic compartment (i.e., alveoli) is frequently used to describe pulmonary mechanics (Figure 1.9). In this model, the lungs are considered as a homogeneous assembly of units with uniform pressure–volume (compliance) and pressure–low (resistance) characteristics derived from this single representative unit. To achieve inflation, a transrespiratory pressure (P_{tr})

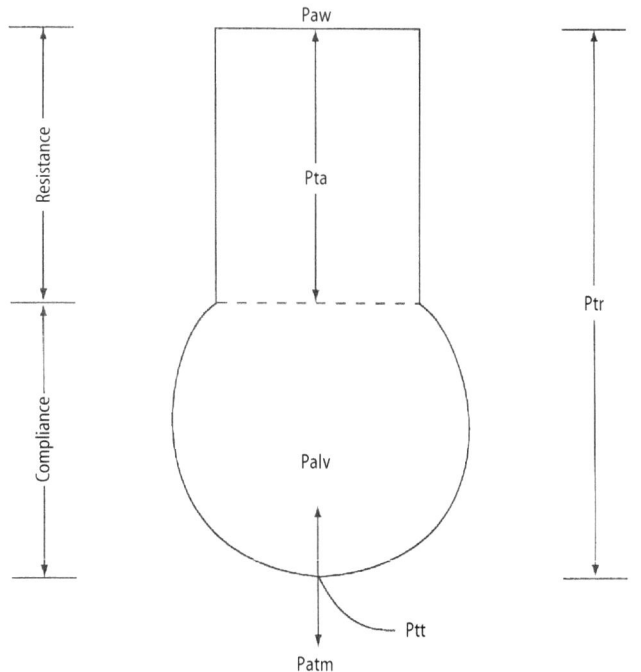

Figure 1.9. The simplified single-compartment model of the lungs composed of a flow-resistive element adjoined in series with a compliance element. P_{aw} is airway pressure; P_{alv} is alveolar pressure; P_{atm} is atmospheric pressure; P_{ta} is transairway ($P_{aw} - P_{alv}$) pressure; P_{tt} is transthoracic ($P_{alv} - P_{atm}$) pressure; and P_{tr} is transrespiratory ($P_{aw} - P_{atm}$) pressure. Ventilator manometers are equivalent to P_{tr}. (From Martin L. Mechanical ventilation, respiratory monitoring and the basics of pulmonary physiology. In: Tobias JD, ed. Pediatric Critical Care: The Essentials. Armonk, NY: Futura; 1999:60.)

composed of two components is required. The first component, the transthoracic pressure (P_{tt}), is defined as the pressure required to deliver the tidal volume against the elastic recoil of the lungs and chest wall, and the second component, the transairway pressure (P_{ta}), is the pressure necessary to overcome air flow resistance. This is described mathematically by the equation $P_{tr} = P_{tt} + P_{ta}$, where P_{tr} is airway minus body surface pressure, Ptt is alveolar minus body surface pressure, and P_{ta} is airway minus alveolar pressure. The pressure required for inspiration may come from the respiratory muscles (P_{rm}) and/or the ventilator (P_{tr}):$P_{rm} + P_{tr} = P_{tt} + P_{ta}$. Because the ventilator measures pressure relative to atmosphere, P_{tr} is equal to P_{aw} displayed by the ventilator, allowing the substitution: $P_{rm} + P_{aw} = P_{tt} + P_{ta}$.

The single-compartment model assumes a linear relationship between pressure and volume and between pressure and flow. The change in P_{tr} is directly proportional to the corresponding change in lung volume and the constant of proportionality is the slope ($\Delta P/\Delta V$) of the pressure–volume curve (i.e., reciprocal of compliance [C]). Similarly, the change in P_{ta} is proportional to the change in flow rate (F), and the constant of proportionality ($\Delta P/\Delta F$) is resistance (R). Substituting $\Delta P/\Delta V$ for P_{tr} and $\Delta P/\Delta F$ for P_{ta} yields the equation of motion of the respiratory system for inspiration: $P_{rm} + P_{aw} = V/C + (F)(R)$, where V is the volume inspired or expired, C is the compliance of the respiratory system, F is the inspiratory or expiratory flow rate, and R is the resistance of the respiratory system. For passive expiration, the equation of motion of the respiratory system is defined as: $V/C = -(F)(R)$, where the elastic components of the lungs ($P_A=V/C$) provides the pressure to drive the expiratory flow rate. In situations where respiratory muscles are relaxed, measurement of pressure, volume, and flow allow calculation of total respiratory system compliance and resistance.

The relationships represented in the equation of motion can be graphically represented for both constant inspiratory flow (i.e., volume-limited ventilation) and constant inspiratory pressure (i.e., pressure-limited ventilation) as shown in Figure 1.10. During constant inspiratory flow ventilation (Figure 1.10, left), the initial rise in pressure is related to the resistance and flow rate, whereas the slope of the pressure rise is inversely proportional to compliance, tidal volume, resistance, and inspiratory flow rate. Lung pressure (P_L) is expressed as $P_L = (F)(t)/C$, where F is inspiratory flow rate, t is the inspiratory time, and C is the compliance of the respiratory system. Lung volume (V_L) can be represented as $V_L = (F)(t)$. During constant inspiratory pressure ventilation (Figure 1.10, right), the P_L, V_L, and F during inspiration are exponential functions of time derived from the equation of motion as $P_L = \Delta P(1 - e^{-t/T})$, $V_L = C(\Delta P)(1 - e^{-t/T})$, and $F = \Delta P/R\ (e^{-t/T})$, where ΔP is equal to peak inspiratory pressure minus end-expiratory pressure, t is the inspiratory time, e is the natural logarithm (≈ 2.72), and T is the time constant of the respiratory system. The time constant (T) is the product of compliance (volume/pressure) and resistance (pressure $\times$ time/volume) and is measured in seconds. Exhalation during any form of mechanical ventilation is passive. Therefore, the P, V, and F can also be derived from the equation of motion as: $P_L = \Delta P(e^{-t/T})$, $V_L = C(\Delta P)(e^{-t/T})$, and $F = -\Delta P/R\ (e^{-t/T})$, where t is the expiratory time and T is the expiratory time constant. Note that all variables are measured relative to their value at end-expiration, the P_L is pressure above positive-end expiratory pressure (PEEP), and V_L is the volume above end-expiratory volume. When inspiratory and expiratory times are between zero and infinity, the shapes of the lung pressure and lung volume curves are defined by the T. By plotting these curves over time in units of T, clinically useful principles emerge (Figure 1.11). Irrespective of the specific values of resistance and compliance, after 1 T 63% of lung inflation or deflation occurs,

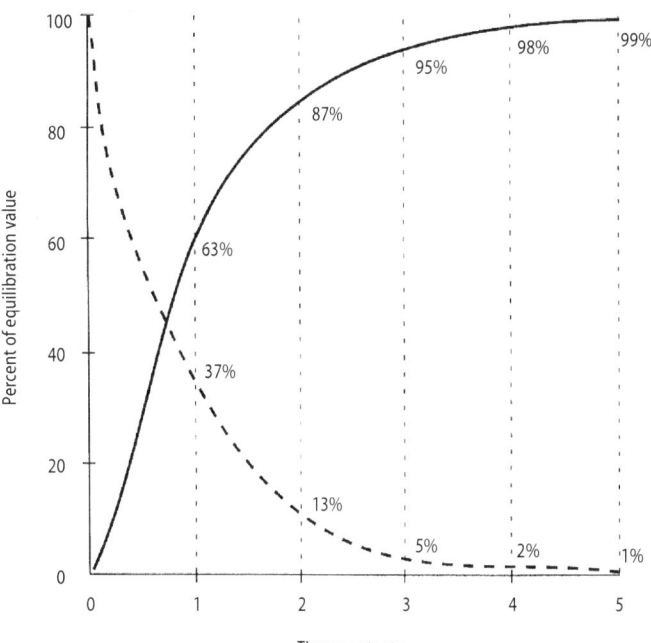

FIGURE 1.11. Exponential lung pressure or volume curves as a function of time constant during inspiration (solid line) and expiration (dashed line). (From Martin L. Mechanical ventilation, respiratory monitoring and the basics of pulmonary physiology. In: Tobias JD, ed. Pediatric Critical Care: The Essentials. Armonk, NY: Futura; 1999:63.)

95% after 3 T, and for all practical purposes, complete equilibration after 5 T.

The equation of motion is a useful means to more closely examine the differences between constant flow volume-limited ventilation and constant pressure ventilation with a decelerating inspiratory flow waveform. Peak airway pressures are higher for a constant flow pattern than for the constant pressure pattern. However, peak alveolar pressures depend on only the compliance and tidal volume, thereby making peak lung pressures independent of the pattern of ventilation. Second, at any point in time, airway pressure is equal to the volume/compliance plus the resistance/flow. The pressure required to overcome flow resistance (shaded area in Figure 1.10) is constant with fixed inspiratory flow, whereas it decreases exponentially with the decelerating flow pattern. In the example depicted, the area is equal for both patterns, because tidal volume and inspiratory times are equal. Third, the more rapid approach to the pressure limit during constant pressure decelerating flow ventilation leads to a higher P_{aw} compared with constant flow ventilation. Because all shaded areas are equal, the total area under the airway curve is equal to the total area under the lung pressure curve for each pattern. Therefore, the P_{aw} is equal to mean P_L, a finding that has been verified in animals [35].

The final feature of pulmonary mechanics that must be appreciated is the sigmoidal shape of the static pressure–volume (compliance) relationship of the respiratory system (Figure 1.12). The respiratory system is most compliant in the mid-volume range, becoming progressively less compliant at high (near total lung capacity) and low (approaching residual volume) volume extremes. Tidal ventilation near total lung capacity occurs under two conditions: (2) when total lung volume and/or vital capacity is decreased secondary to intrinsic lung disease and (2) when end-expiratory volume is decreased. Conversely, ventilation near residual volume

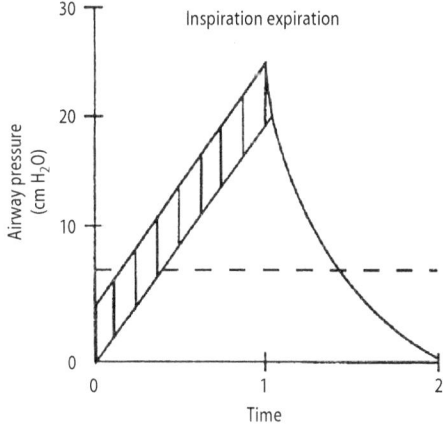

FIGURE 1.10. Graphic representation of the equation of motion for constant inspiratory flow (left) and constant inspiratory pressure (right) breaths. Pressure, volume, and flow are measured relative to their respective end-expiratory values. The shaded areas represent equal geometric areas proportional to the pressure required to overcome lung elastic recoil. The dashed line represents mean airway and lung pressure. Note the higher peak and lower mean airway pressures with the constant inspiratory flow breath (left) compared with the constant inspiratory pressure breath (right). (From Martin L. Mechanical ventilation, respiratory monitoring and the basics of pulmonary physiology. In: Tobias JD, ed. Pediatric Critical Care: The Essentials. Armonk, NY: Futura; 1999:62.)

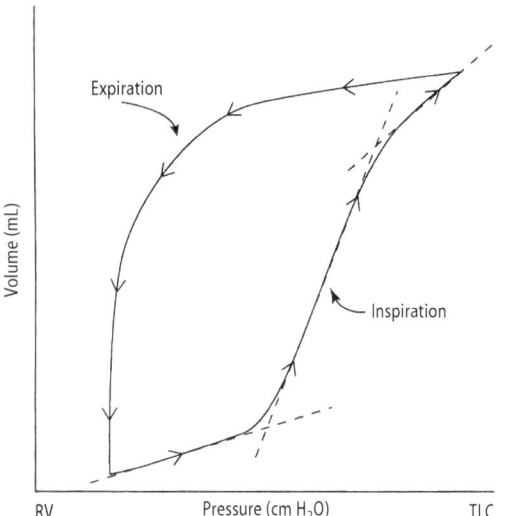

Figure 1.12. A hypothetical static pressure–volume curve of the respiratory system. Note the sigmoidal shape of the inspiratory limb with high compliance in the midvolume range and low compliance at either high or low lung volumes. Inflection points denote the change from low to high compliance regions. (From Martin L. Mechanical ventilation, respiratory monitoring and the basics of pulmonary physiology. In: Tobias JD, ed. Pediatric Critical Care: The Essentials. Armonk, NY: Futura; 1999:64.)

Table 1.2. Conditions predisposing to convergence of closing and functional residual capacities.

Elevation of closing capacity
   Infancy
   Bronchiolitis
   Asthma
   Bronchopulmonary dysplasia
   Smoke inhalation (thermal airway injury)
   Cystic fibrosis
Reduction of functional residual capacity
   Supine position
   Abdominal distention
   Thoracic or abdominal surgery/trauma
   Atelectasis
   Pulmonary edema
   Acute lung injury/acute respiratory distress syndrome
   Near drowning
   Diffuse pneumonitis
      Aspiration pneumonitis
      Idiopathic interstitial pneumonitis
      Bacterial pneumonia
      Viral pneumonia
      Opportunistic organism (i.e., *Pneumocystis carinii*)
      Radiation

Source: Adapted from Martin L. Mechanical ventilation, respiratory monitoring and the basics of pulmonary physiology. In: Tobias JD, ed. Pediatric Critical Care: The Essentials. Armonk, NY: Futura; 1999:58.

with a decrease in compliance also occurs under two conditions: (1) when obesity and/or abdominal distention increase residual volume and encroach on the lower range of vital capacity and (2) when intrinsic lung disease results in airway or alveolar closure at end-expiratory volume.

The relationship between end-expiratory lung volume and closing capacity is critical. Conditions that decrease FRC below closing capacity or increase closing capacity above FRC result in maldistribution of ventilation and perfusion and adversely affect the mechanics of breathing (Table 1.2). In the school-aged child and in the adult, FRC is normally well above closing capacity. However, the relationship is more precarious in young infants, as noted previously, in whom studies suggest that closing capacity exceeds FRC [38]. A primary goal of mechanical ventilation is the restoration of the normal relationship between FRC and closing capacity. Conditions associated with a decrease in FRC (e.g., pulmonary edema, pneumonitis, infant respiratory distress syndrome [(IRDS]] and acute respiratory distress syndrome [(ARDS)] are treated with PEEP to increase FRC back to normal levels. Situations associated with increased closing capacity, such as bronchiolitis and reactive airway disease, are treated with bronchodilators and measures to control secretions in order to reduce closing capacity and maintain airway patency.

Work of Breathing

The pressure–volume (compliance) and pressure–flow (resistance) characteristics of the respiratory system determine the work of breathing, which, in reality, represents the afterload on the respiratory muscles [39]. The work of breathing overcomes two major sources of impedance: (1) elastic recoil of the lung and chest wall (Figure 1.13, areas A, C, and D) and (2) the frictional resistance to gas flow in the airways (Figure 1.13, areas A, B, and C). The total work of breathing (Figure 1.13, areas A through D) is increased by a decrease in respiratory compliance and/or an increase in respira-

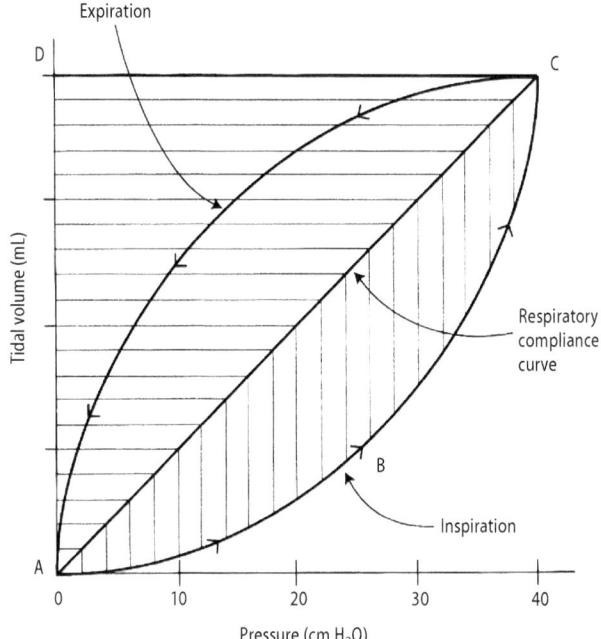

Figure 1.13. Inspiratory and expiratory pressure–volume curve recorded during a complete respiratory cycle. Total work of breathing (pressure X volume) is defined as the sum of resistive work (area defined by ABC) plus the elastic work (area defined by ACD). Total work (defined by area ABCD) is increased by either an increase in resistive properties of the respiratory system or a decrease in compliance (slope of line between A and C). (From Martin L. Mechanical ventilation, respiratory monitoring and the basics of pulmonary physiology. In: Tobias JD, ed. Pediatric Critical Care: The Essentials. Armonk, NY: Futura; 1999:66.)

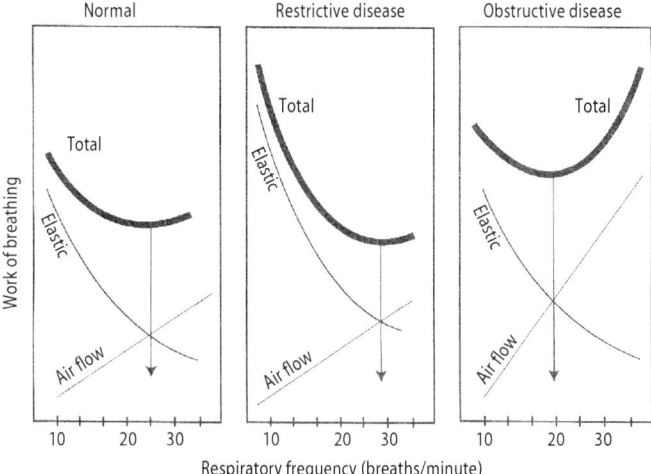

FIGURE 1.14. Hypothetical diagrams showing work done against elastic and resistance, separately, and summated to indicate total work at different respiratory frequencies. For a constant minute volume, minimum work is performed at higher frequencies with restrictive (low compliance) disease and at lower frequencies when airflow resistance is increased. (From Martin L. Mechanical ventilation, respiratory monitoring and the basics of pulmonary physiology. In: Tobias JD, ed. Pediatric Critical Care: The Essentials. Armonk, NY: Futura; 1999:67.)

tory resistance properties. When total work of breathing against compliance and resistance is summated and plotted against respiratory frequency, an optimal respiratory frequency exists that minimizes the total work of breathing (Figure 1.14). In patients with low lung compliance (restrictive lung diseases) such as pulmonary edema, IRDS, or ARDS, the optimal frequency is increased, leading to rapid, shallow breathing. In contrast, in obstructive lung diseases with increased resistance, such as bronchiolitis and asthma, the optimal frequency is decreased with slow, deep breathing.

Developmental Anatomy and Physiology of the Pulmonary Circulation

Development of the lungs and development of the pulmonary vasculature are closely related, as adequate blood flow is essential for the formation of the lungs and preacinar arteries develop in utero with conducting airways [40]. The arterial tree undergoes complex remodeling in the peripheral portions of the pulmonary circulation, following changes in wall stress [41]. Muscularization of the pulmonary vasculature occurs throughout infancy and reaches adult levels by adolescence. Pulmonary vascular muscle thickness is a function of gestational age and blood flow. For example, congenital heart disease with increased pulmonary blood flow leads to long-standing pulmonary hypertension because of smooth muscle proliferation in the pulmonary vessels [42]. Premature infants are born with less arterial smooth muscle than are full-term infants; this muscle in premature infants regresses earlier and is therefore predisposed to early congestive heart failure in the setting of left–right shunts.

Pulmonary Vascular Pressures

Pressures within the pulmonary circulation are quite low despite the fact that the entire cardiac output is designed to flow through

it. Following the initial fall after birth, pulmonary arterial pressures remain fairly constant in the disease-free state throughout life, with systolic, diastolic, and mean pressures of 25, 8, and 15 mm Hg, respectively. Pulmonary venous pressure is routinely just higher than the left atrial pressure, near 5 mm Hg. The transpulmonary pressure is determined by subtracting the left atrial pressure from the mean pulmonary arterial pressure and is approximately 10 mm Hg in the healthy subject. The pressure within the pulmonary capillaries is uncertain, although experimental animal evidence suggests it may range from 8 to 10 mm Hg. The pulmonary vascular pressures vary based on gravity and may range from near 0 mm Hg at the apex of the lung and rise to 25 mm Hg at the base [43]; the consequences that result from this gradient are discussed later.

The pressure that surrounds the pulmonary capillaries plays an important role in their patency, as they are surrounded by gas and are not supported by the alveolar epithelial cells. The pressure within the capillaries is fairly close to alveolar, and ,when the transmural pressure is positive, the capillaries collapse. As the lung expands, the extraalveolar vessels are pulled open by the radial traction of the elastic lung parenchyma. In addition, this expansion results in a negative intrapleural pressure that also maintains the patency of the alveolar vessels (Figure 1.15).

Pulmonary Vascular Resistance

The resistance within any system may be described by a variation of the previously described Ohm's law, where

$$Resistance = \frac{Input\ presure - Output\ pressure}{Blood\ flow}$$

Decreased pulmonary vascular resistance (PVR) can only occur if there is an increase in the diameter of the blood vessels or there is an increase in the number of blood vessels. This is a key concept to understanding the ability of the pulmonary vasculature to drop its resistance in response to increases in arterial or venous pressure (Figure 1.16). During increases in blood flow, the initial mechanism to reduce resistance is the recruitment of capillaries with low or no blood flow. If this mechanism is not sufficient and pressures begin to rise, the pulmonary capillaries then distend, which increases the surface area that blood may pass through, thereby decreasing the pressure.

An additional mechanism that alters pulmonary resistance is the volume of the lung, although its relationship is complex. A change

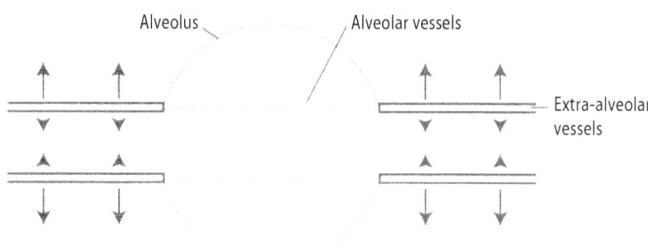

FIGURE 1.15. Alveolar and extraalveolar vessels. Alveolar vessels are predominantly capillaries exposed to alveolar pressure. Extraalveolar vessels are pulled open by the radial traction of the lung parenchyma, resulting in a lower external pressure that promotes vascular patency. (From West JB. Respiratory Physiology—The Essentials. Philadelphia: Lippincott Williams & Wilkins; 2000:31, with permission.)

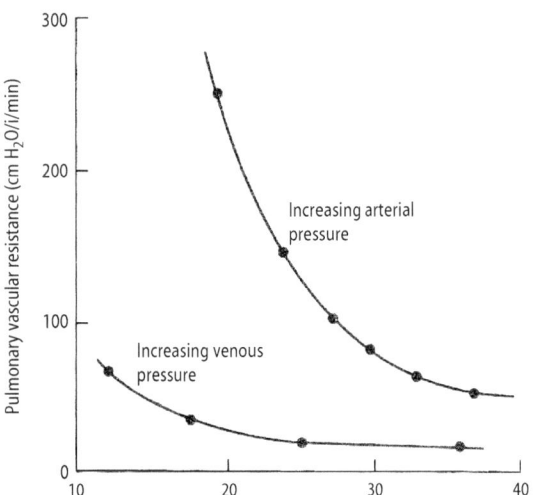

FIGURE 1.16. Pulmonary vascular resistance decreases with increases in either pulmonary arterial or venous pressure. During decreases in arterial pressure, venous pressure was held constant and vice versa. (From West JB. Respiratory Physiology—The Essentials. Philadelphia: Lippincott Williams & Wilkins; 2000:33, with permission.)

is lung volume has opposite effects on the resistances of extraalveolar and alveolar vessels. During lung inflation, the radial traction as noted earlier opens extraalveolar vessels; however, the same increase in lung volume increases the resistance to flow through alveolar vessels (Figure 1.17). It can be seen from Figure 1.11 that there is a lung volume where pulmonary resistance is at a minimum. It has been concluded that this lung volume, where pulmonary resistance nadirs, is FRC [44].

Neurogenic stimuli, vasoactive compounds, and chemical mediators have been demonstrated to alter PVR in the setting of elevated PVR in adults. However, in adults with normal PVR, these agents do not appear to significantly alter resistance. Interestingly, the neonate appears to respond to a variety of dilating agents, including acetylcholine, β-adrenergic agonists, bradykinin, prostaglan-

din E_1, prostacyclin, bosentan, calcium channel blockers, and nitric oxide. The ability of the pulmonary vasculature to constrict is not age dependent, and even newborns with only a small amount of arterial muscularization are able to induce significant pulmonary vasoconstriction, as noted in neonates with persistent pulmonary hypertension (PPHN). There are numerous vasoconstrictors, including endothelin, carbon dioxide, thromboxanes, hypoxia, and platelet activating factor.

Distribution of Blood Flow

Blood flow in the lung, whether supine or upright, is influenced by gravity. In the upright lung, blood flow decreases almost linearly from the base to the apex. The uneven distribution is explained by the hydrostatic pressure differences within blood vessels. In order to understand the effects of the hydrostatic forces, one may consider the lung as being composed of three distinct units or zones (Figure 1.18). At the apex of the lung, zone 1, alveolar pressure exceeds both pulmonary arterial and venous pressures, resulting in collapse of the alveolar vessels. This zone is ventilated, but not perfused, and is termed *alveolar dead space*. In the midregion of the lung is zone 2, where pulmonary arterial pressure exceeds alveolar pressure. Blood flow is determined by the difference between alveolar and arterial pressures in this zone and is not impacted by venous pressure. At the base of the lung, zone 3, venous pressure exceeds alveolar pressure, and flow is determined by the usual arterial-venous pressure difference.

Ventilation–Perfusion Relationships

Matching ventilation to perfusion (V/Q) depends to some extent on gravity. Both ventilation and perfusion rise with increasing distance toward the base of the lung; however, perfusion increases more than ventilation, which accounts for the variability in V/Q from apex to base (Figure 1.19). The apical regions are usually underperfused, V/Q = 3, while the base is underventilated in relation to perfusion, V/Q = 0.6 [45]. In the discussion and explanation to follow, it is important to recognize the difference between shunt and venous admixture.

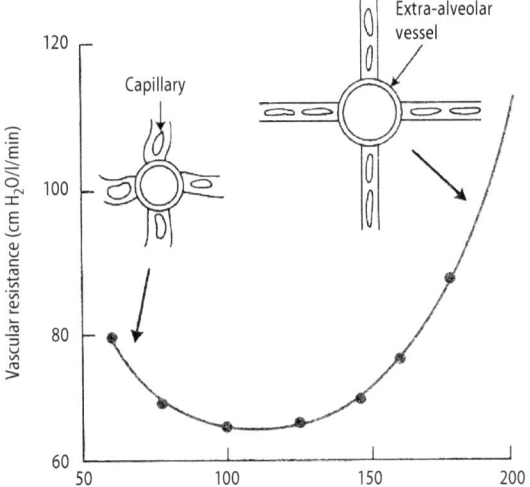

FIGURE 1.17. Effects on pulmonary vascular resistance as lung volume changes. At low lung volumes the extraalveolar vessels are narrow, and at high volumes the capillaries are stretched, reducing their caliber. Both of these effects increase pulmonary vascular resistance. (From West JB. Respiratory Physiology—The Essentials. Philadelphia: Lippincott Williams & Wilkins; 2000:35, with permission.)

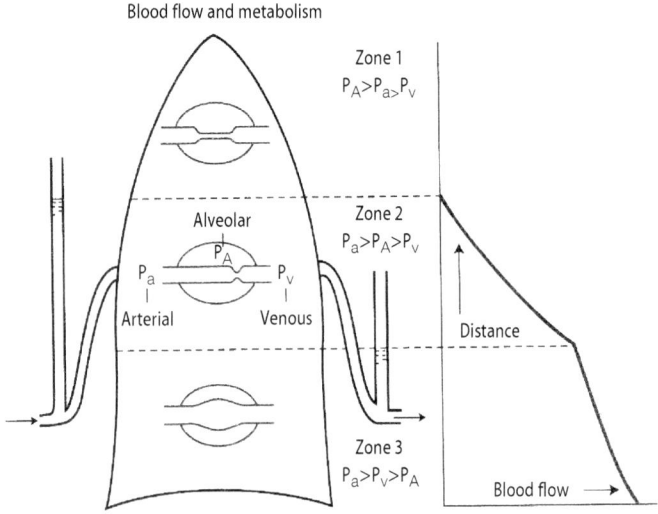

FIGURE 1.18. West lung zones. Explanation of uneven distribution of blood flow. (From West JB. Respiratory Physiology—The Essentials. Philadelphia: Lippincott Williams & Wilkins; 2000:37, with permission.)

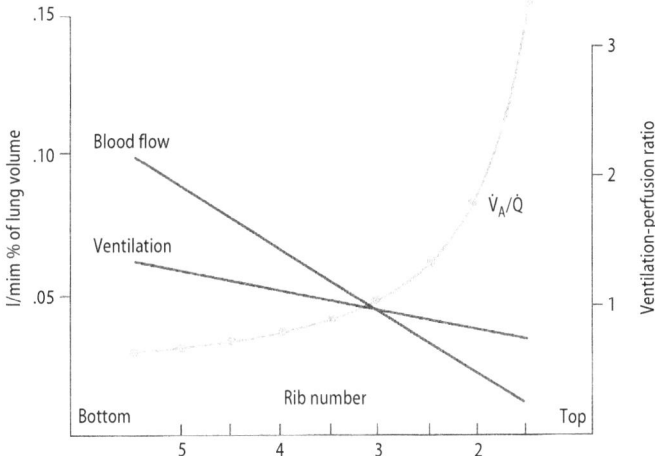

FIGURE 1.19. The distribution of pulmonary blood flow, ventilation, and the ventilation/perfusion ratio as found between apex and base in an upright lung. (From West JB. Respiratory Physiology—The Essentials. Philadelphia: Lippincott Williams & Wilkins; 2000:54, with permission.)

Shunt refers to the anatomic shunt that occurs when venous blood travels to the arterial side of the circulation without contacting ventilated lung. Examples include bronchial and thebesian circulation, right-to-left shunting in cyanotic congenital heart disease, and blood flow through completely atelectatic lung segments. Venous admixture is the amount of venous blood that needs to be added to the pulmonary end-capillary blood to produce the actual arterial oxygen content. Venous admixture is a calculated value and not an anatomic construct. Lung units with low V/Q ratios contribute to venous admixture. They are differentiated from lung units with V/Q ratios of 0 by the fact that the administration of supplemental oxygen will increase the saturation of blood emerging from their end capillaries.

V/Q mismatching lowers arterial PO_2 and results in desaturation through the addition of mixed venous blood to pulmonary end-capillary blood. There are two additional reasons that V/Q mismatching results in lower arterial PO_2. (1) More blood will flow through lung units with low V/Q ratios than through high V/Q units, resulting a greater amount of venous admixture. (2) Because of the sigmoidal shape of the oxyhemoglobin dissociation curve, lung units with low V/Q ratios have lower PO_2 values and accordingly lie on the steep portion of the curve and will have a disproportionately greater drop in saturation. This is in contrast to high V/Q units, which reside on the flat part of the curve, and even large increases in PO_2 will have minimal impact on saturation. The net result is arterial desaturation, as slightly higher oxygen contents from high V/Q units cannot counteract the significantly lower oxygen contents from the low V/Q units.

The difference between mixed venous PCO_2 (46 mm Hg) and pulmonary end-capillary PCO_2 (40 mm Hg) is not very great. Accordingly, even a significant amount of venous admixture will only produce a very small increase in arterial PCO_2. The presence of dead space ventilation, on the other hand, will have a much larger impact on arterial PCO_2. For example, an infant with bronchiolitis may have a large portion of his lung composed of lung units with high V/Q ratios. In this setting, additional increases in ventilation will be ineffective at eliminating PCO_2, as these units are already maximally ventilated in relation to their perfusion.

References

1. O'Brodovich HM, Haddad GG. The functional basis of respiratory pathology and disease. In: Chernick V, Boat TF, eds. Kendig's Disorders of the Respiratory Tract in Children, 6th ed. Philadelphia: WB Saunders; 1998:34.
2. Gautier C. Developmental anatomy and physiology of the respiratory system. In: Taussig LM, Landau LI, eds. Pediatric Respiratory Medicine. St. Louis: Mosby; 1999:24.
3. O'Brodovich HM, Haddad GG. The functional basis of respiratory pathology and disease. In: Chernick V, Boat TF, eds. Kendig's Disorders of the Respiratory Tract in Children, 6th ed. Philadelphia: WB Saunders; 1998:36.
4. O'Brodovich HM, Haddad GG. The functional basis of respiratory pathology and disease. In: Chernick V, Boat TF, eds. Kendig's Disorders of the Respiratory Tract in Children, 6th ed. Philadelphia: WB Saunders; 1998:37.
5. Boyden EA, Tompsett DH. The changing patterns in the developing lungs of infants. Acta Anat (Basel) 1965;61:164.
6. Dunnil MS. Postnatal growth of the lung. Thorax 1962;17:329.
7. Macklem PT. Airway obstruction and collateral ventilation. Physiol Rev 1971;51:368.
8. Bodeyn EA. Development and growth of the airways. In: Hodson WA, ed. Development of the Lung. New York: Marcel Dekker; 1977:3.
9. Halfaer MA, Nichols DG, Rogers MC. Developmental physiology of the respiratory system. In: Rogers MC, Nichols DG, eds. Textbook of Pediatric Intensive Care, 3rd ed. Baltimore: Williams & Wilkins; 1996:100.
10. O'Brodovich HM, Haddad GG. The functional basis of respiratory pathology and disease. In: Chernick V, Boat TF, eds. Kendig's Disorders of the Respiratory Tract in Children, 6th ed. Philadelphia: WB Saunders; 1998:39.
11. Zapletal A, Paut T, Samanek M. Pulmonary elasticity in children and adolescents. J Appl Physiol 1976;40:953–959.
12. Keely FW, Fagan DG, Webster SI. Quantity and character of elastin in developing human lung parenchymal tissues of normal infants and infants with respiratory distress syndrome. J Lab Clin Med 1977;90: 982–989.
13. West JB. Respiratory Physiology—The Essentials. Philadelphia: Lippincott Williams & Wilkins; 2000:83.
14. O'Brodovich HM, Haddad GG. The functional basis of respiratory pathology and disease. In: Chernick V, Boat TF, eds. Kendig's Disorders of the Respiratory Tract in Children, 6th ed. Philadelphia: WB Saunders; 1998:41.
15. Marchal F, Crance JP. Measurement of ventilatory system compliance in infants and young children. Respir Physiol 1987;68:311–318.
16. Halfaer MA, Nichols DG, Rogers MC. Developmental physiology of the respiratory system. In: Rogers MC, Nichols DG, eds. Textbook of Pediatric Intensive Care, 3rd ed. Baltimore: Williams & Wilkins; 1996:121.
17. Guslits BG, Gaston SE, Bryan MH, England SJ, Bryan AC. Diaphragmatic work of breathing in premature human infants. J Appl Physiol 1987;62:1410–1415.
18. Muller N, Volgyesi G, Calle D, Whitton J, Froese AB, Bryan MH, Bryan AC. Diaphragmatic muscle fatigue in the newborn. J Appl Physiol 1979;46:688.
19. Levitsky MG. Pulmonary Physiology. New York: McGraw-Hill; 1991:33.
20. West JB. Respiratory Physiology—The Essentials. Philadelphia: Lippincott Williams & Wilkins; 2000:92.
21. Hogg JC, Williams J, Richardson JB, Macklem PT, Thurlbeck WM. Age as factor in the distribution of lower airway conductance and in the pathologic anatomy of obstructive lung disease. N Engl J Med 1970; 282:1283.
22. West JB. Respiratory Physiology—The Essentials. Philadelphia: Lippincott Williams & Wilkins; 2000:94.
23. Halfaer MA, Nichols DG, Rogers MC. Developmental physiology of the respiratory system. In: Rogers MC, Nichols DG, eds. Textbook of Pediatric Intensive Care. Baltimore: Williams & Wilkins; 1996:105.

24. Merritt TA. Oxygen exposure in the newborn guinea pig-lung lavage cell populations, chemotactic and elastase response: a possible relationship to neonatal broncho-pulmonary dysplasia. Pediatr Res 1982; 16:798.

25. O'Brodovich HM, Haddad GG. The functional basis of respiratory pathology and disease. In: Chernick V, Boat TF, eds. Kendig's Disorders of the Respiratory Tract in Children, 6th ed. Philadelphia: WB Saunders; 1998:41.

26. Agostoni E. Volume–pressure relationships to the thorax and lung in the newborn. J Appl Physiol 1959;14:909–913.

27. Gaultier CL, Boule M, Allaire Y, Clement A, Girard F. Growth of lung volumes during the first three years of life. Bull Eur Physiopathol Respir 1979;15:1103–1116.

28. Le Souef PN, Endlgand SJ, Bryan AC. Passive respiratory mechanics in newborns and children. Am Rev Respir Dis 1984;129:552–556.

29. Mortola JP, Milic-Emili J, Noworaj A, Smith B, Fox G, Weeks S. Muscle pressure and flow during expiration in infants. Am Rev Respir Dis 1984;129:49–53.

30. Kosch PC, Hutchison AA, Wozniak JA, Carlo WA, Stark AR. Posterior cricoarytenoid and diaphragm activities during tidal breathing in neonates. J Appl Physiol 1988;64:1968–1978.

31. Stark AR, Cohlan BA, Waggener TB, Frantz ID III, Kosch PC. Regulation of end-expiratory lung volume during sleep in premature infants. J Appl Physiol 1987;62:1117–1123.

32. Harding R, Johnson P, McClelland ME. Respiratory function of the larynx in developing sheep and the influence of sleep state. Respir Physiol 1980;40:165–179.

33. Mansell A, Bryan C, Levison H. Airway closure in children. J Appl Physiol 1972;33:711.

34. Dantzker DR, Brook CJ, Dehart P, et al. Ventilation–perfusion distributions in the adult respiratory distress syndrome. Am Rev Respir Dis 199;120:1039–1052.

35. Marini JJ, Ravenscraft SA. Mean airway pressure: physiologic determinants and clinical importance—parts 1 and 2. Crit Care Med 1992;20:1604–1616.

36. Boros SJ, Matalon SV, Ewald R, et al. The effect of independent variations in inspiratory–expiratory ration and end-expiratory pressure during mechanical ventilation in hyaline membrane disease: the significance of mean airway pressure. J Pediatr 1977;91:794–798.

37. Weisman IM, Rinaldo JE, Rogers RM, Sanders MH. Intermittent mandatory ventilation. Am Rev Respir Dis 1983;127:641–647.

38. Mansell A, Bryan C, Levison H. Airway closure in children. J Appl Physiol 1972;33:711–714.

39. Banner MJ, Jaegar MJ, Kirby RR. Components of the work of breathing and implications for monitoring ventilator-dependent patients. Crit Care Med 1994;22:515–523.

40. Halfaer MA, Nichols DG, Rogers MC. Developmental physiology of the respiratory system. In: Rogers MC, Nichols DG, eds. Textbook of Pediatric Intensive Care, 3rd ed. Baltimore: Williams & Wilkins; 1996:106.

41. Belik J, Keeley FW, Baldwin F, Rabinovitch M. Pulmonary hypertension and vascular remodeling in fetal sheep. Am J Physiol 1994;266: H2303–H2309.

42. Rabinovitch M, Keane JF, Norwood WI, Castaneda AR, Reid L. Vascular structure in lung tissue obtained at biopsy correlated with pulmonary hemodynamic findings after repair of congenital heart defects. Circulation 1984;69:655–667.

43. O'Brodovich HM, Haddad GG. The functional basis of respiratory pathology and disease. In: Chernick V, Boat TF, eds. Kendig's Disorders of the Respiratory Tract in Children, 6th ed. Philadelphia: WB Saunders; 1998:47.

44. O'Brodovich HM, Haddad GG. The functional basis of respiratory pathology and disease. In: Chernick V, Boat TF, eds. Kendig's Disorders of the Respiratory Tract in Children, 6th ed. Philadelphia: WB Saunders; 1998:49.

45. Halfaer MA, Nichols DG, Rogers MC. Developmental physiology of the respiratory system. In: Rogers MC, Nichols DG, eds. Textbook of Pediatric Intensive Care, 3rd ed. Baltimore: Williams & Wilkins; 1996:109.

2
Disorders of the Pediatric Chest

Margaret A. Chase and Derek S. Wheeler

Introduction

The lungs are unique in that they are internal organs, yet they are constantly exposed to a barrage of foreign substances from both the internal environment—at any one point in time, they receive approximately half of the cardiac output—and the external environment—with each breath, they are exposed to pollens, viruses, bacteria, smoke, and so forth. There is a virtual cornucopia of diseases that affect the human respiratory tract, many of which are specific to the pediatric chest. According to the Centers for Disease Control and Prevention, chronic respiratory tract diseases and pneumonia were the seventh and eighth leading causes of deaths in children aged 1–19 years in 2002 [1]. Dr. George A. Gregory, one of the founding fathers of pediatric critical care medicine, once stated that acute respiratory failure accounts for approximately 50% of all admissions to the pediatric intensive care unit (PICU) [2]. Just as important are the myriad of respiratory disease processes that are not associated with acute respiratory failure but nevertheless constitute a major portion of the practice of pediatric critical care medicine, some of which result in significant morbidity and mortality [3]. In this chapter, we review some of these disease processes as a general introduction to the respiratory system in critical illness, and the remainder of these disorders are discussed in greater detail in subsequent chapters.

Congenital Anomalies of the Tracheobronchial Tree

Congenital anomalies of the trachea (e.g., tracheomalacia, tracheal stenosis, tracheoesophageal fistula) are described in subsequent chapters in this textbook and are not discussed further here.

Bronchomalacia

Bronchomalacia frequently coexists with tracheomalacia (some authors prefer the term *tracheobronchomalacia*) [4–8]. *Malacia* refers to an intrinsic defect of the cartilaginous support of the airway, causing the affected portion of the airway to collapse whenever the extraluminal pressure exceeds the intraluminal pressure (e.g., during forced exhalation, crying). Primary (congenital) and secondary (acquired) forms exist. Tracheobronchomalacia is frequently found in association with gastroesophageal reflux, cardiovascular anomalies (especially vascular rings, pulmonary slings, etc.), and tracheoesophageal fistula [5,7,8]. Affected children typically present with respiratory distress, wheezing, chronic cough, and recurrent pneumonia. Historically, tracheotomy and long-term mechanical ventilatory support have been the mainstays of treatment, although recent technologic improvements in noninvasive positive pressure ventilation will likely improve the outcome of children with this disease. Surgical treatment options include resection of affected segments, pexy procedures (aortopexy, bronchopexy, etc.), and stenting [9–13].

Tracheal Bronchus

The *tracheal bronchus* (also commonly referred to as a *pig bronchus*) encompasses a variety of congenital bronchial anomalies, although an anomalous right upper lobe bronchus arising from the lateral wall of the trachea is most commonly described [14–16]. This anomaly occurs in 0.1%–5% of the population [17–19] and is frequently associated with other congenital anomalies, such as tracheoesophageal fistula, tracheal stenosis, and Down's syndrome [15,16,20–23]. Affected children are usually asymptomatic, although the diagnosis should be entertained for critically ill children with persistent or recurrent upper-lobe pneumonia, atelectasis, or air-trapping on chest radiograph [20]. Although most children can be managed conservatively, surgical resection of the involved lung segment may be necessary when symptoms are severe [14,16,20].

Bronchial Atresia

Congenital bronchial atresia (CBA) is rare and most commonly affects the upper lobes of the lung. In most cases, the atresia affects either a proximal segmental or subsegmental bronchus. Development of the structures distal to the affected segment is unaffected, however, and mucus often accumulates in the affected lung segments, leading to the formation of a bronchocele with surrounding areas of hyperinflation [24,25]. Although frequently detected as an incidental finding on chest radiograph, CBA occasionally results in recurrent infections of affected lung segments [24]. Lobectomy or segmentectomy of the affected areas is curative but only occasionally necessary [26,27].

Bronchogenic Cysts

Bronchogenic cysts arise from abnormal budding of tracheobronchial tissue during embryogenesis. The respiratory system develops as an outpouching of the embryonic foregut. Therefore, histologically, bronchogenic cysts are lined with ciliated epithelium and frequently contain cartilage, smooth muscle, mucous glands, nerve tissue, and occasionally gastric epithelium. They may be air filled, mucus filled, or both [16,28]. These cysts are single, unilocular, and spherical in shape and are usually classified by their location in the thorax (central or mediastinal bronchogenic cysts and peripheral or pulmonary bronchogenic cysts) [16,28]. Most bronchogenic cysts are asymptomatic and are detected as an incidental finding on chest radiograph [16,28]. However, respiratory distress may be precipitated by enlargement of the cyst with subsequent airway compromise. Additional complications include rupture of the cyst into a bronchus or the pleura with hemorrhage, recurrent infections, and abscess formation. Surgery is indicated when these cysts are symptomatic, and most authors advocate surgical resection upon diagnosis because of the risk of associated complications [16,28–30].

Congenital Anomalies of the Lung

Congenital Lobar Emphysema

Congenital lobar emphysema (CLE) is characterized by massive distension of one or more affected lobes of the lung, most commonly the left upper lobe [16,28,30–33]. Congenital lobar emphysema is the most common congenital lung anomaly and is thought to arise from a ball-valve type of bronchial obstruction resulting in progressive air trapping and hyperinflation [16,28,33]. This bronchial obstruction is idiopathic in most cases, although extrinsic vascular compression and bronchomalacia have occasionally been implicated [34–38]. Congenital heart disease is present in 10% of affected infants [28]. Congenital lobar emphysema appears to be more common in males than in females and typically presents before 6 months of age. Respiratory distress is the most common clinical presentation [16,28,33,37,38]. Chest radiography will demonstrate hyperinflation of affected lobes, and CLE is frequently confused with pneumothorax [39]. Surgical resection of the affected lobe is curative [16,28–33,39].

Congenital Cystic Adenomatoid Malformation

Congenital cystic adenomatoid malformations (CCAM) are the second most common congenital lung anomalies and represent maldevelopment of the terminal bronchiolar structures during early lung embryogenesis. Congenital cystic adenomatoid malformation consists of a multicystic, dysplastic mass of pulmonary tissue and typically presents either prenatally on routine ultrasound or during the neonatal period with severe respiratory dis-

tress. Management depends on the extent of disease, and prognosis is variable [16,26,28–31,33,36,40]. Malignant transformation of CCAM (high incidence of rhabdomyosarcoma) has been described such that surgical resection is probably indicated even when the lesion is asymptomatic [41–44].

Congenital Diaphragmatic Hernia

Congenital diaphragmatic hernia results from a defect in the diaphragm that allows evisceration of abdominal contents into the thorax (the left hemithorax in the vast majority of cases) (Figure 2.1). Congenital diaphragmatic hernia is frequently detected on prenatal ultrasound, and severely affected fetuses often die before birth. More than 50% of cases have additional congenital anomalies (i.e., cardiac, genitourinary, and chromosomal anomalies). Although the majority of cases present with severe respiratory compromise immediately after birth, late presentation beyond the immediate neonatal period occasionally occurs and is typically milder [16,28,45,46]. Definitive surgery includes decompression of the lungs by reduction of the abdominal viscera and primary closure of the diaphragmatic defect. The majority of affected children will have some degree of pulmonary hypoplasia as well as pulmonary artery hypertension resulting from increased muscularization of the intraacinar pulmonary arteries, a small cross-sectional area of the pulmonary vascular bed, and abnormal pulmonary vasoconstriction, all of which will impact long-term outcome [16,28,47,48].

Pulmonary Sequestration

Pulmonary sequestration is defined as a lung segment that receives its blood supply from an anomalous systemic artery and does not communicate with the tracheobronchial tree [16,26,28,29,31,33,

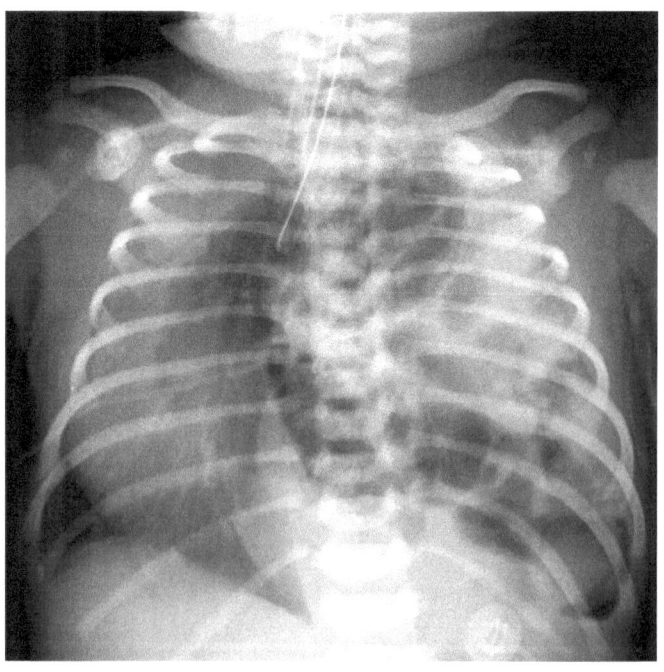

FIGURE 2.1. .Congenital diaphragmatic hernia in a term male newborn admitted to the neonatal intensive care unit with respiratory failure. (Courtesy of Corning Benton, MD, Cincinnati Children's Hospital Medical Center.)

49–51]. Traditionally, sequestrations are divided into *extralobar*, in which the abnormal lung segment lies within its own pleura and is located more posteriorly in the chest, and *intralobar*, in which the abnormal lung segment lies within the pleural cavity in close contact with the normal lung. Venous drainage of intralobar sequestrations is usually via the pulmonary veins, whereas extralobar sequestrations drain to the systemic venous circulation via the azygos vein, hemiazygos vein, or vena cava. The vast majority of sequestrations affect the lower lobes, usually on the left. Intralobar sequestrations are frequently acquired anomalies that arise from recurrent infections or bronchial obstruction. Extralobar sequestrations, on the other hand, are congenital and usually diagnosed at an earlier age because of a higher incidence of associated anomalies. There is a 4:1 male:female preponderance for extralobar sequestrations, whereas intralobar sequestrations affect both equally. Infants present with recurrent lower respiratory infections, reactive airway disease, and, occasionally, hemoptysis. Treatment of pulmonary sequestration is resection; extralobar tissue can be treated with resection alone, and intralobar lesions will usually require lobectomy [16,26,28,29,31,33,49–51].

Scimitar Syndrome

The scimitar syndrome, also called *congenital venolobar syndrome*, is a rare congenital anomaly classically described by (1) partial or complete anomalous pulmonary venous drainage of the right lung to the inferior vena cava, (2) hypoplasia of the right lung, (3) hypoplasia of the right pulmonary artery, (4) dextrocardia, and (5) anomalous systemic arterial supply of the right lower lobe of the lung from the subdiaphragmatic descending aorta or its branches [16,52–55]. The majority of children are symptomatic; however, clinical presentation depends to a great extent on significance of the resulting left-to-right shunt. Two forms are commonly described [56–59]. The infantile form is usually associated with a variety of congenital anomalies, including additional congenital heart defects such as coarctation of the aorta, tetralogy of Fallot, and ventricular septal defect. Affected children are prone to recurrent pneumonia, congestive heart failure, and pulmonary hypertension [57–59]. The adult form is characterized by a small left-to-right shunt with minor symptoms and lack of associated anomalies [56,59]. Surgical management of the scimitar syndrome is often dependent on the clinical presentation and is therefore age dependent [59–61]. Indications for surgery include (1) the presence of a large left-to-right shunt with consequent pulmonary hypertension and heart failure and (2) recurrent pneumonia caused by pulmonary sequestration [61]. Surgical management includes ligation of the anomalous systemic artery, reimplantation of the scimitar vein to the left atrium, and resection of the sequestration [59–62]. Postoperative pulmonary venous obstruction or pulmonary hypertension is frequent and greatly impacts outcome.

Pulmonary Agenesis, Aplasia, and Hypoplasia

Pulmonary underdevelopment is commonly classified into three groups: (1) pulmonary agenesis (complete absence of bronchus and lung), (2) pulmonary aplasia (rudimentary bronchus ends blindly without lung tissue), and (3) pulmonary hypoplasia (incomplete development of the bronchus with variable reduction in lung tissue) [16,26,28,47,48,63–69]. Associated congenital anomalies are frequently present [63,64,66,68]. Compensatory hyperinflation of the contralateral lung with herniation across the midline is typically noted on chest radiograph. Additional findings include mediastinal shift toward the affected hemithorax, which is usually accentuated during inspiration. Management is largely supportive, as there are currently no acceptable long-term surgical options for management of these children [16,26,28,47,48]. Expandable prosthetic devices (including saline-filled prostheses, ping pong ball plombage, etc.) used for the postpneumonectomy syndrome (dyspnea and respiratory distress occurring secondary to mediastinal shift into the empty hemithorax) [70–72] have been attempted recently with some success [73].

Atelectasis

The term *atelectasis* is derived from the Greek words *ateles* and *ektasis*, which literally mean *incomplete expansion*. Atelectasis is associated with a variety of respiratory diseases and may be identified in as many as 15% of children admitted to the PICU [74–77]. Atelectasis occurs by three mechanisms: (1) compression of lung parenchyma by intrathoracic, chest wall, or extrathoracic disease processes (*compression atelectasis*); (2) obstruction of airways with subsequent gas resorption (*resorption atelectasis*); and (3) increased surface tension in small airways and alveoli (Table 2.1) [78–80]. *Compression atelectasis* occurs when the distending pressure (i.e., transmural pressure) that keeps an alveolus open is reduced below a certain threshold, allowing the alveolus to collapse. The dependent lung regions are the areas most commonly affected by this type of atelectasis.

Resorption atelectasis occurs via one of two possible mechanisms. In the first, complete airway obstruction creates a pocket of trapped gas in the alveoli distal to the obstruction. As the affected lung region is perfused, but not ventilated, gas is absorbed and the alveoli eventually collapse. The second mechanism is a conse-

TABLE 2.1. Causes of atelectasis in infants and children.

Compression atelectasis
  Extrinsic bronchial compression
    Tumors
    Lymph nodes
    Cardiomegaly (e.g., congenital heart disease, congestive heart failure)
    Vascular rings
    Congenital lobar emphysema
  Compression of lung parenchyma
    Chylothorax
    Hemothorax
    Pneumothorax
    Tumors
Resorption atelectasis
  Intrabronchial obstruction
    Obstructive airways disease (e.g., asthma, cystic fibrosis, bronchiolitis)
    Foreign body
    Inspissated secretions and/or mucous plugs
    Cystic fibrosis
    Sickle cell disease and acute chest syndrome
  Administration of High FiO_2 in the setting of low V_A/Q
Surfactant deficiency or dysfunction
  Infant respiratory distress syndrome (hyaline membrane disease)
  Acute respiratory distress syndrome
  Pneumonia
  Pulmonary edema
  Near-drowning

quence of oxygen being more readily absorbed than nitrogen. As a result, the rate of absorption of the gas increases with the fractional concentration of oxygen in the alveoli. Administration of either supplemental oxygen or mechanical ventilation with high fractional inspired oxygen (FiO_2) can result in resorption atelectasis, especially in lung zones with low ventilation to perfusion (V_A/Q) ratios. Finally, loss or dysfunction of surfactant results in increased surface tension in small airways and alveoli, leading to lung collapse. All three mechanisms likely contribute to atelectasis in acute lung injury and its more severe form, the acute respiratory distress syndrome [78–80].

Young children are particularly susceptible to atelectasis compared with older children and adults [74,75,77,78,80]. As previously discussed, the child's airways are smaller than the adult's and have a higher peripheral airways resistance [81,82]. The child's airways are therefore more susceptible to obstruction by inspissated secretions or mucus. In addition, children are more susceptible to dynamic airway compression because of weak cartilaginous support [83,84]. Finally, the collateral pathways of ventilation (pores of Kohn and Lambert's canals) are less well developed in children than adults [78,80,83–86] such that airway obstruction leads to air trapping and subsequent collapse via *resorption atelectasis*. Children also appear to differ from adults with respect to the distribution of atelectasis as well. The upper lobes, especially the right upper lobe, appear to be more commonly affected in critically ill children admitted to the PICU [74–77]. Collapse of the lower lobes, especially the left lower lobe, appears to be more common in critically ill adults.

Atelectasis compromises pulmonary function by affecting both mechanical properties of the lung as well as gas exchange According to the Laplace relationship, smaller alveoli (e.g., collapsed or atelectatic areas of lung) require a greater opening pressure to reinflate and reexpand. As the lung now requires higher pressures to inflate, atelectasis causes a significant reduction in lung compli-

ance. Atelectasis also leads to ventilation–perfusion mismatch, leading to gas exchange abnormalities and hypoxemia. Atelectasis may also result in a compensatory overdistention of adjacent alveoli, especially in the setting of airways obstruction and obstructive atelectasis [78,80,86]. Additional consequences of atelectasis can include bronchiectasis, pneumonia, and lung abscess, which result from retained, infected secretions within the collapsed lung and not atelectasis per se.

A chest radiograph is often required to document the presence, extent, and distribution of atelectasis (Figure 2.2). Opacification may represent areas of either collapse or consolidation. However, loss of lung volume with movement of the diaphragm, mediastinum, and major fissures toward the affected areas are highly suggestive of collapse (discussed later in the chapter on respiratory monitoring).

The management of atelectasis is tailored to the etiology as well as the prevention of subsequent complications (e.g., inspissated secretions and worsening airways obstruction, hypoxemia, infection). Several new modalities to facilitate reexpansion of atelectatic alveoli in the PICU are available, although few randomized, controlled clinical trials exist to support the merits of one modality over another [78,80,86,87]. Vigorous coughing, the use of incentive spirometry, and chest physiotherapy are frequently employed [88–91]. In recalcitrant cases, or those associated with neuromuscular disease or cystic fibrosis (CF), assisting devices such as intermittent positive pressure breathing [90,91], cough-assist insufflation/exsufflation therapy [92,93], or noninvasive bilevel positive pressure ventilation (BiPAP) [92–97] may be helpful. The use of recombinant DNase (rhDNase), which is approved for use in CF patients, has also been employed in persistent atelectasis, especially in those cases that are caused by resorption atelectasis secondary to obstruction by inspissated secretions. DNase is thought to improve atelectasis by decreasing the viscosity of secretions and assisting mucociliary clearance, thereby relieving airways obstruction [98–

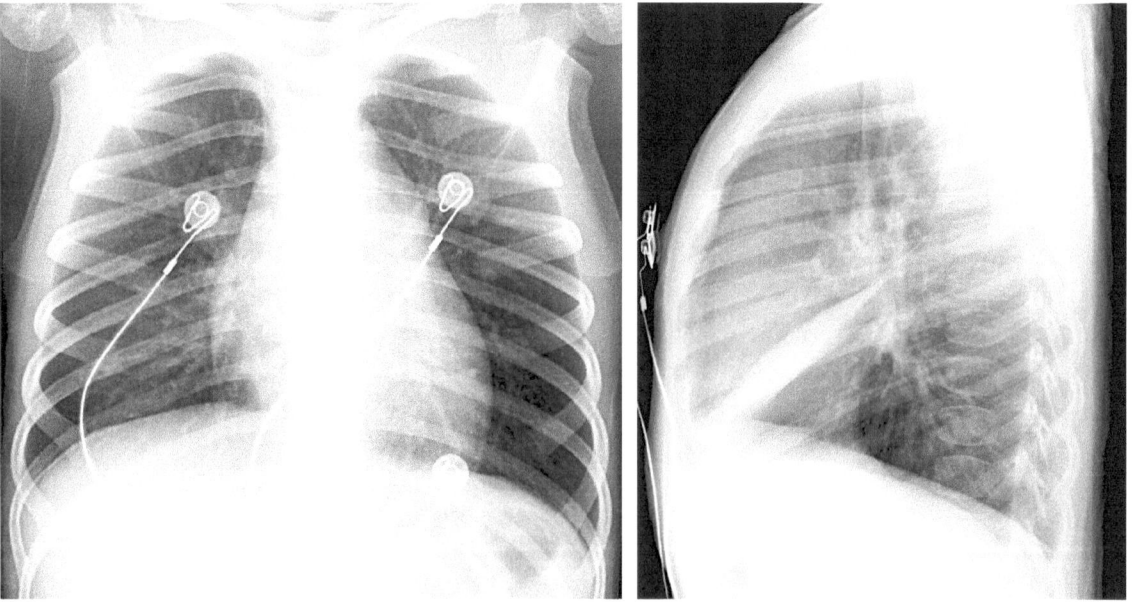

FIGURE 2.2. Right middle lobe atelectasis in a 3-year-old child admitted to the pediatric intensive care unit with status asthmaticus. (**A**) Anteroposterior view. (**B**) Lateral view. (Courtesy of Corning Benton, MD, Cincinnati Children's Hospital Medical Center.)

107]. Finally, for those patients requiring ventilator support, atelectasis can necessitate a prolonged course on the ventilator and thus has increased risks of associated complications. For these patients, the use of positive end-expiratory pressure, often in increased levels, as well as increased inspiratory times may be necessary. If atelectasis is not resolved with these interventions, flexible bronchoscopy may be helpful for diagnosis as well as removal of inspissated secretions and reexpansion of collapsed alveoli [108–111].

Pulmonary Edema

Pathophysiology

Pulmonary edema is defined simply as an abnormal accumulation of fluid in the lung. The net flow of fluid across the alveolar-capillary membrane is generally expressed using the Starling equation, as follows:

$$Q_f = K_f \left[(P_C - P_T) - \sigma (\pi_C - \pi_T) \right]$$

where Q_f is equal to the net flow across the alveolar–capillary membrane; K_f is the filtration coefficient, which takes into account the contribution of the permeability and surface area of the alveolar-capillary membrane; P_C is equal to the capillary hydrostatic pressure; P_T is equal to the interstitial fluid hydrostatic pressure; σ is the reflection coefficient of the alveolar–capillary membrane ($\sigma = 1$ if the membrane is completely impermeable to protein, and $\sigma = 0$ if the membrane is completely permeable to protein); π_C is the capillary oncotic pressure; and π_T is the interstitial oncotic pressure.

Under normal physiologic conditions, P_C is gravity dependent and ranges from 8 to 12 mm Hg, whereas P_T is estimated at –2 to –10 mm Hg. The balance of hydrostatic pressures therefore overwhelmingly favors net fluid movement *out* of the pulmonary capillary. Normally, π_C approximates 25 mm Hg, and π_T ranges between 10 and 15 mm Hg. Given that σ is between 0.7 and 0.95, the balance of oncotic pressures tends to favor a relatively small amount of net fluid movement into the pulmonary capillary. Therefore, under normal conditions, the balance of Starling forces across the alveolar–capillary membrane favors a net flow of fluid out from the microvascular space into the interstitium (Figure 2.3) [reviewed in 112–116].

Several factors protect against the development of pulmonary edema. If the alveolar–capillary membrane is able to retard the movement of proteins (i.e., σ remains unchanged), the increased

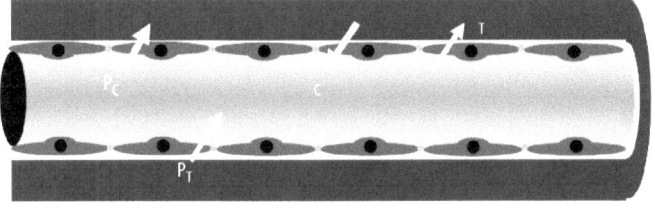

$$Q_f = K_f [(P_C - P_T) - \sigma (\pi_C - \pi_T)]$$

FIGURE 2.3. Starling forces across the pulmonary capillary endothelium. Q_f is net flow across the alveolar–capillary membrane; K_f is filtration coefficient; P_C is capillary hydrostatic pressure; P_T is interstitial fluid hydrostatic pressure; σ is reflection coefficient of the alveolar–capillary membrane ($\sigma = 1$ if the membrane is completely impermeable to protein, and $\sigma = 0$ if the membrane is completely permeable to protein); π_C is capillary oncotic pressure; and π_T is interstitial oncotic pressure.

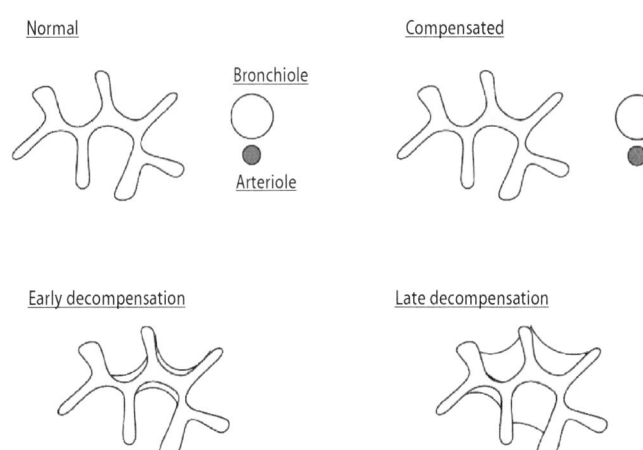

FIGURE 2.4. Pattern of alveolar fluid accumulation. (Adapted from Staub et al. [117].)

fluid that enters the interstitium will lower the interstitial osmotic pressure and thereby oppose interstitial fluid accumulation. In addition, the increased interstitial hydrostatic pressure that results from this fluid accumulation will abolish the normal hydrostatic pressure gradient and further oppose fluid movement into the interstitium. Finally, the lymphatics have a tremendous capacity to clear any fluid that accumulates within the lung interstitium. Once these defensive mechanisms are overcome, fluid begins to accumulate in a relatively predictable manner [117]. Fluid first accumulates in the loose interstitial tissue surrounding small blood vessels and airways. Alveolar fluid next accumulates in the corners of the alveolus, and, if edema persists, fluid eventually completely fills the alveolus (Figure 2.4).

The last decade has witnessed a dramatic increase in our understanding of the normal fluid clearance mechanisms of the lung. Importantly, the lung's ability to clear pulmonary edema (regardless of mechanism) correlates with improved survival in critical illnesses such as sepsis, acute lung injury, and congestive heart failure [118–120]. Under normal conditions, alveolar fluid clearance is dependent on the active transport of Na^+ and Cl^- (with water following) across the lung epithelium, a process that depends on Na^+/K^+ ATPase, intercellular tight junctions, and Na^+ ion channels [reviewed in 115,116,121,122]. Recent evidence suggests that alveolar lung clearance is partly regulated by endogenous β-adrenergic receptors, leading some investigators to suggest that aerosolized β-adrenergic agonists may be helpful in patients with acute lung injury and acute respiratory distress syndrome [120,122–126].

Etiology

Factors that increase the pulmonary capillary pressure, such as left ventricular failure or valvular regurgitation, serve to increase the driving force through the capillary wall into the interstitium and lead to fluid accumulation. This aspect of fluid accumulation, however, is not limited to cardiogenic causes and can also be seen in pulmonary veno-occlusive disease and other processes impairing pulmonary venous drainage (Figure 2.5A). Plasma oncotic pressure, often reflected in the child's serum albumin level, can also play a role in the accumulation of pulmonary edema (Figure 2.5B). In illnesses such as protein losing enteropathy or nephrotic syndrome, with increased protein losses, or those with decreased

Three forms of pulmonary edema:

1. ⬆ P_{MV} (cardiogenic pulmonary edema)

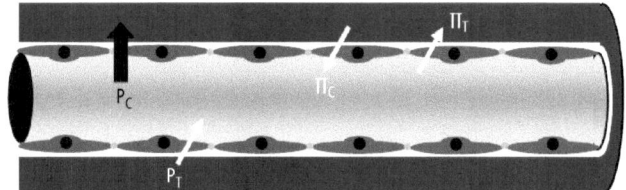

A

Three forms of pulmonary edema:

2. ⬇ π_C (osmotic pulmonary edema)

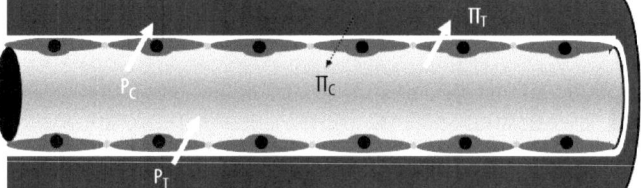

B

Three forms of pulmonary edema:

3. ⬇ σ (capillary leak pulmonary edema)

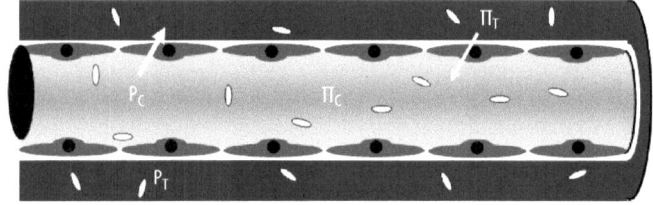

C

FIGURE 2.5. Mechanisms of pulmonary edema. (A) ↑ P_C. (B) ↓ π_C. (C) ↓ σ.

protein production, such as hepatic disease or malnutrition, the forces promoting return of fluid into the vascular space are decreased. These children develop systemic extravascular fluid overload, of which pulmonary edema can be the most clinically significant. In general, alteration of capillary membrane permeability is seen as a result of insult to the membrane itself (Figure 2.5C). In the PICU population, this is frequently a consequence of infection (either pulmonary or systemic) or acute respiratory distress syndrome. *Leaky* capillaries can also be attributed to circulating toxins such as chemotherapy or even endogenous mediators of the immune system such as leukotrienes, tumor necrosis factor-α, or histamine. Similarly, direct toxins, such as smoke, chemical irritants, or even water in near-drowning can injure the endothelium and alter permeability, predisposing to pulmonary edema.

An additional but poorly understood mechanism of pulmonary edema is that resulting from increased negative interstitial pressure or *postobstructive pulmonary edema*. It is most often seen in those disorders associated with upper airway obstruction such as croup, foreign body aspiration, severe acute asthma, or laryngospasm after the obstruction is relieved. High negative intrathoracic pressure causes increases in cardiac preload, afterload, and pulmonary blood flow, which in turn increase the microvascular pressure driving fluid into the interstitium. This may be an additional etiology of edema in those children experiencing smoke inhalation or near-drowning.

Neurogenic pulmonary edema is similarly not fully understood but may be associated with a massive sympathetic discharge. This release in catecholamines and the subsequent increase in sympathetic tone that follows may increase pulmonary and systemic vasoconstriction, shifting blood to the pulmonary vasculature, increasing capillary pressure, and leading to edema formation. There may also be a component of increased capillary permeability from stress failure or hypoxia-related injury of the capillary endothelium contributing to pulmonary edema formation.

Clinical Consequences

The presence of fluid in the interstitial and alveolar spaces serves to decrease lung compliance and increase atelectasis. Most commonly, children with pulmonary edema develop some component of respiratory distress. This may be seen through increased work of breathing in an attempt to maintain minute ventilation or desaturations as V/Q mismatch progresses or to increase ventilator requirements in those already with respiratory failure. Physical examination of the lung fields may reveal wheezing and fine crackles. Chest radiograph serves as the main diagnostic tool (Figure 2.6). Early in the process, peribronchial and perivascular cuffing may be observed, resulting from interstitial edema. Lung fields demonstrating increased pulmonary vascular markings and cardiomegaly may be seen with edema arising from left ventricular dysfunction. Progressively, as edema begins to fill the alveolar spaces, diffuse patchy densities may be appreciated.

Management

Primary management of pulmonary edema should be directed at correcting the underlying disturbance that led to pulmonary edema. Often this is easier said than done, and supportive care of the patient focusing on respiratory stabilization and decreasing pulmonary edema is pursued. Removal of excessive interstitial and alveolar fluid can be attempted with diuretics [127]. However, diuretics such as furosemide probably work because of their effects on venous capacitance and not via the induced diuresis [112–116].

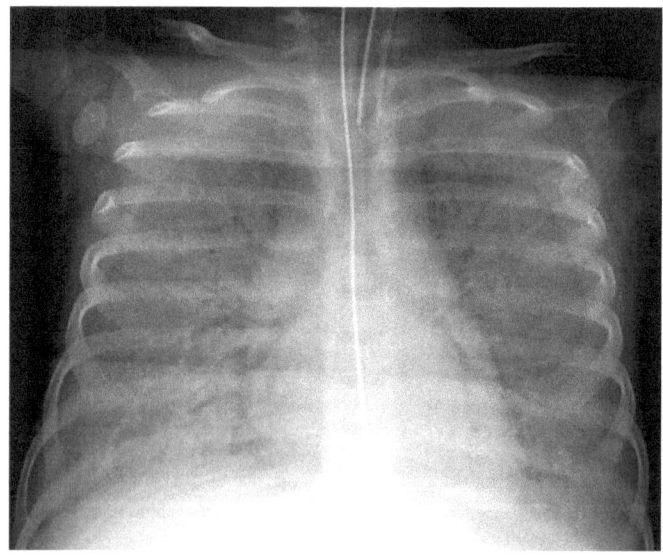

FIGURE 2.6. Pulmonary edema in an 11-month-old child with congestive heart failure. (Courtesy of Corning Benton, MD, Cincinnati Children's Hospital Medical Center.)

Supportive care with noninvasive ventilation is often helpful, as it decreases the work of breathing and provides a constant level of positive end-expiratory pressure, stenting open alveoli and forcing out excess fluid—although efforts to minimize further ventilator-induced lung injury are crucial as well. For those patients on the ventilator or with severe distress requiring ventilation, increased levels of positive end-expiratory should be employed for the same reasons. Additionally, dependent areas of the lung are at increased risk of developing pulmonary edema, and therefore frequent changes in patient position or even prone ventilation may help to mobilize fluid, resolve associated atelectasis, and redistribute areas of V/Q mismatch. For those patients with hypoalbuminemia and pulmonary edema, there may be some benefit of albumin supplementation in decreasing edema fluid [127]. Finally, as discussed earlier, aerosolized β-adrenergic agonists may help augment alveolar fluid clearance and relieve pulmonary edema [120,122–126].

Diseases of the Pleural Space

Pleural Effusions

The pleural membrane is a thin, double-layered membrane that separates the lung from the chest wall, diaphragm, and mediastinum. The outer layer, called the *parietal pleura*, covers the inner surface of the chest wall, including the mediastinum, diaphragm, and ribs. The inner layer, called the *visceral pleura*, covers the entire surface of the lungs, including the interlobar fissures, except for the hilus, where the pulmonary blood vessels, bronchi, and nerves enter the lung tissue. The mediastinum completely separates the right and left pleural spaces. Under normal conditions, the two pleurae are separated by a thin space (pleural space) that contains a small amount of serous fluid. This fluid provides a frictionless surface between the two pleurae in response to changes in lung volume with respiration. Essentially an ultrafiltrate of plasma, normal pleural fluid is clear in appearance, with a pH of 7.60–7.64,

a protein content less than 2% (1–2 g/dL), fewer than 1,000 WBCs per cubic millimeter, a glucose content similar to that of plasma, and a lactate dehydrogenase level less than 50% of plasma [128,129].

A pleural effusion (Figure 2.7) is broadly defined as an abnormal collection of fluid in the space between the parietal and visceral pleurae and may arise from a variety of processes that alter the normal flow and absorption of pleural fluid. These can include changes in the permeability of the pleural membrane (e.g., pneumonia, malignancy), reduction in intravascular oncotic pressure (e.g., hypoalbuminemia), increased capillary hydrostatic pressure (e.g., congestive heart failure, SVC syndrome), or decreased lymph drainage or lymphatic obstruction (e.g., thoracic duct trauma) [128,129]. The most common causes of pleural effusions in children are pneumonia (parapneumonic effusion), congenital heart disease, and malignancy [128,129]. A diagnostic or therapeutic thoracentesis is usually indicated to determine the nature of the effusion as well as to relieve associated dyspnea and respiratory compromise.

When performing a thoracentesis, the child is seated, leaning over a table or supine if that is not possible. The preferred entry is at the seventh intercostal space along the posterior axillary line. This area is cleaned and draped in sterile fashion and local anesthesia provided to the subcutaneous tissue, rib periosteum, and pleura with 1% lidocaine. An 18–22 gauge intravenous catheter over a needle or large-bore needle is attached to a syringe and advanced with steady negative pressure through the skin, onto the rib, and guided over the superior aspect of the rib, taking care to avoid the neurovascular bundle running beneath. Advancement of the needle is halted once fluid is obtained, and, if an intravenous or pigtail catheter with guidewire is used, the catheter may be advanced into the pleural space. Fluid is removed, and, once drainage is complete, the needle or catheter is removed and an occlusive dressing placed over the site. A chest radiograph should be obtained after the procedure to rule out pneumothorax.

Depending on analysis of the fluid obtained, pleural effusions may be classified into either transudates or exudates. In transuda-

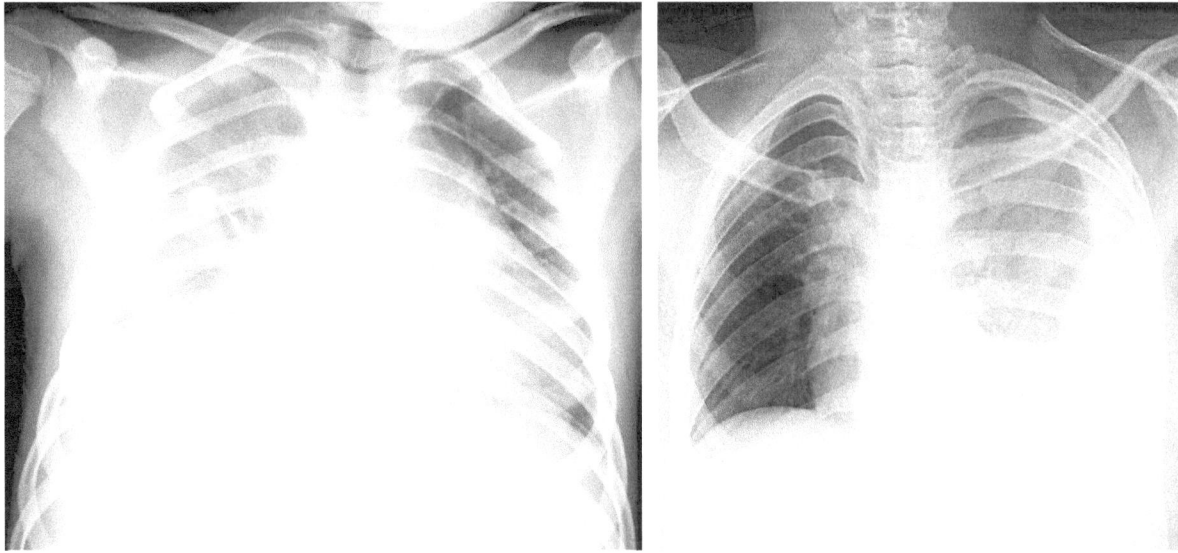

A   B

FIGURE 2.7. (**A**) Pleural effusion in a 9-year-old child with pneumonia (i.e., parapneumonic effusion). (**B**) Pleural effusion in a 19-year-old adolescent. (Courtesy of Corning Benton, MD, Cincinnati Children's Hospital Medical Center.)

TABLE 2.2. Evaluation of a pleural effusion: transudate versus exudates.

	Transudate	Exudate
pH	>7.4	<7.3
Protein (g/dL)	<3.0	>3.0
Lactate dehydrogenase (LDH)	<2/3 serum level	>2/3 serum level
Pleural fluid: serum protein	<0.5	>0.5
Pleural fluid: serum LDH	<0.6	>0.6
Red blood cell	<5,000	>5,000
White blood cell	<1,000	>1,000
Glucose	Equal to serum	Less than serum

tive effusions, the pleural membranes are intact and pleural permeability is normal. There is instead an imbalance of Starling forces along the pleural membrane from increased capillary hydrostatic pressure, decreased colloid oncotic pressure, or both. Examples of transudative effusions are those associated with congestive heart failure, cirrhosis, and nephrotic syndrome. Alternately, in exudative effusions, there is a disruption in the permeability of the pleural membrane, occasionally with coexisting lymphatic obstruction. This leads to a more viscous and tenacious fluid collection such as that associated with infection, malignancy, collagen vascular disease, or trauma. Transudative and exudative effusions are compared in Table 2.2. Distinguishing between transudative and exudative effusions can be helpful from a diagnostic standpoint and may also impact management of the effusion, as exudative fluid collections often need chest tube drainage, whereas transudates can often be managed without further invasive procedures.

Parapneumonic Effusions and Empyema

Nearly one-half of all children with pneumonia will develop a parapneumonic effusion, although less than 5% of these effusions progress to empyema (see Chapter 17 for additional discussion). An otherwise uncomplicated parapneumonic effusion does not usually warrant immediate drainage. However, if the effusion persists despite antibiotic therapy, or certainly if the effusion is associated with respiratory compromise, drainage via tube thoracostomy is generally indicated.

Historically, the microorganisms most commonly isolated from parapneumonic effusions and empyemas during childhood have been *Staphylococcus aureus, Streptococcus pneumoniae, Streptococcus pyogenes*, and *Haemophilus influenzae*. Multiple modalities exist for the treatment of empyema, including thoracentesis, chest tube drainage, instillation of fibrinolytic therapy into the pleural cavity, video-assisted thoracic surgery (VATS), and open thoracotomy with decortication. Prospective studies evaluating the use of fibrinolytic therapy in the management of parapneumonic effusion in children suggest that treatment with fibrinolytic therapy increases pleural drainage and decreases the need for surgical intervention (via thoracotomy) [129–132], although a recent Cochrane Database review suggested that VATS may be superior to even fibrinolytic therapy [133]. If surgery is required, the less invasive nature of VATS coupled with excellent published results have led many experts to recommend this approach over thoracentesis, chest tube drainage, and open thoracotomy [128,133].

Bronchopleural Fistula

A potential complication of empyema and lung abscess is the development of an abnormal connection between the airway and pleural cavity, called a *bronchopleural fistula* (BPF). A BPF may result from the rupture of a lung abscess, cyst, or bulla or from injury to the bronchus or lung parenchyma from trauma or mechanical ventilation. Additional sources include erosion of the bronchus by carcinoma or chronic inflammation as well as the breakdown of suture lines after pulmonary resection (more common in adults). The presence of a BPF is typically heralded by the return or increase in the air leak of the chest tube system or, in the absence of a chest tube, the occurrence of a pneumothorax. Diagnosis may be confirmed by bronchoscopy, but occasionally additional radiologic or contrast studies are used. Bronchopleural fistulae are difficult to manage and are associated with a poor prognosis. Typically, patients are treated aggressively with antibiotics and continued drainage, but often surgical closure is required.

Chylothorax

A chylothorax is defined as the accumulation of chyle within the pleural space, usually occurring because of injury to the thoracic duct or a derangement of lymphatic flow within the thorax. Chylothorax is the most common type of neonatal pleural effusion, often resulting from birth trauma, congenital malformations, or increased venous pressure from thrombosis of central venous catheters. Chyle is classically described as a white, milky, opaque fluid, although this appearance is seen in less than half of all patients with a chylothorax. In children, chylothorax is commonly iatrogenic, following surgical correction or palliation of congenital heart disease. Treatment includes drainage (via tube thoracostomy) and the institution of a low-fat (or medium-chain triglyceride)/high-protein diet. There are reports of successful treatment of chylothorax with the somatostatin analog octreotide; however, no controlled trials exist to document benefit [134–141]. For refractory cases, surgical ligation of the thoracic duct is indicated [142].

Hemothorax

The presence of blood in the pleural space with a hematocrit equal to 50% of that of peripheral blood constitutes a hemothorax. Extensive bleeding into the pleural cavity is rare in children but may be seen after trauma or as a complication of surgery. Chest tube placement and surgical intervention to control active bleeding are required.

Pneumothorax

A pneumothorax is defined as an accumulation of air in the pleural space. By convention, a small pneumothorax occupies 15% or less of the pleural space, a moderate pneumothorax occupies 15%–60% of the pleural space, and a large pneumothorax occupies more than 60% of the pleural space. Pneumothoraces are commonly classified into three types (*simple, communicating,* and *tension*). A simple (also called *closed* or *noncommunicating*) pneumothorax exists when there is no direct communication with the atmosphere. Additionally, there is no mediastinal shift resulting from the accumulated air (Figure 2.8). A simple pneumothorax is a common complication of nonpenetrating trauma to the chest in which one or more fractured ribs lacerates or punctures the visceral pleura and lung parenchyma, causing an escape of air from the lung into the pleural space. A pneumothorax in this setting may also occur in the absence of rib fracture when the impact is delivered at a full inspiration with the glottis closed, leading to a drastic increase in

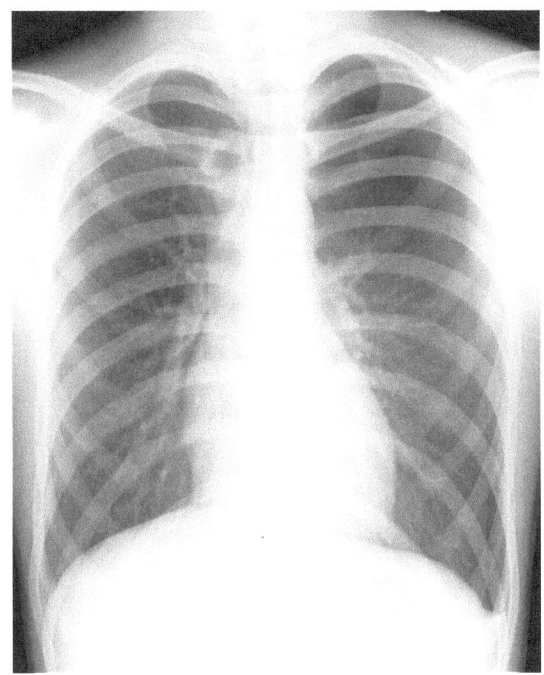

FIGURE 2.8. Simple pneumothorax in a 15-year-old male (spontaneous pneumothorax). (Courtesy of Corning Benton, MD, Cincinnati Children's Hospital Medical Center.)

intraalveolar pressure and subsequent rupture of the alveoli. Finally, a simple pneumothorax may occur as a consequence of barotrauma or volutrauma during positive pressure mechanical ventilatory support.

A communicating or open pneumothorax is associated with an open defect in the chest wall, most commonly occurring as a complication of penetrating chest trauma. As intrathoracic pressure is always less than atmospheric pressure (i.e., negative intrathoracic pressure) during spontaneous breathing, air rapidly accumulates in the pleural space. Loss of negative intrathoracic pressure results in varying degrees of lung collapse and further respiratory compromise.

A tension pneumothorax is caused by progressive accumulation of air in the pleural space (Figure 2.9). This collection of air shifts the mediastinum to the contralateral hemithorax and compresses the contralateral lung and great vessels, compromising both cardiovascular and respiratory function. Whether the air enters the pleural space through a defect in the chest wall, a lacerated or ruptured bronchus, or a ruptured alveolus, a one-way valve effect is created such that air enters during inhalation but cannot exit during exhalation. Accumulation of air continues until the intrathoracic pressure of the affected hemithorax equilibrates with atmospheric pressure. At this point, the accumulation of pressure within the thorax leads to depression of the ipsilateral hemidiaphragm and displacement of the mediastinum (and associated great vessels) toward the contralateral hemithorax. While the superior vena cava (SVC) is able to move to some extent, the inferior vena cava (IVC) is relatively fixed within the diaphragm and will be compressed (*kinked*). As two-thirds of the venous return in children comes from below the diaphragm, compression of the IVC leads to a drastic and profound reduction in venous return to the heart, leading to cardiovascular collapse (obstructive shock) [143].

The clinical presentation of a pneumothorax will depend on its size, how rapidly it has accumulated, and whether or not it is under tension. Classic signs and symptoms include chest pain (often radiating to the tip of the ipsilateral shoulder), dyspnea, tachypnea, tachycardia, and cyanosis. Diminished or absent breath sounds on the involved side with displacement of the trachea toward the contralateral side are often detected on physical examination. A tension pneumothorax will present with cardiovascular collapse and profound respiratory distress. The chest radiograph is the preferred imaging study and should be obtained unless the clinical condition warrants immediate treatment, although small pneumothoraces are often missed on initial chest x-ray. Computed tomography is superior to plain x-ray for detecting small pneumothoraces, although many of these are clinically insignificant and do not require intervention. Decompression via needle thoracentesis or tube thoracostomy is the treatment of choice (see later).

Pneumomediastinum

A pneumomediastinum is an abnormal collection of air within the mediastinal space. Most commonly, pneumomediastinum results from microscopic alveolar rupture. There is some evidence that this may occur earlier in the continuum of pressure-induced injury, with the majority of ventilated patients developing pneumomediastinum before pneumothorax. As with pneumothorax, those patients receiving high peak pressures on the ventilator are most at risk, but there may be spontaneous development as well [144–146]. Aside from alveolar disruption, however, pneumomediastinum can also result from air escaping from the esophagus, trachea, or upper respiratory tract. This free air may be the result of trauma [147–149], surgery, or iatrogenic injury during medical procedures such as tracheal intubation, upper GI endoscopy, and

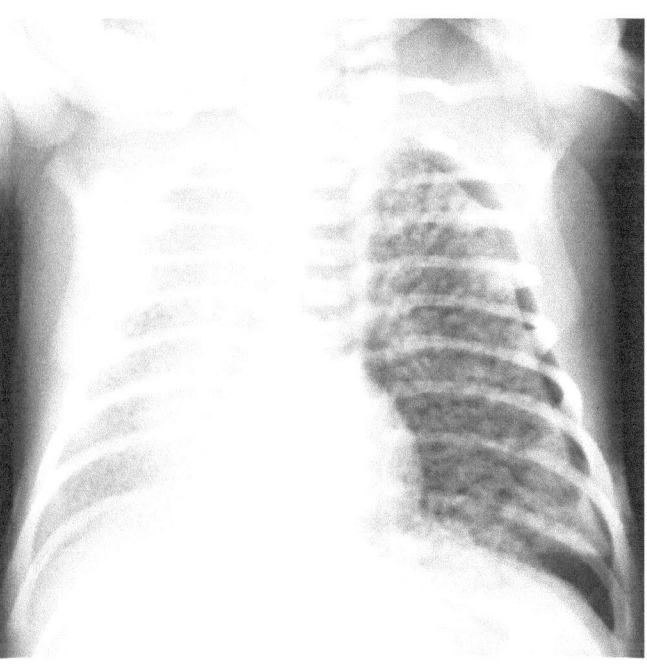

FIGURE 2.9. Tension pneumothorax in a 9-day-old premature infant with pulmonary interstitial emphysema and iatrogenic barotraumas from ventilator-induced lung injury. (Courtesy of Corning Benton, MD, Cincinnati Children's Hospital Medical Center.)

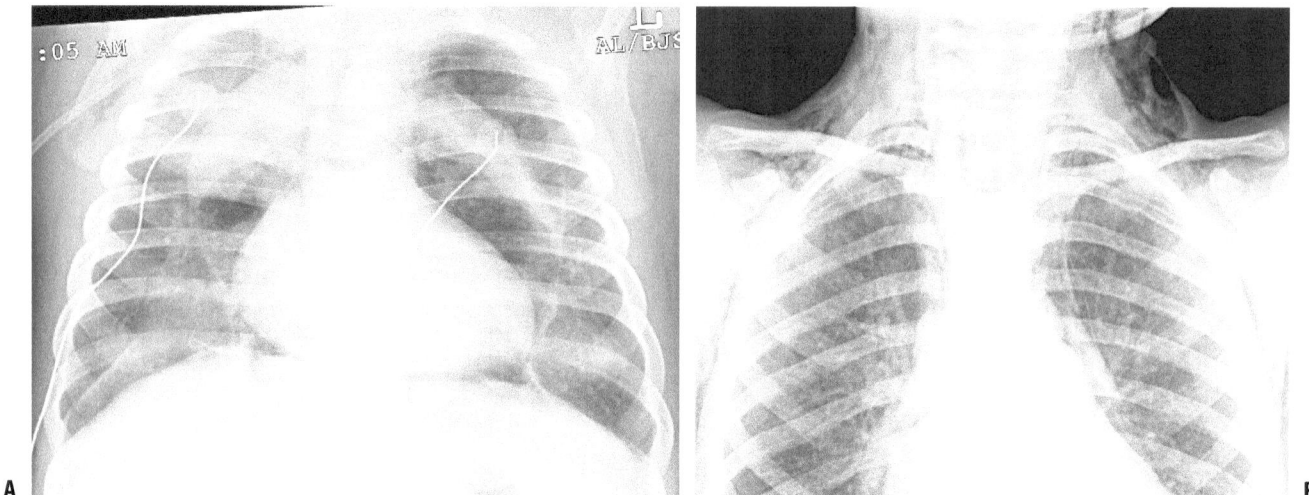

FIGURE 2.10. (A) Pneumomediastinum in a 6-month-old baby with acute respiratory failure (secondary to bacterial pneumonia) and ventilator-induced lung injury. (B) Pneumomediastinum in an 8-year-old boy admitted to the pediatric intensive care unit with status asthmaticus. (Courtesy of Corning Benton, MD, Cincinnati Children's Hospital Medical Center.)

so forth. Pneumomediastinum may also result from retropharyngeal abscesses or other dental or oropharyngeal infections, especially those from gas-producing bacteria [144].

Pneumomediastinum is often asymptomatic, but, as mediastinal air may track into the subcutaneous tissues of the neck and chest, crepitus may develop. The patient may complain of chest pain, neck pain, or dyspnea. Diagnosis is typically made by chest x-ray (Figure 2.10). Isolated pneumomediastinum usually resolves without treatment, but, if severe, with cardiac compromise, or as a consequence of tracheal or esophageal rupture, surgical intervention is required. Turlapati et al. described a technique for placement of mediastinal tubes at the bedside for emergency decompression of hemodynamically significant pneumomediastinum [150].

Chest Tubes

The Physics of Chest Tubes

Chest tubes have been employed since the days of Hippocrates. The chest tube and collecting system have undergone some changes since then, with the closed tube thoracostomy being put into widespread use for hemothorax following the Korean conflict. Currently, the indications for chest tube use include significant pleural effusion, hemothorax, chylothorax, pneumothorax, empyema, and malignant effusion. Although these conditions can occasionally be managed through observation and thoracentesis, often chest tube placement is required.

The closed tube system consists of three chambers. The collection chamber is connected to the patient through the chest tube and is also connected to a water seal chamber. A water seal chamber serves as a one-way valve, preventing return of the drained fluid to the patient. The water seal chamber is then connected to a third chamber that controls the amount of suction applied to the pleural space (Figure 2.11) [151,152].

Placement of Chest Tubes

The placement of a thoracotomy tube varies somewhat on the medium that is to be drained. Pigtail catheters placed via Seldinger technique in the midaxillary line of the fifth intercostal space have become a common alternative to traditional, more invasive chest tubes, especially for the pediatric population [153]. These tubes are very useful in draining transudative effusions or air and can be placed with minimal sedation. Pigtail tubes, in general, are more comfortable for the patient while in place. They are, however, limited by their caliber and are more prone to clogging, especially with chylous, grossly bloody, or purulent pleural fluid collections. In those circumstances when pigtail catheters fail or are inappropriate because of more viscous media in the pleura, a traditional thoracostomy tube should be placed. Here, the patient is placed supine with the involved side elevated 10°–20° from the bed. The lateral chest wall is prepped and draped in a sterile fashion, and, after local anesthesia is administered, a small transverse incision is made at the intercostal space below that selected for the chest tube (typically the fifth intercostal space). With a clamp or scissors, blunt dissection is used to separate skin and chest wall. The intercostal muscles are then separated over the edge of the fifth rib with a blunt clamp, and the parietal pleura is penetrated. With the tip of a gloved finger, the tract and penetration of the pleural space is verified. The tip of the plastic catheter (size ranging from 20 to 36 F) is then inserted through the tract and directed toward the most dependent portion of the lung. The tube is then secured in place and attached to the collecting system as described earlier.

Chest Tube Management

After insertion, chest tubes should be monitored daily to evaluate the amount and quality of the drainage, the presence of bubbling (i.e., air leak), and movement of the fluid with respiration to ensure patency and correct positioning. Reexpansion pulmonary edema has been reported after drainage of large effusions or

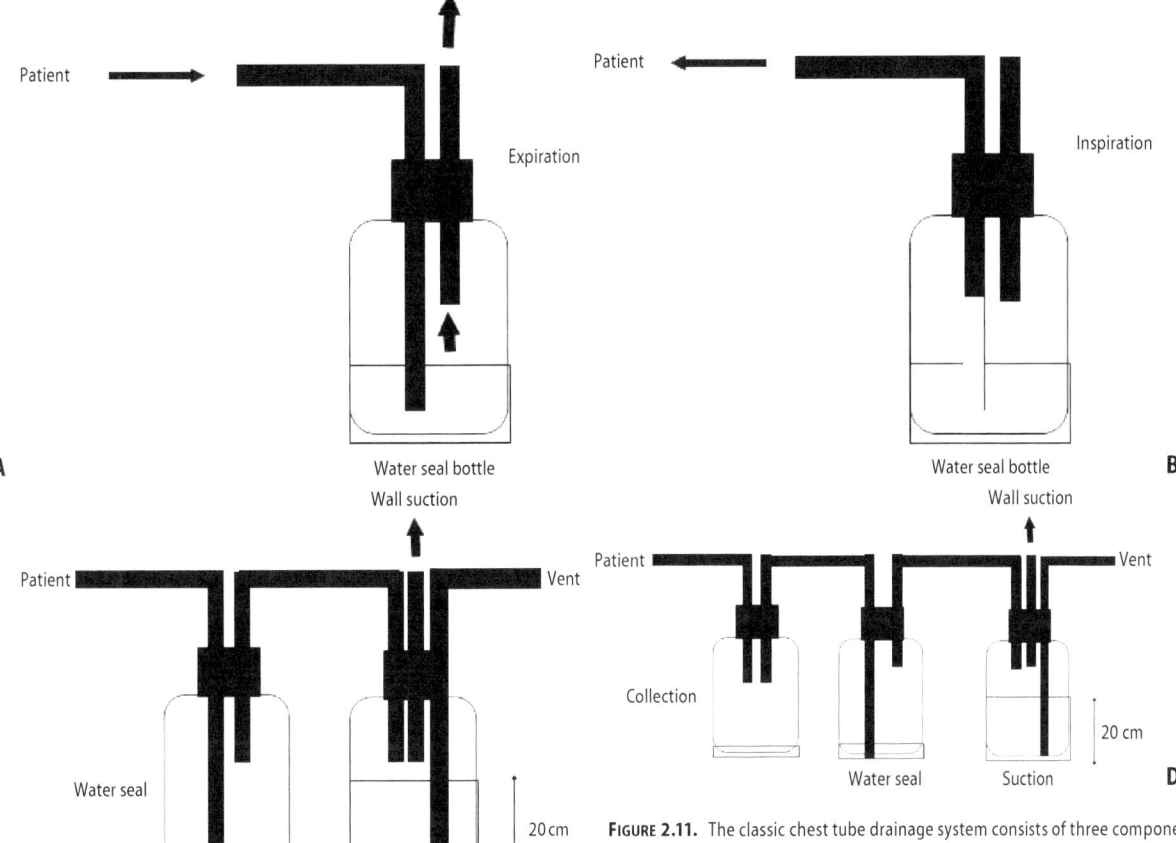

FIGURE 2.11. The classic chest tube drainage system consists of three components: (1) water seal, (2) a mechanism to control suction, and (3) a collection reservoir. The first bottle is a water seal bottle and serves as a one-way valve. Air can bubble out through the water during expiration or coughing (**A**), but cannot return to the chest during inspiration (**B**). An *air leak* (air bubbling out from the patient during expiration or coughing) is present with residual pneumothorax or bronchopleural fistula. The same principle can be accomplished by placing the end of the chest tube in an open bottle of sterile water or with the use of a Heimlich valve. A second bottle is added in order to control the amount of negative pressure in the patient's pleural cavity (**C**). Suction applied directly to the water seal bottle (and without a vent) would result in excessive negative pressure and subsequent tissue damage. The underwater distance of the third tube in the suction bottle (vented on the other end) determines the amount of negative pressure in the system (in this case, −20 cm H₂O). Wall suction at −10 cm H₂O will result in a negative pressure in the bottle of −10 (and −20 wall suction = −20 in the bottle, but the negative pressure in the bottle will never exceed 20!). Negative pressure applied to the patient will equal the difference between the underwater distance of the water seal and the underwater distance in the suction bottle. Evaporative losses in the suction bottle or pleural fluid drainage into the water seal bottle will decrease negative pressure in the chest tube. The third bottle (**D**) therefore serves only to collect fluid draining from the patient and is connected as a fluid trap between the patient and water seal bottle. The concept of the three-bottle system is used in most chest tube drainage systems in the pediatric intensive care unit today (**E**). The chamber on the far left is the suction control chamber—this chamber is filled with sterile water to the desired amount of suction (usually −10 to −20 cm H₂O). The middle chamber (denoted by the letter *C*) is the water seal chamber—bubbling in the water seal chamber indicates the presence of an air leak (persistent pneumothorax, bronchopleural fistula, etc.). When the water seal chamber is filled to 2 cm as shown, a 2-cm water seal is established. The air leak meter indicates the approximate degree of air leak from the chest cavity—the higher the numbered column through which bubbling occurs, the greater the degree of air leak. The chamber denoted by the letter *B* is a safety mechanism that maintains an effective water seal in the event of excessive negative pressure. The calibrated manometer between the water seal chamber (*C*) and the safety chamber (*B*) measures the amount of negative pressure within the pleural cavity. As intrapleural pressure becomes more negative, the water level in this manometer rises. In the absence of an air leak, the water level here will rise and fall with the child's respirations, reflecting normal pressure changes in the pleural cavity (i.e., with spontaneous respiration, the water level will rise during inhalation and fall during exhalation—the converse is true with positive pressure ventilation). The chamber on the far right is the collection (chest tube drainage) chamber, denoted by the letter *D*.

pneumothoraces in both adults and children [154–156]. This potentially lethal complication of thoracostomy tube placement is fortunately quite rare. Young patients, especially those with spontaneous pneumothorax, appear to be at a greater risk [155,156]. Suggestions that have been proposed to minimize the risk of this rare complication include slow drainage of large pleural effusions, use of supplemental oxygen (if the patient is not on positive pressure ventilation), and avoiding or minimizing suction until the lung has reexpanded following placement of a chest tube for pneumothorax [155–157].

If the fluid drainage ceases suddenly, the tube may be kinked or blocked by exudative drainage. Evaluation of the drain especially at the exit site may alleviate the problem of kinking, and flushing the tube with a small amount (10 mL) of sterile normal saline may relieve blockage of pus or debris. If this does not restore fluid drainage and fluid persists by chest radiography, it may be that the tube has shifted, with its drainage ports resting outside the pleura, or that the fluid has become loculated and sequestered from drainage. In these instances the tube may need to be replaced or, in the case of loculations, fibrinolytics or VATS considered.

The timing of chest tube removal should be determined clinically, by resolution of symptoms and minimal chest tube drainage, commonly defined as 10–15 mL over 24 hr. Complete cessation of drainage should not be anticipated, as the presence of the chest tube itself may serve as a stimulus for fluid production. For those chest tubes placed for accumulation of air or pneumothorax, a period of observation after chest tube clamping is recommended to observe for reaccumulation of air or bronchopleural leak. It is often advisable to maintain pleural drainage in those patients who remain on positive pressure ventilation until they are weaned from the ventilator because of the increased risk of reaccumulation of air.

Once the decision to remove the chest tube has been made, the child should be provided with analgesia and sedation. Chest tube removal should be completed briskly, during the expiratory phase or with a Valsalva maneuver in a cooperative child. The site should be covered with an occlusive dressing and a chest x-ray obtained to evaluate for residual or recurrent pneumothorax.

References

1. Martin JA, Kochanek KD, Strobino DM, Guyer B, MacDorman MF. Annual summary of vital statistics—2003. Pediatrics 2005;115:619–634.
2. Gregory GA, ed. Clinics in Critical Care Medicine: Respiratory Failure in the Child. New York: Churchill Livingstone; 1981:vii.
3. Vidyasagar D. Clinical diagnosis of respiratory failure in infants and children. In: Gregory GA, ed. Clinics in Critical Care Medicine: Respiratory Failure in the Child. New York: Churchill Livingstone; 1981:1.
4. Finder JD. Primary bronchomalacia in infants and children. J Pediatr 1997;130:59–66.
5. Masters IB, Chang AB, Patterson L, et al. Series of laryngomalacia, tracheomalacia, and bronchomalacia disorders and their associations with other conditions in children. Pediatr Pulmonol 2002;34:189–195.
6. Austin J, Ali T. Tracheomalacia and bronchomalacia in children: pathophysiology, assessment, treatment, and anaesthesia management. Paediatr Anaesth 2003;3–11.
7. Boogard R, Huiksmans SH, Pijnenburg MW, Tiddens HA, de Jongste JC, Merkus PJ. Tracheomalacia and bronchomalacia in children: Incidence and patient characteristics. Chest 2005;128:3391–3397.
8. Yalcin E, Dogru D, Ozcelik U, Kiper N, Aslan AT, Gozacan A. Tracheomalacia and bronchomalacia in 34 children: clinical and radiologic profiles and associations with other diseases. Clin Pediatr (Phila) 2005;44:777–781.
9. Mair EA, Parsons DS, Lally KP. Treatment of severe bronchomalacia with expanding endobronchial stents. Arch Otolaryngol Head Neck Surg 1990;116:1087–1090.
10. Mutabagani KH, Menke JA, McCoy KS, Besner GE. Bronchopexy for congenital bronchomalacia in the newborn. J Pediatr Surg 1999;34:1300–1303.
11. Ahel V, Banac S, Rozmanic V, Vukas D, Drescik I, Ahel VA Jr. Aortopexy and bronchopexy for the management of severe tracheomalacia and bronchomalacia. Pediatr Int 2003;45:104–106.
12. Pillai JB, Smith J, Hasan A, Spencer D. Review of pediatric airway malacia and its management, with emphasis on stenting. Eur J Cardiothorac Surg 2005;27:35–44.
13. Valerie EP, Durrant AC, Forte V, Wales P, Chait P, Kim PC. A decade of using intraluminal tracheal/bronchial stents in the management of tracheomalacia and/or bronchomalacia: is it better than aortopexy? J Pediatr Surg 2005;40:904–907.
14. Doolittle AM, Mair EA. Tracheal bronchus: classification, endoscopic analysis, and airway management. Otolaryngol Head Neck Surg 2002;126:240–243.
15. Sanchez I, Navarro H, Mendez M, Holmgren N, Caussade S. Clinical characteristics of children with tracheobronchial anomalies. Pediatr Pulmonol 2003;35:288–291.
16. Berrocal T, Madrid C, Novo S, Gutierrez J, Arjonilla A, Gomez-Leon N. Congenital anomalies of the tracheobronchial tree, lung, and mediastinum: embryology, radiology, and pathology. Radiographics 2004;24:e17.
17. Le Roux BT. Anatomical abnormalities of the right upper lobe bronchus. J Thorac Cardiovasc Surg 1962;44:225–227.
18. Atwell SW. Major anomalies of the tracheobronchial tree: with a list of minor abnormalities. Dis Chest 1967;52:611–615.
19. Barat M, Konrad HR. Tracheal bronchus. Am J Otolaryngol 1987;8:118–122.
20. O'Sullivan BP, Frassica JJ, Rayder SM. Tracheal bronchus: a cause of prolonged atelectasis in intubated children. Chest 1998;113:537–540.
21. Siegel MJ, Shackelford FG, Francis RS, et al. Tracheal bronchus. Radiology 1979;130:353–355.
22. McLaughlin FJ, Strieder DJ, Harris GBC, et al. Tracheal bronchus: association with respiratory morbidity in childhood. J Pediatr 1985;106:751–755.
23. Bertrand P, Navarro H, Caussade S, Holmgren N, Sanchez I. Airway anomalies in children with Down syndrome: endoscopic findings. Pediatr Pulmonol 2003;36:137–141.
24. Jederlinic PJ, Sicilian LS, Baigelman W, Gaensler EA. Congenital bronchial atresia. A report of 4 cases and a review of the literature. Medicine (Baltimore) 1987;66:73–83.
25. Ward S, Morcos SK. Congenital bronchial atresia—presentation of three cases and a pictorial review. Clin Radiol 1999;54:144–148.
26. Shanmugam G, MacArthur K, Pollock JC. Congenital lung malformations—antenatal and postnatal evaluation and management. Eur J Cardiothorac Surg 2005;27:45–52.
27. Morikawa N, Kuroda T, Honna T, et al. Congenital bronchial atresia in infants and children. J Pediatr Surg 2005;40:1822–1826.
28. Krummel TK. Congenital malformations of the lower respiratory tract. In: Chernick V, Boat TF, eds. Kendig's Disorders of the Respiratory Tract in Children, 6th ed. Philadelphia: WB Saunders; 1998:305–307.
29. Schwartz MZ, Ramachandran P. Congenital malformations of the lung and mediastinum—a quarter century of experience from a single institution. J Pediatr Surg 1997;32:44–47.
30. Laberge JM, Puligandla P, Flageole H. Asymptomatic congenital lung malformations. Semin Pediatr Surg 2005;14:16–33.
31. Ayed AK, Owayed A. Pulmonary resection in infants for congenital pulmonary malformations. Chest 2003;124:98–101.

32. Ozcelik U, Gocmen A, Kiper N, Dogru D, Dilber E, Yalcin EG. Congenital lobar emphysema: Evaluation and long-term follow-up of thirty cases at a single center. Pediatr Pulmonol 2003;35:384–391.

33. Mendeloff EN. Sequestrations, congenital cystic adenomatoid malformations, and congenital lobar emphysema. Semin Thorac Cardiovasc Surg 2004;16:209–214.

34. Sagy M, Silver P, Nimkoff L, Zahtz G, Amato JJ, Bierman FZ. Pediatric intrathoracic large airway obstruction: diagnostic and therapeutic considerations. Pediatr Emerg Care 1994;10:351–358.

35. Doull IJ, Connett GJ, Warner JO. Bronchoscopic appearance of congenital lobar emphysema. Pediatr Pulmonol 1996;21:195–197.

36. Al-Bassam A, Al-Rabeeeah A, Al-Nassar S, et al. Congenital cystic disease of the lung in infants and children (experience with 57 cases). Eur J Pediatr Surg 1999;9:364–368.

37. Yoshioka H, Aoyama K, Iwamura Y, et al. Case of congenital lobar emphysema in an 18-month-old boy and review of earlier cases. Pediatr Int 2003;45:587–589.

38. Chao MC, Karamzdeh AM, Ahuja G. Congenital lobar emphysema: an otolaryngologic perspective. Int J Pediatr Otorhinolarnygol 2005;69:549–554.

39. Powers JE, Counselman FL. Congenital lobar emphysema: tube thoracostomy not the treatment. Pediatr Emerg Care 2005;21:760–762.

40. Khosa JK, Leong SL, Borzi PA. Congenital cystic adenomatoid malformation of the lung: indications and timing for surgery. Pediatr Surg Int 2004;20:505–508.

41. Ueda K, Gruppo R, Unger F, Martin L, Bove K. Rhabdomyosarcoma of lung arising in congenital cystic adenomatoid malformation. Cancer 1977;40:383–388.

42. Granata C, Gambini C, Balducci T, et al. Bronchioloalveolar carcinoma arising in congenital cystic adenomatoid malformation in a child: a case report and review on malignancies originating in congenital cystic adenomatoid malformation. Pediatr Pulmonol 1998;25:62–66.

43. Ozcan C, Celik A, Ural Z, Veral A, Kandiloglu G, Balik E. Primary pulmonary rhabdomyosarcoma arising within cystic adenomatoid malformation: a case report and review of the literature. J Pediatr Surg 2001;36:1062–1065.

44. Pai S, Eng HL, Lee SY, Hsiao CC, Huang WT, Huang SC. Rhabdomyosarcoma arising within congenital cystic adenomatoid malformation. Pediatr Blood Cancer 2005;45:841–845.

45. Singh S, Bhende MS, Kinnane JM. Delayed presentations of congenital diaphragmatic hernia. Pediatr Emerg Care 2001;17:269–271.

46. Elhalaby EA, Abo Sikeena MH. Delayed presentation of congenital diaphragmatic hernia. Pediatr Surg Int 2002;18:480–485.

47. Smith NP, Jesudason EC, Featherstone NC, Corbett HJ, Losty PD. Recent advances in congenital diaphragmatic hernia. Arch Dis Child 2005;90:426–428.

48. Gosche JR, Islam S, Boulanger SC. Congenital diaphragmatic hernia: searching for answers. Am J Surg 2005;190:324–332.

49. John PR, Beasley SW, Mayne V. Pulmonary sequestration and related congenital disorders. A clinico-radiological review of 41 cases. Pediatr Radiol 1989;20:4–9.

50. Horak E, Bodner J, Gassner I, et al. Congenital cystic lung disease: diagnostic and therapeutic considerations. Clin Pediatr (Phila) 2003;42:251–261.

51. Corbett HJ, Humphrey GM. Pulmonary sequestration. Paediatr Respir Rev 2004;5:59–68.

52. Woodring JH, Howard TA, Kanga JF. Congenital pulmonary venolobar syndrome revisited. Radiographics 1994;14:349–369.

53. Holt PD, Berdon WE, Marans Z, Griffiths S, Hsu D. Scimitar vein draining to the left atrium and a historical review of the scimitar syndrome. Pediatr Radiol 2004;34:409–413.

54. Rokade ML, Rananavare RV, Shetty DS, Saifi S. Scimitar syndrome. Indian J Pediatr 2005;72:245–247.

55. Sehgal A, Loughran-Fowlds A. Scimitar syndrome. Indian J Pediatr 2005;72:249–251.

56. Dupuis C, Charaf LA, Breviere GM, Abou P, Remy-Jardin M, Helmius G. The "adult" form of the scimitar syndrome. Am J Cardiol 1992;70:502–507.

57. Dupuis C, Charaf LA, Breviere GM, Abou P. "Infantile" form of the scimitar syndrome with pulmonary hypertension. Am J Cardiol 1993;71:1326–1330.

58. Gao YA, Burrows PE, Benson LN, Rabinovitch M, Freedom RM. Scimitar syndrome in infancy. J Am Coll Cardiol 1993;22:873–882.

59. Najm HK, Williams WG, Coles JG, Rebeyka IM, Freedom RM. Scimitar syndrome: twenty years' experience and results of repair. J Thorac Cardiovasc Surg 1996;112:1161–1169.

60. Torres AR, Dietl CA. Surgical management of the scimitar syndrome: an age-dependent spectrum. Cardiovasc Surg 1993;1:432–438.

61. Schramel FM, Westermann CJ, Knaepen PJ, van den Bosch JM. The scimitar syndrome: clinical spectrum and surgical treatment. Eur Respir J 1995;8:196–201.

62. Brown JW, Ruzmetov M, Minnich DJ, et al. Surgical management of scimitar syndrome: an alternative approach. J Thorac Cardiovasc Surg 2003;125:238–245.

63. Hoffman MA, Superina R, Wesson DE. Unilateral pulmonary agenesis with esophageal atresia and distal tracheoesophageal fistula: report of two cases. J Pediatr Surg 1989;24:1084–1085.

64. Kitagawa H, Nakada K, Fujioka T, et al. Unilateral pulmonary agenesis with tracheoesophageal fistula: a case report. J Pediatr Surg 1995;30:1523–1525.

65. Nowotny T, Ahrens BC, Bittigau K, et al. Right-sided pulmonary aplasia: longitudinal lung function studies in two cases and comparison to results from term healthy neonates. Pediatr Pulmonol 1998;26:138–144.

66. Thomas RJ, Lathif HC, Sen S, Zachariah N, Chacko J. Varied presentations of unilateral lung hypoplasia and agenesis: a report of four cases. Pediatr Surg Int 1998;14:94–95.

67. Bentsianov BL, Goldstein NA, Giuste R, Har-El G. Unilateral pulmonary agenesis presenting as an airway lesion. Arch Otolaryngol Head Neck Surg 2000;126:1386–1389.

68. Ootaki Y, Yamaguchi M, Yoshimura N, Oka S. Pulmonary agenesis with congenital heart disease. Pediatr Cardiol 2004;25:145–148.

69. Abrams ME, Ackerman VL, Engle WA. Primary unilateral pulmonary hypoplasia: Neonate through early childhood—case report, radiographic diagnosis, and review of the literature. J Perinatol 2004;24:667–670.

70. Rasch DK, Grover FL, Schnapf BM, Clarke E, Pollard TG. Right pneumonectomy syndrome in infancy treated with an expandable prosthesis. Ann Thorac Surg 1990;50:127–129.

71. Morrow SE, Glynn L, Ashcraft KW. Ping-pong ball plombage for right postpneumonectomy syndrome in children. J Pediatr Surg 1998;33:1048–1051.

72. Podevin G, Larroquet M, Camby C, Audry G, Plattner V, Heloury Y. Postpneumonectomy syndrome in children: advantages and long-term follow-up of expandable prosthesis. J Pediatr Surg 2001;36:1425–1427.

73. Dobremez E, Fayon M, Vergnes P. Right pulmonary agenesis associated with remaining bronchus stenosis, an equivalent of postpneumonectomy syndrome. Treatment by insertion of tissue expanders in the thoracic cavity. Pediatr Surg Int 2005;21:121–122.

74. Finer NN, Moriartey RR, Boyd J, Phillips HJ, Stewart AR, Ulan O. Postextubation atelectasis: a retrospective review and a prospective controlled study. J Pediatr 1979;94:110–113.

75. Rivera R, Tibballs J. Complications of endotracheal intubation and mechanical ventilation in infants and children. Crit Care Med 1992;20:193–199.

76. Boothroyd AE, Murthy BV, Darbyshire A, Petros AJ. Endotracheal suctioning causes right upper lobe collapse in intubated children. Acta Paediatr 1996;85:1422–1425.

77. Thomas K, Habibi P, Britto J, Owens CM. Distribution and pathophysiology of acute lobar collapse in the pediatric intensive care unit. Crit Care Med 1999;27:1594–1597.

78. Duggan M, Kavanagh BP. Pulmonary atelectasis: a pathogenic perioperative entity. Anesthesiology 2005;102:838–854.

79. Massard G, Wihlm JM. Postoperative atelectasis. Chest Surg Clin North Am 1998;8:503–528.

80. Peroni DG, Boner AL. Atelectasis: mechanisms, diagnosis, and management. Paediatr Respir Rev 2000;1:274–278.

81. Hogg JC, Williams J, Richardson JB, Macklem PT, Thurlbeck WM. Age as a factor in the distribution of lower-airway conductance and in the pathologic anatomy of obstructive lung disease. N Engl J Med 1970;282: 1283–1287.

82. Mansell A, Bryan C, Levison H. Airway closure in children. J Appl Physiol 1972;33:711–714.

83. Berry FA, Yemen TA. Pediatric airway in health and disease. Pediatr Clin North Am 1994;41:153–180.

84. Stocks J. Respiratory physiology during early life. Monaldi Arch Chest Dis 1999;54:358–364.

85. Menkes H, Traystman R, Terry P. Collateral ventilation. Fed Proc 1979;38:22–26.

86. Hazinski TA. Atelectasis. In: Chernick V, Boat TF, eds. Kendig's Disorders of the Respiratory Tract in Children, 6th ed. Philadelphia: WB Saunders; 1998:634–641.

87. Krause MF, Hoehn T. Chest physiotherapy in mechanically ventilated children: a review. Crit Care Med 2000;28:1648–1651.

88. Krastins I, Corey ML, McLeod A, Edmonds J, Levison H, Moes F. An evaluation of incentive spirometry in the management of pulmonary complications after cardiac surgery in a pediatric population. Crit Care Med 1982;10:525–528.

89. Bellet PS, Kalinyak KA, Shukla R, Gelfand MJ, Rucknagel DL. Incentive spirometry to prevent acute pulmonary complications in sickle cell diseases. N Engl J Med 1995;333:699–703.

90. Reardon CC, Christiansen D, Barnett ED, Cabral HJ. Intrapulmonary percussive ventilation vs incentive spirometry for children with neuromuscular disease. Arch Pediatr Adolesc Med 2005;159:526–531.

91. Hsu LL, Batts BK, Rau JL. Positive expiratory pressure device acceptance by hospitalized children with sickle cell disease is comparable to incentive spirometry. Respir Care 2005;50:624–627.

92. Chatwin M, Ross E, Hart N, Nickol AH, Polkey MI, Simonds AK. Cough augmentation with mechanical insufflation/exsufflation in patients with neuromuscular weakness. Eur Respir J 2003;21:502–508.

93. Miske LJ, Hickey EM, Kolb SM, Weiner DJ, Panitch HB. Use of the mechanical in-exsufflator in pediatric patients with neuromuscular disease and impaired cough. Chest 2004;125:1406–1412.

94. Friedman O, Chidekel A, Lawless ST, Cook SP. Postoperative bilevel positive airway pressure ventilation after tonsillectomy and adenoidectomy in children—a preliminary report. Int J Pediatr Otorhinolaryngol 1999;51:177–180.

95. Jaarsma AS, Knoester H, van Rooyen F, Bos AP. Biphasic positive airway pressure ventilation (PeV+) in children. Crit Care 2001;5:174–177.

96. Padman R, Henry M. The use of bilevel positive airway pressure for the treatment of acute chest syndrome of sickle cell disease. Del Med J 2004;76:199–203.

97. Tokuda Y, Matsumoto M, Sugita T, Nishizawa J. Nasal mask bilevel positive airway pressure ventilation for diaphragmatic paralysis after pediatric open-heart surgery. Pediatr Cardiol 2004;25:552–553.

98. Shah PL, Scott SF, Hodson ME. Lobar atelectasis in cystic fibrosis and treatment with recombinant human DNase I. Respir Med 1994;88:313–315.

99. Gershan WM, Rusakow LS, Chetty A, Splaingard ML. Resolution of chronic atelectasis in a child with asthma after aerosolized recombinant human DNase. Pediatr Pulmonol 1994;18:268–269.

100. Touleimat BA, Conoscenti CS, Fine JM. Recombinant human DNase in management of lobar atelectasis due to retained secretions. Thorax 1995;50:1319–1323.

101. Voelker KG, Chetty KG, Mahutte CK. Resolution of recurrent atelectasis in spinal cord injury patients with administration of recombinant human DNase. Intensive Care Med 1996;22:582–584.

102. Boeuf B, Prouix F, Morneau S, Marton D, Lacroix J. Safety of endotracheal rh DNase (Pulmozyme) for treatment of pulmonary atelectasis in mechanically ventilated children. Pediatr Pulmonol 1998;26:147.

103. Durward A, Forte V, Shemie SD. Resolution of mucus plugging and atelectasis after intratracheal rhDNase therapy in a mechanically ventilated child with refractory status asthmaticus. Crit Care Med 2000;28:560–562.

104. El Hassan NO, Chess PR, Huysman MW, Merkus PJ, de Jongste JC. Rescue use of DNase in critical lung atelectasis and mucus retention in premature neonates. Pediatrics 2001;108:468–470.

105. Merkus PJ, de Hoog M, van Gent R, de Jongste JC. DNase treatment for atelectasis in infants with severe respiratory syncytial virus bronchiolitis. Eur Respir J 2001;18:734–737.

106. Kupeli S, Teksam O, Dogru D, Yurdakok M. Use of recombinant human DNase in a premature infant with recurrent atelectasis. Pediatr Int 2003;45:584–586.

107. Riethmueller J, Borth-Bruhns T, Kumpf M, et al. Recombinant human deoxyribonuclease shortens ventilation time in young, mechanically ventilated children. Pediatr Pulmonol 2006;41:61–66.

108. Barbato A, Novello A Jr, Tormena F, Carra S, Malocco F. Use of fiberoptic bronchoscopy in asthmatic children with lung collapse. Pediatr Med Chir 1995;17:253–255.

109. Wood RE. The emerging role of flexible bronchoscopy in pediatrics. Clin Chest Med 2001;22:311–317.

110. Scolieri P, Adappa ND, Coticchia JM. Value of rigid bronchoscopy in the management of critically ill children with acute lung collapse. Pediatr Emerg Care 2004;20:384–386.

111. Bar-Zohar D, Sivan Y. The yield of flexible fiberoptic bronchoscopy in pediatric intensive care patients. Chest 2004;126:1353–1359.

112. Demling RH, LaLonde C, Ikegami K. Pulmonary edema: pathophysiology, methods of treatment, and clinical importance in acute respiratory failure. New Horiz 1993;1:371–380.

113. O'Brodovich H, Mellins RB. Pulmonary edema. In: Chernick V, Boat TF, eds. Kendig's Disorders of the Respiratory Tract in Children, 6th ed. Philadelphia: WB Saunders; 1998:653–675.

114. Deshpande JK, Wetzel RC, Rogers MC. Unusual causes of myocardial ischemia, pulmonary edema, and cyanosis. In: Rogers MC, ed. Textbook of Pediatric Intensive Care, 3rd ed. Baltimore: Williams & Wilkins; 1996:432–442.

115. Rosenberg AL. Fluid management in patients with acute respiratory distress syndrome. Respir Care Clin North Am 2003;9:481–493.

116. O'Brodovich H. Pulmonary edema in infants and children. Curr Opin Pediatr 2005;17:381–384.

117. Staub NC, Nagano H, Pearce ML. Pulmonary edema in dogs, especially the sequence of fluid accumulation in the lungs. J Appl Physiol 1967;22:227–240.

118. Verghese GM, Ware LB, Matthay BA, Matthay MA. Alveolar epithelial fluid transport and the resolution of clinically severe hydrostatic pulmonary edema. J Appl Physiol 1999;87:1301–1312.

119. Ware LB, Matthay MA. Alveolar fluid clearance is impaired in the majority of patients with acute lung injury and the acute respiratory distress syndrome. Am J Respir Crit Care Med 2001;163:1376–1383.

120. Flori HR, Glidden DV, Rutherford GW, Matthay MA. Pediatric acute lung injury: prospective evaluation of risk factors associated with mortality. Am J Respir Crit Care Med 2005;171:995–1001.

121. Berthiaume Y, Folkesson HG, Matthay MA. Lung edema clearance: 20 years of progress: invited review: alveolar fluid clearance in the injured lung. J Appl Physiol 2002;93:2207–2213.

122. Mehta D, Bhattacharya J, Matthay MA, Malik AB. Integrated control of lung fluid balance. Am J Physiol Lung Cell Mol Physiol 2004;287: L1081–L1090.

123. Morina P, Herrera M, Venegas J, Mora D, Rodriguez M, Pino E. Effects of nebulized salbutamol on respiratory mechanics in adult respiratory distress syndrome. Intensive Care Med 1997;23:58–64.

124. Atabai K, Ware LB, Snider ME, et al. Aerosolized beta(2)-adrenergic agonists achieve therapeutic levels in the pulmonary edema fluid of ventilated patients with acute respiratory failure. Intensive Care Med 2002;28:705–711.

125. McAuley DF, Frank JA, Fang X, Matthay MA. Clinically relevant concentrations of beta2-adrenergic agonists stimulate maximal cyclic adenosine monophosphate-dependent airspace fluid clearance and decrease pulmonary edema in experimental acid-induced lung injury. Crit Care Med 2004;32:1470–1476.

126. Perkins GD, McAuley DF, Thickett DR, Gao F. The beta-agonist lung injury trial (BALT): a randomized placebo controlled trial. Am J Respir Crit Care Med 2006;173:281–287.

127. Martin GS, Moss M, Wheeler AP, Mealer M, Morris JA, Bernard GR. A randomized, controlled trial of furosemide with or without albumin in hypoproteinemic patients with acute lung injury. Crit Care Med 2005;33:1681–1687.

128. Mocelin HT, Fischer GB. Epidemiology, presentation, and treatment of pleural effusion. Paediatr Respir Rev 2002;3:292–297.

129. Boyer DM. Evaluation and management of a child with a pleural effusion. Pediatr Emerg Care 2005;21:63–68.

130. Hawkins JA, Scaife ES, Hillman ND, Feola GP. Current treatment of pediatric empyema. Semin Thorac Cardiovasc Surg 2004;16:196–200.

131. Gates RL, Hogan M, Weinstein S, Arca MJ. Drainage, fibrinolytics, or surgery: a comparison of treatment options in pediatric empyema. J Pediatr Surg 2004;39:1638–1642.

132. Jaffe A, Balfour-Lynn IM. Management of empyema in children. Pediatr Pulmonol 2005;40:148–156.

133. Coote N, Kay E. Surgical versus non-surgical management of pleural empyema. Cochrane Database Syst Rev 2005;4:CD001956.

134. Chan EH, Russell JL, Williams WG, Van Arsdell GS, Coles JG, McCrindle BW. Postoperative chylothorax after cardiothoracic surgery in children. Ann Thorac Surg 2005;80:1864–1870.

135. Campbell RM, Benson LN, Williams WW, Adatia I. Chylopericardium after cardiac operations in children. Ann Thorac Surg 2001;72: 193–196.

136. Le Coultre C, Oberhans I, Mossaz A, Bugmann P, Faidutti B, Belli DC. Postoperative chylothorax in children: differences between vascular and traumatic origin. J Pediatr Surg 1991;26:519–523.

137. Pratap U, Slavik Z, Ofoe VD, Onuzo O, Franklin RC. Octreotide to treat postoperative chylothorax after cardiac operations in children. Ann Thorac Surg 2001;72:1740–1742.

138. Rosti L, Bini RM, Chessa M, Butera G, Drago M, Carminati M. The effectiveness of octreotide in the treatment of post-operative chylothorax. Eur J Pediatr 2002;161:149–150.

139. Mohseni-Bod H, Macrae D, Slavik Z. Somatostatin analog (octreotide) in management of neonatal postoperative chylothorax: is it safe? Pediatr Crit Care Med 2004;5:356–357.

140. Beghetti M, La Scala G, Belli D, Bugmann P, Kalangos A, Le Coultre C. Etiology and management of pediatric chylothorax. J Pediatr 2000;136:653–658.

141. Mohan H, Paes ML, Haynes S. Use of intravenous immunoglobulins as an adjunct in the conservative management of chylothorax. Paediatr Anaesth 1999;9:89–92.

142. Marts BC, Naunheim KS, Fiore AC, Pennington DG. Conservative versus surgical management of chylothorax. Am J Surg 1992;164:532–535.

143. Salim MA, DiSessa TG, Arheart KL, Alpert BS. Contribution of superior vena caval flow to total cardiac output in children: a Doppler echocardiographic study. Circulation 1995;92:1860–1865.

144. Damore DT, Dayan PS. Medical causes of pneumomediastinum in children. Clin Pediatr (Phila) 2001;40:87–91.

145. Newcomb AE, Clarke CP. Spontaneous pneumomediastinum: a benign curiosity or a significant problem? Chest 2005;128:3298–3302.

146. Nounla J, Trobs R, Bennek J, Lotz I. Idiopathic spontaneous pneumomediastinum: an uncommon emergency in children. J Pediatr Surg 2004;39:E23–E24.

147. Cooper A. Thoracic injuries. Semin Pediatr Surg 1995;4:109–115.

148. Inci I, Ozcelik C, Nizam O, Eren N, Ozgen G. Penetrating chest injuries in children: a review of 94 cases. J Pediatr Surg 1996;31: 673–676.

149. Cotton BA, Nance ML. Penetrating trauma in children. Semin Pediatr Surg 2004;13:87–97.

150. Turlapati KM, Spear RM, Peterson BM. Mediastinal tube placement in children with pneumomediastinum: hemodynamic changes and description of technique. Crit Care Med 1996;24:1257–1260.

151. von Hippel A. Chest Tubes and Chest Bottles. Springfield, IL: Charles C. Thomas; 1970:1–96.

152. Brandt ML, Luks FI, Lacroix J, Guay J, Collin PP, Dilorenzo M. The paediatric chest tube. Clin Intensive Care 1994;5:123–129.

153. Roberts JS, Bratton SL, Brogan TV. Efficacy and complications of percutaneous pigtail catheters for thoracostomy in pediatric patients. Chest 1998;114:1116–1121.

154. Jardine OS. Reexpansion pulmonary edema. Am J Dis Child 1991;145:1092–1094.

155. Dubin JS. Reexpansion pulmonary edema. J Emerg Med 2000;19: 377–378.

156. Sherman SC. Reexpansion pulmonary edema: a case report and review of the current literature. J Emerg Med 2003;24:23–2427.

157. Baumann MH, Strange C, Heffner JE, et al. Management of spontaneous pneumothorax—an American College of Chest Physicians Delphi Consensus Statement. Chest 2001;119:590–602.

3

Respiratory Monitoring

John Marcum and Christopher J.L. Newth

Introduction

Respiratory failure is one of the leading reasons for admission to the pediatric intensive care unit (PICU) (Figure 3.1). Respiratory monitoring assists the clinician in the early detection of acute respiratory failure and provides valuable data that guide therapeutic decision making. The term *monitoring* is derived from the Latin word *monere*, which means *to warn*. Respiratory monitoring in the PICU serves as an *early warning system* that continuously measures key indices that enhance our understanding of underlying pathology; aid with diagnosis and guide management; provide alarms that alert the physicians, nurses, and respiratory therapists to significant changes in the child's condition; and create trends that assist in assessing the therapeutic response and predicting prognosis [1].

Physical Examination and Assessment

Despite recent advances in technological monitoring devices, physical examination remains a vital aspect of the evaluation and management of the critically ill or injured child. The importance of a thorough physical examination, which necessarily includes observation, palpation, and auscultation, cannot be overemphasized. As such, there are a number of overt or subtle signs of serious respiratory compromise that should not be ignored (Table 3.1). When observing a child's respiratory status, the clinician should pay particular attention to the respiratory rate and pattern. Respiratory rate varies inversely with age, and normal values as a function of age have been reported (Table 3.2) [2]. Tachypnea is often the first sign of respiratory distress, and respiratory rate, if carefully measured, is a sensitive and reasonably specific marker of acute respiratory dysfunction [3]. Although tachypnea is the usual compensatory response to hypoxia, bradypnea in the context of marked respiratory distress is an ominous finding. A quick assessment of the child's neurologic status may demonstrate early signs of hypoxia and/or hypercarbia, which include restlessness, irritability, confusion, anxiety, and an inability to recognize parents. Conversely, the child who is awake, alert, and cooperative is less likely to deteriorate acutely. Nasal flaring, retractions, and use of the accessory muscles of breathing are often present [4].

The examiner should closely inspect the symmetry of the chest and the degree of chest wall excursion. A large anteroposterior (AP) diameter, or *barrel chest*, may indicate an increased total lung volume (consistent with hyperinflation or obstructive pulmonary disease), whereas a narrow AP diameter may indicate a decreased total lung volume (consistent with restrictive pulmonary disease). The presence of dyscoordinate, *seesaw* breathing, which if severe will manifest as paradoxical movement of the thoracic cage during breathing (i.e., the chest moves inward during inspiration), is often a harbinger of impending respiratory failure [5,6]. The *Hoover sign* is an easily recognized and reproducible abnormality of chest wall motion that consists of the paradoxical inspiratory indrawing of the lateral rib margin [7,8] and is a useful sign of either obstructive airways disease or unilateral diaphragmatic paralysis [8–10]. Inspection of the skin color, especially the lips and buccal mucosa, may reveal cyanosis—the presence of cyanosis is frequently associated with oxyhemoglobin saturations of 80% or less [11]. However, cyanosis in certain situations is a very unreliable marker of hypoxemia, particularly when anemia is present. Similarly, cyanosis will appear at higher oxyhemoglobin saturations when polycythemia is present. Cyanosis usually appears when the absolute concentration of deoxyhemoglobin in the arterial blood is greater than 3–5 g/dL. The oxygen saturation at which cyanosis is present therefore ranges from approximately 62% (at hemoglobin 8 g/dL) to 88% (at hemoglobin 24 g/dL) [12]. The presence of digital clubbing is associated with chronic hypoxemia and may imply a chronic pulmonary or cardiac disease process. Jugular venous distension or a deviated trachea also indicates severe underlying pathology (e.g., cardiac tamponade, tension pneumothorax).

Palpation of the chest wall, axillae, and cervical region may reveal the presence of crepitus or subcutaneous emphysema arising from air leak syndrome (e.g., pneumothorax, pneumomediastinum). A deviated trachea or displaced cardiac impulse may indicate the presence of a tension pneumothorax. A palpable thrill or friction rub indicates potentially serious cardiac pathology. Percussion of the chest wall may also provide valuable diagnostic information. Hyperresonance suggests the presence of

D.S. Wheeler et al. (eds.), The *Respiratory Tract in Pediatric Critical Illness and Injury*,
DOI 10.1007/978-1-84800-925-7_3, © Springer-Verlag London Limited 2009

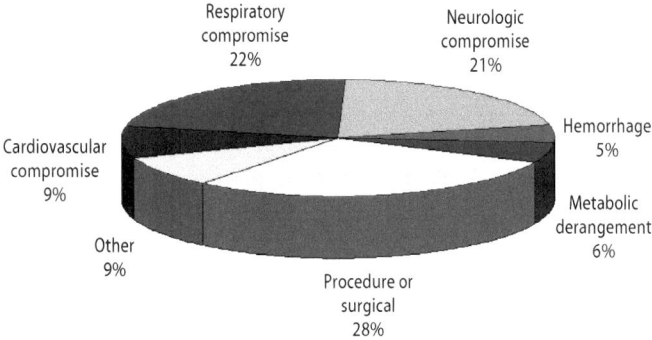

FIGURE 3.1. Admissions to the pediatric intensive care unit at Children's Hospital of Los Angeles, 2004–2005.

hyperinflation, consistent with an obstructive disease process. Dullness to percussion, on the other hand, suggests the presence of consolidation, atelectasis, or pleural effusion.

Auscultation of the chest can provide valuable information but may be particularly challenging in the infant, as the thorax is quite small and many lung sounds are easily transmitted throughout the chest wall. The examiner should listen for the presence of grunting, wheezing, stridor, rales, or rhonchi. The presence of grunting usually occurs in restrictive disease processes and represents the child's attempt to increase intrinsic positive end-expiratory pressure (PEEP) and maintain functional residual capacity (FRC) [13]. Unequal breath sounds or absent breath sounds suggest a tension pneumothorax, whereas diminished or muffled heart sounds suggest the presence of a pericardial effusion with possible cardiac tamponade. Wheezing is a sign of airway narrowing in the large- and medium-sized airways. Although wheezing is usually associated with asthma, other causes for wheezing must be considered. When lower airway obstruction is present, the length of the expiratory time may help guide ongoing therapeutic interventions. Stridor, also a result of airway obstruction, is harsher or lower pitched than wheezing and is predominantly heard on inspiration. Inspiratory stridor suggests extrathoracic or upper airway obstruction, whereas biphasic or expiratory stridor indicates intrathoracic or lower airway obstruction [14].

Imaging Modalities for the Pediatric Chest

There are multiple imaging modalities available to help with the diagnosis and care of the critically ill or injured child. Imaging should be utilized as a complement to the physical examination and as a guide to therapeutic decision making in the PICU. Common modalities employed in the PICU include plain radiography, ultrasonography, computed tomography (CT), magnetic resonance imaging (MRI), and fluoroscopy.

Plain Radiographs

Plain x-ray films are the most commonly obtained imaging study in the PICU, although the accuracy and efficacy of plain radiography in the pediatric population have not been well studied. Multiple studies have shown the benefit of routine radiographs for critically ill adults [15–18]. When interpreting chest radiographs in the PICU, it is important to have a systematic approach. First, the position of all catheters (e.g., central venous catheter, pulmonary artery catheter), tubes (e.g., tracheal tube, nasogastric tube, chest tubes), and support devices (e.g., pacemaker wires, intraaortic balloon pump, pacemaker) should be assessed, followed by assessment of the heart size, pulmonary vascularity, and lung parenchyma. Finally, the presence of any abnormal air (e.g., pneumothorax, pneumomediastinum) or fluid collections (e.g., pleural effusion, chylothorax, pericardial effusion) should be noted.

Confirmation of tracheal tube position remains one of the most important uses of routine chest radiographs. Multiple adult studies have shown that between 12% and 15% of tracheally intubated patients have significant tracheal tube malposition that is not recognized by either physical examination or clinical assessment [15,17,19]. In the critically ill pediatric patient, increased activity level and a shorter trachea provide further challenges to maintaining proper position of the tracheal tube. Unplanned extubations and bronchial intubations may be prevented by confirming correct placement of tracheal tubes with the use of daily plain chest radiographs [20,21].

The value of the daily chest radiograph may be more apparent for critically ill children with acute pulmonary or cardiac disease [21]. Atelectasis may be detected on chest radiographs with a vari-

TABLE 3.1. Signs of possible serious respiratory compromise.

Inspection	Palpation	Auscultation
Evidence of increased work of breathing	Crepitus	Unequal breath sounds
Tachypnea (bradypnea is an ominous finding in this setting)	Subcutaneous air	Shift in heart sounds
Nasal flaring	Deviation of the trachea	Muffled heart sounds
Chest wall retractions	Absent or displaced cardiac impulse	Pericardial or pleural rub
Paradoxical breathing (Hoover sign)		
Agitation		
Malformations of the chest wall	Precordial rub	
Large anteroposterior (AP) diameter (*barrel chest*)	Localized tenderness and/or instability of the chest wall	
Narrow AP diameter		
Evidence of hypoxemia or hypercarbia		
Agitation, confusion	Dullness to percussion	
Somnolence	Hyperresonance to percussion	
Cyanosis		
Chest wall mass		
Digital clubbing		
Cyanosis		
Jugular vein distension		

TABLE 3.2. Normal respiratory rates by age.

Age (years)	Mean breaths/min	Standard deviation
2	25	17–33
4	23	18–28
6	21	17–27
8	20	15–26
10	18	15–25
12	18	14–26
14	17	15–23
16	17	12–22

Source: Adapted from Iliff and Lee [2].

TABLE 3.3. Hydrostatic versus increased capillary permeability edema: distinguishing radiographic features.

Radiographic feature	Hydrostatic edema	Increased permeability edema
Cardiomegaly	+	−
Widened vascular pedicle	+	−
Increased vascularity	+	−
Kerley lines	+	−
Peribronchial cuffing	+	−
Pleural effusion	+	−
Air space consolidation	+	+

Source: Reprinted from Boiselle PM. Radiologic imaging in the critically ill patient. In: Criner GJ, D'Alonzo GE, eds. Critical Care Study Guide: Text and Review. New York: Springer; 2002:164. Reproduced with kind permission of Springer Science+Business Media.

able radiographic appearance ranging from linear, platelike, and patchy opacities to total lobar consolidation [18,21,22–24]. For critically ill adults, atelectasis occurs most frequently in the left lower lobe (66%), followed by the right lower lobe (22%) and right upper lobe (11%) [17,23,25]. Conversely, in critically ill children atelectasis more commonly involves the upper lobes, especially the right upper lobe [26]. The reasons for these differences are unclear, although children may be more prone to atelectasis because of the lack of collateral pathways of ventilation (pores of Kohn, Lambert's canals) and a greater susceptibility to dynamic compression. When compared with chest CT, chest radiography has 74% sensitivity and 100% specificity for detection of consolidation or atelectasis [26].

Pneumonia is difficult to differentiate from atelectasis using chest radiographs alone. Generally, chest radiograph changes because of pneumonia appear later and resolve more slowly than changes caused by atelectasis [27]. Additional features that favor the diagnosis of atelectasis include a displaced hilum, displaced fissures, mediastinal shift toward the side of collapse, loss of volume on ipsilateral hemithorax, and elevation of ipsilateral diaphragm (all of these features are indicative of volume loss). However, portable chest radiography is a very poor test for the identification of pneumonia, with a sensitivity of only 62% and a specificity of 28% [28]. Chest radiographs should therefore be used only in conjunction with other clinical data such as fever, leukocytosis, increased oxygen requirement, decreased pulmonary compliance, changes in sputum production or color, isolation of organisms from the lower respiratory tract, and the presence of white cells in the sputum sample.

Although chest radiography has poor sensitivity and specificity when used in isolation to diagnose pneumonia, it is relatively accurate at defining the presence of pulmonary edema [28]. It is important to differentiate between hydrostatic pulmonary edema (e.g., congestive heart failure, acute renal failure, nephrotic syndrome) from increased capillary permeability (noncardiogenic) pulmonary edema. Several features may aid this distinction (Table 3.3), although it is important to bear in mind that this distinction may not be possible based on chest radiograph alone. In addition, both types of edema can occur in the same child, making such a distinction superfluous.

An enlarged cardiac silhouette and increased pulmonary vascularity are consistent with hydrostatic pulmonary edema. The most common method of assessing heart size on chest radiographs is the cardiothoracic ratio, which is determined by dividing the widest transverse diameter of the heart by the widest transverse diameter of the thoracic cavity, and a cardiothoracic ratio greater than 0.5 is usually consistent with the presence of cardiomegaly. The vascular pedicle may be found between the thoracic inlet and the top of the

heart on chest radiograph and consists of the right brachiocephalic vein, superior vena cava, and left subclavian artery. An increase in the width of the vascular pedicle is also suggestive of hydrostatic pulmonary edema.

Hydrostatic pulmonary edema follows a typical progression. Increased pulmonary vascularity is followed by accumulation of fluid within the interstitial space, the peribronchovascular sheath, and the interlobular septa. As fluid accumulates within the peribronchovascular sheath, the pulmonary vessels become indistinct and peribronchial cuffing is found on chest radiograph. Kerley lines refer to the linear opacities that are best visualized in the lung periphery (Figure 3.2), which represent fluid accumulation within the interlobular septa. As hydrostatic pulmonary edema worsens, fluid accumulates within the interlobar fissures and may eventually extend into the alveolar spaces of the lung. Air space consolidation from hydrostatic pulmonary edema is typically bilateral, symmetric, and centrally located in the perihilar region. Pleural effusions are also commonly observed in children with hydrostatic pulmonary edema.

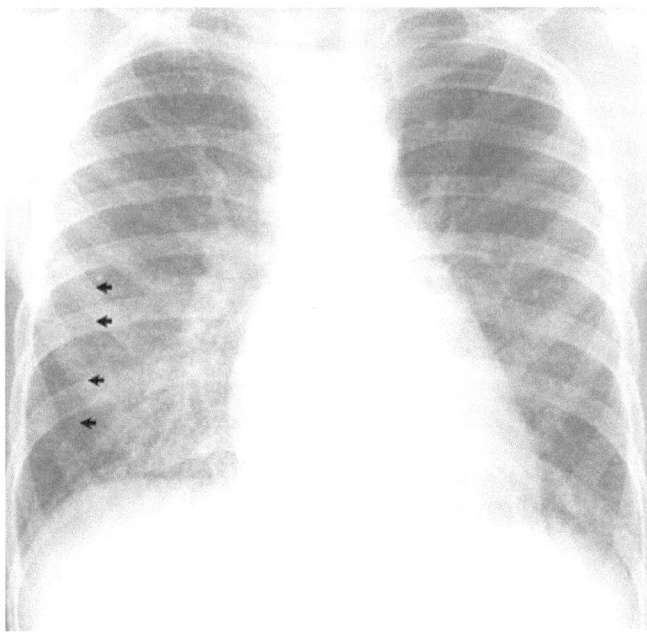

FIGURE 3.2. Kerley lines are best visualized in the lung periphery and represent fluid accumulation within the interlobular septa (i.e., hydrostatic pulmonary edema).

Children with noncardiogenic or increased capillary permeability pulmonary edema, on the other hand, typically have a normal cardiothoracic ratio and vascular pedicle width. Kerley lines, peribronchial cuffing, and pleural effusions are notably absent. Although air space consolidation may be observed with both types of pulmonary edema, the presence of patchy, peripherally distributed air space opacities is more commonly associated with increased alveolar–capillary permeability pulmonary edema [29].

Pleural effusions, like atelectasis, pneumonia, and pulmonary edema, are common in the PICU. Pleural effusions are often not large enough to be clinically significant or readily apparent on chest radiograph. However, larger pleural effusions can affect oxygenation and respiratory mechanics, and their prompt detection is necessary. Lateral and upright chest films are preferred over supine films for detecting a pleural effusion. Supine chest films are not as sensitive in detecting free pleural fluid, whereas lateral decubitus films are able to detect even small effusions [30]. However, in the critically ill child, upright and lateral films may be difficult to obtain, and supine films often must suffice. Signs of pleural effusion on supine films include a diffuse ground-glass appearance of one or both hemithoraces, pulmonary vessels visible through the hazy density, and the absence of air bronchograms (Figure 3.3) [31]. The sensitivity of detecting a pleural effusion on a supine chest film increases with the size of the pleural effusion [32]. It is important for the clinician to remember that a supine chest film does not rule out the possibility of a small- to moderate-sized pleural effusion.

Pneumothorax, the abnormal collection of air within the thoracic cavity, is a life-threatening condition that requires immediate recognition and prompt treatment. The size of a pneumothorax observed on a chest radiograph correlates poorly with the size of the air collection as measured by CT scan, which explains, in part,

TABLE 3.4. Signs of pneumothorax on supine chest radiographs.

Anteromedial pneumothorax
  Sharp outline of mediastinal vascular structures, heart border, and cardiophrenic angles
Subpulmonic pneumothorax
  Hyperlucent upper quadrant of abdomen
  Deep costophrenic sulcus
  Sharp hemidiaphragm despite lung opacification in lower lobe
  Visualization of inferior surface of consolidate lung in lower lobe

Source: Reprinted from Boiselle PM. Radiologic imaging in the critically ill patient. In: Criner GJ, D'Alonzo GE, eds. Critical Care Study Guide: Text and Review. New York: Springer; 2002:170. Reproduced with kind permission and Springer Science+Business Media.

why the size of the pneumothorax on a chest radiograph correlates poorly with clinical severity [18]. A pneumothorax is usually easily identified on an upright chest radiograph by the presence of an apicolateral white line (representing the visceral pleura) with an absence of pulmonary vessels beyond it. However, the supine chest radiograph poses further challenges to the clinician, as air may preferentially collect in the anteromedial and subpulmonic regions of the chest (Table 3.4), and the classic apicolateral pleural line is not observed until the pneumothorax is quite large. Radiographic features that suggest the presence of a tension pneumothorax include mediastinal shift, diaphragmatic inversion, and flattening of the heart border and adjacent vascular structures (e.g., the superior and inferior venae cavae) [33,34].

Computed Tomography

Computed tomography is a valuable tool in the PICU. The major advantage of chest CT over plain chest films is greater resolution of anatomic structures, which makes chest CT valuable in the diagnosis of interstitial lung disease, chest masses, vascular malformations, pulmonary embolus, and empyemas. Chest CT has even recently been used to evaluate and study the severity of acute respiratory distress syndrome (ARDS) [35,36]. With the advent of high-resolution chest CT (1–2 mm slices vs. the traditional 5–8 mm slices), even more intricate pathology can be detected. With high-resolution CT, the severity and progression of interstitial lung disease can be accurately monitored [37,38]. Additionally, the diagnosis of a pulmonary vascular thrombus can be made utilizing contrast-enhanced high-resolution chest CT. Using this modality, one can reliably detect a thrombus from the proximal pulmonary arteries out to the fourth order branched vessels [39,40]. Although chest CT is potentially beneficial in elucidating disease processes, the risks of sedation, intravenous contrast, and interhospital transport should be carefully weighed.

Magnetic Resonance Imaging

Magnetic resonance imaging can also delineate fine anatomic details of the chest, although the information provided is rarely beyond that provided by chest CT. Compared with chest CT, MRI is a much lengthier procedure that requires that a patient be away from the PICU for a longer period of time. Additionally, MRI requires a deeper level of sedation than CT. Given the limited potential benefits and increased risks, MRI of the chest has limited practicality or applicability in the monitoring of critically ill children with respiratory disease.

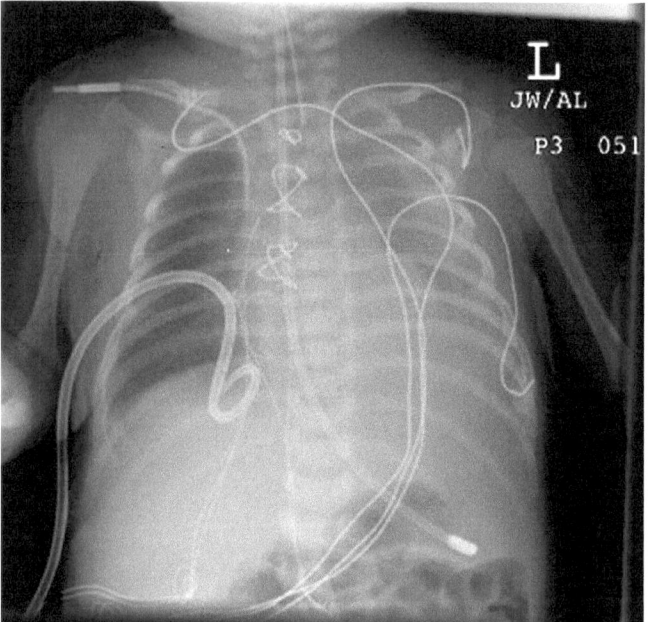

FIGURE 3.3. Chest radiograph demonstrating a rather large left-sided pleural effusion—in this case a chylothorax—in a 1-month-old infant following repair of tetralogy of Fallot. Note also the right pigtail catheter that has drained a right-sided pleural effusion.

Ultrasonography

Ultrasonography has gained increasing acceptance in the PICU for the diagnosis and treatment of respiratory diseases. The ability to perform bedside examinations and its noninvasive nature help make ultrasonography an attractive tool for the pediatric intensivist. Real-time images can be particularly valuable in assisting with diagnosis and guiding treatment. Ultrasonography can accurately measure diaphragmatic excursion, and in some centers it is the preferred modality for the diagnosis of diaphragmatic paralysis [41,42]. Ultrasonography can also effectively identify pleural effusions and can further delineate the presence of loculated fluid collections (i.e., empyema). During thoracentesis or chest tube placement, ultrasound can safely guide the drainage of pleural fluid and placement [43–45]. With a skilled practitioner, ultrasonography can be of great assistance in the diagnosis and management of pediatric respiratory disease.

Fluoroscopy

Like ultrasonography, fluoroscopy is a portable, noninvasive mode of chest imaging that is capable of producing real-time images. Unlike ultrasonography, fluoroscopy does expose the patient to non-negligible levels of ionizing radiation. In the pediatric population, fluoroscopy has been effectively utilized to diagnose defects in diaphragmatic movement. The accuracy depends heavily on the skill of the operator and the ability to correctly interpret the results.

Monitoring of Oxygenation

Hypoxemia is usually defined as a $PaO_2 \leq 60\,mm\,Hg$ and most often results from ventilation–perfusion mismatching, the presence of either fixed or physiologic shunts, and global hypoventilation (see Chapter 1). The early and accurate detection of hypoxemia is critical for the prevention of hypoxia and eventual cellular death. Monitoring of oxygenation is also important to detect hyperoxemia. Hyperoxemia may lead to free-radical formation, and its contribution to tissue destruction should not be neglected.

Invasive Forms of Oxygenation Monitoring

One of the most frequently ordered tests in the PICU is measurement of the arterial blood gas. For the purposes of oxygenation monitoring, only arterial samples suffice because capillary PO_2 values correlate poorly with arterial PO_2 values [46–49]. Blood gas samples should be freshly drawn from an arterial source, and the syringe should be free of air bubbles. An air bubble will have a PO_2 of $158\,mm\,Hg$ and when present will equilibrate with the sample. If the sample PO_2 is less than $158\,mm\,Hg$, then the measured PO_2 in the sample will be artificially elevated. Likewise, if the sample PO_2 is greater than $158\,mm\,Hg$, the sample PO_2 will be falsely lowered. For the sake of accuracy, all samples should be immediately processed, as red blood cells continue to consume oxygen and a delay in running specimens may result in falsely decreased PO_2 values. It is important to remember that routine blood gas analysis measures PO_2 directly and uses temperature, pH, PCO_2, and PO_2 to calculate the percent oxyhemoglobin saturation. Therefore, the percent oxyhemoglobin saturation in most blood gases is entirely inaccurate.

Although pulse oximetry and routine blood gas analyses are very useful monitoring devices for blood oxygenation, co-oximetry remains the *gold standard* for oxygenation monitoring in the PICU.

In contrast to pulse oximetry, which utilizes only two wavelengths of light, a co-oximeter employs four to six wavelengths of light that can more accurately quantify the fractional composition of hemoglobin (see later). Co-oximetry has many practical roles in the intensive care unit. Pulse oximetry values and calculated oxygen saturations from routine blood gas analyses should be compared periodically with co-oximetry values to ensure good correlation. Because co-oximetry is the only monitoring device that can detect methemoglobin or carboxyhemoglobin, a co-oximeter must be utilized when one suspects either of these entities to be present.

Noninvasive Forms of Oxygenation Monitoring

Transcutaneous oxygen monitoring and pulse oximetry are now widely available in the vast majority of PICUs. Transcutaneous oxygen monitoring was introduced by neonatologists in the early 1980s. Transcutaneous oxygen monitors electrochemically measure the amount of oxygen diffused through the dermal and epidermal skin layers. Because the electrodes measure diffused gas from the tissue bed, transcutaneous oxygen monitors more accurately reflect tissue oxygen levels than true arterial PO_2. In states of hypoperfusion, transcutaneous oxygen monitors may detect abnormally low partial pressures of oxygen when in fact arterial levels may be normal or elevated. Further limitations of transcutaneous oxygen monitors have been well documented [50,51]. Overall, transcutaneous oxygen monitors are not as accurate or reliable as pulse oximetry [52,53] and have very limited utility in the modern PICU.

Pulse oximetry was also developed in the 1980s and has greatly impacted respiratory monitoring in the PICU as it is noninvasive, continuous, accurate, and relatively inexpensive. Pulse oximetry detects the percentage of hemoglobin bound to oxygen by measuring the amounts of oxyhemoglobin (hemoglobin bound to oxygen) and deoxyhemoglobin (hemoglobin not bound to oxygen). Understanding this technology is an important aspect of critical care that enables the intensivist to interpret pulse oximetry data correctly.

Pulse oximetry depends on two principles. The first principle is based on the fact that oxygenated and reduced hemoglobin have different absorption spectra. The second principle is called the Beer-Lambert law and states that the unknown concentration of a solute (i.e., oxyhemoglobin) can be determined by measuring the amount of light absorbed by the solution. The pulse oximeter probe is composed of two light-emitting diodes and a photodetector. The diodes emit light through a capillary bed at wavelengths of 660 nm (red) and 940 nm (infrared). Each wavelength of light is absorbed differently by oxy- and deoxyhemoglobin. Figure 3.4 reflects the unique absorption properties of oxyhemoglobin and deoxyhemoglobin at 660 and 940 nm, respectively. Deoxygenated blood absorbs 660 nm well but absorbs 940 nm (infrared [IR] light) poorly. Conversely, oxygenated blood absorbs 660 nm poorly but absorbs 940 nm (IR light) well [54–56]. During an arterial pulsation, oxyhemoglobin perfuses into the capillary bed, and the absorbance of red light decreases while the absorbance of IR light increases. The photodetector measures the amount of light transmitted during baseline (diastole) and during an arterial pulsation. The data are sent to a microprocessor that calculates the percentage of oxyhemoglobin. Importantly, pulse oximeters, which employ two light-emitting diodes, measure *functional oxygen saturation*, which is the percentage of oxyhemoglobin relative to the sum of oxyhemoglobin and deoxyhemoglobin. Conversely, co-oximeters (discussed above) employ between four to six light-emitting diodes and measure *fractional oxygen saturation*, that is, the percentage of

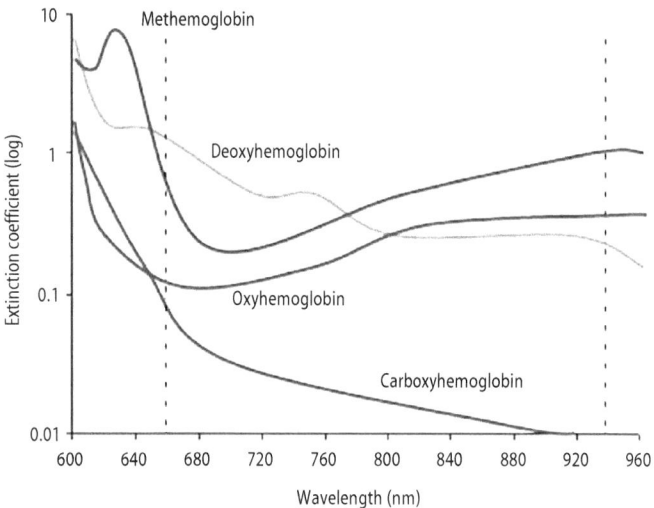

Figure 3.4. The unique absorption properties of oxyhemoglobin and deoxyhemoglobin at 660 nm and 940 nm, respectively. Deoxygenated blood absorbs 660 nm (red light) well but absorbs 940 nm (infrared [IR] light) poorly. Conversely, oxygenated blood absorbs 660 nm (red light) poorly but absorbs 940 nm (IR light) well. (Reprinted from Schnapp and Cohen [69]. Copyright 1990 from American College of Chest Physicians. Reprinted with permsssion.)

oxyhemoglobin relative to the sum of oxyhemoglobin, deoxyhemoglobin, carboxyhemoglobin, and methemoglobin. Pulse oximeters are calibrated in healthy volunteers without producing severe hypoxemia and are usually accurate to an oxyhemoglobin saturation ≥60%. However, below 60%, the readings are often falsely elevated [57].

Proper site selection of the pulse oximeter probe is essential to help ensure a meaningful signal. The pulse oximeter probe should be attached to a site that is sufficiently thin to allow light to be transmitted through the capillary bed. These sites include a finger or a toe in older patients and the palm or the heel in the infant. During states of hypoperfusion, the ear lobe or nasal septum may retain more pulsatile blood flow and are acceptable alternative sites for monitoring [58,59]. Newer generation pulse oximetry monitors are purported to accurately measure oxyhemoglobin saturation even during states of poor peripheral perfusion (e.g., shock) [60–63].

Although pulse oximetry remains the most accepted noninvasive form of oxygenation monitoring, the technology has several limitations (Table 3.5). Because other forms of hemoglobin can absorb light similar to deoxyhemoglobin and oxyhemoglobin, pulse oximetry cannot accurately measure the true percent oxygen saturation when these other forms of hemoglobin are present. For instance, when carboxyhemoglobin is present in the blood, the pulse oximeter cannot differentiate it from oxyhemoglobin, and an incorrectly high oxyhemoglobin value results [64–66]. Figure 3.4 details the nearly identical absorption of oxyhemoglobin and carboxyhemoglobin at 660 nm. The photodetector erroneously reports increased amounts of oxyhemoglobin when carboxyhemoglobin is present [54–56,65]. This results in a patient with hypoxemia and normal oxygen saturations. Similarly, the presence of methemoglobin also causes erroneous pulse oximetry measurements [54–56,67]. Methemoglobin absorbs light well at both 660 nm and 940 nm. At 660 nm, methemoglobin absorbs light similar to deoxyhemoglobin while at 940 nm methemoglobin absorbs light similar to oxyhemoglobin. Therefore, when methemoglobin is present, the photodetec-

tor reports the methemoglobin as both deoxyhemoglobin and oxyhemoglobin. For this reason, pulse oximetry detects desaturation and an erroneously elevated level of oxyhemoglobin [68]. In the clinical setting, this results in an oxygen saturation of 85%, which may mask profound desaturation. Carboxyhemoglobinemia and methemoglobinemia are two potentially fatal disorders, and, if either is suspected, an arterial blood sample should be examined by co-oximeter analysis.

Further limitations of pulse oximetry exist and can lead to potentially erroneous readings. Motion artifact is common in the PICU, particularly in the pediatric population. Motion causes variance in light transmission and detection, which leads to inaccurate oximetry reading. To ensure accuracy of the pulse oximeter, the clinician should confirm that the heart rate measured by the pulse oximeter approximates the heart rate measured by electrocardiography. Hypoperfused states are common in the PICU and can lead to increased background noise in the pulse oximeter sensor. Vasopressors such as dopamine and epinephrine may exacerbate this situation. Some authors recommend warming the extremity and using local vasodilators to increase blood flow to the desired area [69]. Severe peripheral edema or peripheral vascular disease can also limit the usefulness of pulse oximetry. Placing the sensor on the nasal septum may be beneficial when an arterial pulse cannot otherwise be detected [58]. Less commonly, venous pulsations may be detected by the pulse oximeter probe and can lead to an overestimation of deoxygenated hemoglobin [69]. Another source of inaccuracy is optical shunting or detection of emitted light that has not passed through the arteriolar bed. This optical *chatter* prevents the probe from detecting the arterial pulse and can be minimized by ensuring the probe is fresh and properly fitting. External optical interference can affect photodetection, and, if bright fluorescent lights, bilirubin lights, infrared heating lamps, or direct sunlight is present, the probe should be covered with an opaque material to prevent optical interference [70].

Table 3.5. Causes of inaccurate pulse oximeter readings of oxyhemoglobin saturation.

Condition	Cause	Effects on pulse oximeter
Dyshemoglobinemia		
Carbon monoxide	Smoke inhalation	Falsely elevated
Methemoglobin	Local anesthetics, nitrates, sulfa drugs, ethylenediaminetetraacetic acid	Initially decreased, but falsely elevated at higher levels of methemoglobinemia
Dyes and pigments		
Methylene blue	Antidote for methemoglobinemia	Falsely low
Bilirubin	Hyperbilirubinemia	Inaccurate reading
Poor peripheral perfusion	Hypothermia	Inaccurate reading
	Shock	Inadequate pulse signal
	Peripheral vascular disease	
	Vasopressors	
Anemia	Bleeding, hemolysis	Inaccurate at hemoglobin <5 g/dL
Increased venous pulsation	Right heart failure	Any pulsatile flow is interpreted as an arterial signal
	Tricuspid regurgitation	
External light source	Excessive light interference	Inaccurate reading

Source: Reprinted from Cordova FC, Marchetti N. Noninvasive monitoring in the intensive care unit. In: Criner GJ, D'Alonzo GE, eds. Critical Care Study Guide: Text and Review. New York: Springer; 2002:132. Reproduced with kind permission of Springer Sicence+Business Media.

Monitoring of Ventilation

Carbon dioxide clearance is directly related to alveolar minute ventilation. Careful monitoring of $PaCO_2$ levels is essential in the PICU. Elevated $PaCO_2$ levels (hypercarbia) are commonly detected in critically ill patients and usually indicate the presence of respiratory compromise. Low $PaCO_2$ levels (hypocarbia) are less commonly encountered, but their detection is critical in preventing cerebral hypoperfusion and subsequent central nervous system compromise, particularly in children with traumatic brain injury.

Invasive Forms of Ventilation Monitoring

The gold standard of CO_2 determination remains the arterial blood gas. Routine blood gas analysis directly measures the pH and the CO_2 level in the blood (PCO_2). Arterial specimens are preferred, but free-flowing capillary specimens will accurately approximate $PaCO_2$ values [46,48,71,72]. Venous samples drawn from free-flowing blood through a central line may accurately reflect arterial pH values as well [72–74]. Some authors have even suggested that central venous pH and PCO_2 better reflect the acid–base status at the cellular and tissue levels, especially in states of hypoperfusion [75–78]. Peripheral venous samples appear to correlate reasonably well with arterial samples [72,79–82].

Noninvasive Forms of Ventilation Monitoring

Acceptable noninvasive forms of ventilation monitoring consist of end-tidal carbon dioxide ($etCO_2$) monitors and transcutaneous carbon dioxide ($tcPCO_2$) monitors [83,84]. Whereas transcutaneous O_2 monitors correlate poorly with PaO_2, $tcPCO_2$ more accurately reflect $PaCO_2$ [50,83,85–90]. Similar to the transcutaneous O_2 monitor, the transcutaneous CO_2 monitor heats the skin from 41° to 43°C to cause vasodilation and diffusion of CO_2 into the dermal and epidermal layers. CO_2 then diffuses across the membrane of the probe and into the reservoir where the partial pressure of the gas is detected electrochemically. Probes should be attached to well-perfused, non-bony surfaces. Acceptable sites include the abdomen, chest, and lower back [91]. Transcutaneous CO_2 monitoring provides continuous data and allows for trending of $tcCO_2$ levels over time. In infants and younger children, $tcCO_2$ closely approximates $PaCO_2$ levels to within 6–10 mm Hg [92]. The technology is particularly useful in nonintubated patients or whenever $etCO_2$ monitoring is not possible, such as in high-frequency oscillatory ventilation. In fact, some studies suggest that $tcCO_2$ more accurately reflects $PaCO_2$ than does $etCO_2$ [87–90,93]. Therefore, transcutaneous CO_2 monitoring can be a very useful tool to monitor children with acute respiratory failure, especially when used in conjunction with arterial CO_2 monitoring.

However, transcutaneous CO_2 monitoring does have significant limitations. The accuracy of these devices is complicated by drifting, and the probes require frequent calibration to address this issue. Additionally, the accuracy of the probe is affected by skin temperature and tissue perfusion. The heated probe may locally increase the metabolic rate of the skin and yield a falsely elevated CO_2 level. Additionally, during hypoperfusion, CO_2 levels increase in the tissue, and the $tcCO_2$ may overestimate the true $PaCO_2$. Skin thickness also limits the accuracy of the $tcCO_2$ and likely explains the decreasing accuracy of this modality in older children and

adults [50,51]. Despite the theoretical advantages of transcutaneous CO_2 monitoring, it is not widely used in the PICU setting because of its high cost and slow response time, the need to heat the skin to 43°C, and the need to frequently relocate the electrodes to prevent skin burn.

Capnography and $etCO_2$ monitors have become an integral part of the daily management of tracheally intubated patients in the PICU. Capnography is defined as the graphic waveform produced by variations in CO_2 concentration throughout the respiratory cycle as a function of time [94,95]. Capnography detects exhaled CO_2 levels by using three components—an IR light source, an exhalation gas chamber, and a light detector. Because each exhaled gas possesses unique IR absorption characteristics, the concentration of exhaled CO_2 can be determined. The capnograph is connected inline to the end of the tracheal tube and secured such that the device does not cause traction or kinking of the airway. When properly connected, capnography has many uses, which include $etCO_2$ monitoring, evaluation of respiratory rate and rhythm, quantification of dead space (which can provide information regarding cardiac output), confirmation of tracheal tube placement, and detection of mechanical ventilator failures or patient–ventilator asynchrony [94,95]. Additionally, capnography can be utilized to detect the presence of obstructive airways disease and help guide medical therapy.

Capnometry, on the other hand, is the quantitative measurement of the CO_2 concentration in exhaled gases. Capnometry is currently considered the standard of care for confirming proper placement of the tracheal tube following elective or emergency tracheal intubation [97–100]. Disposable, portable, colorimetric $etCO_2$ monitors are now available for confirming tracheal tube placement during cardiopulmonary resuscitation and should be a standard in *every code cart* [97–99]. Following tracheal intubation, the device is connected to the tracheal tube, and the capnometer changes color when exposed to exhaled CO_2. Although this method provides a rapid and accurate assessment of tracheal tube placement, there are a few situations that may lead to erroneous measurements with this technique. For example, low cardiac output states may lead to low exhaled CO_2 and a falsely negative capnometer reading (see later). Although there is usually no CO_2 in the gastrointestinal tract, ingestion of carbonated beverages before tracheal intubation may result in a high enough CO_2 level to produce a falsely positive capnometer reading despite esophageal intubation (the so-called cola effect) [101,102].

The principle of bedside capnometry and capnography is based on IR spectroscopy or calorimetry. Similar to pulse oximetry, capnometers utilize the unique light absorption characteristics of CO_2—specifically, CO_2 is measured by quantifying the absorption of IR light at a wavelength of 4.3 μm as it passes through the exhaled gas. Oxygen, helium, and nitrogen do not absorb IR light and therefore do not interfere with the measurement of CO_2. Capnometers are generally classified into two types, mainstream and sidestream, on the basis of the gas sampling method. Mainstream analyzers are attached inline to the tracheal tube and directly sample exhaled gas, whereas sidestream analyzers continuously withdraw a sample of exhaled gas from the breathing circuit into the analyzer. There are advantages and disadvantages to both methods, although generally the choice of which method to utilize is a matter of personal preference. Sidestream analyzers can be used in nonintubated children and are particularly useful in closely monitoring the respiratory status during procedural sedation [103,104].

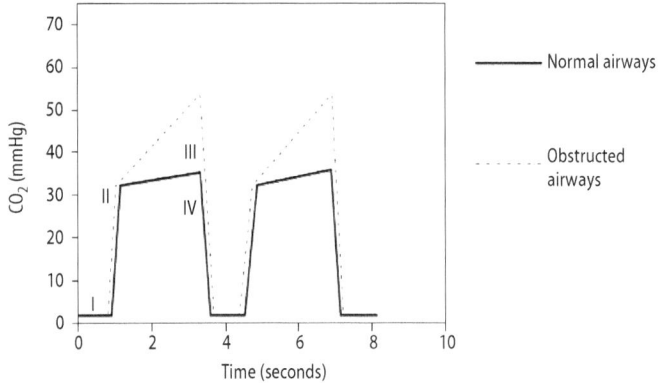

FIGURE 3.5. Capnograph of normal airways and obstructed airways.

The normal capnograph consists of four phases (Figure 3.5). Phase I begins with exhalation and the release of dead space gas from the trachea with a CO_2 content near zero. When the CO_2 level begins to rise, this indicates detection of alveolar gas and the beginning of phase II. During phase II, the fraction of alveolar gas mixed with dead space gas increases and corresponds to an increasing CO_2 level on the capnograph. Finally, when predominantly alveolar gas is being analyzed, the capnograph plateaus and phase III begins. As phase III continues, the CO_2 value infinitesimally approaches $PaCO_2$ but never actually reaches this value, as there is always a finite amount of dead space gas present. Phase IV begins with inhalation and is marked by a rapid fall in detected CO_2.

In healthy children, the $etCO_2$, measured at the peak of phase III, is generally 1–3 mm Hg lower than the $PaCO_2$, mainly as a result of normal physiologic ventilation–perfusion (V_A/Q) mismatching in the upper regions of the lung (ventilation is greater relative to perfusion in the upper, nondependent regions of the lung as a result of gravitational effects that influence blood flow). When the V_A/Q ratio approaches 1.0, $etCO_2$ correlates reasonably well with $PaCO_2$. If the V_A/Q ratio is greater than 1.0, as occurs with an increase in dead space ventilation, the $etCO_2$ will be much lower than $PaCO_2$. In fact, the etCO2 can be used to estimate dead space ventilation (V_D/V_T) by the following equation:

$$V_D/V_T = (PaCO_2 - etCO_2)/PaCO_2 = 1 - (PaCO_2 - etCO_2)$$

Therefore, conditions that alter dead space ventilation will be easily detected by changes in $etCO_2$ (Table 3.6).

The shape of the capnograph can provide useful information about the underlying disease pathology. A prolongation of phase I indicates an increased time of dead space sampling, which may result from increased anatomic dead space or decreased expiratory flow. Decreased expiratory flow may be a consequence of conducting airway obstruction distal to the tracheal tube. A normally sloped phase II is steep and represents a rapidly increasing concentration of CO_2 in the exhaled alveolar gas. A flattened phase II occurs when CO_2 concentration reaches its peak value more slowly and can be seen in severe obstructive airways disease [105]. During phase III, upsloping of the capnograph indicates delayed emptying of alveolar gas, which in turn indicates the presence of obstructive airways disease. The degree of upsloping has been shown to correlate with the degree of airways obstruction [105]. Continuous monitoring of the phase III slope can be utilized to trace the progression of the disease and help guide therapeutic decision making.

Monitoring of Respiratory Mechanics

Increased airways resistance or decreased pulmonary compliance can ultimately lead to decompensated ventilatory failure and the need for mechanical ventilatory support. The pediatric intensivist should focus on reversing the child's underlying pulmonary pathology while minimizing damage to the remainder of the lung. These goals are achieved through accurate monitoring of respiratory mechanics and proper interpretation of the collected data. Monitoring of respiratory mechanics helps diagnose the type of pulmonary pathology present, assists in recognizing the progression of disease, helps trace the response to treatment, and guides the ventilatory weaning strategy. For these reasons, careful and accurate monitoring of respiratory mechanics is essential in the PICU [106].

Monitoring of Flow–Volume Loops

With volume-limited ventilation, the clinician sets the desired tidal volume and the ventilator delivers this volume with a constant inspiratory flow rate. Figure 3.6 compares a flow–volume loop from a patient with normal lungs receiving volume-limited mechanical ventilation with a patient with normal lungs receiving pressure-limited mechanical ventilation. The y-axis represents ventilatory flow rates, and the x-axis represents the tidal volume. The loop begins at zero flow and zero volume and moves clockwise through inspiration and then exhalation. By convention, inspiration is denoted as negative flow, and exhalation is denoted as positive flow. With volume-limited ventilation, the inspiratory flow is constant until the ventilator reaches a preset tidal volume, at which time flow terminates and exhalation begins. In infants and young children, care must be taken to prevent inaccurate measurements of flow and volume (and hence tidal volume, resistance, and dynamic compliance) by placing the measurement device at the tracheal tube connector and not back in the ventilator.

With pressure-limited ventilation, the clinician sets the desired peak airway pressure, and the ventilator delivers a tidal volume with a decelerating flow. Figure 3.6 depicts an example of a flow–volume loop of pressure-limited mechanical ventilation (dashed line). Compared with volume-limited ventilation, pressure-limited

TABLE 3.6. Conditions associated with alterations in end-tidal carbon dioxide ($etCO_2$).

Increase in etCO$_2$	
Acute	Increase in cardiac output
	Administration of sodium bicarbonate
Gradual	Hypoventilation increased CO$_2$ production
Decrease in etCO$_2$	
Acute	Sudden hyperventilation
	Decrease in cardiac output
	Pulmonary embolism
	Air embolism
	Tracheal tube obstruction
Gradual	Hyperventilation
	Decrease in oxygen consumption
	Increase in dead space ventilation
Absent etCO$_2$	Esophageal intubation
	Accidental extubation
	Ventilator disconnect

Source: Adapted from Martin LD. Mechanical ventilation, respiratory monitoring, and the basics of pulmonary physiology. In: Tobias JD, ed. Pediatric Critical Care—The Essentials. Armonk, NY: Futura; 1999:99.

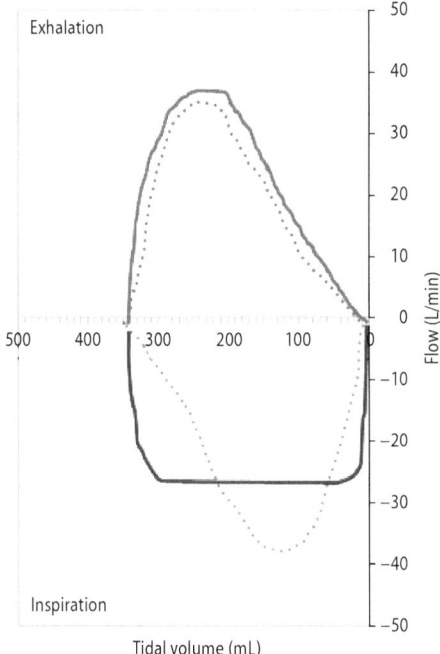

Figure 3.6. Flow–volume loop of normal lung. Dotted lines represent pressure control, and solid lines represent volume control.

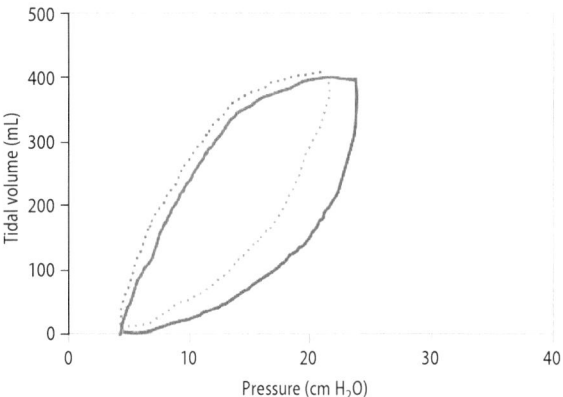

Figure 3.7. Pressure–volume loop of normal lung. Dotted lines represent pressure control, while solid lines represent volume control.

ventilation initially generates a greater peak inspiratory flow that represents the filling of the most compliant alveoli. Subsequently, as less compliant alveoli with longer time constants are recruited, flow decelerates to maintain the set peak inspiratory pressure. In diseased lung, pressure-limited ventilation helps ensure that the most compliant (least diseased) alveoli are preferentially ventilated over the least compliant (most diseased) alveoli. Furthermore, pressure-limited ventilation serves to limit flow (and overdistention) to the most diseased portions of the lung.

Monitoring of Pressure–Volume Loops

Figure 3.7 compares a pressure–volume loop from a child with normal lungs receiving volume-limited mechanical ventilation versus a child with normal lungs receiving pressure-limited ventilation. The y-axis depicts the tidal volume, and the x-axis represents airway pressure. The loop begins at a tidal volume of zero and a pressure equal to the end-expiratory pressure of the airway. As inspiration begins with volume ventilation, airway pressure gradually increases until the preset tidal volume is reached and the exhalation limb begins. In pressure-limited mechanical ventilation, airway pressure rises more rapidly than volume-limited ventilation. Additionally, pressure-limited ventilation generates a lower peak airway pressure for the same tidal volume delivered by volume-limited ventilation. In diseased lung, this important distinction can help limit the degree of ventilator-induced lung injury from barotrauma and overdistention.

Monitoring of Decreased Pulmonary Compliance

Increased work of breathing results from poor pulmonary compliance and/or increased airways resistance. The goal of mechanical ventilatory support is to minimize the work of breathing by increas-

ing pulmonary compliance and decreasing airways resistance. Pressure–volume loops can be utilized to calculate pulmonary compliance and help guide ventilator management. The pressure–volume loops of a patient with normal pulmonary compliance (dotted line) and a patient with decreased pulmonary compliance (solid line) are shown in Figure 3.8. With decreased pulmonary compliance, the slope of the inspiratory limb (solid line) of the pressure–volume curve decreases. Decreased pulmonary compliance may result from overdistention, under-recruitment, or worsening of the underlying disease process. Thus, careful monitoring of pulmonary compliance can be a very useful tool in the care of the critically ill child.

Monitoring of Iatrogenic Overdistention and Under-Recruitment

Ventilator-induced overdistention and under-recruitment lead to decreased pulmonary compliance, increased work of breathing, and increased iatrogenic lung injury. One of the most important advances in the management of ARDS has been the advent of an open-lung, low tidal volume ventilatory strategy [107]. Strong evidence suggests that limiting alveolar recruitment/derecruitment and preventing alveolar overdistention protects the lung from ventilator-induced injury. The pressure–volume loop can play a

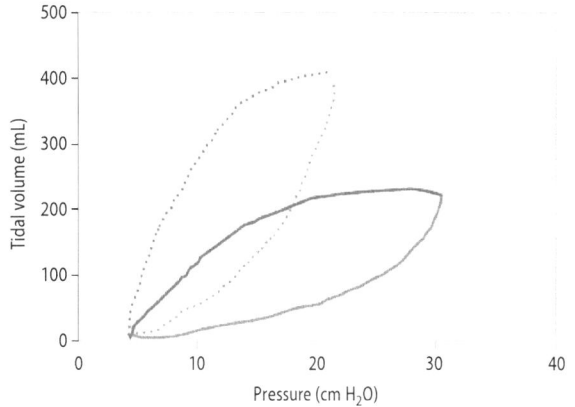

Figure 3.8. Pressure–volume loop of low-compliance lung. Dotted lines represent normal-compliance lung, and solid lines represent low-compliance lung.

critical role in choosing a ventilator strategy that prevents under-recruitment, limits overdistension, and minimizes lung injury.

In restrictive lung disease, derecruitment of alveolar lung units leads to an end-expiratory lung volume less than FRC. The objective of the clinician is to select an appropriate positive PEEP that optimally recruits the lung without overdistending the alveoli. The pressure–volume loop can be an invaluable tool in selecting the appropriate PEEP. Figure 3.9 represents a pressure–volume loop of a patient with ARDS. The curve begins at a pressure equal to the end-expiratory pressure and a volume delivered of zero. As the airway pressure rises, there is minimal increase in lung volume. This represents the zone of under-recruitment (dotted line). Once the airway pressure reaches the critical opening pressure of the alveoli, small changes in airway pressure lead to large changes in lung volume (solid line). The point at which this occurs is called the *lower inflection point (LIP)*. The airway pressure at the lower inflection point denotes the pressure needed to maintain alveolar recruitment. To prevent derecruitment and limit lung injury, the intensivist should take care not to decrease PEEP below this critical pressure.

The pressure–volume loop can also be helpful in selecting a safe peak inspiratory pressure that does not overdistend lung units. In Figure 3.9, as airway pressure continues to increase beyond the zone of maximal compliance, the inspiratory limb flattens into the zone of overdistension (dashed line). This portion of the curve represents alveolar overdistension and decreased compliance. The point at which this occurs is called the *upper inflection point (UIP)*. The airway pressure at the upper inflection point identifies the pressure beyond which alveolar overdistension occurs. To prevent alveolar overdistension and limit lung injury, the intensivist should take care not to increase the peak inspiratory pressure above this critical pressure.

Excessive PEEP, on the other hand, can lead to an elevation in end-expiratory lung volume, alveolar overdistension, and decreased pulmonary compliance. The pressure–volume loops can be instrumental in detecting the application of excessive PEEP. Figure 3.10 compares a pressure–volume loop of normal lung (dotted line) with a pressure–volume loop of overdistended lung secondary to excessive PEEP (solid line). When excessive PEEP is applied to the airway, end-expiratory lung volume increases, and pulmonary compliance decreases. This decrease in pulmonary compliance is represented by flattening of the inspiratory limb of the pressure–volume loop. The intensivist should utilize a PEEP that maintains alveolar recruitment without overdistending lung units and limiting pulmonary compliance.

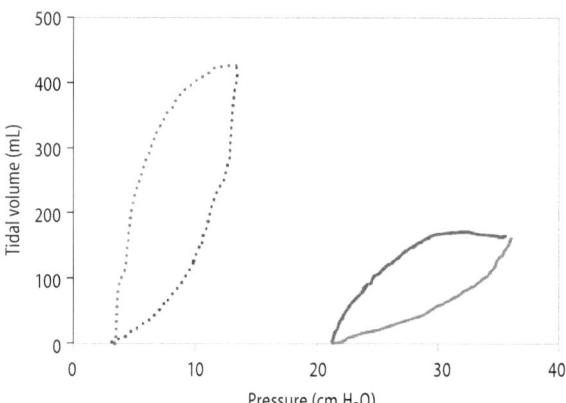

Figure 3.10. Pressure–volume loop of overdistended lung. Dotted lines represent normal lung, and solid lines represent overdistended lung.

Monitoring Increased Airway Resistance

The recognition and treatment of increased airway resistance (obstructed airways disease) is essential in the PICU. Obstructed airway disease may result from extrathoracic or intrathoracic airway obstruction. The flow–volume loops can be diagnostic of obstructed airway disease, and the loops can accurately guide ongoing therapeutic decisions. Variable extrathoracic airway obstruction primarily limits air from entering the lung during inspiration. Examples include croup, laryngomalacia, tracheomalacia, vocal cord dysfunction, epiglottitis, micrognathia, and macroglossia. Figure 3.11 represents a flow–volume loop of a normal lung with normal airway resistance and a flow–volume loop of increased airway resistance secondary to variable extrathoracic airway obstruction. The limitation of inspiratory flow is seen as flattening of the inspiratory limb of the flow–volume loop with markedly diminished peak inspiratory flows. Placement of a tracheal tube through the area of obstruction can normalize the flow–volume loop.

Variable intrathoracic airway obstruction primarily limits gas from exiting the lung during exhalation. An example of variable intrathoracic upper airway obstruction is tracheobronchomalacia. Figure 3.12 represents a flow–volume loop of a normal lung with normal airway resistance and a flow–volume loop of increased airway resistance secondary to variable intrathoracic obstruction. The limitation of expiratory flow is seen as flattening of the expiratory limb of the flow–volume loop with markedly diminished peak expiratory flows. Diseases of the small to medium airways such as asthma and bronchiolitis may also cause variable intrathoracic airway obstruction and lead to distinctive appearing flow–volume loops. Like upper intrathoracic airway obstruction, lower airway obstruction results in flattening of the expiratory flow with diminished peak expiratory flows. The flattening or *scooping* of the expiratory limb of the flow–volume loop is considered a hallmark of lower airway obstruction, and its presence suggests increased lower airways resistance. With bronchodilation, the clinician should see a rise in expiratory flow rates and less flattening (scooping) of the expiratory flow loop (Figure 3.13). These changes in the flow–volume loops can be followed to assess the response to therapy and progression of the disease.

Fixed airway obstruction restricts the flow of gas on inspiration and exhalation. Figure 3.14 represents a flow–volume loop of a normal lung with normal airway resistance and a flow–volume loop of increased airway resistance secondary to fixed airway

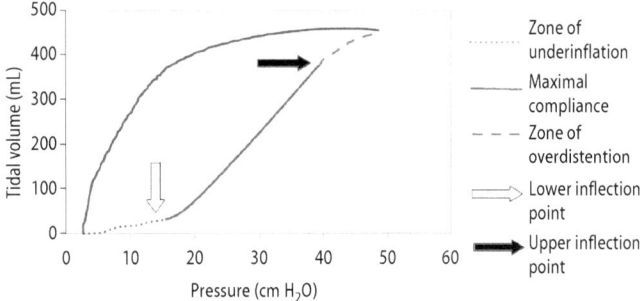

Figure 3.9. Pressure–volume loop of patient's lung with acute respiratory distress syndrome.

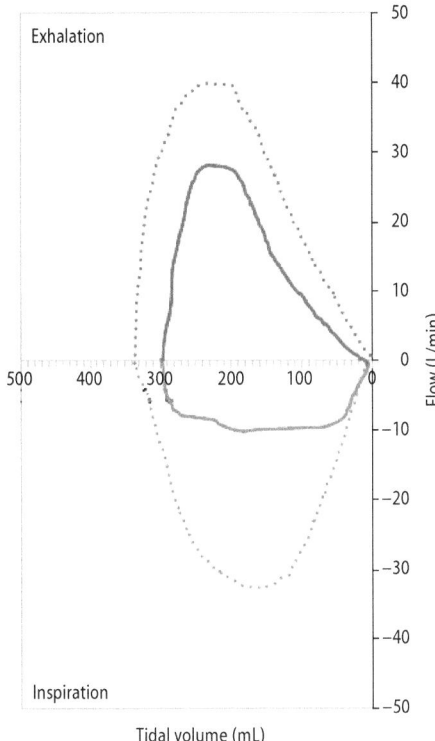

FIGURE 3.11. Flow–volume loop of variable extrathoracic obstruction. Dotted lines represent normal airway resistance, and solid lines represent variable extrathoracic airway obstruction.

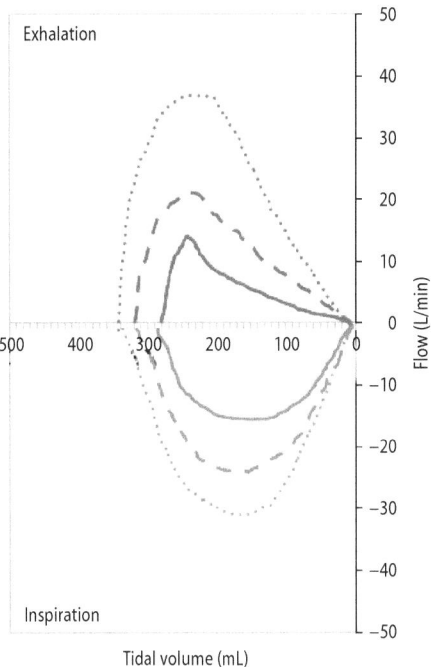

FIGURE 3.13. Flow–volume loop of asthma. Solid lines represent asthma, dashed lines represent asthma after response to repeated administration of bronchodilators (note the sequential improvement in the flow-volume loops.)

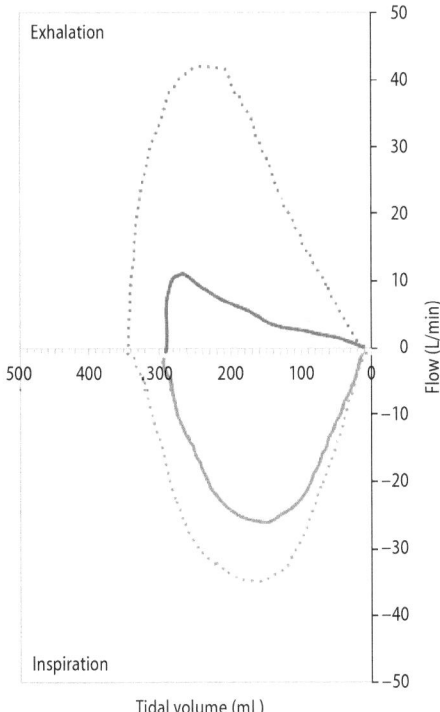

FIGURE 3.12. Flow–volume loop of variable intrathoracic obstruction. Dotted lines represent normal airway resistance, and solid lines represent variable intrathoracic airway obstruction.

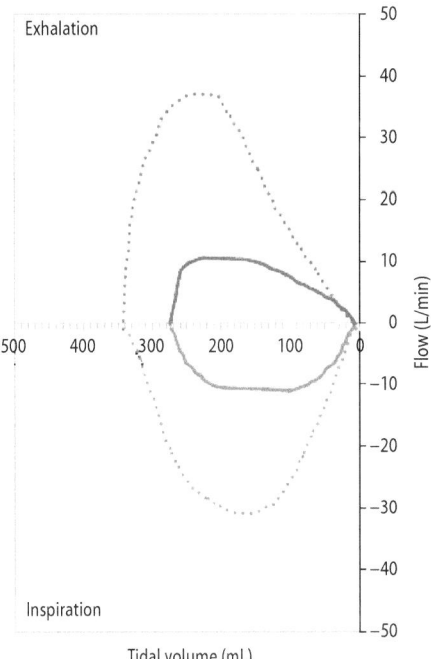

FIGURE 3.14. Flow–volume loop of fixed airway obstruction. Dotted lines represent normal airway resistance, and solid lines represent fixed airway obstruction.

FIGURE 3.15. (A) Flow–volume loop with air leak.
(B) Pressure–volume loop with air leak.

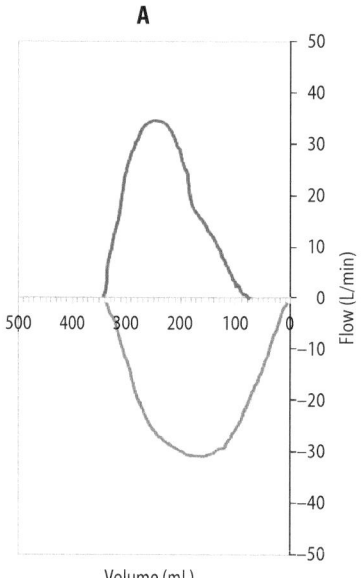

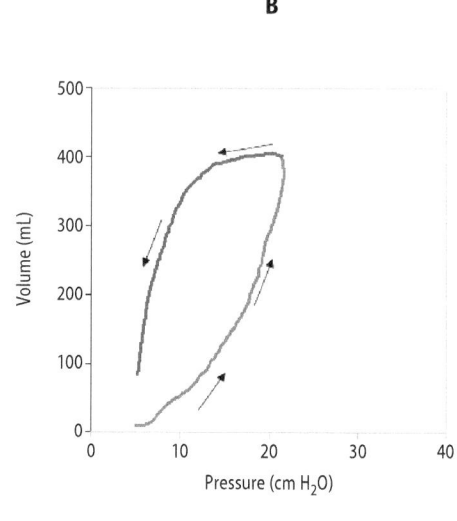

obstruction. Examples of fixed airway obstruction include tracheal stenosis, extratracheal compression, tracheal mass, foreign body, and an occluded or kinked tracheal tube. The flow–volume loop of fixed airway obstruction demonstrates markedly decreased peak expiratory and inspiratory flows with flattening of the expiratory and inspiratory loops. Flow–volume loops can reliably detect the presence of airway obstruction and can be instrumental in identifying the type of obstruction present. Careful monitoring of the flow–volume loops can assist the pediatric intensivist in the recognition and treatment of obstructive airway disease, and pressure-flow loops can demonstrate flow limitation.

Detection of Air Leak

The accurate interpretation of flow–volume and pressure–volume loops may be limited by the presence of an air leak around the tracheal tube or in the ventilator circuit. The sudden development of a large air leak usually represents mechanical failure such as compromised ventilator tubing, a loose connection, or cuff failure. Flow–volume and pressure–volume loops may be helpful in alerting the clinician to the presence of a large air leak, which could lead to diminished airway pressures and decreased minute ventilation. Figure 3.15A represents a flow–volume loop of a circuit with a large air leak. The loop begins at zero flow and zero volume delivered. The inspiratory limb moves clockwise into the expiratory limb. When the expiratory limb terminates before reaching zero volume, an air leak is present. The degree of air leak present can be estimated by the distance the loop terminates from zero volume.

The pressure–volume loop can also be utilized to detect the presence of an air leak. Figure 3.15B represents a pressure–volume loop that begins at the end-expiratory pressure and zero volume. The loop moves counterclockwise into the expiratory limb. When an air leak is present, the expiratory limb terminates before reaching zero. The degree of air leak can also be estimated by assessing the distance the expiratory limb terminates from zero.

Conclusion

Respiratory monitoring is an essential tool in the care of critically ill pediatric patients. The accurate interpretation and integration of data enables the pediatric intensivist to more effectively treat children in the PICU. With the physical examination, radiographic studies, blood gas analyses, capnography, and respiratory mechanics, the pediatric intensivist can greatly ameliorate the deleterious effects of respiratory disease in the pediatric population.

References

1. Weil MH. Patient evaluation, "vital signs," and initial care. In: Shoemaker WC, Thompson WL, eds. Critical Care: State of the Art. Fullerton, CA: Society of Critical Care Medicine;1980:1–31.
2. Iliff A, Lee VA. Pulse rate, respiratory rate, and body temperature in children between two months and eighteen years of age. Child Dev 1952;23:237–245.
3. Gravelyn TR, Weg JT. Respiratory rate as an indicator of acute respiratory dysfunction. JAMA 1980;244:1123–1125.
4. Mezzanotte WS, Tangel DJ, White DP. Mechanisms of control of alae nasi muscle activity. J Appl Physiol 1992;72:925–933.
5. Tobin MJ, Perez W, Guenther SM, Lodato RF, Dantzker DR. Does ribcage abdominal paradox signify respiratory muscle fatigue? J Appl Physiol 1987;63:851–860.
6. Willis BC, Graham AS, Wetzel RL, Newth CJ. Respiratory inductance plethysmography used to diagnose bilateral diaphragmatic paralysis: a case report. Pediatr Crit Care Med 2004;4:399–402.
7. Hoover CF. The diagnostic significance of inspiratory movements of the costal margins. Am J Med Sci 1920;159:633–646.
8. Gilmartin JJ, Gibson GJ. Abnormalities of chest wall motion in patients with chronic airflow obstruction. Thorax 1984;39:264–271.
9. Klein M. Hoover sign and peripheral airways obstruction. J Pediatr 1992;120:495–496.
10. Garcia-Pachon E. Paradoxical movement of the lateral rib margin (Hoover sign) for detecting obstructive airway disease. Chest 2002;122:651–655.
11. Comroe JH Jr, Botelho S. The unreliability of cyanosis in the recognition of arterial anoxemia. Am J Med Sci 1947;214:1–6.

12. Driscoll DJ. Evaluation of the cyanotic newborn. Pediatr Clin North Am 1990;37:1–23.
13. Harrison VC, Heese Hde V, Klein M. The significance of grunting in hyaline membrane disease. Pediatrics 1968;41:549–559.
14. London R. Lung sounds. Am Rev Respir Dis 1984;130:663–673.
15. Henschke CI, Pasternak GS, Schroeder S, Hart KK, Herman PG. Bedside chest radiography: diagnostic efficacy. Radiology 1983;149:23–26.
16. Henschke CI, Pasternak GS, Herman PG. Maximizing the efficacy of chest radiography in the ICU. Appl Radiol 1984;13:139–143.
17. Bekemeyer WB, Crapo RO, Calhoon S, Cannon CY, Clayton PD. Efficacy of chest radiography in a respiratory intensive care unit. A prospective study. Chest 1985;88:691–696.
18. Henschke CI, Yankelevitz DF, Wand A, Davis SD, Shiau M. Accuracy and efficacy of chest radiography in the intensive care unit. Radiol Clin North Am 1996;34:21–31.
19. Brunel W, Coleman DL, Schwartz DE, Peper E, Cohen NH. Assessment of routine chest roentgenograms and the physical examination to confirm endotracheal tube position. Chest 1989;96:1043–1045.
20. Levy FH, Bratton SL, Jardine DS. Routine chest radiographs following repositioning of endotracheal tubes are necessary to assess correct position in pediatric patients. Chest 1994;106:1508–1510.
21. Quasney MW, Goodman DM, Billow M, et al. Routine chest radiographs in pediatric intensive care units. Pediatrics 2001;107:241–248.
22. Redding GJ. Atelectasis in childhood. Pediatr Clin North Am 1984;31:891–905.
23. Duggan M, Kavanagh BP. Pulmonary atelectasis: a pathogenic perioperative entity. Anesthesiology 2005;102:838–854.
24. Shevland JE, Hirleman MT, Hoang KA, Kealey GP. Lobar collapse in the surgical intensive care unit. Br J Radiol 1983;56:531–534.
25. Thomas K, Habibi P, Britto, Owens CM. Distribution and pathophysiology of acute lobar collapse in the pediatric intensive care unit. Crit Care Med 1999;27:1594–1597.
26. Beydon L, Saada M, Liu N, et al. Can portable chest x-ray examination accurately diagnose lung consolidation after major abdominal surgery? A comparison with CT scan. Chest 1992;102:1697–1703.
27. Goodman LR, ed. Intensive Care Radiology. St. Louis, CV Mosby; 1983.
28. Lefcoe MS, Fox GA, Leasa DJ, Sparrow RK, McCormack DG. Accuracy of portable chest radiography in the critical care setting. Diagnosis of pneumonia based on quantitative cultures obtained from protected brush catheter. Chest 1994;105:885–887.
29. Aberle DR, Wiener-Kronish JP, Webb WR, Matthay MA. Hydrostatic versus increased permeability pulmonary edema: diagnosis based on radiographic criteria in critically ill patients. Radiology 1988;168:73–79.
30. Moskowitz H, Platt RT, Schachar R, Mellins H. Roentgen visualization of minute pleural effusion. An experimental study to determine the minimum amount of pleural fluid visible on a radiograph. Radiology 1973;109:33–35.
31. Kohan JM, Poe RH, Israel RH, et al. Value of chest ultrasonography versus decubitus roentgenography for thoracentesis. Am Rev Respir Dis 1986;133:1124–1126.
32. Woodring JH. Recognition of pleural effusions on supine radiographs: how much fluid is required? Am J Roentgenol 1984;142:59–64.
33. Kollef MH. Risk factors for the misdiagnosis of pneumothorax in the ICU. Crit Care Med 1991;197:906–910.
34. Tocino I. Chest Radiography in the critically ill patient. In Greene R, Muhm JR. eds. Syllabus: A Diagnostic Categorical Course in Chest Radiology. Oak Brook, IL: Radiological Society of North America; 1992:311–319.
35. Gattinoni L, Pelosi P, Pesenti A, et al. CT scan in ARDS: clinical and pathophysiological insights. Acta Anaesthesiol Scand Suppl 1991;95:87–96.
36. Pelosi P, Crotti S, Brazzi L, Gattinoni L. Computed tomography in adult respiratory distress syndrome: what has it taught us? Eur Respir J 1996;9:1055–1062.
37. Fan LL. Evaluation and therapy of chronic interstitial pneumonitis in children. Curr Opin Pediatr 1994;6:248–254.
38. McDonagh J, Greaves M, Wright AR, Heycock C, Owen JP, Kelly C. High Resolution computed tomography of the lungs in patients with rheumatoid arthritis and interstitial lung disease. Br J Rheumatol 1994;33:118–122.
39. Primack SL, Muller NL, Mayo JR, Remy-Jardin M, Remy J. Pulmonary parenchymal abnormalities of vascular origin: high resolution CT findings. Radiographics 1994;14:739–746.
40. Patel S, Kazerooni EA. Helical CT for the evaluation of acute pulmonary embolism. AJR Am J Roentgenol 2005;185:135–149.
41. Houston JG, Fleet M, Cowan MD, McMillan NC. Comparison of ultrasound with fluoroscopy in the assessment of suspected hemidiaphragmatic movement abnormality. Clin Radiol 1995;50:95–98.
42. Gottesman E, McCool FD. Ultrasound evaluation of the paralyzed diaphragm. Am J Respir Crit Care Med 1997;155:1570–1574.
43. Kohan JM, Poe RH, Israel RH, et al. Value of chest ultrasonography versus decubitus roentgenography for thoracentesis. Am Rev Respir Dis 1986;133:1124–1126.
44. Laing FC, Filly RA. Problems in the application of ultrasonography for the evaluation of pleural opacities. Radiology 1978;126:211–214.
45. Mayo PH. Safety of ultrasound-guided thoracentesis in patients receiving mechanical ventilation. Chest 2004;125:1059–1062.
46. Courtney SE, Weber KR, Breakie LA, et al. Capillary blood gases in the neonate. A reassessment and review of the literature. Am J Dis Child 1990;144:168–172.
47. Saili A, Dutta AK, Sarna MS. Reliability of capillary blood gas estimation in neonates. Indian Pediatr 1992;29:567–570.
48. Harrison AM, Lynch JM, Dean JM, Witte MK. Comparison of simultaneously obtained arterial and capillary blood gases in pediatric intensive care unit patients. Crit Care Med 1997;25:1904–1908.
49. Ueta I, Jacobs BR. Capillary and arterial blood gases in hemorrhagic shock: a comparative study. Pediatr Crit Care Med 2002;3:375–377.
50. Hamilton PA, Whitehead MD, Reynolds EO. Underestimation of arterial oxygen tension by transcutaneous electrode with increasing age in infants. Arch Dis Child 1985;60:1162–1165.
51. Rome ES, Stork EK, Carlo WA, Martin RJ. Limitations of transcutaneous PO_2 and PCO_2 monitoring in infants with bronchopulmonary dysplasia. Pediatrics 1984;74:217–220.
52. Durand M, Ramanathan R. Pulse oximetry for continuous oxygen monitoring in sick newborn infants. J Pediatr 1986;109:1052–1056.
53. Fanconi S. Pulse oximetry and transcutaneous oxygen tension for detection of hypoxemia in critically ill infants and children. Adv Exp Biol 1987;220:159–164.
54. Wahr JA, Tremper KK, Diab M. Pulse oximetry. Respir Clin North Am 1995;1:77–105.
55. Sinex JE. Pulse oximetry: principles and limitations. Am J Emerg Med 1999;17:59–67.
56. Aoyagi T. Pulse oximetry: its invention, theory, and future. J Anesth 2003;17:259–266.
57. Marini JJ. Monitoring during mechanical ventilation. Clin Chest Med 1988;9:73–100.
58. Scheller J, Loeb R. Respiratory artifact during pulse oximetry in critically ill patients. Anesthesiology 1988;69:602–603.
59. Salyer JW. Neonatal and pediatric pulse oximetry. Respir Care 2003;48:386–398.
60. Goldman JM, Petterson MT, Kopotic RJ, Barker SJ. Masimo signal extraction pulse oximetry. J Clin Monit Comput 2000;16:475–483.
61. Bohnhorst B, Peter CS, Poets CF. Pulse oximeters' reliability in detecting hypoxemia and bradycardia: Comparison between a conventional and two new generation oximeters. Crit Care Med 2000;28:1565–1568.
62. Gehring H, Hornberger C, Matz H, Konecny E, Schmucker P. The effects of motion artifact and low perfusion on the performance of a new generation of pulse oximeters in volunteers undergoing hypoxemia. Respir Care 2002;47:48–60.
63. Hay WW Jr, Rodden DJ, Collins SM, Melara DL, Hale KA, Fashaw LM. Reliability of conventional and new pulse oximetry in neonatal patients. J Perinatol 2002;22:360–366.

64. Barker S, Tremper KK. The effect of carbon monoxide inhalation on pulse oximetry and transcutaneous PO_2. Anesthesiology 1987;66:677–679.

65. Vegfors M, Lennmarken C. Carboxyhaemoglobinaemia and pulse oximetry. Br J Anaesth 1991;66:625–626.

66. Hampson NB. Pulse oximetry in severe carbon monoxide poisoning. Chest 1998;114:1036–1041.

67. Reynolds KJ, Palayiwa E, Moyle JT, Sykes MK, Hahn CE. The effect of dyshemoglobins on pulse oximetry: part i, theoretical approach and part ii, experimental results using an in vitro test system. J Clin Monit 1993;9:81–90.

68. Barker S, Tremper KK, Hyatt J. Effects of methemoglobinemia on pulse oximetry and mixed venous oximetry. Anesthesiology 1989;70:112–117.

69. Schnapp L, Cohen NH. Pulse oximetry: Uses and abuses. Chest 1990;98:1244–1250.

70. Nellcor Inc. Controlling external optical interferences in pulse oximetry. Pulse oximetry Note No. 5, 1986.

71. Escalante-Kanashiro R, Tantalean-Da-Fieno J. Capillary blood gases in a pediatric intensive care unit. Crit Care Med 2000;28:224–226.

72. Yildizdas D, Yapicioglu H, Yilmaz HL, Sertdemir Y. Correlation of simultaneously obtained capillary, venous, and arterial blood gases of patients in a paediatric intensive care unit. Arch Dis Child 2004;89:176–180.

73. Fernandez EG, Green TP, Sweeney M. Low inferior venal caval catheters for hemodynamic and pulmonary function monitoring in pediatric critical care patients. Pediatr Crit Care Med 2004;5:14–18.

74. Malinoski DJ, Todd SR, Slone S, Mullins RJ, Schreiber MA. Correlation of central venous and arterial blood gas measurements in mechanically ventilated trauma patients. Arch Surg 2005;140:1122–1125.

75. Weil MH, Rackow EC, Trevino R, Grundler W, Falk JL, Griffel MI. Difference in acid–base status between venous and arterial blood during cardiopulmonary resuscitation. N Engl J Med 1986;315:153–156.

76. Adrogue HJ, Rashad MN, Gorin AB, Yacoub J, Madias NE. Arteriovenous acid–base disparity in circulatory failure: studies on mechanism. Am J Physiol 1989;257:F1087–F1093.

77. Adrogue HJ, Rashad MN, Gorin AB, Yacoub J, Madias NE. Assessing acid–base status in circulatory failure. Differences between arterial and central venous blood. N Engl J Med 1989;320:1312–1316.

78. Steedman DJ, Robertson CE. Acid base changes in arterial and central venous blood during cardiopulmonary resuscitation. Arch Emerg Med 1992;9:169–176.

79. Tobias JD, Meyer DJ Jr, Helikson MA. Monitoring of pH and PCO_2 in children using the Paratrend 7 in a peripheral vein. Can J Anaesth 1998;45:81–83.

80. Tobias JD, Connors D, Strauser L, Johnson T. Continuous pH and PCO_2 monitoring during respiratory failure in children with the Paratrend 7 inserted into the peripheral venous system. J Pediatr 2000;136:623–627.

81. Kelly AM, McAlpine R, Kyle E. Venous pH can safely replace arterial pH in the initial evaluation of patients in the emergency department. Emerg Med J 2001;18:340–342.

82. Kelly AM, Kyle E, McAlpine R. Venous pCO_2 and pH can be used to screen for significant hypercarbia in emergency patients with acute respiratory disease. J Emerg Med 2002;22:15–19.

83. Sivan Y, Eldadah MK, Cheah TE, Newth CJ. Estimation of arterial carbon dioxide by end-tidal and transcutaneous PCO_2 measurements in ventilated children. Pediatr Pulmonol 1992;12:153–157.

84. Clark JS, Votteri B, Ariagno RL, et al. Noninvasive assessment of blood gases. Am Rev Respir Dis 1992;145:220–232.

85. Monaco F, Nickerson BG, McQuitty JC. Continuous transcutaneous oxygen and carbon dioxide monitoring in the pediatric ICU. Crit Care Med 1982;10:765–766.

86. Palmisano BW, Severinghaus JW. Transcutaneous PCO_2 and PO_2: a multicenter study of accuracy. J Clin Monit 1990;6:189–195.

87. Tobias JD, Meyer DJ. Noninvasive monitoring of carbon dioxide during respiratory failure in toddlers and infants: end-tidal versus transcutaneous carbon dioxide. Anesthesiology 1997;85:55–58.

88. Tobias JD, Wilson WR Jr, Meyer DJ. Transcutaneous monitoring of carbon dioxide tension after cardiothoracic surgery in infants and children. Anesth Analg 1999;88:531–534.

89. Nosovitch MA, Johnson JO, Tobias JD. Noninvasive intraoperative monitoring of carbon dioxide in children: End-tidal versus transcutaneous techniques. Paediatr Anaesth 2002;12:48–52.

90. Berkenbosch JW, Tobias JD. Transcutaneous carbon dioxide monitoring during high-frequency oscillatory ventilation in infants and children. Crit Care Med 2002;30:1024–1027.

91. AARC Clinical Practice Guidelines. Transcutaneous blood gas monitoring for neonates and pediatric patients. Respir Care 1994;39:1176–1179.

92. Epstein MF, Cohen AR, Feldman HA, Raemer DB. Estimation of $PaCO_2$ by two noninvasive methods in the critically ill newborn infant. J Pediatr 1985;106:282–286.

93. Wilson J, Russo P, Russo J, Tobias JD. Noninvasive monitoring of carbon dioxide in infants and children with congenital heart disease: end-tidal versus transcutaneous techniques. J Intensive Care Med 2005;20:291–295.

94. Sullivan KJ, Kissoon N, Goodwin SR. End-tidal carbon dioxide monitoring in pediatric emergencies. Pediatr Emerg Care 2005;21:327–332.

95. Thompson JE, Jaffe MB. Capnographic waveforms in the mechanically ventilated patient. Respir Care 2005;50:100–109.

96. Hoffman RA, Krieger BP, Kramer MR, et al. End tidal carbon dioxide in critically ill patients during changes in mechanical ventilation. Am Rev Respir Dis 1989;140:1265–1268.

97. Bhende MS, Thompson AE, Cook DR, Saville AL. Validity of a disposable end-tidal CO_2 detector in verifying endotracheal tube placement in infants and children. Ann Emerg Med 1992;21:142–145.

98. Bhende MS, Thompson AE, Orr RA. Utility of an end-tidal carbon dioxide detector during stabilization and transport of critically ill children. Pediatrics 1992;89:1042–1044.

99. Bhende MS, Thompson AE. Evaluation of an end-tidal CO_2 detector during pediatric cardiopulmonary resuscitation. Pediatrics 1995;95:395–399.

100. Cumming C, McFadzean J. A survey of the use of capnography for the confirmation of correct placement of tracheal tubes in pediatric intensive care units in the UK. Paediatr Anaesth 2005;15:591–596.

101. Bhende MS, Thompson AE, Howland DF. Validity of a disposable end-tidal carbon dioxide detector in verifying endotracheal tube position in piglets. Crit Care Med 1991;19:566–568.

102. Sum Ping ST, Mehta MP, Symreng T. Accuracy of the FEF CO_2 detector in the assessment of endotracheal tube placement. Anesth Analg 1992;74:415–419.

103. Tobias JD, Flanagan JF, Wheeler TJ, Garrett JS, Burney C. Noninvasive monitoring of end-tidal CO_2 via nasal cannulas in spontaneously breathing children during the perioperative period. Crit Care Med 1994;22:1805–1808.

104. Abramo TJ, Wiebe RA, Scott SM, Primm PA, McIntyre D, Mydler T. Noninvasive capnometry in a pediatric population with respiratory emergencies. Pediatr Emerg Care 1996;12:252–254.

105. Krauss B, Deykin A, Lam A, et al. Capnogram shape in obstructive lung disease. Anesth Analg 2005;100:884–888.

106. Waugh JB, Deshpande VM, Harwood RJ, eds. Rapid Interpretation of Ventilator Waveforms. Upper Saddle River, NJ: Prentice Hall; 1999.

107. ARDS Network: Ventilation with lower tidal volumes as compared with traditional tidal volumes for acute lung injury and the acute respiratory distress syndrome. N Engl J Med 2000;342:1301–1308.

4
Bronchoscopy in the Pediatric Intensive Care Unit

Robert E. Wood

to acquire a suitable working knowledge of the relevant anatomy and pathology likely to be encountered. Finally, physicians performing bronchoscopy must ensure that they have appropriate instruments and that those instruments are properly prepared and cared for. A bronchoscope that has been improperly cleaned can transmit potentially fatal diseases from patient to patient. Inappropriate handling during cleaning or storage can destroy the instrument.

Introduction

Bronchoscopy is the visual examination of the airways and can be an extremely useful tool for the management of patients in the pediatric intensive care unit (PICU). Bronchoscopy is done for both diagnostic and therapeutic indications and can be performed with either rigid or flexible instruments. Because flexible instruments can be passed through artificial airways, they are in most cases the instruments of choice for applications in the PICU. With the proper instrument, there is no patient whose airways cannot be effectively and safely evaluated—age and size are not limitations. Flexible bronchoscopes suitable for use in children are as small as 2.2 mm in diameter (Table 4.1).

The question frequently arises as to who should perform bronchoscopy in the PICU. Clearly, this procedure must be performed by adequately trained physicians—it is not a *throw-away* procedure to be performed by a medical student or an unsupervised first-year resident. Flexible bronchoscopes are expensive, fragile instruments, and they should be used only by properly trained, responsible physicians who are adequately supported by ancillary personnel. An instrument costing more than $20,000 can be destroyed in 20 milliseconds! Furthermore, of all the complications of bronchoscopy, other than death of the patient, the most serious is the failure to arrive at the correct diagnostic answer. Although it is perfectly reasonable for an intensivist to become skilled in the manipulation of a flexible bronchoscope and in the recognition (and management) of abnormal findings, in many cases it may be preferable for the PICU staff to rely on specialists (pulmonology, otolaryngology) who perform bronchoscopy on a daily basis. If an intensivist or anesthesiologist is to perform bronchoscopy, it is important to achieve a suitable baseline skill level and to perform enough procedures to maintain and enhance that skill, as well as

Indications for Bronchoscopy in the Pediatric Intensive Care Unit

What can be done with a bronchoscope? The most obvious answer is, of course, to visually examine the airways. Other applications include the removal of specimens or material (mucus, foreign bodies) obstructing the airways, the delivery of medications or fluid to the airways, and the manipulation of the airways for therapeutic purposes. One of the most useful applications beyond visual inspection is bronchoalveolar lavage (BAL). Bronchoalveolar lavage is a very efficient and effective way to obtain a relatively representative diagnostic specimen from the distal airways and alveoli. This involves the instillation of saline into, and recovery from, the distal airways in such a volume that the recovered fluid contains at least some fluid that was present on the alveolar surface. In pediatric patients, the volumes of saline used per aliquot range from 5 mL in very small infants to 20 mL, and approximately half the volume instilled will be recovered. The care with which the specimen is handled and analyzed should match the care with which it is obtained.

There are two major categories of indications for bronchoscopy, diagnostic and therapeutic. In general, there is only one indication for diagnostic bronchoscopy—bronchoscopy is indicated when there is information in the lungs or airways of the patient, necessary for the care of the patient, that is most appropriately obtained by bronchoscopy. All specific indications stem from this overriding consideration. Therapeutic bronchoscopy, on the other hand, is indicated when it is the most appropriate way to achieve the necessary therapeutic goals.

D.S. Wheeler et al. (eds.), The *Respiratory Tract in Pediatric Critical Illness and Injury*,
DOI 10.1007/978-1-84800-925-7_4, © Springer-Verlag London Limited 2009

TABLE 4.1. Flexible bronchoscopes.*

Diameter (mm)	Suction channel (mm)	Smallest endotracheal tube for intubation (mm)	Smallest endotracheal tube for assisted ventilation (mm)	Smallest endotracheal tube for spontaneous ventilation (mm)	Largest tube that should be used with this instrument for intubation (mm)[†]
2.2	None	2.5	3.0	3.5	4.0
2.8	1.2	3.0	3.5	4.0	4.5
3.5	1.2	4.5	5.0	5.5	6.0
3.8[‡]	1.2	5.0	5.0	5.5	7.5
4.4	2.0	5.0	5.5	6.0	7.5
4.9	2.0	5.5	6.0	6.5	NA

*Olympus Corporation. Instruments by other manufacturers may have similar (but not necessarily identical) characteristics.

[†]Use with larger tubes may result in damage to the instrument.

[‡]True videoscope; tip diameter is actually closer to 4.4 mm.

Diagnostic Bronchoscopy

Bronchoscopy is useful not only for the visualization of the airways but also for the recovery of diagnostic specimens. In some cases, there may be multiple indications for bronchoscopy, as in the patient with recurrent pneumonia in whom it is important not only to exclude anatomic abnormalities or an aspirated foreign body but also to obtain specimens for cytology and microbiologic studies. Radiographic studies can sometimes yield similar information about airway structure but are not capable of yielding specimens for microscopic examination or culture; in general, radiologic procedures are not effective for the demonstration of airway dynamics. There are many specific indications for diagnostic bronchoscopy in pediatric patients; the following discussion focuses on the most common indications in patients likely to be found in the PICU.

Atelectasis usually responds relatively promptly to conventional therapy, and by no means does every patient with atelectasis require bronchoscopy for either diagnosis or therapy. However, if the atelectasis is of sufficient magnitude to significantly interfere with gas exchange, is persistent, or is in some way atypical, diagnostic bronchoscopy can be very useful. In the majority of cases, the bronchial anatomy will be normal, but a variety of abnormalities may be discovered. These include bronchial stenosis, bronchial compression, unsuspected foreign bodies, endobronchial mass lesions, and mucous plugs. For many patients, bronchoscopy is most helpful to definitively *exclude* anatomic abnormalities that might have required a very different approach to therapy. Whenever bronchoscopy is done, it is useful to perform BAL for cytology and microbiologic studies, as these data may lead to significant alterations in therapy.

Radiographic evidence of generalized hyperinflation most often reflects a generalized process such as bronchospasm, but, in patients in whom the response to therapy is unsatisfactory, bronchoscopy can yield important diagnostic clues. In such patients, BAL may give evidence of inflammation or diffuse mucous plugging. The BAL specimen should be examined visually for evidence of bronchial casts, which suggest mucous stasis and bronchial inflammation. The loss of anatomic detail on the mucosa (such as loss of visible tracheal rings or obvious thickening of the minor carinae) suggests mucosal edema, as may be associated with an acute asthmatic episode or infection. Localized hyperinflation may result from localized bronchial compression, stenosis, a foreign body, or dynamic collapse on expiration (bronchomalacia).

Hemoptysis is relatively uncommon in pediatric patients (although perhaps more so in PICU patients) and often generates considerable anxiety on the part of parents and caregivers. In the presence of known lung disease, modest amounts of hemoptysis may not warrant bronchoscopic evaluation, but larger bleeds may require investigation. If bleeding is brisk, it may seriously compromise the ability of the bronchoscopist to visualize the anatomy; some authorities recommend the use of a rigid instrument in the face of significant, active bleeding. On the other hand, if there is no active bleeding at the time of the procedure, it can be challenging to accurately identify the bleeding site. A systematic search should be made, segment by segment, gently suctioning away any visible blood and observing to see if it returns. If saline lavage is needed to help clear the mucosa, the smallest reasonable volume should be used, as drainage of bloody fluid can confuse the interpretation. Children can have significant bleeding from the lungs and exhibit no cough or physical (or even radiographic) signs; the presenting manifestation may be hematemesis. It is not rare for the airways to appear perfectly normal, while BAL yields bloody fluid. In patients who have not bled for several days, the only manifestation of the bleeding may be the presence of significant numbers of hemosiderin-laden macrophages in the BAL specimen. On the other hand, hemoptysis does not necessarily originate from the lungs; a careful search of the oropharynx and the nasopharyngeal airway should also be made (as well as the esophagus and stomach in some patients).

Stridor, whether acute or chronic, often causes considerable concern, even alarm, in the PICU. Flexible bronchoscopy, properly performed, is an infallible technique for the definitive diagnosis of stridor. Stridor is visible—if one can hear the noise, the vibrating structures causing that noise will *always* be visible if one is looking in the right place—there is no such thing as a diagnosis of stridor by exclusion. The patient must, however, be examined at a time or under conditions that allow the stridor to be heard. A flexible instrument should be passed through both nostrils so that the entire airway is examined, and the subglottic space as well as the trachea all the way to the carina should also be included. An advantage of flexible instrumentation for this purpose is that it is not necessary to apply traction to the tongue base and larynx (with a rigid laryngoscope) to visualize the larynx, a move that often masks the true nature of the lesion causing the stridor. Children with stridor often have more than one lesion; it is important to carry out the examination of the airway anatomy and dynamics all the way to the carina, even if a lesion is visualized that appears to adequately explain the stridor. For example, a child with severe subglottic or tracheal stenosis (not visible until the tip of the bronchoscope is at or below the glottis) may also have laryngomalacia, or very large lingual tonsils (which may have appeared to be the site of the airway obstruction causing the stridor). Conversely, examination with a rigid instrument may reveal the subglottic stenosis but fail to visualize the glossoptosis that can obstruct the airway after repair of the subglottis. Table 4.2 shows a partial list of the possible causes of stridor in children.

Table 4.2. Causes of stridor in children.

Laryngomalacia
Vocal cord paralysis
Subglottic stenosis or edema
Subglottic cyst
Subglottic hemangioma
Supraglottic hemangioma
Supraglottic cyst
Tracheomalacia
Tracheal compression
Laryngeal foreign body
Esophageal foreign body
Lingual tonsillar hypertrophy
Glossoptosis
Tonsillar hypertrophy
Adenoidal hypertrophy
Vallecular cyst or mass
Laryngeal papilloma
Laryngeal edema—supraglottic or subglottic
Laryngeal granulation tissue (intubation complications)

Persistent wheezing, unresponsive or poorly responsive to conventional therapy, is a common indication for diagnostic bronchoscopy in children. Other than stridor, this is the indication most commonly associated with the finding of an anatomic abnormality. Wheezing that responds promptly and completely to bronchodilator therapy rarely (but sometimes) warrants endoscopic evaluation. Like stridor, wheezing can result from a variety of causes, and the endoscopic diagnosis may also depend on the technique utilized for the examination. For example, bronchomalacia, the dynamic collapse of a bronchus during expiration, may not be detectable if the patient is too heavily sedated to generate sufficient expiratory effort to collapse the airway or if the procedure is performed with positive pressure ventilation. As with atelectasis, a negative examination often has real value, and evaluation of BAL cytology and culture often gives an important clue to the diagnosis.

Recurrent or persistent pneumonia is a common indication for diagnostic bronchoscopy in pediatric patients, although, in the PICU, bronchoscopy is more likely to be performed as part of the evaluation of pneumonia in a compromised host. In general, the diagnostic value of bronchoscopy and BAL for such a patient is maximized by performing the procedure before the initiation of therapy. However, in real life, it is more frequently the case that the clinical condition of the patient mandates immediate initiation of empirical (usually broad-spectrum) therapy. This may result in a false-negative culture result, although many clinicians theorize that what they are really searching for is an infectious agent that is not affected by the antimicrobial agents being utilized. Nonculture-based methods for detection of infectious agents (i.e., special stains for microorganisms such as *Pneumocystis carinii* and polymerase chain reaction or antibody-based tests) can enhance the yield. Care must be taken to select the most appropriate diagnostic tests to which the BAL specimen will be subjected.

In the evaluation of the patient who is immunocompromised, great care must be taken to minimize the risk of contamination of either the diagnostic specimen or the lower airways with aspirated secretions from the oropharynx. This is most often ensured by

elective tracheal intubation and passing the flexible bronchoscope through the tracheal tube. This should be done without application of topical anesthetic to the larynx (which promptly results in the aspiration of oral secretions). If desired, the supraglottic airway can be examined after the BAL specimen has been obtained. Other techniques to minimize contamination of the specimen include placing the patient in a Trendelenburg position, assiduously avoiding suctioning through the suction channel of the bronchoscope until it is in the position desired for the collection of the BAL specimen, and insufflating oxygen (at no more than 2 L/min) through the suction channel continuously during passage of the bronchoscope.

Children admitted to the PICU are not infrequently suspected of harboring an aspirated foreign body. If there is radiographic evidence of the foreign body, or if the clinical suspicion is quite high (witnessed aspiration with wheezing, for example), bronchoscopy should be performed as soon as feasible with a rigid instrument (or with a rigid instrument immediately available). Removal of foreign bodies with flexible bronchoscopes is almost never a good idea—it accepts all the limitations of flexible instruments (very small working channels and extremely limited forceps, etc.) while rejecting all the advantages of rigid instruments (large working channels, a wide variety of suitable and specially designed forceps). The exceptions to this rule are few and include very small, peripheral objects whose shape allows them to be grasped by small, flexible forceps.

Bronchoscopy is often useful in the evaluation of patients with intrathoracic masses or vascular lesions suspected of compressing the airways. In theory, imaging techniques, such as computed tomography (CT) scan with three-dimensional reconstruction, could substitute for a bronchoscope in such patients. However, the techniques are often complementary, each providing information that the other cannot. Bronchoscopy cannot define the lesion outside the airway as well as a CT scan, but a CT scan will not demonstrate the airway dynamics or give as accurate a demonstration of the degree of obstruction, and it does not provide information obtainable by BAL.

Bronchoscopy is useful for the evaluation of a patient with aspiration. Bronchoalveolar lavage can demonstrate the presence of aspirated material, but, unfortunately, there is no unequivocal marker of aspiration. The demonstration of significant numbers of lipid-laden macrophages is usually thought to be indicative of aspiration, but this test is neither specific nor very sensitive. False-positive results are common with patients who have been given intravenous lipid infusions, for example, whereas false-negative results are common in patients who aspirate oral secretions but are not fed by mouth.

Children in PICUs have a surprisingly high incidence of congenital airway anomalies that may be a reason for bronchoscopy or that may be discovered during bronchoscopy. These include complete tracheal rings (congenital tracheal stenosis) and tracheoesophageal fistulas. If in doubt, take a look. All too often, the initials *WNL* written by a well-meaning physician and thought to mean *within normal limits* actually mean *we never looked*.

Therapeutic Bronchoscopy

The preceding discussion should make it clear that there is a potentially large role for diagnostic bronchoscopy in the PICU. Arguably, however, the therapeutic role may be larger, at least in terms of the number of procedures done in the PICU. In general, bronchoscopes are quite useful in providing relief of airway obstruction by removing endobronchial obstructions of various kinds and by facilitating the management of artificial airways.

Many intensivists and anesthesiologists view flexible bronchoscopes almost entirely in the context of airway management, facilitating difficult intubations and evaluating tube placement and patency. This is surely a very important aspect of flexible bronchoscopy. It is fair to say that there is virtually no patient otherwise capable of extrauterine survival who cannot be tracheally intubated with the aid of a suitable flexible bronchoscope *and an operator skilled in its use.*

Bronchoscopic tracheal intubation is substantially easier when performed transnasally than transorally. A tracheal tube of suitable size is loaded over a flexible bronchoscope of suitable size (see Table 4.1), and the tube is pulled as far proximally on the shaft of the bronchoscope as possible. The bronchoscope is passed via the nostril to the glottis, topical anesthetic is applied, and the tip of the bronchoscope is then advanced to the carina. A variety of anatomic abnormalities may be encountered along the way (perhaps the reason the tracheal intubation was difficult in the first place) and should be recognized and documented by the bronchoscopist. With the tip of the bronchoscope at the carina, the flexible bronchoscope is held vertically so that the shaft is as straight as possible. The tracheal tube is then advanced over the bronchoscope, using a rotating, twisting motion (this motion dramatically reduces friction against the bronchoscope and also facilitates the safe passage of the tube through the turbinates and the glottis). It is critically important that the operator keep the carina in view at all times; it is very easy, especially in small infants, for the tip of the bronchoscope to find its way into the esophagus. The tube is advanced until it can be seen through the bronchoscope and its tip positioned in the desired relation to the carina. The bronchoscope can then be withdrawn. This entire process can usually be accomplished within 30 seconds by an experienced bronchoscopist. If the operator chooses to intubate orally, it is critically important to ensure that the patient does not bite the bronchoscope.

When the tracheal tube is properly positioned, the bronchoscope can be withdrawn and the patient ventilated through the tracheal tube. After securing the tube at the nostril, the bronchoscope should again be passed to evaluate the distal airways and to verify the position of the tip of the tube (thus obviating the need for a chest film for tube placement). It is important to choose the proper flexible bronchoscope for the tracheal tube selected for the patient. See Table 4.1 for minimum tube sizes for the different flexible bronchoscopes available. Note also that the *nominal* diameter of a flexible bronchoscope may be different from the actual diameter, as the diameter may increase where different materials used to cover the instrument are joined.

Flexible bronchoscopes are often utilized to evaluate problems with artificial airways during mechanical ventilation (or in children with tracheostomies). The instruments can be passed through the tube without moving the tube or changing the anatomic relationships, thus revealing the patency of the tube and the airways distal to the tip of the tube as well as the position of the tube. This can have special utility in children with tracheostomies to ensure that the tube is an appropriate length.

Bronchoscopes are employed to remove lesions (and objects) that obstruct the airway, such as foreign bodies, tissue masses, blood clots, and mucous plugs. Flexible instruments are useful for

TABLE 4.3. Contraindications to bronchoscopy.

Absolute contraindication	Relative contraindication
Lack of proper indication(s)	Severe hypoxemia or hypercapnia (may be an indication)
Lack of proper instruments	Coagulopathy (can usually be corrected, at least temporarily)
Lack of suitably trained personnel	Severe airway obstruction (requires extra care with technique and selection of instruments, anesthetic technique, etc.)—may be an important indication!
	Known, active cavitary pulmonary tuberculosis (until appropriate therapy has been initiated and sputum smears are negative)

diagnosis but are of relatively limited value in the *management* of foreign bodies and tissue masses (although the latter can be treated through the flexible instrument with a laser fiber or electrocautery electrode). Discovery of a foreign body or endobronchial tissue mass during flexible bronchoscopy in the PICU should lead to a rigid bronchoscopy (possibly in a more conventional venue). Mucous plugs, however, are usually effectively treated with flexible bronchoscopy, although they may require a prolonged effort if they are tenacious and extensive. Large blood clots can be challenging, especially when fresh; suctioning often results in fibrin strands that still obstruct the peripheral bronchi without removal of the clot itself. Localized instillation of thrombolytic agents may be helpful but has the potential to cause fresh hemorrhage.

Bronchoscopy can be helpful in the management of patients with persistent bronchopleural fistulas. The bronchus leading to the air leak can be selectively obstructed with a Fogarty catheter, thus identifying the site. This bronchus can then be obstructed temporarily with material such as fibrin glue or Gelfoam, stopping the leak long enough to allow tissue repair at the pleura.

Contraindications

There are few absolute contraindications (Table 4.3) to bronchoscopy if the procedure really needs to be done.

Complications

Complications will occur. A complication is defined as an event that is unexpected and that results in injury to the patient, premature termination of the procedure, or a significant alteration of the procedure that results in less than optimal results. In general there are five types of complications: mechanical, physiologic, microbiologic, anesthetic, and cognitive (Table 4.4). In the PICU, disease acuity is high, patients are, almost by definition, less stable, and procedures may be performed by physicians with relatively less experience. Thus, the potential for complications is high. The incidence of complications can be decreased by careful attention to

TABLE 4.4. Potential complications of flexible bronchoscopy.

Mechanical complications
   Pneumothorax, pneumomediastinum
   Hemoptysis, epistaxis
   Mucosal trauma
   Subglottic edema, bronchial edema
   Damage to the bronchoscope (teeth, etc.)
Physiologic complications
   Hypoxemia
   Hypercapnia
   Hypotension/hypertension
   Increased intracranial pressure
   Aspiration
   Hypoglycemia (nothing-by-mouth status)
   Seizure (missed medication)
Microbiologic complications
   Nosocomial pneumonia (introduction of infectious agents into the patient's lungs)
   Spread of infection from one lobe to another
   Spread of infection from patient to hospital staff
   Endocarditis (although risk is thought to be low for flexible bronchoscopy)
Anesthetic complications
   Allergic reaction to agent
   Hypotension, etc.
   Seizures (especially with excessive lidocaine)
   Performing the procedure with excessive sedation, masking airway dynamics that
      may have been the primary diagnostic entity
Cognitive complications
   Failure to perform bronchoscopy when it is indicated and necessary
   Performing the procedure under inappropriate conditions or with inappropriate/
inadequate equipment
   Failure to recognize the pathology
   Failure to examine the appropriate anatomic region

Note: Doing the procedure and obtaining the wrong answer is the most serious complication, other than death of the patient!

detail, adequate patient preparation, use of appropriate instruments and sedation techniques, and practice.

Anesthesia

It is important for patients undergoing bronchoscopy to be safe and comfortable. A significant percentage of PICU patients will already be tracheally intubated and sedated; further sedation may not be needed. However, topical anesthesia of the distal trachea and bronchi may be important. The operator must take care, by placing an appropriate bite block, to ensure that the orally intubated patient does not damage the bronchoscope. The bronchoscopist and the anesthesiologist or intensivist who is supervising the sedation must have effective and continuous communication.

Patients who are not tracheally intubated will usually need some form of sedation, which must be given carefully and with a good working knowledge of the agents employed. A discussion of sedation techniques and drugs is beyond the scope of this chapter, and the reader is referred to subsequent chapters in this textbook. Anesthesia/sedation always places the patient at some degree of risk. The minimal dose of drug(s) should be used to achieve the desired results. The technique chosen for sedation must be appropriate to the diagnostic or therapeutic goals of the procedure. The wrong sedation technique may result in the operator obtaining the wrong diagnostic answer. If the primary goal is to evaluate and hopefully treat atelectasis, for example, intubation with deep sedation or even muscle relaxation may be appropriate. However, if the primary goal is the evaluation of airway dynamics, it will be necessary for the patient to be breathing spontaneously, and it may even be important that some coughing be witnessed. Positive pressure ventilation with or without muscle relaxation will effectively mask airway dynamics.

5
Acute Lung Injury and Acute Respiratory Distress Syndrome

Michael Vish and Thomas P. Shanley

Introduction

Acute lung injury (ALI) is a clinical syndrome of inflammation of the lung resulting in the loss of the capillary–alveolar integrity. Patients suffer from a high-permeability, nonhydrostatic pulmonary edema, reduced lung compliance, alveolar flooding and collapse, ventilation and perfusion (V_A/Q) mismatch, and consequent intrapulmonary shunting leading to hypoxemia. In 1967, Ashbaugh and colleagues described a cohort of 12 patients who had the acute onset of tachypnea, hypoxemia, panlobular infiltrates on chest radiograph, and decreased lung compliance [1]. It was noted that this syndrome was similar to the infant respiratory distress syndrome, and in 1971 the same investigators coined the name *adult respiratory distress syndrome* [2]. Since that time, it was noted that the same condition occurs in children and consequently was renamed the *acute respiratory distress syndrome* (ARDS). In 1988, Murray and colleagues defined ARDS via the Lung Injury Score (LIS) based on chest radiographic findings, the degree of hypoxemia (PaO$_2$/FiO$_2$ ratio), the level of positive end-expiratory pressure (PEEP), and lung compliance (Table 5.1) [3]. Later, in 1994, a joint American-European Consensus Committee (A-ECC) was convened with the goal of developing a universally accepted, consensus definition of ALI and ARDS.

The definition (Table 5.2) included an acute pulmonary or nonpulmonary triggering of the disease process in previously normal lungs, oxygenation abnormalities as defined by the PaO$_2$/FiO$_2$ ≤ 300 for ALI or PaO$_2$/FIO$_2$ ≤ 200 for ARDS, radiographic findings, and the exclusion of left atrial hypertension when measured, but it did not include PEEPs, as described in the LIS [4]. Thus, this description defined ARDS as the most severe manifestation of ALI. Although highly useful in stratifying and identifying patients for clinical studies, it is currently being considered for revision, as the

predictive value of this definition for adults has been questioned. In contrast to adult studies, recent epidemiologic studies in pediatric ALI have demonstrated a correlation between the initial PaO$_2$/FiO$_2$ and mortality [5]. Nevertheless, this definition fails to incorporate any information about the amount of positive pressure ventilation being used to support a patient at a given FiO$_2$. Because the oxygenation index (OI) incorporates the mean airway pressure (MAP) in its equation OI = [(MAP × FiO$_2$)/PaO$_2$] × 100, many clinicians believe this to be a more relevant parameter for stratifying ALI/ARDS patients for clinical studies as well as following the clinical response to therapeutic maneuvers as the amount of PEEP, positive inspiratory pressure, and inspiratory time are incorporated into the determination of the MAP. Acute lung injury/ARDS is perhaps one of the most common and challenging clinical entities pediatric intensivists will face throughout their careers, and, therefore, it is crucial to possess a comprehensive understanding of the epidemiology, pathophysiology, and management of this disease process.

Epidemiology

The exact incidence of ARDS has been relatively difficult to establish. A 1972 population study in the state of New York by the National Heart, Lung, and Blood Institute reported the incidence of ARDS in adults to be approximately 150,000 cases/year [6]. Other investigators have reported an incidence ranging from 1.5 to 75 patients/100,000 inhabitants/year [7–10], for children, the exact incidence has also been difficult to establish [11]. Only recently have prospective epidemiologic studies that made use of the A-ECC definition of ALI/ARDS provided more definitive data regarding the current incidence of ARDS. In a prospective, population-based, cohort study that was centered around Kings County, Washington, Rubenfeld et al. reported a crude incidence of ALI of 79 per 100,000 person-years and an age-adjusted incidence of 86 per 100,000 person-years, with an inhospital mortality rate of 38.5% [12]. Based on these data, they estimated that there are over 190,000 cases of ALI/ARDS per year, which are associated with nearly 75,000 deaths and 3.6 million hospital days—thus supporting the conclusion that ALI has a substantial impact on public health, both in this country and abroad. Unfortunately, as patients under the age of 15 years were excluded from this most recent study, the burden of pediatric ALI/ARDS largely remains unknown.

D.S. Wheeler et al. (eds.), The *Respiratory Tract in Pediatric Critical Illness and Injury*,
DOI 10.1007/978-1-84800-925-7_5, © Springer-Verlag London Limited 2009

TABLE 5.1. Murray lung injury score.

	SCORE
Chest radiograph	
No consolidation	0
1 Quadrant	1
2 Quadrants	2
3 Quadrants	3
4 Quadrants	4
Hypoxemia (PaO_2/FiO_2)	
≥300	0
225–229	1
175–224	2
100–174	3
<100	4
Peep (cm H_2O)	
≤5	0
6–8	1
9–11	2
12–14	3
≥15	4
Compliance (ml/cm H_2O)	
≥80	0
60–69	1
40–59	2
30–39	3
≤29	4

Note: The final value is obtained by dividing the sum of the individual component scores by 4.
Scores: 0 = no injury; 0.1–2.5 = Mild to moderate injury; >2.5 = Severe injury (acute respiratory distress syndrome).

Etiology

The varieties of insults that lead to ALI/ARDS are diverse (Table 5.3). This heterogeneity of several different etiologies leading to a similar end-organ event may relate to the distinct environment of the lungs. The pulmonary surface area that participates in gas exchange totals approximately 50–100 m^2 [13] and by virtue of its function must encounter the particulate and microbiologic environment of the outside world. This intimate connection of the atmosphere to the delicate capillary network of the pulmonary vasculature is separated by only micrometers from the epithelial lining layer, necessitating that the body's defenses be poised to react rapidly to pathogenic challenges. This proximity of the pul-

TABLE 5.2. American-European Consensus Committee definition of acute respiratory distress syndrome (ARDS) and acute lung injury (ALI).

	Timing	Oxygenation	Chest radiograph	Pulmonary artery wedge pressure
ALI	Acute onset	PaO_2/FiO_2 ratio ≤300 mm Hg (regardless of PEEP level)	Bilateral infiltrates seen on frontal chest radiograph	≤18 mm Hg when measured or no clinical evidence of left atrial hypertension
ARDS	Acute onset	PaO_2/FiO_2 ratio ≤200 mm Hg (regardless of PEEP level)	Bilateral infiltrates seen on frontal chest radiograph	≤18 mm Hg when measured or no clinical evidence of left atrial hypertension

TABLE 5.3. Common causes of acute lung injury and acute respiratory distress syndrome.

Pulmonary (direct causes)
    Pneumonia
    Aspiration
    Hydrocarbon aspiration
    Inhalation injury
    Pulmonary contusion
Extrapulmonary (indirect causes)
    Sepsis
    Pancreatitis
    Trauma
    Transfusion
    Near-drowning

monary structures explains in part the common manner by which inflammation can be triggered in this organ and is placed at further risk by the presence of additional factors.

The clinical syndrome of ALI/ARDS may be triggered from either a direct insult to the lungs as in pneumonia or aspiration *(pulmonary ARDS)* or from remote or systemic injuries such as sepsis or trauma *(extrapulmonary ARDS)*. Although physicians initially thought that the clinical presentation in either case resulted from similar pathophysiologic mechanisms, differences in the therapeutic responses have raised the possibility that this assumption is incorrect. Recent publications suggest that the pathophysiology of ARDS caused by pulmonary versus extrapulmonary disease may be different [14,15]. It is intuitive that, depending on the site of triggering insult, the injurious effect on the cell type comprising each component of the epithelial–endothelial barrier capacity may differ. For example, in the setting of a direct insult, alveolar epithelial cellular injury and dysfunction will be associated with an intrapulmonary inflammatory response with the accumulation of intraalveolar fluid, blood, and proteinaceous materials. Conversely, in the setting of a systemic or extrapulmonary trigger, the increase in pulmonary vascular permeability results from injury to the vascular endothelium via systemically released mediators of inflammation [16]. However, the subsequent similarity in the cascade of inflammatory events leading to the common clinical end-point described in ALI/ARDS has led clinical investigators to surmise a common pathway. This is countered by the observation that there are clinically measurable differences in pulmonary versus extrapulmonary ARDS in terms of the response to PEEP, respiratory mechanics, and findings on computed tomography (CT) scans [17]. Overall, however, no significant differences in the responsiveness to ventilation strategies has been observed [18] so that whether or not the two types of triggers should alter the approach to ALI/ARDS and lead to clinically relevant differences in treatment strategies remains to be determined.

Risk Factors and Outcomes

Several risk factors for the development of ALI/ARDS in adults have been consistently identified, including sepsis and pneumonia. Fewer studies have been performed in children [19,20], as the pediatric literature on ALI/ARDS has suffered from relatively small study size, variable exclusion criteria among studies, examination of only individual patient populations [21], and the variable adherence to the current consensus definition. These factors have made comparisons among pediatric studies difficult. However, the presence of sepsis, septic shock, and multiple-organ dysfunction have consistently had a very high association with the development of ALI/ARDS in both adults and children [20,22]. The literature would suggest an approximate 40% incidence of developing ARDS in patients with sepsis [23–26], with the incidence increasing in patients with additional risk factors such as witnessed gastric aspiration, multiple transfusions, and trauma [24]. Sepsis secondary to Gram-negative bacteria portends a particularly high mortality rate in the setting of ARDS. In a series of 86 patients with Gram-negative bacteremia by Kaplan et al., 20 patients developed ARDS (23%) and the mortality rate (90%) was substantially higher than for those who did not develop ARDS (50%) [27]. Historically, prior investigations on the incidence and outcomes from ALI/ARDS reported mortality rates that were substantially higher than more recent reports [28–30]. In one of the most recent epidemiologic studies of ALI in pediatrics, Flori et al. reported on 328 admissions (for 320 patients) for ALI/ARDS as defined by consensus definition at two centers over a nearly 4-year time frame [5]. The most common diagnoses were consistent with historical observations: pneumonia (35%), aspiration (15%), sepsis (13%), near-drowning (9%), and concomitant cardiac disease (7%) [5]. Overall mortality rate of the group was 22% (in contrast to adult outcomes of 35%–55%), with the highest rates observed among near-drowning (54%), associated cardiac disease (39%), and sepsis (31%). Importantly, hypoxemic respiratory failure was an uncommon cause of demise; more frequently, death occurred as a result of either a *do not resuscitate* order or withdrawal of life support in the face of medical futility. Again, as mentioned earlier, in stark contrast to the majority of adult series, mortality did in fact correlate with the initial PaO_2/FiO_2 ratio.

Clinical Course and Histopathology

The initial phase of ARDS (the *acute* or *exudative phase*) is manifested clinically by progressively refractory hypoxemia. The chest radiograph demonstrates bilateral patchy pulmonary infiltrates, similar to that observed during cardiogenic pulmonary edema (Figure 5.1), whereas CT scans of the chest reveal that alveolar filling, consolidation, and atelectasis occur predominantly in the dependent lung zones (Figure 5.2). Histologic examination reveals alveolar epithelial cell damage characterized by cytoplasmic swelling, cell membrane fragmentation, and denudation of the cell lining in severe cases. As a result, the impermeability of the endothelial–epithelial barrier is abrogated, resulting in protein-rich alveolar fluid and parenchymal infiltration by neutrophils and monocytes in association with the loss of type I alveolar epithelial cells.

Although some patients will recover after this acute stage, other patients will enter a second phase, known as the *fibroproliferative phase*. The time of onset of the fibroproliferative phase is highly variable (commonly thought to be 3–7 days after initial onset of ARDS) and is typically characterized by the onset of lung architectural changes and persistent hypoxemia. More recent translational research evidence suggests that the fibroproliferative response is driven by the proinflammatory cytokine interleukin (IL)-1β and begins much sooner than previously believed [31,32]. Histologically this phase is characterized by prominent interstitial infiltration by fibroblasts, myofibroblasts, and inflammatory cells (mostly of the mononuclear lineage) and increased collagen deposition. Of note,

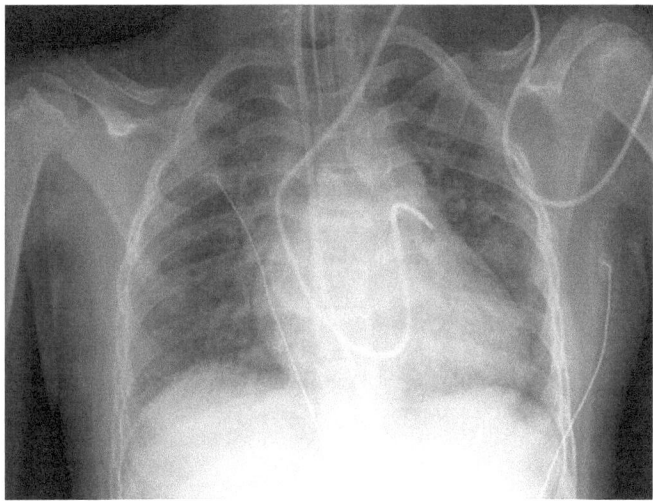

FIGURE 5.1. Chest radiograph of a patient with acute respiratory distress syndrome illustrating bilateral diffuse alveolar infiltrates.

the infiltration of immature monocytes occurs during this phase and may correlate with persistence of hypoxemia [33]. The type II pneumocyte, which is responsible for surfactant production, is the only epithelial cell type that appears capable of mitotic division and replication and must repopulate the alveolar lining and differentiate into type I pneumocytes for the lungs to recover. Clinical features of the fibroproliferative stage include increased alveolar dead space and further decreases in lung compliance. This process of fibroproliferation may be attenuated by the administration of corticosteroid therapy during this phase, as suggested by preliminary observations of Meduri and colleagues [34–36].

The final phase is the *recovery phase*, characterized by gradual resolution of the hypoxemia and improved compliance as the lung architecture is restored to normal. The timing and duration of this stage are also highly variable. Unfortunately, some patients will not recover and have histologic changes showing progressive lung fibrosis and cyst formation with irreversible loss of functional

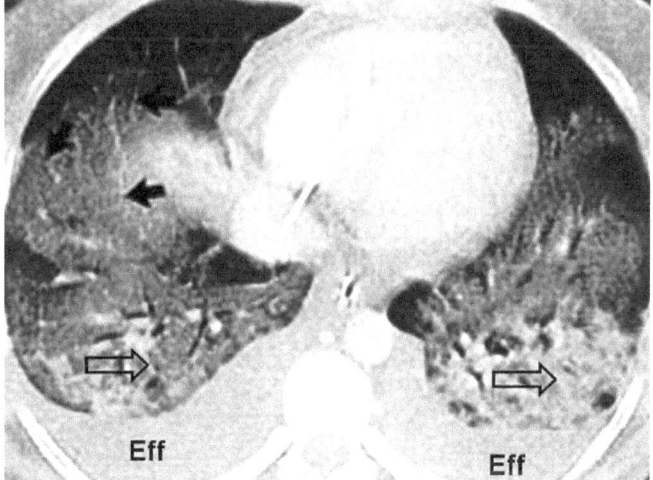

FIGURE 5.2. Chest computed tomography scan of a patient with acute respiratory distress syndrome illustrating bilateral diffuse alveolar consolidation and septal fluid (closed arrow), pronounced dependent edema (open arrows), and pleural effusions (Eff).

alveoli that ultimately leads to death secondary to refractory hypoxemia.

Pathophysiologic Mechanisms

Development of Pulmonary Edema

As reviewed earlier, the hallmark of ARDS is the development of pulmonary edema and flooding of the alveolar space, resulting in either alveolar collapse [37] or alveolar flooding [38,39]. In either case, the result is an impairment of matching between ventilation and perfusion primarily as a result of impaired ventilation of alveolar units. The subsequent intrapulmonary shunt results in clinically significant hypoxemia and is most often refractory to supplemental oxygen. The numerous factors that contribute to the development of pulmonary edema may be best thought of in the context of the Starling equation, which predicts fluid flux into or out of the pulmonary capillary system (Figure 5.3). Intravascular capillary pressure can be an important driving force of fluid transudation into the airs pace and is countered by interstitial pressure. This physiologic effect explains the finding of pulmonary edema that results from elevated left atrial as well as pulmonary venous pressure in the setting of congestive heart failure (CHF). For this reason, an elevated pulmonary wedge pressure remains an exclusion factor in defining ALI/ARDS. In contrast to hydrostatic pressure, increases in pulmonary capillary oncotic pressure serve to retain fluid within the intravascular space. Loss of plasma proteins (e.g., nephrotic

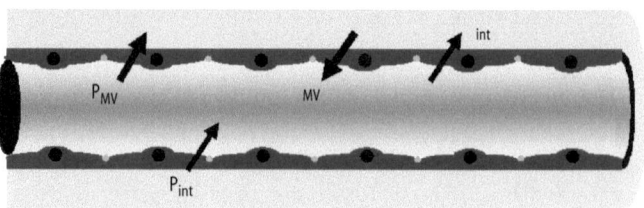

$$J_v = LpA \left[(P_{MV} - P_T) - \sigma (_{MV} - _T) \right]$$

FIGURE 5.3. Factors regulating fluid flux in the lungs as predicted by Starling's equation. LpA = Kf (permeability coefficient; P, hydrostatic pressure; π, oncotic pressure; MV, microvasculature; int, interstitial space).

syndrome) or impaired synthesis (e.g., liver failure) can result in decreased plasma oncotic pressure and increase the flux of fluid into the interstitial space. Importantly, this process can dilute interstitial protein concentration, decrease the interstitial oncotic pressure, and diminish the force driving fluid out of the vascular space. This process may provide a *safety factor* for interstitial fluid flux, although ultimately the capacity to resorb excess fluid is overcome, eventually resulting in alveolar flooding.

In the context of ARDS, perhaps the largest contributor to the development of pulmonary edema is a change in the permeability coefficient, Kf. For reasons elucidated later, numerous mediators affect the barrier function of the endothelium and epithelium, which increases the permeability of these cell layers to both fluid and ultimately circulating proteins (Figure 5.4). In this manner, the effect on

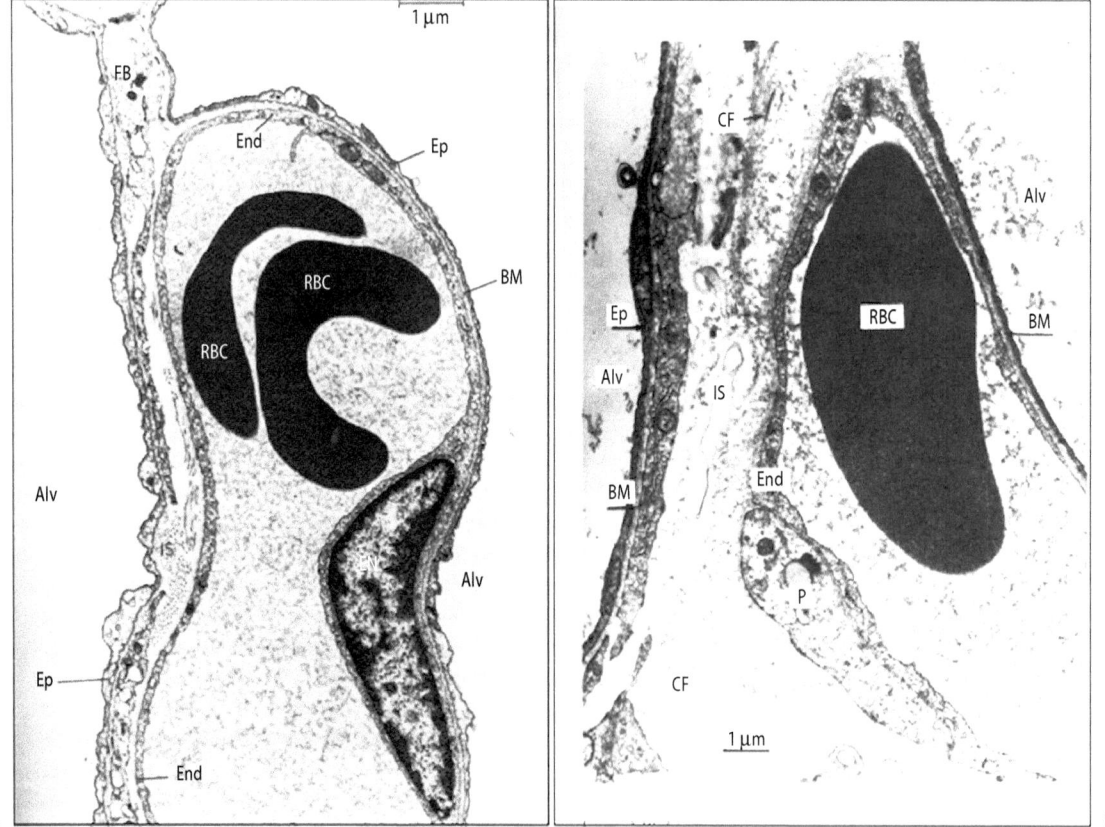

FIGURE 5.4. Ultrastructural changes in the endothelial–epithelial barrier in acute lung injury/acute respiratory distress syndrome. Alv, alveolus; BM, basement membrane; CF, cytokine-mediated fluid extravasation; End, endothelium; Ep, epithelium; FB, fibroblast; P, plasma lemmal vessicles; RBC, red blood cell; S, IS, interstitial space.

the development of pulmonary edema attributed to a small increase in elevated microvascular pressure, denoted P_{mv} (e.g., related to decreased myocardial compliance in sepsis) and/or a decrease in interstitial oncotic pressure will be amplified by increased permeability. The biologic causes of this change in permeability have been extensively studied over the past several years.

Cytokines

The difficulty in elucidating the pathophysiology of ARDS relates to the multiple etiologies that have been associated with its onset. Although initially it was believed that both direct/pulmonary and indirect/extrapulmonary causes of ARDS were characterized by a similar cascade of pathophysiologic events, recent insight into the responses of these different mechanisms to therapeutic interventions suggests they may differ. Nevertheless, the reason for surmising that the two shared a similar pathophysiology related to the consistent observation of increased cytokines measured either locally (from bronchoalveolar lavage [BAL] samples) or systemically (in serum samples) in the setting of ARDS [40]. Because of their presence and multiple effects, cytokines have been extensively investigated as causative mediators in ARDS (Figure 5.5).

Cytokines are soluble proteins synthesized by every cell type in the lung, including the alveolar epithelium, pulmonary vascular endothelium, alveolar macrophages, lymphocytes, and interstitial cells. They comprise a diverse group of peptides and glycoproteins that mediate numerous functions, including intercellular communication, adhesion molecule expression, chemotaxis, leukocyte activation, generation of oxygen- and nitrogen-based radicals, and

de novo gene expression mediated by intracellular signal transduction. Most of the effects of cytokines are mediated via binding to receptors on various target cells. The receptor–ligand interaction initiates any number of signaling cascades that can result in either inhibitory or stimulatory responses by the target cell [41]. In the setting of ARDS, some of the most extensively studied cytokines include tumor necrosis factor-α (TNF-α) [42], interleukin-1β (IL-1β) [43], interleukin-8 (IL-8/CXCL8), and monocyte chemoattractant protein (MCP)-1/CCL2.

Tumor necrosis factor-α and IL-1β are classically described as *early response cytokines* produced by cells of the innate immune system that evolved to protect the host from pathogen invasion. Microorganisms express a series of highly conserved molecular patterns that distinguish them from the host, for example, double-stranded RNA of viruses, unmethylated CpG dinucleotides of bacteria, mannan binding proteins of yeast, glycolipids of mycobacteria, lipoproteins of bacteria and parasites, lipoteichoic acids of Gram-positive bacteria, and lipopolysaccharide (LPS) of Gram-negative bacteria [44–49]. These so-called pathogen-associated molecular patterns (PAMPs) are recognized by members of the toll-like family of receptors (TLRs). As a result of TLR binding, cellular activation results in the expression of these early response cytokines, which appear to be critical to the induction of acute lung inflammation.

Tumor necrosis factor-α is biologically active as a trimer and binds to one of two distinct receptors (55 and 75 kD forms) that exist on nearly every cell type studied. In early preclinical studies, administration of purified TNF-α caused fever, hypotension, and impaired endothelial barrier function characterized by the onset of pulmonary edema. Conversely, anti-TNF-α neutralizing

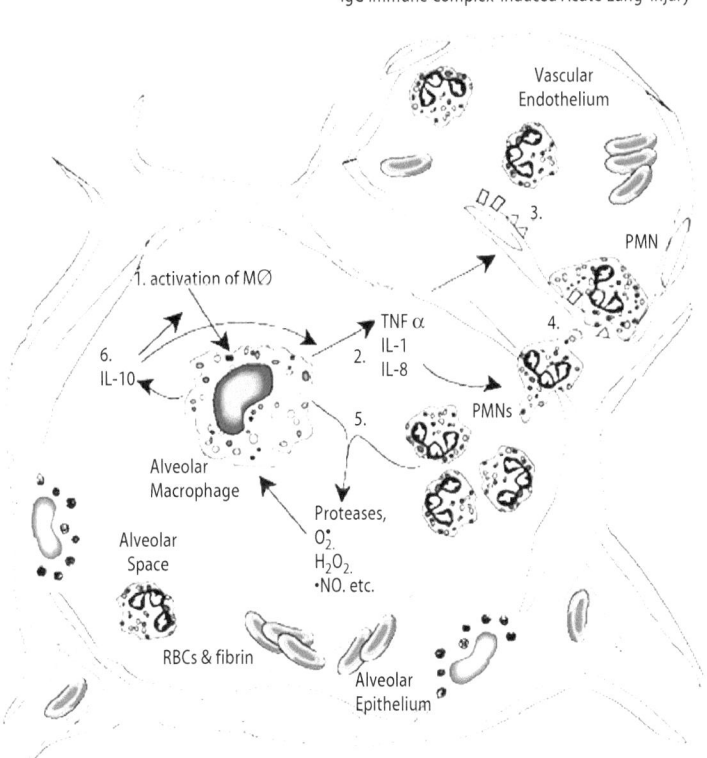

IgG Immune Complex-Induced Acute Lung Injury

1. Local or systemic inflammatory trigger, such as immune complexes ( ), complement activation products ( ), or bacterial products.

2. Activation of NF-κB/AP-1 in alveolar macrophages (MØs) with release of TNFα, IL-1, IL-8

3. Upregulation of endothelial cell adhesion molecules.

4. Sequential engagement of adhesion molecule pathways with expression of IL-8 ... leading to chemotactic transmigration.

5. Damage of alveolar epithelial and vascular endothelial cells as a result of proteases and $O_2^{\bullet}$, H_2O_2, •NO, etc.

6. Release of anti-inflammatory proteins (e.g. IL-10) to regulate pro-inflammatory process.

FIGURE 5.5. Schematic of pathophysiologic mechanisms in acute lung injury/acute respiratory distress syndrome. IL, interleukin; PMN, polymorphonuclear leukocyte; RBC, red blood cell; TNF, tumor necrosis factor.

antibodies prevented signs of sepsis, including ARDS, when Gram-negative bacteria or its toxic moiety endotoxin was administered to animals [42,50–52]. Because of the frequent observation of ARDS in sepsis and increased levels of TNF-α in BAL fluids of ARDS patients, a causative role for TNF-α in ARDS was hypothesized [53,54].

Interleukin-1β is a second early response cytokine whose peak level of expression characteristically follows TNF-α. When referring to IL-1, it is important to note that it can exist as one of two proteins, an α or a β isoform that share little homology. Interleukin-1β is synthesized as a proform that is proteolytically cleaved by the IL-1β converting enzyme (ICE, or caspase-1) to the bioactive form that mediates biologic effects in both the circulation and lung secretions [55,56]. Both TNF-α and IL-1β independently, and synergistically, are capable of regulating expression of subsequent cytokines and other mediators, notably, IL-8 [57], MCP-1, and adhesion molecules (e.g., intercellular adhesion molecule [ICAM]-1). Of note, the induction of both pro- and antiinflammatory cytokines from macrophages by IL-1β differs between children and adults in that there is a substantial antiinflammatory response triggered in children's macrophages whereas only proinflammatory mediators are produced by macrophages from adults [58].

Both IL-8 (CXCL8) and MCP-1 (CCL2) are members of a large family of chemoattractant cytokines, or *chemokines* [reviewed in 59]. Chemokines are divided into four groups on the basis of conserved cysteine motifs, which also form the basis of the newer nomenclature for these molecules: CXC, CC, C, and CX3C chemokine families. Chemokines function as potent chemotactic factors for a variety of leukocytes, including neutrophils, eosinophils, basophils, monocytes, mast cells, dendritic cells, natural killer cells, and T and B lymphocytes [60]. In the setting of a variety of inflammatory challenges in experimental models, CXC chemokines, notably IL-8 (CXCL8), mediate neutrophil infiltration into the lung [61–65]. There is also substantial clinical evidence that IL-8 is present in the lungs of patients with ARDS and that increased BAL fluid levels of IL-8 correlate with the number of lung neutrophils, the severity of injury, and mortality [66]. It remains unclear, however, as to whether neutralization of CXC chemokines may be of benefit, as they are crucial to pathogen clearance. For example, Greenberger and colleagues observed that while depletion of MIP-2 (CXCL2/3) in murine *Klebsiella pneumoniae* pneumonia reduced neutrophil recruitment to the lung, they also observed reduced bacterial clearance and increased bacteremia [61]. In a similar fashion, investigators have attempted to target CXC receptors to determine the importance of CXC chemokine ligand/CXCR biology during bacterial pneumonia. These investigators found marked reductions in lung neutrophils in response to *Pseudomonas aeruginosa*, *Nocardia asteroides*, and *Aspergillus fumigatus*, which were accompanied by reduced clearance of the microorganisms and increased mortality, suggesting that impairing this key component of innate immune response in the setting of bacterial infections may not be of benefit [65]. Nevertheless, as described below, lung injury mediated by noninfectious stimulation of CXC chemokine expression (e.g., lung stretch) may be inhibited with overall favorable outcomes [67].

More recently, the role of CC chemokines in ARDS has been examined, and studies have implicated a key pathophysiologic role for MCP-1. Examination of BAL fluid cellular infiltration over time in patients with ARDS noted increased monocytes recruited to the air space. Importantly, there was a correlation between the number of these cells and MCP-1 BAL fluid levels, suggesting that MCP-1 may mediate the recruitment of this cellular population in ARDS [33]. In a murine model of sepsis, the presence of MCP-1 was also noted to mediate recruitment of neutrophils to the lungs that was attenuated by neutralization of MCP-1 [68,69]. Thus, CC chemokines appear to be important contributors to the pathophysiology of ARDS.

All the cytokines described have a variety of biologic activities that modulate the inflammatory response of the lungs in a number of ways. For example, cytokines can function as key amplifiers of inflammation through synergistic activity [70–72]. As an example, in an immune complex–mediated model of lung inflammation, blocking the CC chemokine MIP-1α decreased BAL fluid TNF-α content, suggesting that MIP-1α might function as an autocrine activator of TNF-α expression [73]. Therefore, targeting proximal cytokine mediators may dampen this autoamplification observed during the acute inflammatory response. One of the most important roles for cytokines is their facilitation of the endothelial cell–leukocyte adhesion cascade (Figure 5.6).

One of the pathologic hallmarks observed in lungs from patients succumbing to ALI/ARDS is neutrophil infiltration. The mechanism by which leukocytes are recruited from the blood to the lung has been extensively studied and is well understood [reviewed in 72]. The initial phase of leukocyte adhesion begins with a process called *rolling* in which members of the selectin family of adhesion molecules (e.g., E-selectin) are upregulated on the endothelium and mediate an interaction with sialylated oligosaccharides that are constitutively expressed on neutrophils [74,75]. In the second phase of adhesion, a firm interaction develops between cytokine-activated β2-integrins (e.g., CD11a,b,c/CD18) expressed on neutrophils and their counterreceptors (e.g., ICAM-1) expressed on the endothelial cell surface that anchors the neutrophil to the pulmonary vascular endothelium [76]. Finally, neutrophils (or other adherent leukocytes) migrate into the alveolar space via chemotactic gradients created by chemokine expression (discussed later) [77]. Once in the interstitial and/or alveolar space, leukocytes release a series of oxygen- and nitrogen-based radical species, proteases, and arachidonic acid metabolites all of which can contribute to impaired endothelial barrier function and the pathognomonic development of noncardiogenic pulmonary edema. Despite initial consideration of a therapeutic strategy aimed at blocking adhesion molecule function, the appreciation that this biologic response remains key to host pathogen clearance has dampened enthusiasm for this approach.

Leukocyte Chemotaxis Related to Acute and Transitional Inflammation

A key characteristic of the acute inflammation associated with the development of ARDS is the recruitment of leukocytes from the blood to the air spaces of the lung [78]. Although this response is critical to eradication of an offending pathogen, an overexuberant cellular response combined with the release of mediators may instead amplify acute inflammation resulting in tissue injury. In addition, the maintenance of leukocyte recruitment necessitates intercellular communication between leukocytes and other structural cell types, including the endothelial and parenchymal cells. This intercellular communication is mediated not only by cytokines and adhesion molecules but also by the production of chemokines.

Early investigations identified a series of nonspecific chemotactic molecules such as N-formylmethionyl peptides from bacterial cell

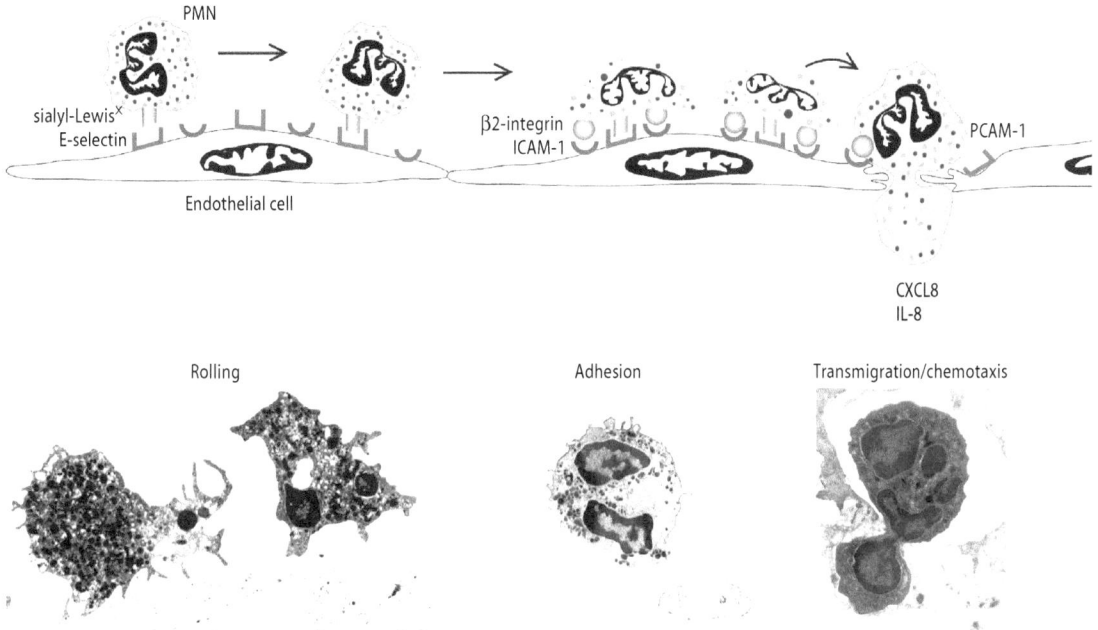

FIGURE 5.6. Schematic depicting the leukocyte–endothelial cell adhesion cascade mediated by cytokine upregulation of both endothelial cell and leukocyte adhesion molecules. Once adhesion has occurred, chemokine expression creates a chemotactic gradient to facilitate leukocyte homing and emigration to the site of inflammation. IL, interleukin; ICAM, intercellular adhesion molecule; PCAM, platelet endothelial cell adhesion molecule; PMN, polymorphonuclear leukocyte.

walls—the anaphylatoxin C5a, leukotriene B4 (LTB4), and platelet activating factor (PAF)—that were principally chemotactic for neutrophils [79]. Although these molecules are critical to leukocyte extravasation, they do not exhibit the degree of specificity for leukocyte subsets. It has become apparent that the nature of the stimulus triggering lung inflammation variably determines the subpopulation of leukocytes recruited to the lungs. Thus, it was hypothesized that a more diverse set of chemokines existed that possess specific activity for subsets of leukocytes. The CXC chemokines (e.g., IL-8/CXCL8, MIP-2/GROα/CXCL2), so designated because the first two cysteine residues are interrupted by a nonconserved amino acid, are principally neutrophil chemoattractants. In contrast, CC chemokines (e.g., MIP-1α/CCL3, MCP-1/CCL2), have their first two cysteine residues adjacent and are the principal mononuclear cell chemoattractants. In ARDS, the acute infiltration of neutrophils is temporally followed by migration of mononuclear cells into the lung. Both T cells and monocytes may contribute to persistent lung inflammation and mediate subsequent fibrosis as observed in animal models of chronic lung inflammation. Recent clinical data suggest that this late mononuclear cell recruitment, or so-called transitional inflammation, is critical to the outcome of patients with ARDS [33]. Further understanding of the regulation of the expression of these chemokines may identify potential therapeutic targets for interrupting the inflammatory process in ARDS.

Role of Antiinflammatory Cytokines in Regulating Acute Respiratory Distress Syndrome

Following their initial discovery, cytokines were principally described as proinflammatory molecules based on their causal association with sepsis and ARDS. Subsequently, it became clear that a counterregulatory response is mounted by the host, characterized by a number of cytokines possessing antiinflammatory properties. Included among this group of cytokines are IL-10, IL-13, transforming growth factor-β (TGF-β), and, in some circumstances, IL-6 and a related cytokine, IL-11. Among the most well characterized of these cytokines is IL-10, which possesses potent antiinflammatory effects by its ability to downregulate cytokine production by macrophages in a myriad of ways [80]. In a rat model of ALI, blocking endogenous IL-10 caused increased inflammation and pulmonary edema in association with increased levels of TNF-α and IL-1β [81]. This finding is further supported by the observation that IL-10 knockout mice are exquisitely sensitive to inflammation as reflected by their response to sublethal endotoxin injection that results in 100% mortality [82]. A correlative finding has been observed in humans in that patients who mounted the lowest levels of IL-10 in their BAL fluid displayed the highest mortality rate from ARDS [83]. Similar findings have been observed in studies examining TGF-β and IL-13 as *monocyte deactivating agents*, suggesting that these molecules also serve as important counterregulatory molecules in the setting of acute inflammatory disease states such as ARDS.

It is important to note that the biologic effects orchestrated by proinflammatory cytokines are critical to mounting an appropriate innate immune response directed against host invasion. In contrast, an overexuberant antiinflammatory response my lead to acquired host immunosuppression, thus impairing pathogen clearance—the so-called compensatory anti-inflammatory response syndrome (CARS) [84]. This inability to regulate both necessary responses associated with the pathologic syndromes of ALI/ARDS and sepsis has been described as *immune dissonance*. Accordingly, as the field of critical care contemplates ongoing interventional studies, it is imperative to not presume that all ARDS patients exhibit any one particular immunologic phenotype. The multitude of clinical investigators who have witnessed the failings of proinflammatory cytokine inhibition to favorably impact clinical outcomes in ARDS are realizing this concept [85,86]. It may in fact be that some patients overexpress antiinflammatory cytokines that contribute unfavorably to overall outcome by impairing pathogen clearance. As a result, it is crucial for the host to maintain a homeostatic cytokine balance in its response to any number of inflammatory challenges. More importantly, future clinical studies may need to better stratify patients by immune status in order to strike the appropriate balance between pro- and antiinflammatory cytokines.

Molecular Regulation of Cytokine Gene Expression

Because of the important role cytokines play in the development, propagation, and eventual resolution of ARDS, their molecular regulation has been a target of active investigation over the past decade. In this era of molecular biology and genomic science, it is necessary to achieve a fundamental understanding of the mechanisms of gene expression and relevant signal transduction pathways that play fundamental roles in the expression of genes contributing to the pathobiology of ARDS. These aspects have been recently reviewed in great detail [87].

Conventional Therapeutics

Therapy for ARDS begins by addressing any treatable, underlying cause of ARDS, such as sepsis, pneumonia, or pancreatitis [reviewed in 26]. Beyond this, with a few exceptions, most therapies specifically directed at the pathophysiologic mechanisms described above remain experimental or have not shown any benefit in clinical trials [reviewed in 9]. Thus, at present, the majority of therapies for ARDS are primarily supportive in nature. Further consideration of any therapy for ARDS must take into account the fact that most patients with ARDS do not die from respiratory failure. Rather, as mentioned previously, most patients with ARDS die as a result of sepsis or multiple-organ failure. Nevertheless, it is expected that therapy specifically directed toward ARDS has the potential to reduce the incidence of all causes of death associated with ARDS.

Conventional Mechanical Ventilation

As is the case for all patients with critical illnesses, maintaining adequate oxygen delivery is an important therapeutic goal in the management of ARDS. For the patient with ARDS, this goal is achieved with the usual strategies of fluid management, achievement of adequate hematocrit, achievement of adequate oxygen saturation, and the use of appropriate inotropes and vasopressors to maintain adequate cardiac output. Of particular importance to the patient with ALI/ARDS is the need for respiratory support, most typically in the form of mechanical ventilation. Mechanical ventilatory support should be targeted toward achieving the greatest benefit while minimizing potential harm.

A select group of patients with respiratory failure have the potential to be managed with noninvasive positive pressure ventilation (NPPV). The most common indication for NPPV appears to be acute hypercapnic respiratory failure, particularly in the setting of chronic obstructive pulmonary disease [88,89]. Additionally, it has been suggested that patients with hypoxemic respiratory failure do not receive the same benefit from NPPV as do patients with hypercapnic respiratory failure [90]. Nevertheless, there are reports of

successful NPPV in the setting of ARDS [91,92]. Thus, NPPV may be considered for some select patients with ARDS (i.e., patients with obstructive pulmonary disease and patients with milder forms of ARDS), but it should be understood that the vast majority of patients with ARDS require tracheal intubation and mechanical ventilation.

Increasing mean alveolar pressure (mPalv) is currently considered the key component of mechanical ventilation for ARDS. Increased mPalv allows for recruitment of alveoli and for reduction of FiO_2 to *nontoxic* levels (still arbitrarily agreed to be <0.6). There are several ways to increase mPalv, but PEEP appears to be the most effective with respect to lung mechanics and perhaps avoidance of ventilator-induced lung injury (VILI). Typically, PEEP levels are increased incrementally until the FiO_2 can be reduced below 0.6 while maintaining a systemic oxygen saturation >90%. It has been advocated to use pressure–volume loops for the optimal setting of PEEP [93]. In this strategy, PEEP is set at or above the *lower inflection point* of the pressure–volume curve (Figure 5.7) with the goal of maintaining alveolar patency and eliminating repeated closure and opening of alveoli consistent with what has been coined as the *open lung approach*. Thus, most patients with ARDS will require PEEP levels in the range of 10 to 15 cm H_2O. The efficacy of this approach was rigorously tested in a recent clinical trial (ALVEOLI Trial) conducted by the ARDS Clinical Network, by comparing a higher end-expiratory lung volume/lower FiO_2 versus a lower end-expiratory lung volume/higher FiO_2 ventilation strategy in patients with ARDS (see www.ardsnet.org) [94]. The study was stopped early after enrolling 549 patients because of futility—an interim analysis suggested that the trial, if continued until completion, would ultimately fail to show any difference in mortality. The reasons for these findings remain unclear, although there can be harmful effects of too high a PEEP.

Negative consequences of PEEP include barotrauma, alveolar overdistension with CO_2 retention, and decreased cardiac output secondary to increased intrathoracic pressure and, as a result, impaired venous return and preload. Fear of barotrauma and VILI should not preclude the aggressive use of PEEP a priori, given the potential benefits of PEEP. Increases of $PaCO_2$ secondary to alveolar distension can be well tolerated physiologically *(permissive hypercapnia)*, or, when excessive, can be corrected by lowering PEEP as long as it does not compromise oxygenation. Finally, reductions in

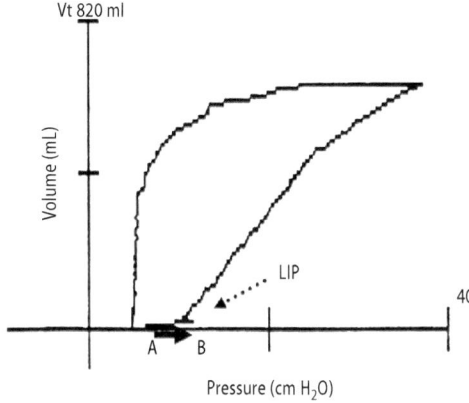

FIGURE 5.7. Pressure–volume loop demonstrating the lower inflection point (LIP). Pressure is applied (A to B) without volume expansion of the lung. The *open lung approach* advocates setting PEEP 1–2 cm H_2O above this point to avoid significant re-collapse upon exhalation, thereby avoiding atelectrauma.

cardiac output can be overcome by appropriate augmentation of preload and appropriate use of intravenous inotropes. In this setting, data derived from a pulmonary artery catheter or a less precise, but potentially useful method of monitoring superior vena cava oxygen saturation might provide valuable guidance in understanding the ramifications of PEEP changes on the overall oxygen delivery as reflected by a mixed-venous oxygen saturation measurement.

Inverse Ratio Ventilation and High-Frequency Ventilation

Apart from PEEP, there are other available modalities for increasing mean airway pressure in the setting of ARDS. Inverse ratio ventilation (IRV) is a strategy that makes use of supraphysiologic, prolonged inspiratory times such that the ratio of inspiratory time to expiratory time is greater than 1:1 [95]. This strategy substantially increases mPalv, thereby increasing alveolar recruitment and improving oxygenation. Whether improvements in oxygenation are caused by increased inspiratory time per se or by increased intrinsic PEEP is a matter of debate. Studies using historical controls suggest that IRV can improve the outcome of ARDS [96–98]; however, when considering the use of IRV, it should be kept in mind that there are no large, prospective randomized trials comparing IRV to conventional ventilation in ARDS.

High-frequency oscillatory ventilation (HFV), in the form of either high-frequency jet ventilation (HFJV) or high-frequency oscillatory ventilation (HFOV), is another alternative means of increasing mPalv in the treatment of ARDS [99]. High-frequency ventilation has theoretical appeal for ARDS because it makes use of small tidal volumes while maintaining alveolar recruitment, thus potentially reducing VILI. A large experience in adults with HFJV ventilation suggests that there is no benefit with respect to mortality [99]. Experience in pediatric patients, however, suggests that HFOV may provide some benefit [100,101], particularly when instituted early in the disease course [102]. Overall, there is continued enthusiasm for the use of HFV in the setting of ARDS, but its true benefit remains to be established.

Lung Protective Strategies

The use of mechanical ventilation presents a clinical paradox. On the one hand, it provides life-sustaining support to allow sufficient time for recovery. On the other hand, the use of high concentrations of oxygen and the stretching forces of positive pressure ventilation can be directly injurious to the lung. Lung toxicity related to high concentrations of oxygen (hyperoxia) has been recognized for many years. Hyperoxia is directly toxic to lung parenchymal cells by the generation of oxygen-related radicals and by impacting the signal transduction pathways of lung parenchymal cells [103]. Although the *safe* level of oxygen during ARDS is not known, a reasonable goal appears to be achieving an $FiO_2 < 0.6$, which is why the recommendation of titrating PEEP to a level that allows reduction of FiO_2 below this level is espoused. Whether this concept will extend to the practice of allowing the systemic arterial oxygen saturation to fall to 85%–90% in order to avoid prolonged exposure to high FiO_2 levels (so-called permissive hypoxemia) remains to be seen.

The concept of VILI secondary to mechanical forces has generated a great deal of clinical and investigative interest in the last decade. Ventilator-induced lung injury is a manifestation of direct physical damage to lung parenchyma, as well as stretch-induced changes in lung parenchymal signal transduction pathways. This latter concept is embodied in the term *mechanotransduction*, which describes how physical forces change gene expression patterns in the lung, thus leading to potentially important negative consequences such as increased inflammation and alterations of ion channels [104]. Multiple experimental models and clinical studies have documented the physiologic relevance of VILI [105–117] and raised the likelihood that the mode of ventilation ultimately impacts the development of organ injury remote from the lungs [104,111,118].

As a result of the recognition of the influence of VILI on the course of ARDS, physicians have mandated the clinical use of lung protective strategies that attempt to use minimal forces (whether pressure or volume triggered) in a manner that limits VILI. Examples described earlier include use of an appropriate level of PEEP to prevent cyclic opening and collapse of alveoli (so-called atelectrauma) and the use of HFOV. Much of the clinical support for this approach stems from the successful implementation of a lung protective strategy in which tidal volume was reduced to 6 mL/kg in contrast to a tidal volume of 12 mL/kg as reported in a study conducted by the ARDS Network. This study has provided the most definitive evidence that a high tidal volume (12 mL/kg) is harmful to patients with ARDS (see www.ardsnet.org) [119]. Because half of the patients in this trial were randomized to a conventional ventilation group in which the preset tidal volumes were often increased to 12 mL/kg tidal volume from the more *conventional* 8–10 mL/kg, it remains unclear as to what is the safest, minimal tidal volume for adults and—with greater uncertainty—children. Nevertheless, although this study was perhaps the largest trial to test this hypothesis, numerous studies had suggested clinical benefits of a low tidal volume strategy [113,120–122].

Permissive Hypercapnia

Although hypercapnia can cause pulmonary hypertension, increased intracranial pressure, and cardiovascular dysfunction, hypercapnia appears to be well tolerated in patients with ALI similar to what has been observed for years in neonatal respiratory distress syndrome [122–125]. In fact, several studies have suggested a possible protective role for hypercarbia in models of ALI/ARDS [123,126–129]. Although most clinicians tolerate a pH of ~7.25, below this level there is considerably less consensus. When pH drops below this level, clinicians choose a myriad of approaches, including tolerating the lower pH, increasing minute ventilation by increasing frequency, or administering intravenous base agents (e.g., sodium bicarbonate) to raise the pH. Which of these three approaches is most appropriate remains to be determined, and the choice of one method over another currently is generally dictated by individual patient scenario and physician experience or preference.

Prone Positioning

Chest CT scans illustrate how heterogeneously the lung parenchyma is affected in patients with ARDS (see Figure 5.2). When in a supine position, the dependent areas (dorsal) tend to be fluid filled and/or collapsed, while the nondependent areas (ventral) tend be well ventilated, thus causing significant mismatch of ventilation and perfusion. Various mechanical factors have been identified to suggest that changing the position of the patient may facilitate the recruitment of these air spaces. Prone positioning has been considered as an inexpensive, noninvasive, and generally safe approach for improving lung physiology for patients with ALI and is reviewed in greater detail in subsequent chapters of this textbook. Although there can be complications from prone positioning (e.g., accidental extubation, pressure sores, catheter dislodgement, and in some cases worsening oxygenation), prone positioning is generally well tolerated and clinically feasible for nearly any patient (Figure 5.8).

Lung collapse is predominant in the dependent regions (zone III), and ventilation is preferentially distributed to the nondependent regions (zone I). Furthermore, perfusion to the air spaces is lowest in the nondependent regions and increases progressively in dependent regions. As a result, patients with ARDS and in a supine position have maximal maldistribution (or mismatch) of ventilation and perfusion with subsequent physiologic shunt and resultant hypoxemia, as reviewed earlier. Conversely, it is now appreciated that placing a patient in the prone position may be associated with a reduction of perfusion to collapsed regions, providing a noninvasive means to improve V/Q matching. Redirection of perfusion from nonventilated regions to newly recruited areas of lung regions in the prone position has been demonstrated in initial studies [130]. Several subsequent studies have shown similar physiologic reduction of perfusion to low V/Q regions and resultant increase in the V/Q ratio with improved oxygenation.

These observations led to additional studies in which prone positioning was found to (1) improve V/Q matching, (2) decrease heterogeneity in the transpulmonary gradient related to heterogeneous lung diseases, (3) improve alveolar recruitment, (4) influence chest wall compliance, and (5) potentially prevent VILI by decreasing the expand/collapse interface between recruited and derecruited air spaces.

Curly et al. demonstrated an immediate improvement in oxygenation as measured by either P/F ratio or OI at various time points during the first 24 hours of prone positioning [131], and this improvement was maintained in immediate responders upon returning to the supine position. In contrast, Casado-Flores et al. showed that the improved oxygenation was not sustained after a return to the supine position [132]. These seemingly discordant data are typical of the reported variability in the response to prone positioning such that predicting who will respond and derive benefit from the prone position is difficult. Unfortunately, despite evidence to show that prone positioning can be applied to improve oxygenation and respiratory mechanics, given the inherent complexity of ARDS studies, proving this to be a therapeutic intervention that alters mortality (and other end-points) in this patient population has been challenging, as none of the large trials in either pediatric or adult ARDS patients demonstrated clear benefit beyond improved oxygenation [133,134]. Although various reasons for this have been the subject of great speculation, one important confounder remains the heterogeneous patient population captured in large ARDS studies. Regardless of the reason, it is becoming increasingly clear that oxygenation and mortality may be insufficient outcomes to exclusively exam in interventional ALI/ARDS studies. From a practical standpoint, most intensivists' clinical experiences indicate that the response to prone positioning is variable from patient to patient, with some patients achieving greater improvements in oxygenation than others. As a result, it remains a reasonable recommendation that the prone position be considered for most patients with severe and/or refractory ALI/ARDS.

Fluid Management

Titrating preload and concomitant hemodynamic variables to supraphysiologic values for patients with ALI/ARDS cannot be recommended based on the current literature; however, titrating these variables to normal levels in the setting of ALI/ARDS is prudent. Furthermore, because alveolar edema is a key component of ARDS, significantly reducing extravascular lung water, with fluid restriction and administration of diuretics, may occasionally be of benefit

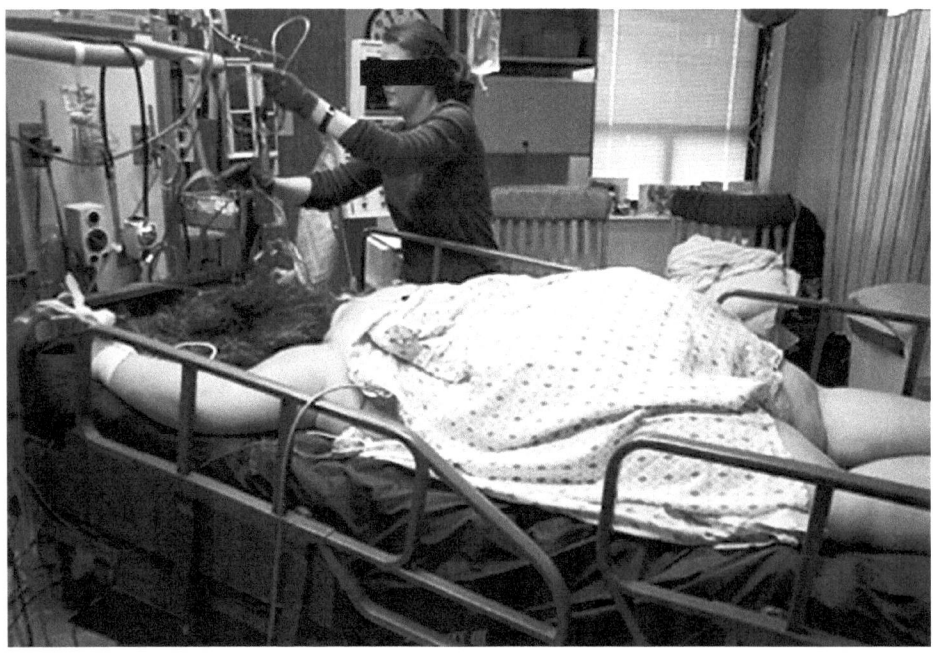

FIGURE 5.8. A 180-kg patient in the prone position, illustrating that the prone position is feasible for nearly every patient with acute respiratory distress syndrome.

for patients with ARDS. The literature supporting or refuting this approach remains controversial and relies heavily on the use of pulmonary artery catheters, which has also come under strong criticism recently with regard to demonstrating patient benefit.

Recent clinical data suggest that pulmonary edema during ALI/ARDS results from not only an imbalance of alveolar–epithelial permeability but also from impaired alveolar fluid clearance by the alveolar epithelium [135,136]. In addition, patients with ARDS who have relatively normal alveolar fluid clearance have a better survival rate than patients who have a lower than normal clearance rates [136]. Based on the available data, the *best* approach seems to be avoidance of hypervolemia and an attempt to reduce extravascular lung water to a level that does not compromise cardiac output. Admittedly, judging the latter can be problematic and is often subjective. Future noninvasive diagnostics capable of better predicting extravascular fluid status and future therapies aimed at restoring normal alveolar fluid clearance (e.g., β-adrenergic receptor agonists) may hold the promise of more specifically managing the pulmonary edema associated with ARDS.

Corticosteroids

There has been interest in the therapeutic use of corticosteroids in ARDS and septic shock since the early 1960s. This strategy is based on the pathophysiologic concept that the organ injury observed in these clinical syndromes is a manifestation of dysregulated inflammation. Because corticosteroids are potent antiinflammatory agents, it has been postulated that they might attenuate organ injury associated with ALI/ARDS. Despite this sound hypothesis, a consistently beneficial effect of corticosteroids had not been established in earlier ARDS studies [137–139]. However, more recently, there has been renewed interest in the use of corticosteroids by patients with so-called late or unresolving ARDS, defined by a failure to demonstrate clinical improvement over the course of the illness [34–36]. This newer strategy employed a longer course of therapy, at lower doses, than the original trials in ARDS. Meduri and colleagues performed a randomized trial involving 24 patients with *unresolving* ARDS and observed that administration of corticosteroids to these patients had several benefits, including improved lung injury score, improved PaO₂/FiO₂ ratio, decreased multiple-organ dysfunction, and decreased mortality [34]. As a result, this approach was subjected to a larger, multiinstitutional study called the Late Steroid Rescue Study or *LsSRS* Trial conducted by the ARDS Network (http://www.ardsnet.org/lasrs.php). Until the full results of this study are disseminated, the ongoing use of corticosteroids for unresolving ARDS is likely to be considered in most intensivists' clinical practices.

Experimental Therapies

Targeting Cytokine Production

Although a number of cells produce cytokines, those of mononuclear-leukocyte lineage, such as the peripheral blood monocyte (in indirect lung injury) and the alveolar macrophage (in direct lung injury), appear to be principal sources. A number of agents have shown promise in *deactivating* these cells as a means of inhibiting cytokine production. Antiinflammatory cytokines such as IL-10 [140] and TGF-β [141] and other pharmacologic agents such as ketoconazole [142,143] and lisofylline [144] display potent

monocyte deactivating properties and have been touted as potential therapeutic candidates in ARDS. Interleukin-10 has demonstrated particular promise as it inhibits a variety of biologic functions that are fundamental to the development and propagation of ARDS. Interleukin-10 inhibits the synthesis of a number of cytokines [145], impairs the endothelial cell–leukocyte adhesion cascade [146], attenuates NFκB activation [147,148], increases the expression of endogenous cytokine antagonists (e.g., IL-1 receptor antagonist protein) [149], and destabilizes cytokine mRNA, resulting in decreased translational expression [150]. In light of the multiple mechanisms by which IL-10 and other regulatory cytokines can regulate inflammation, exogenous administration of these molecules may be a potentially promising strategy, although this potential has not been realized in the studies performed to date.

Cytokine Neutralization

Following their discovery, cytokines were considered as strictly proinflammatory molecules on the basis of their contribution to this pathophysiology of sepsis and ALI/ARDS. In addition, because of the proximal role cytokines play in the inflammatory cascade and their autocrine amplification effects, investigators have attempted to directly block their activity by either antibody neutralization (e.g., anti-TNF-α antibody) or receptor blockade (e.g., IL-1Ra), as reviewed earlier. Although these strategies proved promising in preclinical trials, their ultimate clinical efficacy in human trials has been disappointing [reviewed in 85,151].

There are many reasons for this observation, including inaccurate modeling of the human disease, poor identification of underlying risk factors, and limitations of statistical power analysis [152]. Other factors weighing against the success of this strategy include the fact that cytokines are likely to be increased before the clinical presentation of a critically ill patient. In addition, the cytokine cascade has been discovered to be highly redundant and interlinked, making it unlikely that inhibition of any single mediator will prove beneficial in the context of the clinical trials that are limited by size. Finally, given the heterogeneity of both the triggering insults and the patients' co-morbid conditions and immune responses, it is unlikely that all patients with ALI/ARDS are battling uncontrolled proinflammation. It is likely that a subset of individuals exist in a relatively immunocompromised state as a result of overexpression of antiinflammatory molecules, rendering the patient at substantial risk for overwhelming infection as the cause of respiratory failure.

One notable exception to this approach has been the success observed with the use of the anti-TNF agent etanercept in idiopathic pneumonia syndrome (IPS) following bone marrow transplantation. When etanercept is applied early to patients with this form of acute, noninfectious lung injury, remarkable success has been achieved in decreasing radiologic evidence of lung edema and clinical resolution of ALI sufficient to warrant a phase II/III trial sponsored by the national Bone Marrow Transplant Trials Network and Children's Oncology Group.

Modulating the Regulation of Lung Edema Clearance

An important component of maintaining homeostasis of lung function is the ability to continuously clear alveolar lining fluid. This process becomes more imperative for patients with ALI/ARDS in whom a progressive increase in interstitial fluid occurs early in the illness. Furthermore, because it has been observed that patients who have higher alveolar fluid clearance rates have improved survival than patients with a lower than normal alveolar fluid clearance rate [136], it is critical to ascertain the important factors regulating this biology. Although a detailed, molecular understanding of this process is beyond the scope of this chapter, the reader is referred to several seminal reviews by the pioneers in this field [153,154]. In work derived principally from the Matthay laboratory, it has been established that resolution of alveolar fluid is dependent on active ion transport by the lung epithelial cells [155]. The most important factor that preserves the alveolar space from flood is the resistance of the epithelial cells to injury. Even in the setting of endothelial barrier injury, preservation of epithelial function serves to keep extravasated fluid in the interstitium where lymphatic drainage can accommodate an increased need for fluid removal, thus sparing the air space from edema formation. In experimental settings of endothelial injury (e.g., systemic endotoxemia) not only is alveolar fluid clearance not impaired, but it may in fact be augmented [156]. This observed increase in fluid clearance has subsequently been shown to be inhibited by amiloride and propranolol instillation. These data support the conclusion that this epithelial function is dependent on β-adrenergic agonist stimulation of Na^+-K^+/ATPase–dependent sodium transport [156]. Thus, if the integrity of the alveolar epithelium is maintained, fluid clearance can be augmented in the setting of interstitial and/or mild pulmonary edema, although this process is modulated by various factors. For example, in the context of raised left atrial pressure, fluid clearance is attenuated even with β-adrenergic stimulation because of excess production of atrial natriuretic factor (ANF) [157].

Depending on the trigger used to induce lung injury, numerous mechanisms augment the capacity for fluid transport. In hyperoxia, increased expression of Na^+-K^+/ATPase correlated with increased sodium transport in respiratory epithelial cells [158]. In experimental models of sepsis-induced or hemorrhagic shock–induced lung injury, increased clearance appears to be mediated by catecholamine-dependent stimulation of cAMP and subsequently sodium pump activity. Data have implicated multiple biochemical mechanisms, including increased expression, activity, and/or epithelial membrane insertion of Na^+-K^+/ATPase, as well as increased expression of the epithelial sodium channel (ENaC) [159]. More recent data have suggested that glucocorticoids and other stress hormones may modulate expression of ENaC and/or Na^+-K^+/ATPase, resulting in increased fluid clearance rates [160].

Thus, there are a number of factors that can upregulate the rate of fluid clearance in the injured lung. As a result, future therapies aimed at restoring normal alveolar fluid clearance may hold the promise of more specifically managing the pulmonary edema associated with ARDS. To date, studies have examined the beneficial role of employing a β-adrenergic agonist on alveolar fluid clearance in numerous models of lung injury [153]. However, inhibition by ANF, β-receptor desensitization, or downregulation and endogenous inhibitors of cAMP may all impact on the eventual clinical utility of this approach. Other agents that have been examined include certain growth factors (e.g., keratinocyte growth factor) that have been shown to increase fluid clearance and synergize with β-agonist effects [161]. Finally, future directions may consider application of gene therapy, as preclinical studies have shown that overexpression of the α- and β-subunits of Na^+-K^+/ATPase can decrease lung edema formation in mouse models [162].

Blocking Adhesion Molecules

As our understanding of the role of adhesion molecule expression has unfolded, the goal of antiadhesion molecule therapy has become an intriguing pursuit. Numerous preclinical animal trials have demonstrated that antiadhesion molecule antibodies such as anti-ICAM-1 [163,164], anti-E-selectin [••], anti-L-selectin [166], and anti-P-selectin [164,167] were able to inhibit neutrophil accumulation in the lung and subsequent tissue injury. Despite these encouraging results, to date no human trials have successfully used antiadhesion molecule strategies. It is important to recall that the leukocyte–adhesion molecule cascade is highly conserved, and an adaptive host response is necessary for pathogen clearance as evidenced by individuals who suffer recurrent bouts of infection as a result of leukocyte adhesion deficiency (LAD) syndromes 1 and 2 and the more recently described LAD-3 (although this defect is restricted to platelet aggregation). The molecular basis of the defects associated with LAD-1 and LAD-2 are absent expression of the β-integrins (the counterreceptors for ICAM-1) and absence of sialyl-Lewis X (the carbohydrate ligand for selectins), respectively [168,169]. In light of these observations from *nature's* experiments, investigators must approach the strategy aimed at disrupting this cascade carefully, especially in the setting of an invading pathogen.

Blocking of Chemokines or Chemokine Receptors

As mentioned earlier, chemokines appear to play a central role in the activation and recruitment of neutrophils to the lung in ALI/ARDS, and as a result chemokines have become important therapeutic targets in many inflammatory states, including ALI/ARDS. Monoclonal antibodies directed against IL-8 have been shown to decrease neutrophil influx and tissue injury in a number of animal models of lung injury [170–172]. Because of these encouraging preclinical results, anti-IL-8 antibody has been considered for testing in human ARDS; however, it has come to light that antigen–antibody complex formation between IL-8 and anti-IL-8 may trigger an increased inflammatory response and has been associated with higher mortality [173,174]. Thus, whether this approach will continue to have merit is debated, and alternative approaches to attenuating the effects of chemokines such as IL-8 have been suggested. Besides antibody neutralization, targeting the chemokine receptors has become a novel therapeutic target for clinical investigators [175]. As a result, it is possible that chemokines may be successfully inhibited in a selective and effective manner in the near future.

Application of Genomics

Acute respiratory distress syndrome is a highly heterogenous disease process with respect to both etiology and outcome. Variable outcomes are particularly frustrating to the pediatric intensivist who is faced with the reality that one patient with ARDS may survive, whereas another patient of similar age, having an identical trigger with seemingly similar co-morbidities, may die. These highly divergent outcomes may at times be explained by management strategies. However, recent progress in genomics suggests that part of the basis of these variable outcomes may lie in the genetic background of the child who possesses a predisposition to a more severe manifestation of ALI/ARDS.

The evolving field of genomics holds the promise of elucidating a *genetic predisposition* to ARDS and other diseases afflicting critically ill children [176–178]. Although no clear *ARDS gene* or marker has been established to date, there is good evidence that mutations, or polymorphisms, in surfactant protein genes can impart a phenotype characterized by the propensity to develop interstitial lung disease and/or ARDS [179,180]. In addition, polymorphisms of cytokine genes have been associated with increased mortality in sepsis, a primary cause of indirect ALI [181,182]. Because the development of sepsis is so closely linked, clinically and pathophysiologically, to the development of ARDS, it is expected that similar associations will be found between cytokine gene polymorphisms and the course of ARDS. Additional clinical investigations into candidate ALI/ARDS genes have included an examination of the role of aquaporin (AQP). Aquaporins play a key role in water transport in several tissues, including the lung. Aquaporin-1 (AQP1) is expressed on apical and basolateral membranes of pulmonary microvascular endothelial cells of the lung and has been implicated in the regulation of lung vascular permeability [183]. In animal models of lung injury, AQP1 is substantially increased whereas null mutations in AQP1 in mice have been associated with protection from the development of lung edema fluid [184], although it was interesting to note that AQP1-/- mice were not protected from acute lung edema formation triggered by an inflammatory stimulus [185,186]. Work from the HopGene Program in Genomics supported by the NHLBI has identified two single nucleotide polymorphisms in the 3′-untranslated region of the AQP1 gene (http://www.hopkins-genomics.org/ali/abstracts/aqp1.html). In these studies, higher proportions of the C allele substitutions at positions 525 and 578 were found in patients with sepsis than in controls. Taken together, these data support the concept that AQP1 plays a role in regulating pulmonary vascular permeability. Similar efforts to link polymorphisms in selected genes with ARDS by this group are summarized on the program's Web site (http://www.hopkins-genomics.org/ali/ali_snp.html).

Important tools for the application of genomics to the study of ARDS include the recent sequencing of the human genome, evolution of microarray technology, and expansion of powerful bioinformatics. With these tools it may become possible to further characterize the host response during ARDS at the genomic level. These studies are eagerly awaited, as they hold the promise of increasing our understanding of ARDS and with that hope that individual patient responses can be more thoroughly characterized such that therapies can be more specifically tailored to the needs of individual patients.

Conclusion

Acute lung injury and ARDS continue to be major causes of mortality in pediatric populations. It is clear that cytokines contribute to this pathophysiologic state via receptor-mediated signaling pathways that affect target cell responses. The application of molecular biology techniques to the field of critical care has both improved our understanding of biologic responses and identified a number of potential therapeutic targets. Although in vitro and animal model data have demonstrated amelioration of the inflammatory response and lung injury by these strategies, the modalities that have been tested in humans thus far have proven ineffective. It is hoped that further understanding of the fundamental biology, improved identification of the patient's inflammatory state, and application of therapies directed at multiple sites of action will ultimately prove beneficial for patients suffering from ALI/ARDS.

References

1. Ashbaugh DG, Bigelow DB, Petty TL. Acute respiratory distress in adults. Lancet 1967;2:319–323.
2. Petty TL, Ashbaugh DG. The adult respiratory distress syndrome. Clinical features, factors influencing prognosis and principles of management. Chest 1971;60(3):233–239.
3. Murray JF, Matthay MA, Luce JM, Flick MR. An expanded definition of the adult respiratory distress syndrome. Am Rev Respir Dis 1988;138(3):720–723.
4. Bernard GR, Artigas A, Brigham KL, Carlet J, Falke K, Hudson L, et al. The American-European Consensus Conference on ARDS. Definitions, mechanisms, relevant outcomes, and clinical trial coordination. Am J Respir Crit Care Med 1994;149(3 Pt 1):818–824.
5. Flori HR, Glidden DV, Rutherford GW, Matthay MA. Pediatric acute lung injury: prospective evaluation of risk factors associated with mortality. Am J Respir Crit Care Med 2005;171(9):995–1001.
6. National Heart Lung Institute: Task force report on problems, research approaches, needs. NIH Publication No. 73-432. Washington, DC: National Heart Lung Institute; 1972:165–180.
7. Lewandowski K. Epidemiological data challenge ARDS/ALI definition. Intensive Care Med 1999;25(9):884–886.
8. Valta P, Uusaro A, Nunes S, Ruokonen E, Takala J. Acute respiratory distress syndrome: frequency, clinical course, and costs of care. Crit Care Med 1999;27(11):2367–2374.
9. McIntyre RC Jr, Pulido EJ, Bensard DD, Shames BD, Abraham E. Thirty years of clinical trials in acute respiratory distress syndrome. Crit Care Med 2000;28(9):3314–3331.
10. Villar J, Slutsky AS. The incidence of the adult respiratory distress syndrome. Am Rev Respir Dis 1989;140(3):814–816.
11. Goh AY, Chan PW, Lum LC, Roziah M. Incidence of acute respiratory distress syndrome: a comparison of two definitions. Arch Dis Child 1998;79(3):256–259.
12. Rubenfeld GD, Caldwell E, Peabody E, Weaver J, Martin DP, Neff M, et al. Incidence and outcomes of acute lung injury. N Engl J Med 2005;353(16):1685–1693.
13. West J. Respiratory Physiology: The Essentials. Baltimore, MD: Williams & Wilkins; 1991.
14. Pelosi P, Caironi P, Gattinoni L. Pulmonary and extrapulmonary forms of acute respiratory distress syndrome. Semin Respir Crit Care Med 2001;22(3):259–268.
15. Gattinoni L, Pelosi P, Suter PM, Pedoto A, Vercesi P, Lissoni A. Acute respiratory distress syndrome caused by pulmonary and extrapulmonary disease. Different syndromes? Am J Respir Crit Care Med 1998;158(1):3–11.
16. Pelosi P, Gattinoni L. Acute respiratory distress syndrome of pulmonary and extra-pulmonary origin: fancy or reality? Intensive Care Med 2001;27(3):457–460.
17. Pelosi P, Goldner M, McKibben A, Adams A, Eccher G, Caironi P, et al. Recruitment and derecruitment during acute respiratory failure: an experimental study. Am J Respir Crit Care Med 2001;164(1):122–130.
18. Eisner MD, Thompson T, Hudson LD, Luce JM, Hayden D, Schoenfeld D, et al. Efficacy of low tidal volume ventilation in patients with different clinical risk factors for acute lung injury and the acute respiratory distress syndrome. Am J Respir Crit Care Med 2001;164(2):231–236.
19. Paret G, Ziv T, Barzilai A, Ben-Abraham R, Vardi A, Manisterski Y, et al. Ventilation index and outcome in children with acute respiratory distress syndrome. Pediatr Pulmonol 1998;26(2):125–128.
20. Davis SL, Furman DP, Costarino AT, Jr. Adult respiratory distress syndrome in children: associated disease, clinical course, and predictors of death. J Pediatr 1993;123(1):35–45.
21. Bojko T, Notterman DA, Greenwald BM, De Bruin WJ, Magid MS, Godwin T. Acute hypoxemic respiratory failure in children following bone marrow transplantation: an outcome and pathologic study. Crit Care Med 1995;23(4):755–759.

22. Fein AM, Lippmann M, Holtzman H, Eliraz A, Goldberg SK. The risk factors, incidence, and prognosis of ARDS following septicemia. Chest 1983;83(1):40–42.

23. Hudson LD, Milberg JA, Anardi D, Maunder RJ. Clinical risks for development of the acute respiratory distress syndrome. Am J Respir Crit Care Med 1995;151(2 Pt 1):293–301.

24. Pepe PE, Potkin RT, Reus DH, Hudson LD, Carrico CJ. Clinical predictors of the adult respiratory distress syndrome. Am J Surg 1982;144(1):124–130.

25. Doyle RL, Szaflarski N, Modin GW, Wiener-Kronish JP, Matthay MA. Identification of patients with acute lung injury. Predictors of mortality. Am J Respir Crit Care Med 1995;152(6 Pt 1):1818–1824.

26. Ware LB, Matthay MA. The acute respiratory distress syndrome. N Engl J Med 2000;342(18):1334–1349.

27. Kaplan RL, Sahn SA, Petty TL. Incidence and outcome of the respiratory distress syndrome in Gram-negative sepsis. Arch Intern Med 1979;139(8):867–869.

28. Timmons OD, Dean JM, Vernon DD. Mortality rates and prognostic variables in children with adult respiratory distress syndrome. J Pediatr 1991;119(6):896–899.

29. DeBruin W, Notterman DA, Magid M, Godwin T, Johnston S. Acute hypoxemic respiratory failure in infants and children: clinical and pathologic characteristics. Crit Care Med 1992;20(9):1223–1234.

30. Holbrook PR, Taylor G, Pollack MM, Fields AI. Adult respiratory distress syndrome in children. Pediatr Clin North Am 1980;27(3):677–685.

31. Bowler RP, Duda B, Chan ED, Enghild JJ, Ware LB, Matthay MA, et al. Proteomic analysis of pulmonary edema fluid and plasma in patients with acute lung injury. Am J Physiol Lung Cell Mol Physiol 2004;286(6):L1095–L1104.

32. Olman MA, White KE, Ware LB, Simmons WL, Benveniste EN, Zhu S, et al. Pulmonary edema fluid from patients with early lung injury stimulates fibroblast proliferation through IL-1β–induced IL-6 expression. J Immunol 2004;172(4):2668–2677.

33. Rosseau S, Hammerl P, Maus U, Walmrath HD, Schutte H, Grimminger F, et al. Phenotypic characterization of alveolar monocyte recruitment in acute respiratory distress syndrome. Am J Physiol Lung Cell Mol Physiol 2000;279(1):L25–L35.

34. Meduri GU, Headley AS, Golden E, Carson SJ, Umberger RA, Kelso T, et al. Effect of prolonged methylprednisolone therapy in unresolving acute respiratory distress syndrome: a randomized controlled trial. JAMA 1998;280(2):159–165.

35. Meduri GU, Chinn AJ, Leeper KV, Wunderink RG, Tolley E, Winer-Muram HT, et al. Corticosteroid rescue treatment of progressive fibroproliferation in late ARDS. Patterns of response and predictors of outcome. Chest 1994;105(5):1516–1527.

36. Meduri GU, Tolley EA, Chinn A, Stentz F, Postlethwaite A. Procollagen types I and III aminoterminal propeptide levels during acute respiratory distress syndrome and in response to methylprednisolone treatment. Am J Respir Crit Care Med 1998;158(5 Pt 1):1432–1441.

37. Gattinoni L, Carlesso E, Valenza F, Chiumello D, Caspani ML. Acute respiratory distress syndrome, the critical care paradigm: what we learned and what we forgot. Curr Opin Crit Care 2004;10(4):272–278.

38. Mendez JL, Hubmayr RD. New insights into the pathology of acute respiratory failure. Curr Opin Crit Care 2005;11(1):29–36.

39. Marini JJ, Hotchkiss JR, Broccard AF. Bench-to-bedside review: microvascular and airspace linkage in ventilator-induced lung injury. Crit Care 2003;7(6):435–444.

40. Rosenthal C, Caronia C, Quinn C, Lugo N, Sagy M. A comparison among animal models of acute lung injury. Crit Care Med 1998;26(5):912–916.

41. Abbas AK, Lichtman AH, Pober JS. Cellular and Molecular Immunology: Cytokines. Philadelphia: WB Saunders; 1994.

42. Tracey KJ, Lowry SF, Cerami A. Cachetin/TNF-alpha in septic shock and septic adult respiratory distress syndrome. Am Rev Respir Dis 1988;138(6):1377–1379.

43. Okusawa S, Gelfand JA, Ikejima T, Connolly RJ, Dinarello CA. Interleukin 1 induces a shock-like state in rabbits. Synergism with tumor necrosis factor and the effect of cyclooxygenase inhibition. J Clin Invest 1988;81(4):1162–1172.

44. Krieg AM, Love-Homan L, Yi AK, Harty JT. CpG DNA induces sustained IL-12 expression in vivo and resistance to *Listeria monocytogenes* challenge. J Immunol 1998;161(5):2428–2434.

45. Brightbill HD, Modlin RL. Toll-like receptors: molecular mechanisms of the mammalian immune response. Immunology 2000;101(1):1–10.

46. Medzhitov R, Janeway CA, Jr. Innate immune recognition and control of adaptive immune responses. Semin Immunol 1998;10(5):351–353.

47. Medzhitov R, Janeway C Jr. Innate immune recognition: mechanisms and pathways. Immunol Rev 2000;173:89–97.

48. Medzhitov R, Janeway C Jr. The toll receptor family and microbial recognition. Trends Microbiol 2000;8(10):452–456.

49. Medzhitov R, Janeway CA Jr. How does the immune system distinguish self from nonself? Semin Immunol 2000;12(3):185–188, 257–344.

50. Beutler B, Milsark IW, Cerami AC. Passive immunization against cachectin/tumor necrosis factor protects mice from lethal effect of endotoxin. Science 1985;229(4716):869–871.

51. Beutler B, Cerami A. The biology of cachectin/TNF—A primary mediator of the host response. Annu Rev Immunol 1989;7:625–655.

52. Tracey KJ, Fong Y, Hesse DG, Manogue KR, Lee AT, Kuo GC, et al. Anti-cachectin/TNF monoclonal antibodies prevent septic shock during lethal bacteraemia. Nature 1987;330(6149):662–664.

53. Millar AB, Foley NM, Singer M, Johnson NM, Meager A, Rook GA. Tumour necrosis factor in bronchopulmonary secretions of patients with adult respiratory distress syndrome. Lancet 1989;2(8665):712–714.

54. Hyers TM, Tricomi SM, Dettenmeier PA, Fowler AA. Tumor necrosis factor levels in serum and bronchoalveolar lavage fluid of patients with the adult respiratory distress syndrome. Am Rev Respir Dis 1991;144(2):268–271.

55. Pugin J, Ricou B, Steinberg KP, Suter PM, Martin TR. Proinflammatory activity in bronchoalveolar lavage fluids from patients with ARDS, a prominent role for interleukin-1. Am J Respir Crit Care Med 1996;153(6 Pt 1):1850–1856.

56. Dinarello CA. Interleukin-1. Cytokine Growth Factor Rev 1997;8(4):253–265.

57. Kunkel SL, Standiford T, Kasahara K, Strieter RM. Interleukin-8 (IL-8): the major neutrophil chemotactic factor in the lung. Exp Lung Res 1991;17(1):17–23.

58. Barsness KA, Bensard DD, Partrick DA, Calkins CM, Hendrickson RJ, Banerjee A, et al. IL-1beta induces an exaggerated pro- and anti-inflammatory response in peritoneal macrophages of children compared with adults. Pediatr Surg Int 2004;20(4):238–242.

59. Oppenheim JJ, Zachariae CO, Mukaida N, Matsushima K. Properties of the novel proinflammatory supergene "intercrine" cytokine family. Annu Rev Immunol 1991;9:617–648.

60. Zlotnik A, Yoshie O. Chemokines: a new classification system and their role in immunity. Immunity 2000;12(2):121–127.

61. Greenberger MJ, Strieter RM, Kunkel SL, Danforth JM, Laichalk LL, McGillicuddy DC, et al. Neutralization of macrophage inflammatory protein-2 attenuates neutrophil recruitment and bacterial clearance in murine Klebsiella pneumonia. J Infect Dis 1996;173(1):159–165.

62. Mehrad B, Standiford TJ. Role of cytokines in pulmonary antimicrobial host defense. Immunol Res 1999;20(1):15–27.

63. Standiford TJ, Strieter RM, Greenberger MJ, Kunkel SL. Expression and regulation of chemokines in acute bacterial pneumonia. Biol Signals 1996;5(4):203–208.

64. Mehrad B, Strieter RM, Moore TA, Tsai WC, Lira SA, Standiford TJ. CXC chemokine receptor-2 ligands are necessary components of neutrophil-mediated host defense in invasive pulmonary aspergillosis. J Immunol 1999;163(11):6086–6094.

65. Tsai WC, Strieter RM, Mehrad B, Newstead MW, Zeng X, Standiford TJ. CXC chemokine receptor CXCR2 is essential for protective innate

host response in murine *Pseudomonas aeruginosa* pneumonia. Infect Immun 2000;68(7):4289–4296.

66. Miller EJ, Cohen AB, Nagao S, Griffith D, Maunder RJ, Martin TR, et al. Elevated levels of NAP-1/interleukin-8 are present in the airspaces of patients with the adult respiratory distress syndrome and are associated with increased mortality. Am Rev Respir Dis 1992;146(2):427–432.

67. Belperio JA, Keane MP, Burdick MD, Londhe V, Xue YY, Li K, et al. Critical role for CXCR2 and CXCR2 ligands during the pathogenesis of ventilator-induced lung injury. J Clin Invest 2002;110(11):1703–1716.

68. Speyer CL, Gao H, Rancilio NJ, Neff TA, Huffnagle GB, Sarma JV, et al. Novel chemokine responsiveness and mobilization of neutrophils during sepsis. Am J Pathol 2004;165(6):2187–2196.

69. Guo RF, Riedemann NC, Ward PA. Role of C5a-C5aR interaction in sepsis. Shock 2004;21(1):1–7.

70. Kunkel SL, Strieter RM. Cytokine networking in lung inflammation. Hosp Pract (Off Ed) 1990;25(10):63–66, 69, 73–76.

71. Arai KI, Lee F, Miyajima A, Miyatake S, Arai N, Yokota T. Cytokines: coordinators of immune and inflammatory responses. Annu Rev Biochem 1990;59:783–836.

72. Shanley TP, Warner RL, Ward PA. The role of cytokines and adhesion molecules in the development of inflammatory injury. Mol Med Today 1995;1(1):40–45.

73. Shanley TP, Schmal H, Friedl HP, Jones ML, Ward PA. Role of macrophage inflammatory protein-1 alpha (MIP-1 alpha) in acute lung injury in rats. J Immunol 1995;154(9):4793–4802.

74. Hogg JC, Doerschuk CM. Leukocyte traffic in the lung. Annu Rev Physiol 1995;57:97–114.

75. Donnelly SC, Haslett C, Dransfield I, Robertson CE, Carter DC, Ross JA, et al. Role of selectins in development of adult respiratory distress syndrome. Lancet 1994;344(8917):215–219.

76. Zimmerman GA, Prescott SM, McIntyre TM. Endothelial cell interactions with granulocytes: tethering and signaling molecules. Immunol Today 1992;13(3):93–100.

77. Albelda SM, Smith CW, Ward PA. Adhesion molecules and inflammatory injury. FASEB J 1994;8(8):504–512.

78. Lukacs NW, Ward PA. Inflammatory mediators, cytokines, and adhesion molecules in pulmonary inflammation and injury. Adv Immunol 1996;62:257–304.

79. Ford-Hutchinson AW, Bray MA, Doig MV, Shipley ME, Smith MJ. Leukotriene B, a potent chemokinetic and aggregating substance released from polymorphonuclear leukocytes. Nature 1980;286(5770):264–265.

80. Grutz G. New insights into the molecular mechanism of interleukin-10–mediated immunosuppression. J Leukocyte Biol 2005;77(1):3–15.

81. Shanley TP, Schmal H, Friedl HP, Jones ML, Ward PA. Regulatory effects of intrinsic IL-10 in IgG immune complex–induced lung injury. J Immunol 1995;154(7):3454–3460.

82. Rennick DM, Fort MM, Davidson NJ. Studies with IL-10-/- mice: an overview. J Leukocyte Biol 1997;61(4):389–396.

83. Donnelly SC, Strieter RM, Reid PT, Kunkel SL, Burdick MD, Armstrong I, et al. The association between mortality rates and decreased concentrations of interleukin-10 and interleukin-1 receptor antagonist in the lung fluids of patients with the adult respiratory distress syndrome. Ann Intern Med 1996;125(3):191–196.

84. Bone RC. Sir Isaac Newton, sepsis, SIRS, and CARS. Crit Care Med 1996;24(7):1125–1128.

85. Bone RC. Why sepsis trials fail. JAMA 1996;276(7):565–566.

86. Zeni F, Freeman B, Natanson C. Anti-inflammatory therapies to treat sepsis and septic shock: a reassessment. Crit Care Med 1997;25(7):1095–1100.

87. Angus DC, Fink MPE. Cellular and molecular biology for intensivists: a primer. Crit Care Med 2005;33(12):S399–S560.

88. Ambrosino N. Noninvasive mechanical ventilation in acute respiratory failure. Monaldi Arch Chest Dis 1996;51(6):514–518.

89. Abou-Shala N, Meduri U. Noninvasive mechanical ventilation in patients with acute respiratory failure. Crit Care Med 1996;24(4):705–715.

90. Wysocki M, Tric L, Wolff MA, Millet H, Herman B. Noninvasive pressure support ventilation in patients with acute respiratory failure. A randomized comparison with conventional therapy. Chest 1995;107(3):761–768.

91. Rocker GM, Mackenzie MG, Williams B, Logan PM. Noninvasive positive pressure ventilation: successful outcome in patients with acute lung injury/ARDS. Chest 1999;115(1):173–177.

92. Patrick W, Webster K, Ludwig L, Roberts D, Wiebe P, Younes M. Noninvasive positive-pressure ventilation in acute respiratory distress without prior chronic respiratory failure. Am J Respir Crit Care Med 1996;153(3):1005–1011.

93. Amato MB, Barbas CS, Medeiros DM, Schettino Gde P, Lorenzi Filho G, Kairalla RA, et al. Beneficial effects of the "open lung approach" with low distending pressures in acute respiratory distress syndrome. A prospective randomized study on mechanical ventilation. Am J Respir Crit Care Med 1995;152(6 Pt 1):1835–1846.

94. Brower RG, Lanken PN, MacIntyre N, Matthay MA, Morris A, Ancukiewicz M, et al. Higher versus lower positive end-expiratory pressures in patients with the acute respiratory distress syndrome. N Engl J Med 2004;351(4):327–336.

95. Marcy TW, Marini JJ. Inverse ratio ventilation in ARDS. Rationale and implementation. Chest 1991;100(2):494–504.

96. Armstrong BW Jr, MacIntyre NR. Pressure-controlled, inverse ratio ventilation that avoids air trapping in the adult respiratory distress syndrome. Crit Care Med 1995;23(2):279–285.

97. Lessard MR, Guerot E, Lorino H, Lemaire F, Brochard L. Effects of pressure-controlled with different I:E ratios versus volume-controlled ventilation on respiratory mechanics, gas exchange, and hemodynamics in patients with adult respiratory distress syndrome. Anesthesiology 1994;80(5):983–991.

98. Mercat A, Titiriga M, Anguel N, Richard C, Teboul JL. Inverse ratio ventilation (I/E = 2/1) in acute respiratory distress syndrome: a six-hour controlled study. Am J Respir Crit Care Med 1997;155(5):1637–1642.

99. Krishnan JA, Brower RG. High-frequency ventilation for acute lung injury and ARDS. Chest 2000;118(3):795–807.

100. Arnold JH, Hanson JH, Toro-Figuero LO, Gutierrez J, Berens RJ, Anglin DL. Prospective, randomized comparison of high-frequency oscillatory ventilation and conventional mechanical ventilation in pediatric respiratory failure. Crit Care Med 1994;22(10):1530–1539.

101. Arnold JH, Anas NG, Luckett P, Cheifetz IM, Reyes G, Newth CJ, et al. High-frequency oscillatory ventilation in pediatric respiratory failure: a multicenter experience. Crit Care Med 2000;28(12):3913–3999.

102. Fedora M, Klimovic M, Seda M, Dominik P, Nekvasil R. Effect of early intervention of high-frequency oscillatory ventilation on the outcome in pediatric acute respiratory distress syndrome. Bratisl Lek Listy 2000;101(1):8–13.

103. Wispe JR, Roberts RJ. Molecular basis of pulmonary oxygen toxicity. Clin Perinatol 1987;14(3):651–666.

104. dos Santos CC, Slutsky AS. Mechanotransduction, ventilator-induced lung injury and multiple organ dysfunction syndrome. Intensive Care Med 2000;26(5):638–642.

105. Lee WL, Slutsky AS. Ventilator-induced lung injury and recommendations for mechanical ventilation of patients with ARDS. Semin Respir Crit Care Med 2001;22(3):269–280.

106. Lin CY, Zhang H, Cheng KC, Slutsky AS. Mechanical ventilation may increase susceptibility to the development of bacteremia. Crit Care Med 2003;31(5):1429–1434.

107. Imai Y, Parodo J, Kajikawa O, de Perrot M, Fischer S, Edwards V, et al. Injurious mechanical ventilation and end-organ epithelial cell apoptosis and organ dysfunction in an experimental model of acute respiratory distress syndrome. JAMA 2003;289(16):2104–2112.

108. Plotz FB, Vreugdenhil HA, Slutsky AS, Zijlstra J, Heijnen CJ, van Vught H. Mechanical ventilation alters the immune response in

children without lung pathology. Intensive Care Med 2002;28(4):486–492.

109. Slutsky AS. The acute respiratory distress syndrome, mechanical ventilation, and the prone position. N Engl J Med 2001;345(8):610–612.

110. Veldhuizen RA, Slutsky AS, Joseph M, McCaig L. Effects of mechanical ventilation of isolated mouse lungs on surfactant and inflammatory cytokines. Eur Respir J 2001;17(3):488–494.

111. Ranieri VM, Giunta F, Suter PM, Slutsky AS. Mechanical ventilation as a mediator of multisystem organ failure in acute respiratory distress syndrome. JAMA 2000;284(1):43–44.

112. Slutsky AS. Lung injury caused by mechanical ventilation. Chest 1999;116(1 Suppl):9S–15S.

113. Ranieri VM, Suter PM, Tortorella C, De Tullio R, Dayer JM, Brienza A, et al. Effect of mechanical ventilation on inflammatory mediators in patients with acute respiratory distress syndrome: a randomized controlled trial. JAMA 1999;282(1):54–61.

114. Mehta S, Slutsky AS. Mechanical ventilation in acute respiratory distress syndrome: evolving concepts. Monaldi Arch Chest Dis 1998;53(6):647–653.

115. Slutsky AS, Tremblay LN. Multiple system organ failure. Is mechanical ventilation a contributing factor? Am J Respir Crit Care Med 1998;157(6 Pt 1):1721–1725.

116. Slutsky AS. Mechanical ventilation. American College of Chest Physicians' Consensus Conference. Chest 1993;104(6):1833–1859.

117. Kolobow T, Moretti MP, Fumagalli R, Mascheroni D, Prato P, Chen V, et al. Severe impairment in lung function induced by high peak airway pressure during mechanical ventilation. An experimental study. Am Rev Respir Dis 1987;135(2):312–315.

118. Chiumello D, Pristine G, Slutsky AS. Mechanical ventilation affects local and systemic cytokines in an animal model of acute respiratory distress syndrome. Am J Respir Crit Care Med 1999;160(1):109–116.

119. The Acute Respiratory Distress Syndrome Network. Ventilation with lower tidal volumes as compared with traditional tidal volumes for acute lung injury and the acute respiratory distress syndrome. N Engl J Med 2000;342(18):1301–1308.

120. Brochard L, Roudot-Thoraval F, Roupie E, Delclaux C, Chastre J, Fernandez-Mondejar E, et al. Tidal volume reduction for prevention of ventilator-induced lung injury in acute respiratory distress syndrome. The Multicenter Trail Group on Tidal Volume reduction in ARDS. Am J Respir Crit Care Med 1998;158(6):1831–1838.

121. Brower RG, Shanholtz CB, Fessler HE, Shade DM, White P Jr, Wiener CM, et al. Prospective, randomized, controlled clinical trial comparing traditional versus reduced tidal volume ventilation in acute respiratory distress syndrome patients. Crit Care Med 1999;27(8):1492–1498.

122. Hickling KG, Henderson SJ, Jackson R. Low mortality associated with low volume pressure limited ventilation with permissive hypercapnia in severe adult respiratory distress syndrome. Intensive Care Med 1990;16(6):372–377.

123. Ni Chonghaile M, Higgins B, Laffey JG. Permissive hypercapnia: role in protective lung ventilatory strategies. Curr Opin Crit Care 2005;11(1):56–62.

124. Laffey JG, O'Croinin D, McLoughlin P, Kavanagh BP. Permissive hypercapnia—role in protective lung ventilatory strategies. Intensive Care Med 2004;30(3):347–356.

125. Sevransky JE, Levy MM, Marini JJ. Mechanical ventilation in sepsis-induced acute lung injury/acute respiratory distress syndrome: an evidence-based review. Crit Care Med 2004;32(11 Suppl):S548–S553.

126. Broccard AF, Hotchkiss JR, Vannay C, Markert M, Sauty A, Feihl F, et al. Protective effects of hypercapnic acidosis on ventilator-induced lung injury. Am J Respir Crit Care Med 2001;164(5):802–806.

127. Sinclair SE, Kregenow DA, Lamm WJ, Starr IR, Chi EY, Hlastala MP. Hypercapnic acidosis is protective in an in vivo model of ventilator-induced lung injury. Am J Respir Crit Care Med 2002;166(3):403–408.

128. Laffey JG, Tanaka M, Engelberts D, Luo X, Yuan S, Tanswell AK, et al. Therapeutic hypercapnia reduces pulmonary and systemic injury following in vivo lung reperfusion. Am J Respir Crit Care Med 2000;162(6):2287–2294.

129. O'Croinin D, Ni Chonghaile M, Higgins B, Laffey JG. Bench-to-bedside review: permissive hypercapnia. Crit Care 2005;9(1):51–59.

130. Pappert D, Rossaint R, Slama K, Gruning T, Falke KJ. Influence of positioning on ventilation–perfusion relationships in severe adult respiratory distress syndrome. Chest 1994;106(5):1511–1516.

131. Curley MA, Thompson JE, Arnold JH. The effects of early and repeated prone positioning in pediatric patients with acute lung injury. Chest 2000;118(1):156–163.

132. Casado-Flores J, Martinez de Azagra A, Ruiz-Lopez MJ, Ruiz M, Serrano A. Pediatric ARDS: effect of supine-prone postural changes on oxygenation. Intensive Care Med 2002;28(12):1792–1796.

133. Curley MA, Hibberd PL, Fineman LD, Wypij D, Shih MC, Thompson JE, et al. Effect of prone positioning on clinical outcomes in children with acute lung injury: a randomized controlled trial. JAMA 2005;294(2):229–237.

134. Gattinoni L, Tognoni G, Pesenti A, Taccone P, Mascheroni D, Labarta V, et al. Effect of prone positioning on the survival of patients with acute respiratory failure. N Engl J Med 2001;345(8):568–573.

135. Sznajder JI. Alveolar edema must be cleared for the acute respiratory distress syndrome patient to survive. Am J Respir Crit Care Med 2001;163(6):1293–1294.

136. Ware LB, Matthay MA. Alveolar fluid clearance is impaired in the majority of patients with acute lung injury and the acute respiratory distress syndrome. Am J Respir Crit Care Med 2001;163(6):1376–1383.

137. Weigelt JA, Norcross JF, Borman KR, Snyder WH 3rd. Early steroid therapy for respiratory failure. Arch Surg 1985;120(5):536–540.

138. Bone RC, Fisher CJ Jr, Clemmer TP, Slotman GJ, Metz CA. Early methylprednisolone treatment for septic syndrome and the adult respiratory distress syndrome. Chest 1987;92(6):1032–1036.

139. Bernard GR, Luce JM, Sprung CL, Rinaldo JE, Tate RM, Sibbald WJ, et al. High-dose corticosteroids in patients with the adult respiratory distress syndrome. N Engl J Med 1987;317(25):1565–1570.

140. Bogdan C, Vodovotz Y, Nathan C. Macrophage deactivation by interleukin 10. J Exp Med 1991;174(6):1549–1555.

141. Bogdan C, Paik J, Vodovotz Y, Nathan C. Contrasting mechanisms for suppression of macrophage cytokine release by transforming growth factor-beta and interleukin-10. J Biol Chem 1992;267(32):23301–23308.

142. DeVries A, Semchuk WM, Betcher JG. Ketoconazole in the prevention of acute respiratory distress syndrome. Pharmacotherapy 1998;18(3):581–587.

143. Williams JG, Maier RV. Ketoconazole inhibits alveolar macrophage production of inflammatory mediators involved in acute lung injury (adult respiratory distress syndrome). Surgery 1992;112(2):270–277.

144. Randomized, placebo-controlled trial of lisofylline for early treatment of acute lung injury and acute respiratory distress syndrome. Crit Care Med 2002;30(1):1–6.

145. de Waal Malefyt R, Abrams J, Bennett B, Figdor CG, de Vries JE. Interleukin 10(IL-10) inhibits cytokine synthesis by human monocytes: an autoregulatory role of IL-10 produced by monocytes. J Exp Med 1991;174(5):1209–1220.

146. Krakauer T. IL-10 inhibits the adhesion of leukocytic cells to IL-1-activated human endothelial cells. Immunol Lett 1995;45(1–2):61–65.

147. Wang P, Wu P, Siegel MI, Egan RW, Billah MM. Interleukin (IL)-10 inhibits nuclear factor kappa B (NF kappa B) activation in human monocytes. IL-10 and IL-4 suppress cytokine synthesis by different mechanisms. J Biol Chem 1995;270(16):9558–9563.

148. Lentsch AB, Shanley TP, Sarma V, Ward PA. In vivo suppression of NF-kappa B and preservation of I kappa B alpha by interleukin-10 and interleukin-13. J Clin Invest 1997;100(10):2443–2448.

149. Cassatella MA, Meda L, Gasperini S, Calzetti F, Bonora S. Interleukin 10 (IL-10) upregulates IL-1 receptor antagonist production from lipo-

polysaccharide-stimulated human polymorphonuclear leukocytes by delaying mRNA degradation. J Exp Med 1994;179(5):1695–1699.

150. Brown CY, Lagnado CA, Vadas MA, Goodall GJ. Differential regulation of the stability of cytokine mRNAs in lipopolysaccharide-activated blood monocytes in response to interleukin-10. J Biol Chem 1996;271(33):20108–20112.

151. Fisher CJ, Jr., Agosti JM, Opal SM, Lowry SF, Balk RA, Sadoff JC, et al. Treatment of septic shock with the tumor necrosis factor receptor:Fc fusion protein. The Soluble TNF Receptor Sepsis Study Group. N Engl J Med 1996;334(26):1697–1702.

152. Lemeshow S, Teres D, Moseley S. Statistical issues in clinical sepsis trials. Baltimore, MD: Williams & Wilkins; 1996.

153. Berthiaume Y, Folkesson HG, Matthay MA. Lung edema clearance: 20 years of progress: invited review: alveolar edema fluid clearance in the injured lung. J Appl Physiol 2002;93(6):2207–2213.

154. Matthay MA, Clerici C, Saumon G. Invited review: active fluid clearance from the distal air spaces of the lung. J Appl Physiol 2002; 93(4):1533–1541.

155. Modelska K, Matthay MA, Brown LA, Deutch E, Lu LN, Pittet JF. Inhibition of beta-adrenergic–dependent alveolar epithelial clearance by oxidant mechanisms after hemorrhagic shock. Am J Physiol 1999;276(5 Pt 1):L844–L857.

156. Pittet JF, Wiener-Kronish JP, McElroy MC, Folkesson HG, Matthay MA. Stimulation of lung epithelial liquid clearance by endogenous release of catecholamines in septic shock in anesthetized rats. J Clin Invest 1994;94(2):663–671.

157. Campbell AR, Folkesson HG, Berthiaume Y, Gutkowska J, Suzuki S, Matthay MA. Alveolar epithelial fluid clearance persists in the presence of moderate left atrial hypertension in sheep. J Appl Physiol 1999;86(1):139–151.

158. Carter EP, Duvick SE, Wendt CH, Dunitz J, Nici L, Wangensteen OD, et al. Hyperoxia increases active alveolar Na+ resorption in vivo and type II cell Na,K-ATPase in vitro. Chest 1994;105(3 Suppl):75S–78S.

159. Minakata Y, Suzuki S, Grygorczyk C, Dagenais A, Berthiaume Y. Impact of beta-adrenergic agonist on Na+ channel and Na$^+$-K$^+$/ATPase expression in alveolar type II cells. Am J Physiol 1998;275(2 Pt 1): L414–L422.

160. Folkesson HG, Norlin A, Wang Y, Abedinpour P, Matthay MA. Dexamethasone and thyroid hormone pretreatment upregulate alveolar epithelial fluid clearance in adult rats. J Appl Physiol 2000;88(2):416–424.

161. Viget NB, Guery BP, Ader F, Neviere R, Alfandari S, Creuzy C, et al. Keratinocyte growth factor protects against *Pseudomonas aeruginosa*–induced lung injury. Am J Physiol Lung Cell Mol Physiol 2000;279(6):L1199–L1209.

162. Stern M, Ulrich K, Robinson C, Copeland J, Griesenbach U, Masse C, et al. Pretreatment with cationic lipid-mediated transfer of the Na+K+-ATPase pump in a mouse model in vivo augments resolution of high permeability pulmonary oedema. Gene Ther 2000;7(11):960–966.

163. Kumasaka T, Quinlan WM, Doyle NA, Condon TP, Sligh J, Takei F, et al. Role of the intercellular adhesion molecule-1(ICAM-1) in endotoxin-induced pneumonia evaluated using ICAM-1 antisense oligonucleotides, anti-ICAM-1 monoclonal antibodies, and ICAM-1 mutant mice. J Clin Invest 1996;97(10):2362–2369.

164. Doerschuk CM, Quinlan WM, Doyle NA, Bullard DC, Vestweber D, Jones ML, et al. The role of P-selectin and ICAM-1 in acute lung injury as determined using blocking antibodies and mutant mice. J Immunol 1996;157(10):4609–4614.

165. Ridings PC, Windsor AC, Jutila MA, Blocher CR, Fisher BJ, Sholley MM, et al. A dual-binding antibody to E- and L-selectin attenuates sepsis-induced lung injury. Am J Respir Crit Care Med 1995;152(1):247–253.

166. Mulligan MS, Miyasaka M, Tamatani T, Jones ML, Ward PA. Requirements for L-selectin in neutrophil-mediated lung injury in rats. J Immunol 1994;152(2):832–840.

167. Mulligan MS, Polley MJ, Bayer RJ, Nunn MF, Paulson JC, Ward PA. Neutrophil-dependent acute lung injury. Requirement for P-selectin (GMP-140). J Clin Invest 1992;90(4):1600–1607.

168. Etzioni A, Alon R. Leukocyte adhesion deficiency III: a group of integrin activation defects in hematopoietic lineage cells. Curr Opin Allergy Clin Immunol 2004;4(6):485–490.

169. Kinashi T, Aker M, Sokolovsky-Eisenberg M, Grabovsky V, Tanaka C, Shamri R, et al. LAD-III, a leukocyte adhesion deficiency syndrome associated with defective Rap1 activation and impaired stabilization of integrin bonds. Blood 2004;103(3):1033–1036.

170. Matsumoto T, Yokoi K, Mukaida N, Harada A, Yamashita J, Watanabe Y, et al. Pivotal role of interleukin-8 in the acute respiratory distress syndrome and cerebral reperfusion injury. J Leukocyte Biol 1997;62(5):581–587.

171. Folkesson HG, Matthay MA, Hebert CA, Broaddus VC. Acid aspiration-induced lung injury in rabbits is mediated by interleukin-8–dependent mechanisms. J Clin Invest 1995;96(1):107–116.

172. Mulligan MS, Jones ML, Bolanowski MA, Baganoff MP, Deppeler CL, Meyers DM, et al. Inhibition of lung inflammatory reactions in rats by an anti-human IL-8 antibody. J Immunol 1993;150(12):5585–5595.

173. Kurdowska A, Noble JM, Steinberg KP, Ruzinski JT, Hudson LD, Martin TR. Anti-interleukin 8 autoantibody: interleukin 8 complexes in the acute respiratory distress syndrome. Relationship between the complexes and clinical disease activity. Am J Respir Crit Care Med 2001;163(2):463–468.

174. Krupa A, Kato H, Matthay MA, Kurdowska AK. Proinflammatory activity of anti-IL-8 autoantibody:IL-8 complexes in alveolar edema fluid from patients with acute lung injury. Am J Physiol Lung Cell Mol Physiol 2004;286(6):L1105–L1113.

175. Ponath PD. Chemokine receptor antagonists: novel therapeutics for inflammation and AIDS. Expert Opin Invest Drugs 1998;7(1):1–18.

176. Mehta NM, Arnold JH. Genetic polymorphisms in acute respiratory distress syndrome: new approach to an old problem. Crit Care Med 2005;33(10):2443–2445.

177. Floros J, Pavlovic J. Genetics of acute respiratory distress syndrome: challenges, approaches, surfactant proteins as candidate genes. Semin Respir Crit Care Med 2003;24(2):161–168.

178. Shanley TP, Wong HR. Molecular genetics in the pediatric intensive care unit. Crit Care Clin 2003;19(3):577–594.

179. Lin Z, Pearson C, Chinchilli V, Pietschmann SM, Luo J, Pison U, et al. Polymorphisms of human SP-A, SP-B, and SP-D genes: association of SP-B Thr131Ile with ARDS. Clin Genet 2000;58(3):181–191.

180. Nogee LM, Dunbar AE, 3rd, Wert SE, Askin F, Hamvas A, Whitsett JA. A mutation in the surfactant protein C gene associated with familial interstitial lung disease. N Engl J Med 2001;344(8):573–579.

181. Stuber F, Petersen M, Bokelmann F, Schade U. A genomic polymorphism within the tumor necrosis factor locus influences plasma tumor necrosis factor-alpha concentrations and outcome of patients with severe sepsis. Crit Care Med 1996;24(3):381–384.

182. Mira JP, Cariou A, Grall F, Delclaux C, Losser MR, Heshmati F, et al. Association of TNF2, a TNF-alpha promoter polymorphism, with septic shock susceptibility and mortality: a multicenter study. JAMA 1999;282(6):561–568.

183. King LS, Nielsen S, Agre P. Aquaporin-1 water channel protein in lung: ontogeny, steroid-induced expression, and distribution in rat. J Clin Invest 1996;97(10):2183–2191.

184. Ma T, Fukuda N, Song Y, Matthay MA, Verkman AS. Lung fluid transport in aquaporin-5 knockout mice. J Clin Invest 2000;105(1):93–100.

185. Song Y, Fukuda N, Bai C, Ma T, Matthay MA, Verkman AS. Role of aquaporins in alveolar fluid clearance in neonatal and adult lung, and in oedema formation following acute lung injury: studies in transgenic aquaporin null mice. J Physiol 2000;525 Pt 3:771–779.

186. Song Y, Ma T, Matthay MA, Verkman AS. Role of aquaporin-4 in airspace-to-capillary water permeability in intact mouse lung measured by a novel gravimetric method. J Gen Physiol 2000;115(1): 17–27.

6
Mechanical Ventilation

Alik Kornecki and Brian P. Kavanagh

Introduction

Mechanical ventilation, perhaps the cornerstone of contemporary critical care, can be applied invasively or noninvasively. Although mechanical ventilation is clearly lifesaving, one should remember that it is only a supportive modality; it is not a therapy. Indeed, it is associated with significant adverse effects and may cause important complications when applied improperly. We describe the indications for, classification of, and associated complications and considerations related to weaning from mechanical ventilation.

Indications for Mechanical Ventilation

The need for mechanical ventilation support is the most common reason for admission to a critical care unit. Although explicit indications exist (Table 6.1), they are not well validated. Thus, the decision to institute mechanical ventilation is made by the physician at the bedside on clinical grounds and takes into consideration the underlying condition, the likely course of the disease, and the potential response to medical treatment. The indications for tracheal intubation (e.g., airway protection, relief of airway obstruction) are not the same as for mechanical ventilation and are discussed elsewhere in this textbook. However, children who require tracheal intubation will usually be provided with mechanical ventilation because of the reduction in respiratory drive associated with sedation, the perceived benefits of positive end-expiratory pressure (PEEP), and to counter the resistance to airflow offered by the tracheal tube. In general, institution of mechanical ventilation is indicated when the patient's spontaneous ventilation is threatened or not adequate to sustain life.

Children usually require mechanical ventilation because of respiratory failure or impending respiratory failure that occurs when the system fails to meet the body's requirements in terms of oxygenation and/or elimination of carbon dioxide. It may occur as a result of primary lung disease (e.g., reduction in functional residual capacity [FRC] or compliance, worsened ventilation–perfusion mismatch) or pump dysfunction (e.g., reduced central drive, muscle disease). Beyond these pulmonary indications, mechanical ventilation may be instituted in order to improve left ventricular function in the case of heart failure or to optimize carbon dioxide in the case of increased intracranial pressure. As mechanical ventilation is not without complications, the goal should be to apply it only when necessary and with minimal injury to the lungs and maximal comfort to the patient.

Mechanical Ventilation: Children Versus Adults

Although ventilation has been extensively investigated and characterized for preterm neonates and adults, there have been limited laboratory investigations, and few prospective clinical investigations, of mechanical ventilation for infants or older children. As a result, age-based guidelines for the use of conventional mechanical ventilation in pediatric patients have not been established. Indeed, any recommendations for mechanical ventilation that exist have been extrapolated from adult data. Compared with adults, pediatric patients demonstrate a spectrum of lung and chest wall development. Maturation in the human lung continues well after the neonatal period until between 2 and 8 years of age [1]. There are important morphologic differences among the neonate, the infant, and the adult that may have implications on the way mechanical ventilation should be managed.

The ratio of lung volume, in particular total lung capacity and FRC, to body weight is not constant through development; both ratios are lower in infants than in adults [2,3]. As a result, application of tidal volumes that are based on body weight (i.e., mL per kg) may have a different impact in adults compared with children. Indeed, the susceptibility of adult models to experimental ventilator-induced lung injury (VILI) may be greater than in infant or neonatal models [4], although the relevance of these findings to the clinical context remains to be determined.

D.S. Wheeler et al. (eds.), The *Respiratory Tract in Pediatric Critical Illness and Injury*,
DOI 10.1007/978-1-84800-925-7_6, © Springer-Verlag London Limited 2009

TABLE 6.1. Indications for mechanical ventilation.

Respiratory failure
  Pump failure
    Chest wall dysfunction (e.g., flail chest)
    Neuromuscular disease
    Central nervous dysfunction (decrease in respiratory drive)
      Congenital (e.g., Ondine course)
    Acquired (e.g., trauma, drugs, infectors)
  Pulmonary disease
  Ventilation–perfusion mismatch (e.g., pneumonia)
  Pulmonary shunt (e.g., acute respiratory distress syndrome)
  Reduction in functional residual capacity
Others
  To support an intubated patient (e.g., patient intubated for airway protection)
  To decrease the work of breathing and afterload
  To optimize carbon dioxide levels (e.g., head trauma with increase in intracranial pressure)

TABLE 6.2. Complications and physiologic adverse effects of positive pressure mechanical ventilation.

Respiratory
  Upper airways
    Nasal trauma
    Nasopharyngeal and pharyngeal trauma
    Laryngeal trauma—vocal cord fixation/paralysis
    Subglottic edema/stenosis
  Lower airways
    Air leak
      Pneumothorax
      Pneumomediastinum
      Pulmonary interstitial
    Atelectasis
    Ventilation-associated pneumonia
    Ventilation-associated lung injury
Cardiovascular
  Decrease venous return
  Increase pulmonary vascular resistance
Central nervous system
  Increase intracranial pressure
Renal
  Decrease urine output (direct and indirect effect)

The process of alveolization continues beyond the infant age range until the age of 2–5 years. Approximately 50 million alveoli are present at birth in a term infant, and, by the age of 2–5 years, this number reaches 300 million alveoli [1]. The lung matrix of a neonate contains only small amounts of collagen; the elastin-to-collagen ratio changes during the first months and years of life and affects lung stiffness and potential for overdistension and recoil. Collateral ventilation through the pores of Kohn and Lambert's canal are not well developed in the early years; these collateral pathways may help prevent atelectasis, which is more common in children than in adults.

Considerable structural changes in the chest wall may change infant and childhood predisposition to respiratory failure, lung injury, and ventilation-associated lung injury. The orientation of the ribs is horizontal in the infant; by 10 years of age, the orientation is downward. Ossification of the rib cage, calcification of the costal cartilage, and development of muscular mass develops progressively until adulthood.

Mechanical Ventilation: Invasive Versus Noninvasive

The interface between the ventilator and the patient may be classified into two categories: invasive and noninvasive. Invasive ventilation uses a tracheal or a tracheostomy tube or, for a limited period of time during general anesthesia, a laryngeal mask airway (LMA). Noninvasive ventilation, on the other hand, does not require a tracheal device.

Noninvasive ventilation may be administered with a positive pressure ventilator, sometimes termed noninvasive positive pressure ventilation (NIPPV), or as negative pressure ventilation. The main advantages of noninvasive ventilation are avoidance of tracheal intubation or tracheostomy and thus avoidance of the associated complications (Table 6.2). The presence of a tracheal tube increases the risk of airway trauma and nosocomial pneumonia, as well as the propensity for immobilization, need for sedation, and sometimes paralysis. In addition, important physiologic functions, such as speech, cough, and swallowing, are impaired. Furthermore, noninvasive ventilation may be applied outside the critical care setting and outside the hospital as an optimal home ventilation solution.

Noninvasive Positive Pressure Ventilation

Noninvasive positive pressure ventilation is defined as the use of mask or face mask to provide ventilator support. It was first introduced to provide home ventilation for children with nocturnal hypoventilation caused by neuromuscular disease. Since the early 1990s, NIPPV has gained increased popularity for extended acute and chronic indications. However, as with other modalities of ventilation, there are fewer reports regarding children than adults, and there have been no controlled trials with children. As a result, selection guidelines regarding the use of NIPPV in children are extrapolated from the adult literature (Table 6.3).

Although no randomized, controlled studies regarding the efficacy of NIPPV in children have been performed, there several case series that describe its application in children with mild to moderate acute respiratory failure (e.g., bronchiolitis, asthma, pneumonia) and for chronic home ventilation (e.g., neuromuscular disease) [5]. A trial of NIPPV may be attempted for any child with early respiratory failure; however, one should not persist with its use if it becomes clear that the approach is only deferring the inevitable

TABLE 6.3. Potential applications for noninvasive positive pressure ventilation in children.

More common
  Nocturnal central hypoventilation
  Chronic lung disease
  Neuromuscular disease
  Cystic fibrosis—bridge for transplant
  Cardiac failure
Less common
  Acute respiratory failure—likely to reverse within 24 hr
  Transient postextubation upper airway obstruction
  Pneumonia
  Asthma, bronchiolitis
  Pulmonary edema
  Patients who refuse intubation

need for tracheal intubation. The major contraindications for NIPPV are clinical conditions in which upper airway protective reflexes are compromised, especially with reduced level of consciousness, or recent gastrointestinal surgeries in which increased bowel gas may compromise repair and/or recovery.

Noninvasive positive pressure ventilation may be administered through a nasal mask or an oronasal mask. The nasal mask is available in different sizes but not for very small infants. It is most commonly employed for chronic ventilator support as it is usually better tolerated and allows the child to better communicate and to potentially feed. The oronasal mask covers both the nose and the mouth. It may be less comfortable than the nasal mask; however, it abolishes the potential air leak through the mouth that commonly occurs during nasal mask ventilation. Controlled trials with adults comparing nasal and oronasal masks show inconsistent results regarding the efficacy of gas exchange; however, the nasal mask is generally better tolerated. A relatively new type of mask has been introduced, termed the *helmet* (Figure 6.1) [6]. The helmet covers the patient's entire head, is similar to an over-sized hockey helmet, and is sealed using straps under the shoulder. The patients can better interact with the environment, and the helmet can be applied to any patient regardless of facial contour [7,8].

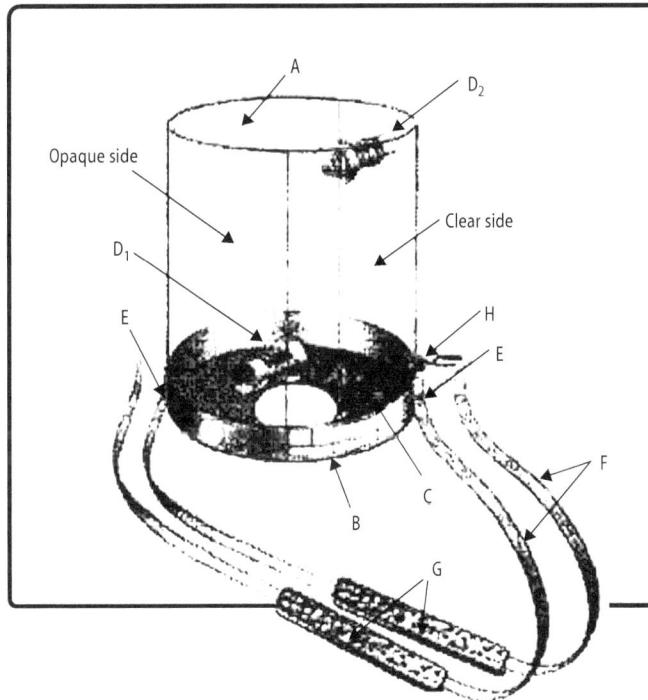

A) Transparent and opaque cylinder
B) Stiff ring
C) Elastic colar
D_1) Connector with pressure monitor port
D_2) 22M connector
E) Securing knob
F) Securing straps
G) Straps guards
H) Straps

Figure 6.1. Illustration of the Castar helmet. The inlet and outlet of the helmet are connected to the inspiratory and expiratory valves through a conventional circuit. (From Starmed, Mirandola, Italy. Reprinted with permission.)

Any ventilator may be used to provide NIPPV. It can be delivered by volume or pressure-preset modes or with a bilevel controlled or continuous positive pressure (CPAP) device. The more commonly used devices are portable bilevel ventilators that are designed for NIPPV and can operate successfully with a relatively large leak, providing high continuous flow. Pressure support ventilation is the most common mode of ventilation used with these devices.

With bilevel devices, the nomenclature may vary, but the inspiratory positive airway pressure (IPAP) and expiratory positive airway pressure (EPAP) are preset. The patient's spontaneous inspiration triggers the machine and the difference between IPAP and EPAP is the magnitude of the pressure support delivered with each breath. Because of the potential leak around the mask with high pressures, 15–20 cm H_2O is generally the highest pressure that usually can be achieved. As certain ventilators do not have an inspiratory time limit, the preset pressure may not be attained in the presence of a significant air leak, and the device will not therefore cycle *off* to expiration. In certain circumstances, only constant CPAP is provided throughout inspiration and expiration.

The old bilevel ventilators lacked an oxygen blender and a sophisticated alarm system, limiting their use to patients without a significant oxygen requirement. The more modern ventilators are equipped with better pressure and FiO_2 monitoring, comprehensive graphic displays, and sophisticated alarms. In addition, they offer volume-controlled, pressure-controlled and proportional assist ventilation options.

The key factor for effective initiation of NIPPV is a cooperative and relaxed patient. Patient coaching and gradual titration of the pressure may improve the rate of success. As a result, initiation of NIPPV is more time consuming for the team than conventional ventilation; this may be the major reason why some clinicians are reluctant to apply it. Noninvasive positive pressure ventilation is safe and can be delivered in any number of settings beyond the pediatric intensive care unit (PICU). However, it can be associated with complications such that it is generally the common practice to initiate NIPPV in the PICU setting where increased personnel and monitoring can provide constant attention to titrating adjustments to the patient's needs. Principal complications include skin ulceration and erosion in the area of contact between the mask and the skin, and, once the skin has become eroded, application of the mask is extremely difficult. Drying of the nasal and pharyngeal mucosa, aspiration, and abdominal distension with gastric dilatation have all been reported also.

Noninvasive Negative Pressure Ventilation

Until the mid-1900s negative pressure ventilation was almost the only method available to provide ventilation for the management of respiratory failure. Today, it is used only on rare occasions. It works by intermittently applying negative (i.e., subatmospheric) pressure to the chest or to the chest and abdomen. This causes expansion of the chest and decreases pleural and alveolar pressure, thereby creating a pressure gradient for inspired gas to move into the alveoli during inspiration. The expiration in most of the ventilators occurs passively by elastic recoil of the lungs. The main two types of ventilators are the traditional *iron lung* in which the torso (i.e., chest and abdomen but not the head) is enclosed in a sealed solid cylinder; and the cuirass system wherein a plastic shell is placed around the chest.

At present, negative pressure ventilation delivers negative pressure by four modes: cyclic negative pressure; so-called negative-positive pressure (where expiration is actively assisted); continuous negative pressure; and negative pressure with an oscillator. Most ventilators have the capacity to independently control the pressure and time during inspiration and expiration. The role of such ventilation is not well established for either adults or children [9,10]. Nonetheless, negative pressure ventilation is routinely used in certain centers for chronic home ventilation when the noninvasive positive pressure is either unavailable or is not tolerated. The main factors that limit its widespread application include large unit size, noise, and potential upper airway collapse during inspiration [11].

When the entire body is exposed to negative pressure, as occurs with the tank ventilators, noninvasive negative pressure ventilation has similar hemodynamic effects to conventional positive pressure ventilation. However, when the negative pressure is confined to the chest alone (e.g., using the cuirass-type, Hayek Oscillator), this modality of ventilation closely mimics the physiologic dynamics of spontaneous ventilation and may have potential hemodynamic advantages over conventional positive pressure ventilation. The deleterious effect of positive pressure ventilation on venous return is not present with negative pressure ventilation; on the contrary, negative pressure ventilation augments venous return, as in spontaneous inspiration. An appealing indication for noninvasive negative pressure ventilation was suggested by Shekerdemian et al. [12]. During inspiration the right atrial pressure decreases, increasing the gradient for venous return. Shekerdemian et al. [12] showed that, following the Fontan operation or repair of tetralogy of Fallot, children had a significantly greater pulmonary blood flow and cardiac output when ventilated with negative versus positive pressure. In conclusion, noninvasive negative pressure ventilation is an attractive mode of ventilation; however, there are not enough physiologic and clinical data to support its use as a first-line approach. It may be applied on individual basis when venous return or pulmonary blood flow is especially tenuous.

Mechanical Ventilation: Classification and Modes

Since the 1960s, when negative pressure ventilation was almost completely abandoned, nearly all mechanical ventilators have employed the principle of intermittent positive pressure ventilation, where the lungs are inflated by applying a positive pressure to the airways. Most modern ventilators are equipped with a piston bellows system or use a high-pressure gas source to drive the gas flow to the lungs. Ventilators used to be classified according to the termination of active inspiration and initiation of passive exhalation. Accordingly, the inspiratory phase may be terminated when a preset pressure is achieved (*pressure-cycled ventilators*), a preset volume is achieved (*volume-cycled ventilators*), or a preset inspiratory time is reached (*time-cycled ventilators*). This classification has become somewhat irrelevant because, with modern ventilators, one may separately control the tidal volume, the pressure delivered, and the inspiratory time (or indirectly with the flow). Some ventilators that are used for transport or for home ventilation are pure pressure-cycled ventilators, where the ventilator produces gas flow to the lungs until it reaches a preset pressure; then inspiration is terminated, and, thereafter, the expiration valve opens and expiration begins. The duration of inspiration and tidal volume varies according to the total respiratory system compliance (chest and lung) and the airway resistance. When lung or chest wall compliance is low or inspiratory time short, then the delivered tidal

volume will be smaller. Furthermore, in case of an air leak, the preset airway pressure may not be reached, thereby preventing the termination of inspiration. The above limitations restrict the use of these ventilators to children with relatively healthy lungs (e.g., neuromuscular disease, central hypoventilation).

Pediatric ventilators are designed differently from adult ventilators. They are designed to minimize the system compliance that includes compression of the gas. In order to reduce the response time of the ventilator and reduce the work of breathing during a spontaneously triggered breath, the ventilators used for children provide a constant flow of fresh gas compared with the adult ventilators that use demand flow, in which the inspiratory valve is opened by patient effort.

The ventilatory cycle during mechanical ventilation is divided into an inspiratory and an expiratory phase. Modes of mechanical ventilation are classified according to the mechanism of the so-called patient–ventilator interaction during inspiration. This ranges from full ventilator control of the tidal volume and frequency, to provision of partial support only during a spontaneous breathing where the patient determines both the tidal volume and the respiratory rate. A classification of common modes of mechanical ventilation follows.

Controlled Mode Mechanical Ventilation

In controlled mode mechanical ventilation (CMV), the ventilator delivers a mechanical breath at a preset interval irrespective of the patient's spontaneous effort (Figure 6.2). The breath is either *volume regulated* or *pressure regulated*. In this mode of ventilation, the patient's spontaneous effort to breathe may interfere with the mandatory breath delivered by the ventilator. To prevent this, the patient's spontaneous breathing may be inhibited by decreasing the respiratory drive either by administering sedative drugs or by hyperventilation to induce respiratory alkalosis. In extreme cases, when the patient's spontaneous breath cannot be eliminated and the patient continues to *fight* with the ventilator (so-called patient–ventilator dysynchrony), neuromuscular blockade is required. This mode of ventilation has almost been completely abandoned for children. It may be used rarely when a high rate of ventilation is required and the specific ventilator is unable to

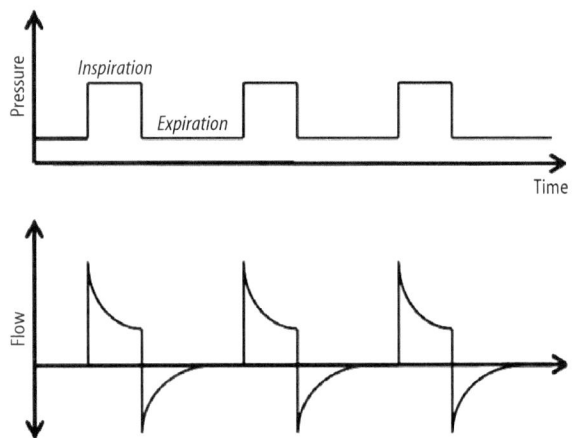

FIGURE 6.2. Controlled ventilation mode. The ventilator delivers preset tidal volume or pressure with a preset inspiratory time and respiratory rate. End expiratory pressure (PEEP) may be kept over zero.

provide synchronized intermittent mandatory ventilation at such respiratory rates.

Assist Control Mechanical Ventilation

Assist control mechanical ventilation (ACMV) is a form of ventilation in which the ventilator provides a preset tidal volume in response to each spontaneous breath, regardless of the size of the tidal volume desired by the patient (Figure 6.3). Where the patient does not trigger the ventilator within the specified time interval, the ventilator will provide the preset tidal volume at the preset respiratory rate.

Synchronized Intermittent Mandatory Ventilation

Synchronized intermittent mandatory ventilation (SIMV) was originally developed as a weaning mode but was quickly adopted as the mainstream mode of ventilation because of its apparent advantages over the control mode. It is a mixed ventilatory mode that allows both mandatory and spontaneous breathing (Figure 6.4). The mandatory breaths can be pressure or volume regulated, and the spontaneous breaths can be pressure supported (or not). The SIMV algorithm is designed to deliver a mandatory breath in each SIMV breathe cycle, where the breath cycle is 60/(number of breaths per minute), in seconds. The mandatory breath is either patient or ventilator initiated.

The SIMV cycle has two periods: The first period is the mandatory period, which is reserved for the mandatory breath. If the patient does not trigger the ventilator during the mandatory period, the machine will deliver the preset mandatory breath at the end of this period. When the patient triggers the ventilator during this period, a preset mandatory breath is delivered and the mandatory period is terminated. The second period is the spontaneous period, which is reserved for the spontaneous breaths. The spontaneous period starts each time a mandatory period terminates. The main advantages of SIMV over CMV are maintenance of spontaneous respiratory activity, which results in continuous use of the respiratory muscle, and improved patient–ventilator synchronization. The result of the latter may be a reduction in the use of excessive sedation and neuromuscular blockade.

Mechanical ventilation can also be classified by whether the ventilator is set to deliver a predetermined tidal volume (volume-preset ventilation) or to achieve a predetermined plateau pressure (pressure-preset ventilation).

Pressure-Preset Ventilation (Pressure-Limited Ventilation)

The breath is delivered at a set rate with a decelerating flow pattern and is terminated when a preset peak inspiratory pressure (PIP) is achieved (Figure 6.5). The tidal volume is determined by the preset PIP and respiratory system mechanics. The inspiratory time is usually set by the operator. Pressure-limited ventilation is usually recommended for patient with leakage around an uncuffed tracheal tube, in cases of obstructive lung disease (e.g., status asthmaticus), for neonates or small infants because measurement of the tidal volume is inherently inaccurate, or, rarely, in the presence of a bronchopleural fistula. When the tidal volume is measured at the ventilator, instead of at the end of the tracheal tube, then changes

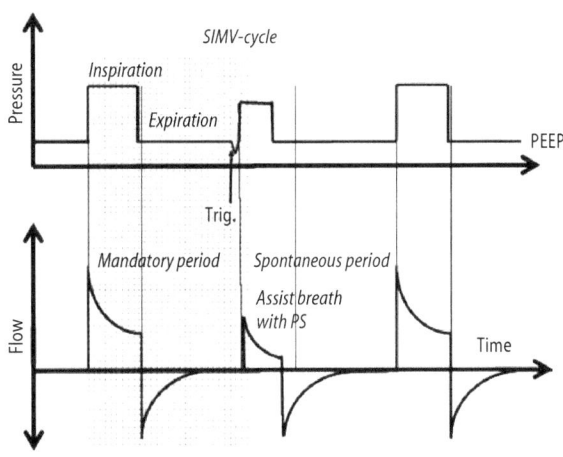

Figure 6.4. Synchronized intermittent mandatory ventilation (SIMV). The SIMV cycle consists of a mandatory period and spontaneous period. A breath effort during the SIMV mandatory period will deliver a breath with a preset volume or pressure. A breath effort during the spontaneous period will deliver spontaneous breath in the absence of pressure support, or pressure/volume supported breath. In case the patient does not take a breath during the mandatory period, the ventilator delivers a mandatory breath (volume limited or pressure limited).

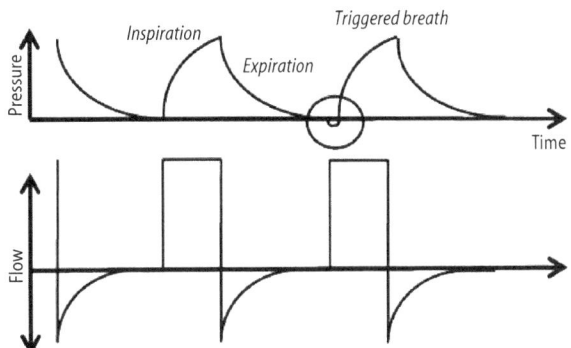

Figure 6.3. Assist control ventilation. When the patient does not trigger the ventilator within the specified time interval, the ventilator will provide the preset tidal volume at the preset respiratory rate (left). When the patient triggered the ventilator, a preset tidal volume in response to each spontaneous breath is delivered by the ventilator (right).

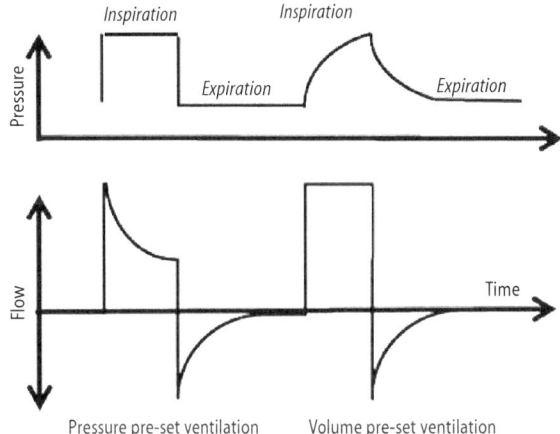

Figure 6.5. Pressure-limited breath (left) versus volume-limited breath (right). The same tidal volume is delivered in both modes. However, there is a decelerating flow in limited pressure mode (left) or a square wave flow in limited volume mode (right).

in circuit compliance significantly influence the data. This is particularly the case with neonates and infants, whose tidal volumes are far smaller than the volume of the ventilator circuit.

The main drawback of pressure-limited ventilation is that tidal volume and minute ventilation are directly influenced by the respiratory system mechanics, and, as these change, so too does the delivered tidal volume. As a result, in cases of rapidly changing respiratory system mechanics (e.g., administration of surfactant), the patient may be at risk of inappropriate levels of ventilation.

Volume-Preset Ventilation

A preset volume is delivered by the ventilator with each breath using a constant flow pattern (see Figure 6.5). The breath is terminated by a preset time (*time cycled*) or after the delivery of the preset tidal volume (*volume cycled*). In the first, the inspiratory flow is regulated in order to deliver the preset tidal volume (*time-cycled ventilation*), and the tidal volume and minute ventilation are guaranteed. This is common for larger infants and children but not recommended for neonates or small infants. The main drawback is variation in tidal volume delivery because of either leaks or inaccurate volume measurement. In modern ventilators, peak pressure can be limited during volume control ventilation.

Pressure-Limited Volume-Controlled Ventilation

Pressure-limited volume-controlled ventilation (PRVC) is strictly a control mode (not an assist mode) of ventilation that is available with most modern ventilators. It combines the purported advantages of a decelerating flow pattern characteristic of the pressure-limited mode with the guaranteed tidal volume associated with volume-preset ventilation. A preset (i.e., chosen) tidal volume is delivered with the lowest pressure possible, using a decelerating flow. After the first volume-limited breath, the plateau pressure measured by the ventilator is used for the next breath; this pattern is continued for each successive breath (Figure 6.6). For each subsequent breath, the ventilator automatically adjusts the minimal inspiratory pressure required to guarantee the preset tidal volume. If the tidal volume increases above the preset value, the next breath

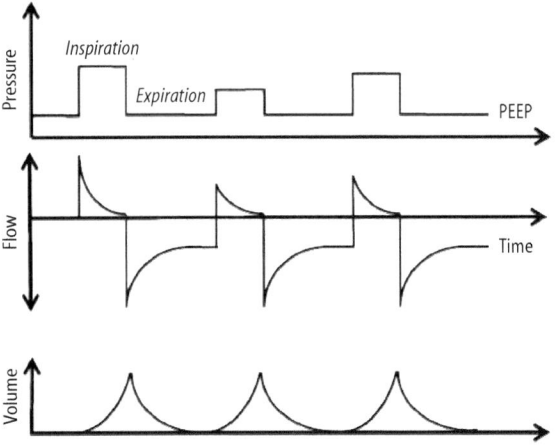

FIGURE 6.6. Pressure-regulated volume control (PRVC) is a mode in which the ventilator delivers a preset tidal volume, with preset frequency and inspiratory time. The ventilator automatically adapts the optimal inspiratory pressure (lowest) in order to deliver the preset tidal volume.

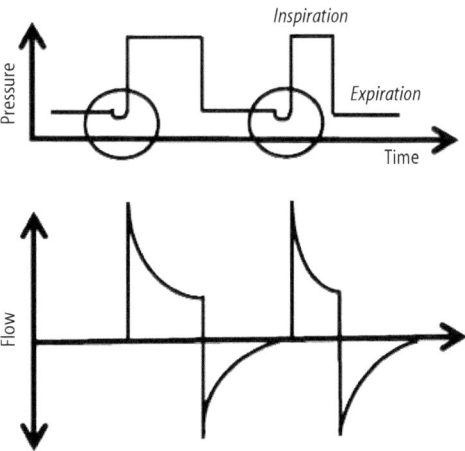

FIGURE 6.7. A combination of control and pressure support ventilation.

is delivered with a lower pressure. Limited clinical trials have documented lower levels of peak airway pressure were required to deliver the same tidal volumes using PRVC compare with volume-control modes [13]. However, it is unclear whether this represents a meaningful advantage in the prevention of ventilator-induced lung injury.

Pressure Support Ventilation

Pressure support was designed as a spontaneous mode of ventilation that augments only spontaneous breaths (Figure 6.7). The idea is that, by doing so, the work of breathing imposed on the patient is reduced. It is a patient-triggered, pressure-limited, flow-cycled mode of ventilation. During pressure support ventilation, the ventilator delivers flow in order to provide a constant preset inspiratory pressure with each spontaneous breath. The patient controls the respiratory rate, inspiratory time, and the tidal volume (unless the preset pressure is extremely high). To trigger the ventilator, the patient has to develop a minimum negative inspiratory effort that exceeds in magnitude the preset sensitivity (*based on either pressure or flow*). To reduce the effort of triggering to a minimum, most modern ventilators are equipped with very sensitive pressure or flow transducers that have a fast demand valve and a continuous flow. Because support ventilation is completely dependent on patient capacity to develop an inspiratory effort when this mode is used in isolation, the patient must have sufficient respiratory drive and muscle strength in order to trigger the ventilator. Furthermore, pressure support ventilation per se does not prevent apnea; however, virtually all modern ventilators have an alarm and backup mechanical support in the event of apnea.

The basis for determining or choosing the optimal preset pressure levels is not well established. In addition, neither the appropriate pulmonary disease states nor the use of adjunct SIMV has been determined for pressure support ventilation. However, in practice, pressure support is usually used in combination with SIMV in order to improve patient comfort or simply because practice has evolved that way. In addition, pressure support is commonly used during the weaning process.

One approach in implementing pressure support ventilation is to adjust the preset pressure to a level appropriate to achieve the desired tidal volume and/or to achieve apparent patient comfort. The major drawback in this mode of ventilation, as with any pressure-preset mode, is that tidal volume is not guaranteed. The delivered tidal volume in pressure support ventilation depends on patient effort, which of course may continuously change. Changes in neurologic status (e.g., increased sedation, which may reduce respiratory drive) or alteration in respiratory mechanics may affect the delivered tidal volume. Furthermore, oxygen demand (i.e., the requirement for O_2 because of fever, stress, or pain) may change over time, and, as a result, minute ventilation may change correspondingly while the preset pressure remains constant.

Volume Support Ventilation

To overcome the major drawbacks of pressure support ventilation (i.e., tidal volume is not guaranteed), some recent models have introduced the concept of volume support ventilation. Basically, this is a pressure support mode in which the inflation pressure changes in order to maintain a constant (i.e., preset) tidal volume. Using a closed-loop control system, the ventilator alters the pressure level to deliver a preset tidal volume. The delivered tidal volume is used as a feedback control for continuous adjustment of the level of pressure. This way the ventilator continuously adapts to the changes in patient effort, respiratory system mechanics, and oxygen requirement. The operator sets the desired tidal volume and also, by choosing the respiratory rate, the minute ventilation.

Airway Pressure Release Ventilation

A continuous relatively high positive airway pressure is applied, which is similar to CPAP, with an intermittent release phase to allow for expiration. Inspiration may be a mechanical preset breath or a spontaneous breath. Most importantly, all spontaneous breaths are unrestricted and are independent of the ventilator. Rather than producing a tidal volume by increasing the airway pressure above a preset PEEP as in the conventional modes of positive pressure ventilation, in airway pressure release ventilation (APRV) the tidal volume is generated when airway pressure is reduced from the preset pressure.

One theoretical advantage of this mode of ventilation may occur in acute respiratory distress syndrome, when FRC is reduced, and potential overdistension of the relatively healthy lung may contribute to the development of VILI. During APRV the FRC increases and inspiration begins from a higher FRC, thereby facilitating the spontaneous breath. In addition, because spontaneous breaths do not trigger the ventilator (as in CPAP), spontaneous inspiration during any phase of APRV results in lower pleural pressure and can therefore augment right ventricular filling. Clinical studies demonstrate improved patient comfort, gas exchange, and cardiac output during spontaneous breaths with APRV. Finally, APRV maintains lung volume (functional residual volume) and thereby may provide an alternative lung protective strategy and minimize the potential for VILI by limiting distension during mechanical ventilation.

Proportional Assist Ventilation

In the conventional mode of pressure support or assist control ventilation the support delivered by the ventilator is fixed as a consequence of patient demand (*triggering*). Thus, whether the patient's demand increases or decreases, the support remains fixed. In contrast, proportional assist ventilation (PAV) is governed by the equation of motion:

$$Pressure = (Elastance \cdot Volume) + (Resistance \cdot Flow)$$

which identifies the necessary pressure to be applied to the respiratory system in order to overcome opposing elastance and resistance forces that exist in proportion to the volume and flow, respectively [14]. During PAV, the ventilator output (i.e., flow and pressure) changes according to changes in the resistance and elastance of the respiratory system, thereby decreasing the work of breathing to a preset level [15].

Neurally Adjusted Ventilatory Assist

In the neurally adjusted ventilatory assist mode of ventilation, continuous detection of the electrical activity of the diaphragm muscles are used as an index of inspiratory drive and the amount of support provided by the ventilator corresponds to the ventilatory demand [16].

Variable Ventilation

The basis of variable ventilation is the hypothesis that loss of physiologic variability in breathing pattern contributes to the deterioration in respiratory mechanics and gas exchange observed over time with controlled mechanical ventilation. Unlike conventional ventilation in which the tidal volume is either constant or it is desired that it be so, in variable ventilation there is breath-to-breath variation in tidal volume. However, the minute ventilation remains constant. Thus, the respiratory rate and tidal volume are constantly varying, with periodically deep inflation that theoretically maintains alveolar recruitment. Studies performed in animals have demonstrated superior gas exchange and lung mechanics, as well as a reduction in the development of lung injury [17]; however, no human trials have yet been performed.

Closed-Loop Ventilation

Closed-loop ventilators are theoretically capable of automatically adjusting ventilator output according to continuous arterial blood gas monitoring. The clinician sets the desired PaO_2 or the hemoglobin saturation, and, by negative feedback, the ventilator adjusts the PEEP and FiO_2. At present, no commercially available system exists.

Automatic Tube Compensation

Although not a mode of ventilation as such, automatic tube compensation is offered by some ventilators as an option in which the ventilator assists a spontaneous breath by delivering positive pressure, the degree of which is proportional to the inspiratory flow. This pressure compensates for the estimated endotracheal resistance via a closed-loop control of the calculated tracheal tube resistance. The theoretical advantage of the system is that the work of breathing imposed by the artificial airway (e.g., tracheal tube, tracheostomy) is overcome. The system uses a known resistive coefficient of the tube, measures the flow through the tube, and then applies a pressure proportional to the resistance throughout the respiratory cycle (inspiration and expiration). It eliminates the imposed work of breathing during inspiration, and, by decreasing the PEEP, it compensates for the flow-dependent pressure drop across the endotracheal tube during expiration. Kinks or bends in the tube as it transverse the upper airway and secretions in the inner lumen may change the tube resistance and result in imperfect compensation. Some investigators have reported that automatic tube compensation improves patient comfort and helps to eliminate dynamic hyperinflation [18].

Determining Initial Ventilator Settings

The overall goal of mechanical ventilation is to provide acceptable gas exchange while causing the least amount of lung injury. Generally speaking, *aggressive* ventilation in terms of airway pressure, tidal volume, and FiO_2 results in better gas exchange but with a higher risk for the development of lung damage. Thus, one should always weigh the benefits of gas exchange against the injury caused to the lung in order to achieve it [19].

The definition of acceptable gas exchange is complex, and there are no validated values for $PaCO_2$ and SaO_2 toward which one should aim. In terms of $PaCO_2$, there has been a gradual acceptance of higher values than clinicians treating neonates [20] and adults with either asthma [21] or acute respiratory distress syndrome have historically practiced [22,23]. In these contexts, the higher levels of $PaCO_2$ are tolerated or *permitted* by the clinician, hence the term *permissive hypercapnia*. Such tolerance is not accepted when elevated $PaCO_2$ could be directly harmful, such as in the presence of intracranial hypertension or acute pulmonary hypertension. In addition, recent experimental work suggests that elevated $PaCO_2$ might be directly beneficial in certain situations [24], although these concepts have not been well tested outside the laboratory. Although the dangers of hypercapnia have received much attention, the dangers of hypocapnia are less well appreciated. In some circumstances hypocapnia is valuable (e.g., evolving brain stem herniation), but in many situations it is either of no benefit or potentially harmful [25].

The lowest acceptable level of oxygenation is even more difficult to define. Although there is no consensus regarding how low one might aim with arterial oxygen saturation (SaO_2), a lower target level of $SaO_2 > 90\%$–92% ($PaO_2 \approx 55\,mm\,Hg$) appears physiologically safe. Indeed, when high levels of PEEP, plateau pressure, and/or FiO_2 are required, clinicians will commonly accept lower target levels of SaO_2 (i.e., 85%–88%) [26].

In cases of parenchymal lung disease, lung compliance and the FRC are usually reduced. Unfortunately, the parenchymal lung disease is usually heterogeneous in nature, and different regions of the lung are differently affected. As a result, the mechanical properties are inhomogenous. The gas delivered will preferentially go to the regions with lower resistance and higher lung compliance. The rationale behind the setting of the ventilator is to homogenize the otherwise inhomogeneous disease (recruitment), to keep the lung open throughout the respiratory cycle (PEEP), and to avoid overdistension (limited tidal volume and/or plateau pressure) of the relatively healthy lung regions.

At this stage the ventilator setting should be tailored to each patient, and there are no proven formulaic guidelines. The basic principles for applying mechanical ventilation in a child with acute respiratory failure include the following:

1. Hemodynamic status should be optimized by ensuring intravascular volume and inotrope support in order to tolerate relative high PEEP.
2. The proportion of nonaerated lung should be minimized by recruitment.
3. The transpulmonary pressure and tidal volume should not be excessive.
4. Patient comfort must be ensured and some ventilatory effort ideally maintained.

The choice of pressure-targeted versus volume-targeted breath is not well established, and it often depends on the type of the ventilator and physician familiarity with the two modes unless the patient is a newborn, in which case pressure-targeted ventilation is preferable.

The optimal tidal volume is not well established, and it is still a matter of considerable debate. However, it is accepted that high tidal volume associated with high end-inspiratory pressure has a negative impact on outcome. Although a precise number for the optimal tidal volume for all critically children has not been identified (it is not likely that one exists), a reasonable approach would be to use the lowest tidal volume necessary to achieve acceptable gas exchange without predisposing to atelectasis. The level of hypercapnia associated with relative low tidal ventilation is usually not significant and it is well tolerated, and experimental evidence suggests that it may exert protective effects against development of VILI [27].

The peak expiratory pressure has a pivotal role in maintaining the unstable lung units open throughout the respiratory cycle and increasing the FRC. The overall effect here may be to limit the risk of VILI and improve oxygenation, thereby allowing the use of a lower FiO_2. However, simultaneously high levels of PEEP have the potential to cause circulatory depression and, by increasing the transpulmonary pressure and lung volume, may in turn contribute to overdistension and VILI. Recently a clinical trial with adults with acute respiratory distress syndrome who were ventilated with low tidal volume (6 mL/kg) and limited plateau pressure (30 cm H_2O) failed to show differences in mortality or length of ventilation between ventilation with high ($13.2 \pm 3.5\,cm\,H_2O$) and low ($8.3 \pm 3.2\,cm\,H_2O$) PEEP [28]. Thus, one could conclude that there are no well-established optimal PEEP levels, nor is there any clear framework with which to establish one. Some suggest determining the optimal PEEP by plotting the semistatic pressure-volume curve and setting the PEEP between the lower and higher inflection points, whereas others suggest increasing PEEP by 2 cm H_2O steps and watching for improvement in oxygenation and lung mechanics (compliance). We suggest optimizing intravascular fluid volume and then assessing the patient for recruitment potential by applying a recruitment maneuver and assessing improvement in oxygenation and lung mechanics (compliance). When the lung is not recruitable, PEEP should be maintained at a low level (5–8 cm H_2O); in contrast, when the lung appears recruitable, the PEEP should be increased gradually by steps of 2 cm H_2O while observing for improvement in oxygenation and lung mechanics. Whether a simultaneous response in improving ventilation associated with a decreased $PaCO_2$ can serve as a secondary indicator of recruitable lungs remains untested in children. Recruitment maneuvers need to be performed routinely, and the PEEP level should be assessed several times per day because the disease changes over time and a previously nonrecruited lung may become recruitable (and vice versa).

The transpulmonary pressure is the idealized pressure that affects the respiratory units. However, it is not normally monitored in the clinical setting, and its measurable analog may be the plateau pressure. Theoretically, in children, because of the higher chest wall compliance, there is a better correlation among the inspiratory pressure, plateau pressure (pressure at the end of inspiration with no flow), and transpulmonary pressure than in the adult. The plateau pressure may be measured in most modern ventilators. The difference between the peak inspiratory pressure measured by the ventilator and the plateau pressure is caused predominately by the tracheal and airway resistance. The transpulmonary pressure is theoretically 10%–30% lower than the plateau pressure. A transpulmonary pressure of 20 cm H_2O is generally safe, and, unless chest wall compliance is very low, plateau pressure should probably be <30 cm H_2O.

Levels of FiO_2 lower than 0.5 are usually considered safe. The initial FiO_2 should be 0.6 unless SaO_2 <92%. After setting the PEEP, FiO_2 should be set to the lowest level required to attain an SaO_2 >92%. In a sick patient, FiO_2 <0.3 is not recommended for safety reasons (e.g., inadvertent extubation). When FiO_2 >0.6 is required despite high levels of PEEP, the tolerated SaO_2 limit may be reduced to 85%–88%, and a trial of prone positioning or nitric oxide may be attempted.

The ventilatory rate is selected according patient age and nature of the disease and is then adjusted according to the $PaCO_2$ and patient comfort. The initial respiratory rate setting is ~40 breaths per minute for a neonate, ~20–25 breaths per minute for an infant, and decreases further with age. The inspiratory time may be selected in order to provide a certain inspiratory:expiratory ratio (usually 1:1.5 or 1:2) or to provide a preset inspiratory time. For neonates, the inspiratory time is usually set to 0.3–0.4 seconds, and this usually increases with age.

In heterogeneous lung disease with low compliance and variable time constants, the inspiratory time is usually longer in order to allow sufficient inflation. In contrast, in the case of obstructive lung disease (e.g., asthma, bronchiolitis), the expiratory time is set longer in order to allow the lung to fully empty, thereby avoiding air trapping and overinflation, which can be confirmed by auscultation, time-flow loops, and auto-PEEP determinations using an expiratory pause.

Triggering the Ventilator

To deliver a triggered breath the ventilator has to sense the patient's inspiratory effort. There are two principal mechanisms by which such sensing occurs—through changes in either pressure or flow. In most modern ventilators designated for pediatric use, a continuous base flow exists in the circuit. Sensors measure the delivered flow and the exhaled flow and continuously calculate the difference between the two. If no leak exists in the system or around the tracheal tube, the flow measured is identical in both sensors unless the patient makes an inspiratory effort. As the patient inspires from the baseline flow, the delivered flow remains unchanged but the exhaled flow is reduced. When the differences between the delivered and exhaled flow equal or are greater than the preset flow sensitivity, the ventilator commences an inspiration. With pressure sensitivity, a drop in pressure below the baseline end-expiratory pressure is the signal to commence a ventilator breath.

Because a noncuffed tube is commonly used in children, particularly in infants and neonates, a leak may exist around the tracheal tube. The leak causes a drop in flow and pressure in the circuit and may be detected as an inspiration; this will cause the ventilator to commence an inspiration, commonly called *auto-cycling* or *auto-triggering*. To compensate for a leak, the operator may attempt to increase the sensitivity to flow or pressure. The differences between flow and pressure sensitivity are subtle. With flow triggering, flow is experienced during the short interval between the start of the effort and the beginning of gas delivery. In contrast, with pressure triggering, a brief isometric effort is experienced. In clinical practice, there may be few significant differences between the two systems.

Complications of Mechanical Ventilation

Mechanical ventilation is a life-saving therapy in many circumstances; however, it is associated with numerous complications and adverse physiologic side effects, which, for the most part, have been studied in adult patients (Table 6.2). In a prospective study conducted by Zwillich et al., a total of 400 complications attributable to mechanical ventilation were observed in 345 consecutive patients [29]. The complications associated with mechanical ventilation can be classified as follows.

Respiratory Effects

Injury to the respiratory system can involve the upper airways and lungs. Airway injury may be caused by laryngoscopy, insertion of the tracheal tube, or presence of the tracheal tube for a prolonged time. Lung injury is due to mechanical stretch caused by the continuous pressure and volume changes associated with positive pressure ventilation. Such injury may be macroscopic (i.e., extraalveolar air leak) or microscopic; the latter is functionally and histologically similar to that observed in acute respiratory distress syndrome and is termed *ventilator-induced lung injury* (VILI). Additional pulmonary complications include ventilator-associated pneumonia and atelectasis.

Upper Airway Injury

Early complications related to tracheal intubation are mostly caused by traumatic intubation and include tooth avulsion or damage, laryngeal trauma, and pharyngeal injury ranging from mild edema to laceration with severe bleeding. Tissue injury secondary to prolonged intubation is likely caused by the pressure and shearing forces that the tube exerts on the surrounding tissues, which may be exacerbated by movement of the head or neck. Nasotracheal intubation may cause pressure sores or necrosis of the ala nasi or nasal septum, and oral intubation may cause similar ulceration at the angle of the mouth. Prolonged ventilation in neonates may cause grooves in the palate and, in extreme cases, a traumatic cleft.

Clinically apparent laryngeal injury is relatively rare and ranges from mild edema to ulceration of the mucosa. Significant vocal cord injury may be minimal or, in extreme cases, involve subluxation of the arytenoid cartilages with subsequent vocal cord fixation. The more frequent and clinically significant complications occur in the subglottic region (i.e., below the vocal cords). This region is a narrower region in children than in adults, and it is the only region with a complete circumferential cartilaginous ring that does not allow for expansion under pressure. Autopsy studies demonstrate the presence of subglottic trauma in over 75% of ventilated children. Infection and ischemic necrosis may develop over time, and, during healing, granulation tissue or, in the absence of resolution, an organized scar may evolve causing subglottic stenosis and clinically significant airway obstruction. Similar injury may develop deeper in the trachea at the tip of the tracheal tube or at the carina as a result of continuous epithelial injury from the suction catheter.

Some of the injuries may be prevented by skillful intubation, with a proper size tube, and taking care with tube repositioning, taping, and carefully measured suctioning lengths. When a cuffed tracheal tube is being used, the cuff should be deflated daily for assessment of a leak and then inflated to a maximal pressure no greater than 25 cm H_2O. Underlying clinical factors that may increase the risk of tissue injury include tissue hypoxia (exacerbated by hypotension or hypoxemia), capillary leak, hypoalbuminemia (causing edema formation), and local infection.

Air Leak

Macroscopic air leak has been reported in up to 40% of children receiving mechanical ventilation [30]. Excessive transpulmonary pressure and overdistension lead to alveolar rupture and escape into the pulmonary interstitium (i.e., pulmonary interstitial emphysema [PIE]). Extension of this may involve the mediastinum (i.e., pneumomediastinum), the pleural space (i.e., pneumothorax), or the pericardium (i.e., pneumopericardium), or it may propagate into the subcutaneous space (i.e., subcutaneous emphysema). Subcutaneous emphysema, pneumopericardium, and PIE are usually not clinically significant, although the former may cause discomfort.

Pneumothorax is generally the most important type of air leak. If continuous, air may enter the pleural space with each inspiration, and, because it cannot exit the space, a net accumulation occurs, with steadily increasing pressure (i.e., tension pneumothorax). Over time, the volume of air and the pressure in the pleural space increase significantly, causing collapse of the ipsilateral lung, shift of the mediastinum, obstruction of the venous return, and compromise of the cardiac output. Tension pneumothorax should be immediately suspected in any mechanically ventilated child who unexpectedly experiences an acute deterioration in oxygenation or cardiac output. Unless it is rapidly diagnosed and drained, it may cause death. Air leak is rare in otherwise healthy lungs, in the absence of excessive airway pressures. Retrospective studies have shown the association of occurrence or air leak with high levels of PIP, PEEP, or tidal volume [31,32]. Application of a protective ventilation strategy that limits plateau pressure and tidal volume may decrease the risk of air leak.

Ventilation-Associated Pneumonia

Pneumonia occurring beyond 48 hours after tracheal intubation is commonly attributed to mechanical ventilation, and is called *ventilator-associated pneumonia* (VAP). Although a common cause of morbidity in adult critical care, it is not well characterized in children. In critically ill adults, the incidence may be as high as 70% overall. Duration of mechanical ventilation, severity of underlying disease, use of neuromuscular blockade, prolonged supine positioning, and head injury all appear to be important risk factors [33].

Ventilator-associated pneumonia is principally a clinical diagnosis based on the appearance of new infiltrates on chest radiography, purulent endotracheal secretions, and the presence of fever or leukocytosis. The microbiologic diagnosis can be confirmed by obtaining a tracheal aspirate for culture during suction, bronchoalveolar lavage (BAL), or bronchoscopic-protected specimen brush sampling, although the latter is rarely performed in children. When the diagnosis of VAP is established on clinical grounds, microbiologic confirmation (i.e., BAL) should be sought and therapy (directed by the local microbial sensitivity profile) commenced pending microbiologic confirmation. The antibiotics should be tailored according to the response and the subsequent microbiologic data.

Aspiration of previously colonized oropharyngeal flora may be the initiating step in development of VAP, and Gram-negative bacilli are the most frequent bacterial causes. After 4 days of mechanical ventilation, the most common organisms include methicillin-resistant *Staphylococcus aureus* and *Pseudomonas aeruginosa*. It is important to recognize the local resistance patterns when making empiric choices about initial antibiotic therapy. Measures that may reduce the risks of VAP include the following: placing patients in a semirecumbent position, establishing a continuous subglottic suctioning routine, changing heat-moisture exchangers, using a nasojejunal instead of a nasogastric tube, and maintaining oral hygiene [34]. The role of prophylactic antibiotics is not well established.

Atelectasis

Injured lungs have a low compliance and a tendency to collapse [35]. Mechanical ventilation increases the risk by direct lung injury, retention of secretions, de-nitrogenation during ventilation with 100% oxygen, endobronchial placement of the endotracheal tube, and intermittent suctioning. Furthermore, neuromuscular blockade, commonly used during mechanical ventilation, abolishes diaphragmatic tone and further decreases FRC. Because infants have a relatively lower FRC and less collateral ventilation than adults, they may be at even greater risk of developing atelectasis [36]. Atelectasis is important because it may compromise oxygenation, increase pulmonary artery pressure, and contribute to VILI by overdistension of the ventilated lung regions. It may be treated with positioning, physiotherapy, increasing the PEEP, and using routine, short recruitment maneuvers. Prolonged ventilation may contribute to *disuse atrophy* of the diaphragm, which has been demonstrated in animal studies but not in humans. However, it seems that maintenance of spontaneous respiratory effort may mitigate against this problem.

Central Nervous System Effects

The effects of positive pressure ventilation have been extensively studied in the context of head trauma, but the effects on intracranial pressure (ICP) and cerebral perfusion pressure are complicated. Some issues are apparent from several studies. The application of PEEP may directly increase ICP by transmission of pleural pressure through vertebral veins toward the cranium. Indirectly, PEEP may increase ICP by increasing the right ventricular afterload, decreasing right ventricular output, and decreasing venous return—including the venous return from the skull. These effects are more prominent in patients with normal ICP and are minimal in the context of modestly elevated ICP [37]. Furthermore, increased PEEP may decrease cardiac output and systemic arterial pressure, thereby reducing cerebral perfusion pressure.

Cardiovascular Effects

The heart is a pressure chamber within another pressure chamber, the thorax. Because the pulmonary vasculature, right ventricle and left atrium all exist in the same pressure chamber (i.e., thorax), changes in pleural and intrathoracic pressures affect them identically. However, intrathoracic pressure will affect the pressure

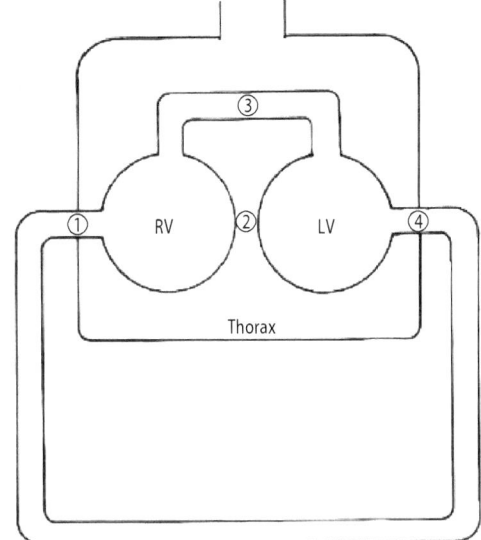

FIGURE 6.8. Schematic model of the cardiovascular effects of mechanical ventilation. (1) Changes in intrathoracic pressure decrease the venous return. (2) Increases in pulmonary vascular resistance may affect the end ventricular diastolic volume and shift the common interventricular septum, affecting the compliance of the other. (3) Changes in lung volume may increase the resistance to pulmonary flow, increasing the afterload for the right ventricle. (4) Changes in intrathoracic pressure may reduce transmural aortic pressure, reducing the afterload for the left ventricle. (From Dantzker DR., Cardiopulmonary Critical Care, 2nd ed. Philadelphia: WB Saunders; 1991:111. Reprinted with permission from Elsevier.)

gradient for both blood draining into the heart (i.e., venous return) and blood leaving the heart (i.e., left ventricle ejection) independent of cardiac function. The overall effects of mechanical ventilation on cardiovascular function are discussed here (Figure 6.8) and in Chapter 45.

During inspiration with positive pressure ventilation, the thorax expands and the lung volume and intrathoracic pressure increase. In contrast, with a negative pressure (or spontaneous) inspiration, the changes are in the opposite direction: the volumes of the thorax and lung increase, but the intrathoracic pressure decreases. It is important to understand that the pressure that the clinician usually observes during mechanical ventilation is the airway pressure, which is that pressure in the proximal trachea, not the pressure transmitted to the lung. During positive pressure ventilation, the volume of the lung increases only by increasing the airway pressure; only part of this pressure is transmitted to the lung. The pleural pressure may be monitored with an esophageal probe, but this is not routine in most centers.

In cases where lung compliance is reduced, as in acute respiratory distress syndrome, or lung resistance is increased, as in asthma, the percentage of airway pressure transferred to pleural pressure is lower than when chest wall compliance is reduced. Generally, when tidal volume is kept constant, the changes in airway pressure reflect mostly the changes in the mechanics of the lung and will not reflect changes in intrathoracic pressure. Additional reviews of cardiorespiratory interaction during positive pressure ventilation are given in Chapter 45 and elsewhere [38,39].

Venous Return

When intrathoracic pressure increases, right atrial atmospheric pressure also increases. The systemic venous return, which is the

principal determinate of cardiac output in the normal heart, depends on the gradient between the upstream mean systemic pressure and the downstream pressure in the right atrium. An increment in the right atrial pressure therefore decreases the venous return to the right atrium, decreasing the filling pressure and stroke volume of the right ventricle. The reduction in venous return caused by an elevation in right atrial pressure may be of a lower magnitude than the increases seen with a reduction in right atrial pressure. This occurs because, during positive pressure ventilation, the intraabdominal pressure increases, increasing the mean systemic pressure.

The hemodynamic effects of increased intrathoracic pressure are, under normal conditions, not clinically significant. However, in certain clinical conditions the effect of elevated intrathoracic pressure may compromise cardiac output. These include hypovolemia, relative hypovolemia (e.g., septic shock), and obstructive right heart lesions and/or right ventricle failure. Often this effect is countered by effects on left ventricular afterload.

Left Ventricular Afterload

The left ventricle and thoracic aorta are also in the thorax, and both are affected by changes in intrathoracic pressure. The pressure that left ventricular work is directed against is the transmural pressure and not the pressure measured outside the thorax. The transmural pressure of the aorta is the difference between the intravascular pressure (positive) and the intrathoracic pressure (negative during spontaneous respiration). During spontaneous inspiration the intrathoracic pressure decreases (becomes more negative) and as a result the transmural pressure increases ($P_{tm} = P_{iv} - P_{it}$), thereby increasing the afterload of the left ventricle. Conversely, during positive pressure ventilation the intrathoracic pressure becomes positive and as a result the transmural pressure decreases, thereby decreasing the afterload of the left ventricle. Thus, the application of positive pressure ventilation with PEEP (or just CPAP) was shown to improve significantly cardiac output in patients with heart failure [40]. Most commonly these swings in intrathoracic pressure are not clinically significant in otherwise healthy children under normal conditions. However, they may become clinically significant in extreme situations, such as severe upper-airway obstruction when the intrathoracic pressure significantly decreases, resulting in a substantial increase in the afterload of the left ventricle and contributing to the development of acute pulmonary edema.

Cardiovascular Effects of Change in Lung Volume

A key effect of altered lung volume is on the pulmonary circulation, a low-resistance, low-pressure system. The pulmonary vessels can be classified to alveolar and extraalveolar vessels. The alveolar vessels are small vessels (i.e., capillaries, arterioles, and venules) that are adjacent to the alveolar wall. The extraalveolar vessels are the larger vessels in the interstitium. The total pulmonary vascular resistance is the sum of the resistance in both the alveolar and the extraalveolar vessels. A change in lung volume has different effects on both systems. In normal lung mechanics, ventilation around FRC is associated with the nadir of pulmonary vascular resistance. However, when the lung is inflated above FRC, the distended alveoli may compress the alveolar vessels and increase the vascular vessels. Similarly, as lung volume falls below FRC, the extraalveolar vessels become more tortuous, the transmural pressure increases, and the vessels tend to collapse, resulting in increased total pulmonary vascular resistance. Thus, at least in the isolated perfused lung (although never conclusively demonstrated in humans), maintenance of the lung volume at physiologic FRC will yield optimal pulmonary vascular resistance. Furthermore, in the case of ventilation with small tidal volumes, certain areas of the lung tend to collapse, causing alveolar hypoxia, which in turn may activate hypoxic pulmonary vasoconstriction. Indeed, in contrast to the traditional beliefs outlined earlier, newer in vivo data suggest that, during atelectasis, alveolar hypoxia, not volume loss, may be the key determinant of increased pulmonary vascular resistance [36].

Ventricular Interdependence

The right and left ventricles pump in series and share a common intraventricular septum. If the right ventricular volume increases, it shifts the septum to the left, reducing left ventricular filling volume and compromising left ventricular diastolic function.

Ventricular interdependence is not a significant factor in positive pressure ventilation unless pulmonary vascular resistance is increased significantly. Some suggest that this phenomenon may become clinically significant in patients with acutely injured lungs whose echocardiographic studies have revealed leftward shift with the application of PEEP, most probably because of the increase in pulmonary vascular resistance and right ventricular afterload.

Renal Effects

Mechanical ventilation with positive pressure induces a reduction in renal water and sodium excretion. This effect appears to be exacerbated by PEEP. The rise in intrathoracic pressure, administration of sedatives and analgesic drugs, and immobility reduce venous return and cardiac output and may eventually lower mean arterial pressure. As a result, renal perfusion decreases, and the renin–angiotensin system is stimulated. Angiotensin II formation stimulates aldosterone production, resulting in increased resorption of water and sodium. Low systemic blood pressure increases the secretion of antidiuretic hormone, which also decreases urinary output. Reduced venous return and decreased right atrial pressure results in reduced levels of atrial natriuretic peptide to further reduce diuresis. These issues are particularly important when discontinuing mechanical ventilation, as, in the presence of good cardiac function, a large diuresis may occur.

The biotrauma hypothesis suggests that nonprotective ventilation may release inflammatory mediators into the systemic circulation that potentially cause renal dysfunction [41]. These effects are not significant in a healthy kidney and usually resolve after administration of extra fluid. However, the clinician must be aware of the phenomenon, especially when significant underlying real disease coexists.

Hepatic Effects

Blood flow to the liver represents the balance of flow through the hepatic artery and portal circulation. The reduction of cardiac output associated with positive pressure ventilation may reduce flow through the hepatic artery. In addition, positive pressure ventilation increases intraabdominal pressure, which may decrease portal vein flow. Many patients receiving positive pressure ventilation demonstrate some degree of hepatic dysfunction; it is not clear whether positive pressure ventilation is causative here or whether the dysfunction represents underlying systemic disease. The precise clinical significance of the positive pressure on liver function in the critically ill is not clear.

Weaning from Mechanical Ventilation

Weaning is the word used to describe termination of mechanical ventilation, because in most adult cases it is a gradual and sometimes long process. However, in children, the more appropriate term would be *liberation* or *termination* of mechanical ventilation, because most children can be easily weaned from the ventilator without either delay or significant problems. Only a small group of children, usually those with underlying chronic pulmonary disease, neurologic disease, or malnutrition are difficult to wean.

One should distinguish between extubation failure and weaning failure. Weaning failure is failure of the patient to maintain ventilation and oxygenation when the ventilatory support is reduced. Extubation failure assumes that the patient has in fact been successfully weaned from ventilatory support and that it is the extubation (i.e., later phase) not the weaning (i.e., earlier phase) that has not been successful. In general, a need for reintubation for any reason within 24 hours after elective extubation is termed *extubation failure*. The major causes of extubation failure include upper airway obstruction from postextubation stridor, poor airway protection, excess secretions, and pulmonary atelectasis. Assessment of the airway for extubation readiness is clinical, and the presence of supraglottic edema, if suspected, most commonly by the absence of an endotracheal leak, can be ascertained by direct laryngoscopy.

For adults the rates of reintubation range from 2% to 20% and are similar for children. The major risk factors associated with extubation failure in children are young age (i.e., <3 years), duration of ventilation, severity of underline lung disease, oxygenation impairment (i.e., oxygenation index >5), and intravenous sedation. The mortality rate increases significantly for children who require reintubation; however, it is impossible to establish whether it is directly attributable to the extubation failure or to the underlying disease. Because of the numerous complications and side effects associated mechanical ventilation, it is widely recognized that it is advantageous to remove the patient from mechanical ventilation as early as it is safe to do so. The duration of mechanical ventilation is known to be an independent risk factor for morbidity, especially VAP; however, premature discontinuation of mechanical ventilation may result in reintubation and additional complications. Thus, the value of removing the ventilator as soon as possible must be balanced against the risks of premature withdrawal.

Termination of mechanical ventilation should always be approached with caution. A rapid approach is possible for children after a short period of intubation (e.g., following surgery) and when the patient has no underlying lung disease. For other patients who have recovered from relatively longer periods of ventilation and potentially severe respiratory failure, a more gradual approach is required. The gradual transition from full or almost full mechanical support to spontaneous breathing may be accomplished by gradually decreasing the mandatory breath rate with SIMV, the level of PEEP, and/or the degree of pressure or volume support. Sedation should be reduced carefully in order not to compromise both the respiratory drive and patient comfort or to precipitate drug withdrawal. During this period, gas exchange and breathing pattern should be assessed. Generally, before discontinuation of mechanical ventilation, patients should be hemodynamically stable, alert, and capable of protecting their airway (i.e., adequate cough and gag) and have no severe metabolic abnormalities that may affect their work of breathing or muscular strength.

The best approach for all patients is to question (perhaps several times) every day: Why are they receiving mechanical ventilation? Do they require the current levels of support? Do they actually still need to be ventilated? There are no well-established methods to predict successful extubation in children, and it unfortunately is impossible to mimic breathing without an endotracheal tube unless an extubation is performed. Purely protocol-directed extubation strategies have yielded inconsistent results. However, it appears that, when clinical standards are reasonable, protocol-directed weaning regimens offer no advantage over usual practice for the weaning of either adults [42] or children [43].

A trial of spontaneous breathing with assessment of the gas exchange and pattern of breathing with minimal pressure support (~10 cm H_2O) or T-tube without pressure support appears to be equally useful approaches in order to evaluate readiness for extubation. Usually levels of PaO_2 <60 mm Hg, where FiO_2 >0.4 constitutes a relative contraindication to extubation. In addition, significantly increased respiratory rate or reduction in tidal volume (or particularly a combination of both) during spontaneous breathing strongly suggests that the patient is not ready for extubation.

The potential for postextubation stridor may be assessed by evaluating the presence of an air leak around the endotracheal tube, although clinical studies do not strongly support this. This may be performed by auscultation after deflation of the cuff in a cuffed endotracheal tube by comparing the inspiratory and expiratory tidal volumes as measured by the ventilator or by manually applying a positive pressure of 25–30 cm H_2O and assessing the leak by auscultation. Administration of corticosteroids before extubation and for a short period following extubation have been demonstrated to confer a minor benefit in terms of a lower rate of reintubation [44]. The administration of inhaled racemic epinephrine or heliox or application of noninvasive positive pressure ventilation for a short period of time may decrease the rate of reintubation in cases of postextubation stridor.

Conclusion

Mechanical ventilation plays a pivotal role in the treatment of critically ill children. Applying knowledge of childhood physiology and ventilation techniques may be among the most important skills a physician will need in critical care medicine. Over time, mechanical ventilators have become more sophisticated, new modes of ventilation have been introduced, and monitoring techniques have undergone dramatic improvements. With the recognition of the complications associated with positive pressure ventilation and the advances in monitoring, it is possible that in the near future we will be able to tailor, in real-time, the modality of ventilation to a specific patient with a specific disease.

References

1. Dunnill MS. Postnatal growth of the lung. Thorax 1962;17:329–333.
2. Thorsteinsson A, Jonmarker C, Larsson A, Vilstrup C, Werner O. Functional residual capacity in anesthetized children: normal values and values in children with cardiac anomalies. Anesthesiology 1990;73(5):876–881.
3. Thorsteinsson A, Larsson A, Jonmarker C, Werner O. Pressure–volume relations of the respiratory system in healthy children. Am J Respir Crit Care Med 1994;150(2):421–430.
4. Copland IB, Martinez F, Kavanagh BP, et al. High tidal volume ventilation causes different inflammatory responses in newborn versus adult lung. Am J Respir Crit Care Med 2004;169(6):739–748.
5. Katz S, Selvadurai H, Keilty K, Mitchell M, MacLusky I. Outcome of non-invasive positive pressure ventilation in paediatric neuromuscular disease. Arch Dis Child 2004;89(2):121–124.
6. Piastra M, Antonelli M, Chiaretti A, Polidori G, Polidori L, Conti G. Treatment of acute respiratory failure by helmet-delivered noninvasive pressure support ventilation in children with acute leukemia: a pilot study. Intensive Care Med 2004;30(3):472–476.
7. Piastra M, Conti G, Caresta E, et al. Noninvasive ventilation options in pediatric myasthenia gravis. Paediatr Anaesth 2005;15(8):699–702.
8. Kavanagh BP, Roy L. Pediatric ventilation—towards simpler approaches for complex diseases. Paediatr Anaesth 2005;15(8):627–629.
9. Samuels MP, Raine J, Wright T, et al. Continuous negative extrathoracic pressure in neonatal respiratory failure. Pediatrics 1996;98(6 Pt 1):1154–1160.
10. Hartmann H, Jawad MH, Noyes J, Samuels MP, Southall DP. Negative extrathoracic pressure ventilation in central hypoventilation syndrome. Arch Dis Child 1994;70(5):418–423.
11. Corrado A, Gorini M, Villella G, De Paola E. Negative pressure ventilation in the treatment of acute respiratory failure: an old noninvasive technique reconsidered. Eur Respir J 1996;9(7):1531–1544.
12. Shekerdemian LS, Schulze-Neick I, Redington AN, Bush A, Penny DJ. Negative pressure ventilation as haemodynamic rescue following surgery for congenital heart disease. Intensive Care Med 2000;26(1):93–96.
13. Guldager H, Nielsen SL, Carl P, Soerensen MB. A comparison of volume control and pressure-regulated volume control ventilation in acute respiratory failure. Crit Care (Lond) 1997;1(2):75–77.
14. Younes M. Proportional assist ventilation, a new approach to ventilatory support. Theory. Am Rev Respir Dis 1992;145(1):114–120.
15. Ambrosino N, Rossi A. Proportional assist ventilation (PAV): a significant advance or a futile struggle between logic and practice? Thorax 2002;57(3):272–276.
16. Navalesi P, Costa R. New modes of mechanical ventilation: proportional assist ventilation, neurally adjusted ventilatory assist, and fractal ventilation. Curr Opin Crit Care 2003;9(1):51–58.
17. Boker A, Graham MR, Walley KR, et al. Improved arterial oxygenation with biologically variable or fractal ventilation using low tidal volumes in a porcine model of acute respiratory distress syndrome. Am J Respir Crit Care Med 2002;165(4):456–462.
18. Fabry B, Haberthur C, Zappe D, Guttmann J, Kuhlen R, Stocker R. Breathing pattern and additional work of breathing in spontaneously breathing patients with different ventilatory demands during inspiratory pressure support and automatic tube compensation. Intensive Care Med 1997;23(5):545–552.
19. Kavanagh BP. Goals and concerns for oxygenation in acute respiratory distress syndrome. Curr Opin Crit Care 1998;4:16–20.
20. Wung JT, James LS, Kilchevsky E, James E. Management of infants with severe respiratory failure and persistence of the fetal circulation, without hyperventilation. Pediatrics 1985;76:488–494.
21. Darioli R, Perret C. Mechanical controlled hypoventilation in status asthmaticus. Am Rev Respir Dis 1984;129(3):385–387.
22. Hickling KG, Walsh J, Henderson S, Jackson R. Low mortality rate in adult respiratory distress syndrome using low-volume, pressure-limited ventilation with permissive hypercapnia: a prospective study. Crit Care Med 1994;22:1568–1578.
23. Hickling KG, Henderson SJ, Jackson R. Low mortality associated with low volume pressure limited ventilation with permissive hypercapnia in severe adult respiratory distress syndrome. Intensive Care Med 1990;16:372–377.
24. Laffey JG, Kavanagh BP. Carbon dioxide and the critically ill—too little of a good thing [hypothesis paper]? Lancet 1999;354:1283–1286.

25. Laffey JG, Tanaka M, Engelberts D, et al. Therapeutic hypercapnia reduces pulmonary and systemic injury following in vivo lung reperfusion. Am J Respir Crit Care Med 2000;162(6):2287–2294.

26. Mao C, Wong DT, Slutsky AS, Kavanagh BP. A quantitative assessment of how Canadian intensivists believe they utilize oxygen in the intensive care unit. Crit Care Med 1999;27(12):2806–2811.

27. Broccard AF, Hotchkiss JR, Vannay C, et al. Protective effects of hypercapnic acidosis on ventilator-induced lung injury. Am J Respir Crit Care Med 2001;164(5):802–806.

28. The National Heart Lung and Blood Institute ARDS Clinical Trials Network. Higher versus lower positive end-expiratory pressures in patients with the acute respiratory distress syndrome. N Engl J Med 2004;351(4):327–336.

29. Zwillich CW, Pierson DJ, Creagh CE, Sutton FD, Schatz E, Petty TL. Complications of assisted ventilation. A prospective study of 354 consecutive episodes. Am J Med 1974;57(2):161–170.

30. Pfenninger J, Gerber A, Tschappeler H, Zimmermann A. Adult respiratory distress syndrome in children. J Pediatr 1982;101(3):352–357.

31. Woodside KJ, vanSonnenberg E, Chon KS, Loran DB, Tocino IM, Zwischenberger JB. Pneumothorax in patients with acute respiratory distress syndrome: pathophysiology, detection, and treatment. J Intensive Care Med 2003;18(1):9–20.

32. Mutlu GM, Factor P. Complications of mechanical ventilation. Respir Care Clin North Am 2000;6(2):213–252, v.

33. Cook DJ, Walter SD, Cook RJ, et al. Incidence of and risk factors for ventilator-associated pneumonia in critically ill patients. Ann Intern Med 1998;129(6):433–440.

34. Dodek P, Keenan S, Cook D, et al. Evidence-based clinical practice guideline for the prevention of ventilator-associated pneumonia. Ann Intern Med 2004;141(4):305–313.

35. Duggan M, Kavanagh BP. Pulmonary atelectasis: a pathogenic perioperative entity. Anesthesiology 2005;102(4):838–854.

36. Duggan M, McNamara PJ, Engelberts D, et al. Oxygen attenuates atelectasis-induced injury in the in vivo rat lung. Anesthesiology 2005; 103(3):522–531.

37. McGuire G, Crossley D, Richards J, Wong D. Effects of varying levels of positive end-expiratory pressure on intracranial pressure and cerebral perfusion pressure. Crit Care Med 1997;25(6):1059–1062.

38. Pinsky MR. The hemodynamic consequences of mechanical ventilation: an evolving story. Intensive Care Med 1997;23(5):493–503.

39. Shekerdemian L, Bohn D. Cardiovascular effects of mechanical ventilation. Arch Dis Child 1999;80(5):475–480.

40. Sin DD, Logan AG, Fitzgerald FS, Liu PP, Bradley TD. Effects of continuous positive airway pressure on cardiovascular outcomes in heart failure patients with and without Cheyne-Stokes respiration. Circulation 2000;102(1):61–66.

41. Ranieri VM, Suter PM, Tortorella C, et al. Effect of mechanical ventilation on inflammatory mediators in patients with acute respiratory distress syndrome: a randomized controlled trial. JAMA 1999;282(1): 54–61.

42. Krishnan JA, Moore D, Robeson C, Rand CS, Fessler HE. A prospective, controlled trial of a protocol-based strategy to discontinue mechanical ventilation. Am J Respir Crit Care Med 2004;169(6):673–678.

43. Randolph AG, Wypij D, Venkataraman ST, et al. Effect of mechanical ventilator weaning protocols on respiratory outcomes in infants and children: a randomized controlled trial. JAMA 2002;288(20):2561–2568.

44. Markovitz BP, Randolph AG. Corticosteroids for the prevention of reintubation and postextubation stridor in pediatric patients: a meta-analysis. Pediatr Crit Care Med 2002;3(3):223–226.

7
Ventilator-Induced Lung Injury

Shinya Tsuchida and Brian P. Kavanagh

Introduction

When considering mechanical ventilation, is it important to avoid an injurious ventilator strategy in the treatment of acute respiratory distress syndrome (ARDS) patients? We believe that the answer is "absolutely yes," because two landmark studies have conclusively demonstrated that how the mechanical ventilator is set has a direct effect on patient mortality [1,2]. Indeed, as reviewed through this chapter, such work represented the clinical confirmation of multiple laboratory studies [3]. Amato and colleagues [1] demonstrated the superiority of a protective strategy comprising low tidal volume, high positive end-expiratory pressure (PEEP), and recruitment maneuvers. Focusing on the tidal volume alone, the investigators from the ARDS Network [2] clearly demonstrated that ventilation with 6 mL/kg predicted body weight resulted in a lower mortality rate than ventilation with 12 mL/kg. Although Eichacker et al. [4] pointed out in their meta-analysis that control groups in these trials might not have reflected the current best standards at that time, it is clear that mechanical ventilation can have an impact on mortality.

The theory of a lung protective strategy is twofold: prevention of atelectasis and prevention of lung overinflation. In fact, there are many practical issues in the application of a lung protective strategy for clinical use. This is further complicated in the pediatric intensive care unit, because the most important data, those studies demonstrating an effect of ventilation on outcome [1,2], are from adult studies only. Furthermore, the accumulating data from the experimental studies, although teaching us to be "gentle" with the injured lung [3], have not elucidated the precise mechanisms of ventilator-induced lung injury, nor have they informed us of the optimal mode of protective ventilation. These "clinical unknowns" are the rationale for reviewing clinical trials and experimental studies in this chapter.

Low Tidal Volume Lessens Ventilator-Induced Lung Injury

In their classic in vivo experiments, Webb and Tierney [5] found that high peak inspiratory pressure combined with zero PEEP was fatally injurious. This was the first demonstration of lethal pulmonary *barotrauma*. Dreyfuss et al. [6] bound the chests, of in vivo anesthetized animals, thereby developing high airway pressures but without high tidal volumes. They found that elevated tidal volume, as opposed to airway pressure per se, was paramount in inducing ventilator-induced lung injury, thus establishing the concept of *volutrauma* [6]. This elegant concept was challenged by Broccard et al. [7], who compared independently the effects of mean airway pressure versus tidal volume under conditions of constant pulmonary blood flow using ex vivo perfused rabbit lungs. They concluded that mean airway pressure contributed more than tidal volume to the increase in pulmonary vascular permeability. They attributed the mechanism whereby high mean airway pressure promoted lung edema formation to the increase of pulmonary vascular resistance and thereby increased (extraalveolar) vascular transmural pressure [7]. Notwithstanding that high stretch has been investigated in terms of the peak airway pressure, tidal volume, and mean airway pressure, it is unclear which of these three factors is most crucial to the progression of ventilator-induced lung injury.

Given that some combination of high tidal volume and elevated airway pressure is harmful, a reasonable supposition might be: "The lower the tidal volume, the better the outcome." Unfortunately, this is also a complex issue. Atelectasis may develop through the use of low tidal volume ventilation and cause *atelectrauma*, especially in the absence of PEEP. Chiumello et al. [8] demonstrated in their studies of rats following acid-aspiration lung injury that, although high tidal volume was adverse (particularly in terms of inflammatory cytokine production), the greatest mortality occurred in those animals ventilated with low tidal volume in the absence of

D.S. Wheeler et al. (eds.), The *Respiratory Tract in Pediatric Critical Illness and Injury*,
DOI 10.1007/978-1-84800-925-7_7, © Springer-Verlag London Limited 2009

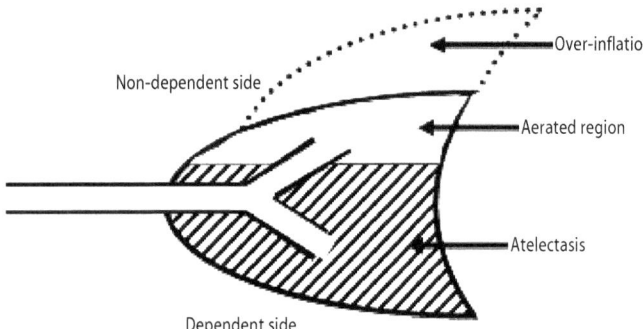

FIGURE 7.1. A schematic illustration of the baby lung concept. In an extensively atelectatic lung, tidal volume will be shifted toward the small aerated lung (baby lung), resulting in overdistention in this region.

PEEP. A similar finding was reported in the absence of preexisting lung injury, wherein a high mortality rate occurred with low tidal volume ventilation (without PEEP or supplemental oxygen) and was attributed to right ventricular failure [9]. On the contrary, in acid-injured in vivo rats, very low tidal volumes (as low as 3 mL/kg) were more protective than higher tidal volumes at the same (elevated) level of PEEP (10 cm H_2O) [10]. Although the atelectasis may partly depend on the PEEP level, it should be elucidated whether low tidal volume is protective against atelectasis-associated lung injury, and, if so, how. Indeed, more questions continue to evolve in this area [11].

A particularly important thesis is the possibility that, because of the heterogeneous nature of the disease, a given tidal volume may ventilate only the healthy portion of the ARDS lungs. This possibility was proposed by Gattinoni et al. [12], who examined the amount of aerated lung tissue and the pressure–volume (PV) curve to different PEEP levels in ARDS patients. As a result, they suggested that the PV curve in ARDS reflects only the residual healthy zones and does not directly estimate the injured zones. Hence, apparently a low tidal volume based on body weight could conceivably be too high for the remaining aerated portion of lung, resulting in ventilator-induced lung injury caused by the overdistention (Gattinoni's so-called baby lung concept; Figure 7.1). Substantiating this concept is the observation that air cysts and bronchiectasis prevail in the nondependent (better-ventilated) areas in ARDS patients [13].

High Positive End-Expiratory Pressure Protects Against Injury with Low Tidal Volumes

A recent clinical trial (i.e., the ALVEOLI study) performed by the ARDS Network [14] was unable to find differences in the clinical outcomes of ARDS patients who were assigned to either the higher PEEP strategy (13.2 ± 3.5 cm H_2O) or the lower PEEP strategy (8.3 ± 3.2 cm H_2O), with the targeted tidal volume being the same in both groups (6 mL/kg). This whole area is problematic, however, as the stated hypothesis was that elevated PEEP may help in some situations and harm in others [14]. Such a dual hypothesis is of course completely defensible on physiologic grounds, as these contrasting effects of PEEP are precisely what is predicted based on many years of physiologic research. However, a fundamental problem with the ALVEOLI study was that, having advanced such

a hypothesis, the investigators then proceeded to randomize patients without attempting to identify those patients who might benefit and/or those who might be harmed by the high PEEP intervention. This negative trial follows another study conducted 20 years earlier [15] that demonstrated that the early application of 8 cm H_2O PEEP was not useful for the prevention of ARDS compared with zero PEEP at the same tidal volume (12 mL/kg). What arises from these clinical studies are the questions of whether the level of PEEP has an impact on outcome and whether PEEP has been subjected to testing with sufficient physiologic stratification.

Important work is, however, available from the laboratory. Muscedere et al. [16] compared 0, 4, and 15 cm H_2O PEEP ventilated with the same low tidal volume (6 mL/kg) in ex vivo, nonperfused saline-lavaged rat lungs. They found that 15 cm H_2O PEEP (i.e., above the inflection point on the PV curve) was protective, and, notably, the injured sites depended on the PEEP level. While 4 cm H_2O PEEP (i.e., below the inflection point on the PV curve) showed mainly alveolar injury, zero PEEP exhibited mostly bronchiolar injury. The investigators attributed these differences to the repetitive opening and closing of airways at different sites (Figure 7.2). According to Tremblay's ex vivo, nonperfused ventilation model in which end-inspiratory lung volume was made equivalent, high tidal volume without PEEP was more injurious, producing more tumor necrosis factor-α (TNF- α) protein and c-*fos* mRNA than the combination of "moderate" tidal volume with high PEEP [17]. Indeed, the progression of ventilator-induced lung injury was reported to be delayed in proportion to the increasing level of PEEP employed in an in vivo rat model, where end-inspiratory lung volume was matched [18]. Additionally, the superiority of high PEEP over low PEEP in in vivo saline-lavaged rabbits has been demonstrated, where mean airway pressure and plateau pressure are similar [19].

However, not all studies are so positive. High PEEP (10 cm H_2O) has been compared with lower PEEP (3 cm H_2O) in an in vivo rabbit model of acid aspiration, demonstrating that there were no significant differences in histologic findings between the two groups [20]. Interestingly, 3 to 4 cm H_2O PEEP is most frequently used for surfactant-treated infants with respiratory distress syndrome (RDS).

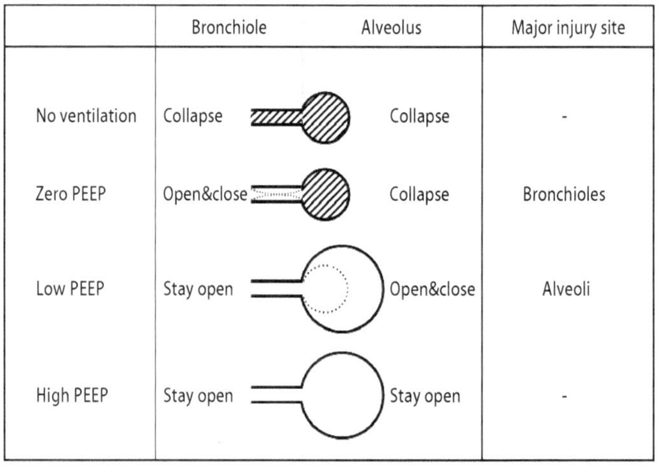

	Bronchiole		Alveolus	Major injury site
No ventilation	Collapse		Collapse	-
Zero PEEP	Open&close		Collapse	Bronchioles
Low PEEP	Stay open		Open&close	Alveoli
High PEEP	Stay open		Stay open	-

FIGURE 7.2. A schematic illustration of repetitive opening and closing of airways as a cause of atelectasis-associated lung injury. The degree of lung recruitment is a determinant of lung injury and its site in an atelectasis-prone lung. The repetitive opening and closing of distal airways is essential in the progression of atelectasis-associated lung injury. PEEP, positive end-expiratory pressure.

A comparison of 0, 4, and 7 cm H_2O PEEP in surfactant-treated preterm lambs that were ventilated with 10 mL/kg tidal volume [21] demonstrated that, whereas both 4 and 7 cm H_2O PEEP were more protective than zero PEEP, the use of 7 cm H_2O PEEP was associated with superior oxygenation but with an adverse increase in pulmonary vascular permeability. Naik et al. [22] also administered surfactant to the preterm lambs and compared the effects of 0, 4, and 7 cm H_2O PEEP on the expression of proinflammatory cytokine production and pulmonary morphometry. Surprisingly, 4 cm H_2O PEEP was most protective among the three different PEEP levels. The morphometry exhibited more atelectatic areas in zero PEEP and a higher proportion of overdistended alveoli in 7 cm H_2O PEEP, suggesting that the injurious mechanism may be different between 0 and 7 cm H_2O PEEP. In addition, the optimal PEEP level may depend on the lung maturity. We know that PEEP is important; however, what the optimal level of PEEP and the associated tidal volume are remain unresolved issues.

Recruitment Is Essential to Lung Protection

The recruitment maneuver has been suggested as a pivotal issue in lung protection. Rimensberger et al. [23] demonstrated that the recruitment maneuver enabled the ventilatory cycles to relocate onto the deflation limb of the PV curve during low tidal volume ventilation, where low tidal volumes (5 mL/kg) were combined with PEEP set to less than the lower inflection point (Figure 7.3). A comparison of the effects of two different maneuvers (i.e., recruitment maneuver and PEEP titration) on the regional aeration of saline-lavaged in vivo dogs using sequential computed tomography demonstrated that the recruitment maneuver resulted in the tidal ventilation being localized on the deflation limb [24]. These were similar in concept to the earlier findings of Rimensberger et al. [23]. However, use of the recruitment maneuver tended to induce a greater increase in hyperaerated lung volume than did use of PEEP titration. Their study shows that alveolar recruitment may occur at the expense of hyperaeration, and, therefore, the advantages of the recruitment maneuver must be weighed against this complication. Using saline-lavaged in vivo sheep, Musch et al. [25] found that

recruitment maneuvers can worsen oxygenation in acute lung injury by diverting pulmonary blood flow from aerated to nonaerated regions.

A recent clinical trial [26], investigators were unable to find sustained improvement in oxygenation or lung mechanics following the recruitment maneuver in ARDS patients ventilated with high PEEP (13.8 cm H_2O) and low tidal volume (6 mL/kg). Indeed, it is possible that the higher PEEP level used in this trial might have concealed the potential for improvements related to recruitment maneuvers [26]. Conversely, others have reported greater effects of recruitment on oxygenation when ARDS patients were ventilated with relatively lower PEEP (9.4 cm H_2O) [27]. In addition to the basal PEEP levels, the effects of a recruitment maneuver may depend on the phase of ARDS. While early ARDS patients mechanically ventilated for less than 3 days showed transient improvements in the lung compliance, venous admixture, and end-expiratory lung volume, patients in later phases of ARDS (i.e., those ventilated for more than 7 days) showed no improvement in these parameters [28]. In both ARDS phases, arterial oxygenation did not change in response to recruitment maneuvers. The investigators pointed out the possibility that alveolar overdistention might redistribute blood flow and increase intrapulmonary shunt. Grasso et al. [29] also found differences in the phases of ARDS between the responders and nonresponders to recruitment maneuvers and attributed the poor responses in late ARDS patients to their impaired chest wall and lung mechanics. Thus, at this time, we should consider the issues of both recruitment maneuvers and optimal level of PEEP to be unresolved in the clinical context.

Susceptibility to Ventilator-Induced Lung Injury: Adults Versus Infants

In the application of noninjurious ventilation to pediatric patients, many intensivists are concerned about ventilator-associated lung injury caused by indiscriminate use of tidal volume based on body weight. Compared with adults, pediatric patients demonstrate a spectrum of lung development, spanning neonatal, infant, juvenile and adult stages. There are important structural and functional differences between infant and adult lungs, thus raising an important question: does the lung maturation have an effect on the susceptibility to ventilator-induced lung injury?

Adkins et al. [30] ventilated in vivo young and adult rabbits with comparable peak inspiratory pressures (pressure-controlled ventilation) and showed that the younger rabbits developed greater microvascular permeability and macroscopic air leak. They speculated that the younger rabbits might have been exposed to disproportionately larger tidal volumes, relative to body weight, because the use of pressure-controlled ventilation might have resulted in far greater tidal volumes in the younger animals, in which respiratory system compliance was clearly greater.

In volume-controlled ventilation, tidal volume is usually expressed based on the body weight. Because the ratio of airway volume to body weight changes with age [31], tidal volume based on body weight might occupy a different fraction of total lung capacity (TLC) in the adult versus the infant, resulting in proportionally more lung stretch and thereby more lung injury. Copland et al. [32] ventilated in vivo neonatal and adult rats with high tidal volume based on the body weight. As a result, all adult rats exposed to a tidal volume of 40 mL/kg developed severe lung injury and died

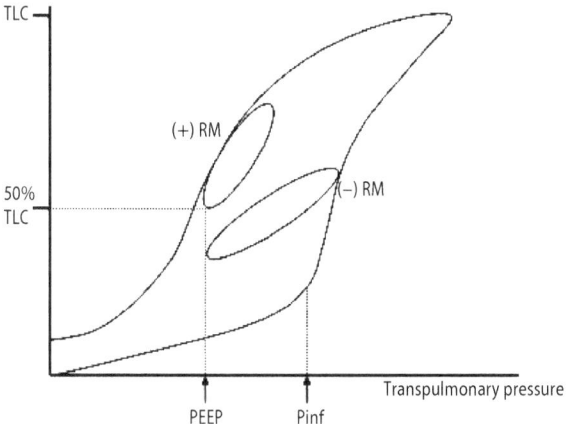

FIGURE 7.3. Effects of a recruitment maneuver (RM) on the ventilatory cycles. The RM enables the ventilatory cycles to relocate onto the deflation limb of the pressure–volume curve, where positive end-expiratory pressure (PEEP) is set to less than the lower inflection point (P_{inf}). TLC, total lung capacity.

within 20 min, but all neonatal rats survived for 3 hr while developing only a small decrement in respiratory system compliance. On the basis of measured compliance, edema formation, and histology, ventilation with 25 mL/kg was also more injurious to adult rats than newborns [32]. Their findings are supported by Kornecki et al. [33], who compared ex vivo, nonperfused infantile and adult lungs ventilated with high tidal volume (30 mL/kg) and found that adult lungs are more susceptible to ventilator-induced lung injury than infantile lungs in terms of lung mechanics and histology. In addition, they performed dynamic subpleural microscopy on the adult and infantile rats, finding greater and more heterogenous alveolar stretch in adult lungs. In summary, great caution should be exercised in the translation to pediatric practice of any recommendations for clinical practice that are based on adult studies.

Stretch Increases Production of Biochemical Mediators (Mechanotransduction)

It has been demonstrated that mechanical ventilation induces the intrapulmonary production of proinflammatory (e.g., interleukin-1β (IL-1β), IL-6, and TNF-α) and antiinflammatory (e.g., IL-10) cytokines, as well as chemokines (e.g., MIP-2) in the presence of underlying lung injury. In patients with ARDS, proinflammatory cytokines (IL-1β, IL-6, and TNF-α) were increased in the bronchoalveolar lavage (BAL) of the control arm but not where protective ventilation (higher PEEP, lower tidal volume) was used [34]. In laboratory studies of conventional versus high-frequency ventilation, Takata et al. [35] reported that intrapulmonary expression of TNF-α mRNA was high with conventional ventilation but not with high-frequency ventilation. Using a comparable model (i.e., the atelectasis-prone, surfactant-depleted rabbit), Imai et al. [36] demonstrated that conventional ventilation increased the production of TNF-α protein in the BAL compared with high-frequency ventilation. Chiumello et al. [8] found the increased TNF-α and MIP-2 protein in the BAL of acid-injured in vivo rats ventilated with high tidal volume (16 mL/kg) and zero PEEP. Most animal studies using "preinjured lungs" show the involvement of proinflammatory cytokines.

In the absence of preceding injury, it is very controversial whether injurious ventilation per se can induce the intrapulmonary production of TNF-α at mRNA and protein levels [37,38]. Injurious ventilation increased TNF-α at both mRNA and protein levels in ex vivo, nonperfused lungs [17] as well as in ventilated ex vivo, perfused mouse lungs [39]. A significant increase in TNF-α protein has been reported in an in vivo rat model ventilated with high tidal volume but without underlying lung injury [40]. Consistent with this, Copland et al. [32] ventilated rats in vivo with high tidal volume (25 mL/kg) and zero PEEP, resulting in the increased expression of TNF-α mRNA at only 30 min. On the contrary, others failed to find a large increase in TNF-α protein in the BAL following high tidal volume ventilation in the ex vivo rat lung [41]. Verbrugge et al. [42] and Imanaka et al. [43] ventilated rats with high peak inspiratory pressure and zero PEEP and found no increase in TNF-α protein and TNF-α mRNA, respectively. In contrast to TNF-α, MIP-2 protein, the murine homolog of IL-8, has been consistently found in most animal studies [17,32,41,44,45]. Quinn et al. [44] ventilated rats with high tidal volume (20 mL/kg) and, interestingly, MIP-2 protein was not increased in the BAL immediately after the

ventilation but was significantly increased at 6 hr after extubation to the room air.

Wilson et al. [45] ventilated in vivo mice in vivo with high tidal volume and exhibited a transient increase in TNF-α protein and more sustained increase in MIP-2 protein in the BAL. Their findings are supported by those of Tremblay et al. [46], who ventilated the ex vivo, nonperfused rats with high tidal volume (40 mL/kg) and demonstrated using in situ hybridization that the proportion of pulmonary epithelial cells expressing TNF-α mRNA peaked at 30 min and returned to baseline thereafter. The transient nature of TNF-α upregulation may help explain the previous controversies regarding the involvement of cytokines in ventilator-induced lung injury.

Copland et al. [32] ventilated newborn rats in vivo with high tidal volume and observed the temporal mRNA expression of several cytokines. They showed that the most prominently upregulated genes were MIP-2 and IL-10 at 30 min, whereas at 3 hr of high tidal volume ventilation IL-6 and MIP-2 were the most strongly induced cytokines. They also referred to the balance between the pro- and antiinflammatory cytokines. With regard to this balance, the compartmentalization of the inflammatory response should be taken into account as well as the temporal factors. Dugernier et al. [47] observed the pro- and antiinflammatory activities in the three different compartments (ascites, lymph, and blood) of patients suffering from severe acute pancreatitis. They concluded that the peritoneal compartment was the site of proinflammatory response and that an early, dominant, and sustained antiinflammatory activity took place in the circulating compartments. Their findings, although obtained from the patients with severe acute pancreatitis, may provide insight into to how a local organ inflammation propagates into an inflammatory response in the systemic circulation.

Does Ventilator-Induced Lung Injury Lead to Multiple-Organ Dysfunction Syndrome?

The leading cause of death in ARDS patients is multiple-organ dysfunction syndrome (MODS) rather than respiratory insufficiency. In the ARDS Network trial [2], plasma IL-6 concentration on day 3 was higher in the ARDS patients of the control group associated with the higher mortality. Ranieri et al. [34] reported an increase in proinflammatory cytokines (IL-6 and TNF-α) not only in the BAL but also in the plasma of ARDS patients in the control arm. Accumulating evidence from multiple experimental studies suggest that ventilator-induced lung injury can lead to systemic inflammation.

Von Bethmann et al. [39] used the isolated, perfused mouse lung in which frequent perfusate sampling allows determination of mediator release into the nonrecirculated perfusate. They demonstrated that hyperventilation increased the mRNA expression of TNF-α and IL-6, peaking at 30 and 150 min, respectively. Furthermore, they found that hyperventilation increased the perfusate concentration of TNF-α and IL-6 protein as ventilation time elapsed, establishing the concept of translocation of proinflammatory cytokine from the lung tissue to the circulation. Held et al. [48] used the same isolated model and found that high stretch and lipopolysaccharide were nearly indistinguishable in terms of their effects on lung nuclear factor-κ B (NFκB) activation and the release of chemokines and cytokines into the perfusate. As lipopolysaccharide is known to elicit inflammation via NFκB activation, they concluded that NFκB activated by the high stretch is associated with the translocation of chemokines and cytokines [48]. Using in vivo saline-lavaged rabbits, Murphy et al. [49] demonstrated that an adverse ventilatory strategy caused pulmonary-to-systemic translocation of endotoxin. They also found that plasma endotoxin levels were higher in eventual nonsurvivors than survivors, suggesting that the poor outcome was associated with systemic spreading of endotoxin [49]. These findings are in line with the results of Chiumello et al. [8], who used in vivo acid-injured rats and demonstrated that high tidal volume ventilation without PEEP gave rise to the greater increases in TNF-α and MIP-2 in both of the BAL and plasma levels. It should be noted that both studies referred to the alveolar capillary stress failure as the translocation mechanism, regardless of whether endotoxin or the cytokine is shifting compartments [8,49].

Another potential mechanism whereby ventilator-induced lung injury might lead to MODS is bacterial translocation from the air spaces into the circulation. Following the tracheal instillation of *Escherichia coli*, Nahum et al. [50] found that an adverse ventilatory strategy caused a higher incidence of bacteremia than the less injurious strategy. Using in vivo saline-lavaged newborn piglets, van Kaam et al. [51] intratracheally instilled group B *Streptococcus*, which is the leading cause of serious infections in human newborns, and induced severe pneumonia. They found that reducing atelectasis by means of exogenous surfactant and open lung ventilation with sufficient PEEP prevented bacterial translocation. However, given that the organisms responsible for the clinical ventilator-associated pneumonia are not usually detectable in the systemic circulation, it seems unlikely that bacterial translocation can account for the chief mechanism of ventilator-induced lung injury spreading to the systemic inflammation.

Finally, injurious mechanical ventilation may induce distal organ dysfunction via circulating soluble factors, such as soluble Fas ligand. Imai et al. [52] ventilated in vivo acid-injured rabbits with injurious or protective ventilatory strategies. They found that the injurious ventilatory strategy led to epithelial cell apoptosis in the kidney and small intestine. They also demonstrated that the induction of apoptosis was increased in the in vitro renal tubular cells incubated with plasma from rabbits treated with the injurious ventilatory strategy, suggesting that distal organ dysfunction is, at least partly, caused by the circulating soluble factors [52].

Conclusion

After numerous studies in both clinical and experimental settings, investigators have recommended the use of low tidal volume and high PEEP for the prevention of ventilator-induced lung injury. However, the optimal levels of PEEP and the associated tidal volume are still unresolved issues. Although the recruitment maneuver has been suggested as a pivotal issue in lung protection, clinical studies have exhibited only the limited advantages of this technique. One should consider the issue of recruitment maneuvers to be unresolved in the clinical context.

Pediatricians often say, "Kids are not small adults," and this holds true in the application of mechanical ventilation to pediatric patients. Indeed, great caution should be exercised in the translation to pediatric practice of any recommendations that are based on adult studies. Several studies have made a breakthrough by showing that mechanical forces such as high stretch can induce biochemical mediators; however, a total understanding of this

mechanism may require more studies elaborating the spatial and temporal dimensions of *mechanotransduction*. The leading cause of death in ARDS patients is MODS rather than respiratory insufficiency. Further studies are required to elucidate the mechanisms whereby a local pulmonary inflammation propagates into an inflammatory response in the systemic circulation and, ultimately, to distal organ dysfunction.

References

1. Amato MB, Barbas CS, Medeiros DM, et al. Effect of a protective-ventilation strategy on mortality in the acute respiratory distress syndrome. N Engl J Med 1998;338:347–354.
2. The Acute Respiratory Distress Syndrome Network. Ventilation with lower tidal volumes as compared with traditional tidal volumes for acute lung injury and the acute respiratory distress syndrome. N Engl J Med 2000;342:1301–1308.
3. Tobin MJ. Culmination of an era in research on the acute respiratory distress syndrome. N Engl J Med 2000;342:1360–1361.
4. Eichacker PQ, Gerstenberger EP, Banks SM, Cui X, Natanson C. Meta-analysis of acute lung injury and acute respiratory distress syndrome trials testing low tidal volumes. Am J Respir Crit Care Med 2002;166: 1510–1514.
5. Webb HH, Tierney DF. Experimental pulmonary edema due to intermittent positive pressure ventilation with high inflation pressures. Protection by positive end-expiratory pressure. Am Rev Respir Dis 1974;110:556–565.
6. Dreyfuss D, Soler P, Basset G, Saumon G. High inflation pressure pulmonary edema. Respective effects of high airway pressure, high tidal volume, and positive end-expiratory pressure. Am Rev Respir Dis 1988;137:1159–1164.
7. Broccard AF, Hotchkiss JR, Suzuki S, Olson D, Marini JJ. Effects of mean airway pressure and tidal excursion on lung injury induced by mechanical ventilation in an isolated perfused rabbit lung model. Crit Care Med 1999;27:1533–1541.
8. Chiumello D, Pristine G, Slutsky AS. Mechanical ventilation affects local and systemic cytokines in an animal model of acute respiratory distress syndrome. Am J Respir Crit Care Med 1999;160:109–116.
9. Duggan M, McCaul CL, McNamara PJ, Engelberts D, Ackerley C, Kavanagh BP. Atelectasis causes vascular leak and lethal right ventricular failure in uninjured rat lungs. Am J Respir Crit Care Med 2003; 167:1633–1640.
10. Frank JA, Gutierrez JA, Jones KD, Allen L, Dobbs L, Matthay MA. Low tidal volume reduces epithelial and endothelial injury in acid-injured rat lungs. Am J Respir Crit Care Med 2002;165:242–249.
11. Kavanagh BP, Slutsky AS. Ventilator induced lung injury: more studies, more questions. Crit Care Med 1999;27:1669–1671.
12. Gattinoni L, Pesenti A, Avalli L, Rossi F, Bombino M. Pressure-volume curve of total respiratory system in acute respiratory failure. Computed tomographic scan study. Am Rev Respir Dis 1987;136:730–736.
13. Treggiari MM, Romand JA, Martin JB, Suter PM. Air cysts and bronchiectasis prevail in nondependent areas in severe acute respiratory distress syndrome: a computed tomographic study of ventilator-associated changes. Crit Care Med 2002;30:1747–1752.
14. Brower RG, Lanken PN, MacIntyre N, et al. Higher versus lower positive end-expiratory pressures in patients with the acute respiratory distress syndrome. N Engl J Med 2004;351:327–336.
15. Pepe PE, Hudson LD, Carrico CJ. Early application of positive end-expiratory pressure in patients at risk for the adult respiratory-distress syndrome. N Engl J Med 1984;311:281–286.
16. Muscedere JG, Mullen JB, Gan K, Slutsky AS. Tidal ventilation at low airway pressures can augment lung injury. Am J Respir Crit Care Med 1994;149:1327–1334.
17. Tremblay L, Valenza F, Ribeiro SP, Li J, Slutsky AS. Injurious ventilatory strategies increase cytokines and c-fos m-RNA expression in an isolated rat lung model. J Clin Invest 1997;99:944–952.

18. Valenza F, Guglielmi M, Irace M, Porro GA, Sibilla S, Gattinoni L. Positive end-expiratory pressure delays the progression of lung injury during ventilator strategies involving high airway pressure and lung overdistention. Crit Care Med 2003;31:1993–1998.

19. Sandhar BK, Niblett DJ, Argiras EP, Dunnill MS, Sykes MK. Effects of positive end-expiratory pressure on hyaline membrane formation in a rabbit model of the neonatal respiratory distress syndrome. Intensive Care Med 1988;14:538–546.

20. Sohma A, Brampton WJ, Dunnill MS, Sykes MK. Effect of ventilation with positive end-expiratory pressure on the development of lung damage in experimental acid aspiration pneumonia in the rabbit. Intensive Care Med 1992;18:112–117.

21. Michna J, Jobe AH, Ikegami M. Positive end-expiratory pressure preserves surfactant function in preterm lambs. Am J Respir Crit Care Med 1999;160:634–639.

22. Naik AS, Kallapur SG, Bachurski CJ, et al. Effects of ventilation with different positive end-expiratory pressures on cytokine expression in the preterm lamb lung. Am J Respir Crit Care Med 2001;164:494–498.

23. Rimensberger PC, Pristine G, Mullen BM, Cox PN, Slutsky AS. Lung recruitment during small tidal volume ventilation allows minimal positive end-expiratory pressure without augmenting lung injury. Crit Care Med 1999;27:1940–1945.

24. Lim CM, Soon Lee S, Seoung Lee J, et al. Morphometric effects of the recruitment maneuver on saline-lavaged canine lungs. A computed tomographic analysis. Anesthesiology 2003;99:71–80.

25. Musch G, Harris RS, Vidal Melo MF, et al. Mechanism by which a sustained inflation can worsen oxygenation in acute lung injury. Anesthesiology 2004;100:323–330.

26. Brower RG, Morris A, MacIntyre N, et al. Effects of recruitment maneuvers in patients with acute lung injury and acute respiratory distress syndrome ventilated with high positive end-expiratory pressure. Crit Care Med 2003;31:2592–2597.

27. Foti G, Cereda M, Sparacino ME, De Marchi L, Villa F, Pesenti A. Effects of periodic lung recruitment maneuvers on gas exchange and respiratory mechanics in mechanically ventilated acute respiratory distress syndrome (ARDS) patients. Intensive Care Med 2000;26:501–507.

28. Villagra A, Ochagavia A, Vatua S, et al. Recruitment maneuvers during lung protective ventilation in acute respiratory distress syndrome. Am J Respir Crit Care Med 2002;165:165–170.

29. Grasso S, Mascia L, Del Turco M, et al. Effects of recruiting maneuvers in patients with acute respiratory distress syndrome ventilated with protective ventilatory strategy. Anesthesiology 2002;96:795–802.

30. Adkins WK, Hernandez LA, Coker PJ, Buchanan B, Parker JC. Age effects susceptibility to pulmonary barotrauma in rabbits. Crit Care Med 1991;19:390–393.

31. Gomes RF, Shardonofsky F, Eidelman DH, Bates JH. Respiratory mechanics and lung development in the rat from early age to adulthood. J Appl Physiol 2001;90:1631–1638.

32. Copland IB, Martinez F, Kavanagh BP, et al. High tidal volume ventilation causes different inflammatory responses in newborn versus adult lung. Am J Respir Crit Care Med 2004;169:739–748.

33. Kornecki A, Tsuchida S, Ondiveeran HK, et al. Lung development and susceptibility to ventilator-induced lung injury. Am J Respir Crit Care Med 2005;171:743–752.

34. Ranieri VM, Suter PM, Tortorella C, et al. Effect of mechanical ventilation on inflammatory mediators in patients with acute respiratory distress syndrome: a randomized controlled trial. JAMA 1999;282:54–61.

35. Takata M, Abe J, Tanaka H, et al. Intraalveolar expression of tumor necrosis factor-alpha gene during conventional and high-frequency ventilation. Am J Respir Crit Care Med 1997;156:272–279.

36. Imai Y, Nakagawa S, Ito Y, Kawano T, Slutsky AS, Miyasaka K. Comparison of lung protection strategies using conventional and high-frequency oscillatory ventilation. J Appl Physiol 2001;91:1836–1844.

37. Slutsky AS, Tremblay LN. Multiple system organ failure. Is mechanical ventilation a contributing factor? Am J Respir Crit Care Med 1998;157:1721–1725.

38. Dreyfuss D, Ricard JD, Saumon G. On the physiologic and clinical relevance of lung-borne cytokines during ventilator-induced lung injury. Am J Respir Crit Care Med 2003;167:1467–1471.

39. von Bethmann AN, Brasch F, Nusing R, et al. Hyperventilation induces release of cytokines from perfused mouse lung. Am J Respir Crit Care Med 1998;157:263–272.

40. Foda HD, Rollo EE, Drews M, et al. Ventilator-induced lung injury upregulates and activates gelatinases and EMMPRIN: attenuation by the synthetic matrix metalloproteinase inhibitor, Prinomastat (AG3340). Am J Respir Cell Mol Biol 2001;25:717–724.

41. Ricard JD, Dreyfuss D, Saumon G. Production of inflammatory cytokines in ventilator-induced lung injury: a reappraisal. Am J Respir Crit Care Med 2001;163:1176–1180.

42. Verbrugge SJ, Uhlig S, Neggers SJ, et al. Different ventilation strategies affect lung function but do not increase tumor necrosis factor-alpha and prostacyclin production in lavaged rat lungs in vivo. Anesthesiology 1999;91:1834–1843.

43. Imanaka H, Shimaoka M, Matsuura N, Nishimura M, Ohta N, Kiyono H. Ventilator-induced lung injury is associated with neutrophil infiltration, macrophage activation, and TGF-beta 1 mRNA upregulation in rat lungs. Anesth Analg 2001;92:428–436.

44. Quinn DA, Moufarrej RK, Volokhov A, Hales CA. Interactions of lung stretch, hyperoxia, and MIP-2 production in ventilator-induced lung injury. J Appl Physiol 2002;93:517–525.

45. Wilson MR, Choudhury S, Goddard ME, O'Dea KP, Nicholson AG, Takata M. High tidal volume upregulates intrapulmonary cytokines in an in vivo mouse model of ventilator-induced lung injury. J Appl Physiol 2003;95:1385–1393.

46. Tremblay LN, Miatto D, Hamid Q, Govindarajan A, Slutsky AS. Injurious ventilation induces widespread pulmonary epithelial expression of tumor necrosis factor-alpha and interleukin-6 messenger RNA. Crit Care Med 2002;30:1693–1700.

47. Dugernier TL, Laterre PF, Wittebole X, et al. Compartmentalization of the inflammatory response during acute pancreatitis: correlation with local and systemic complications. Am J Respir Crit Care Med 2003;168:148–157.

48. Held HD, Boettcher S, Hamann L, Uhlig S. Ventilation-induced chemokine and cytokine release is associated with activation of nuclear factor-kappaB and is blocked by steroids. Am J Respir Crit Care Med 2001;163:711–716.

49. Murphy DB, Cregg N, Tremblay L, et al. Adverse ventilatory strategy causes pulmonary-to-systemic translocation of endotoxin. Am J Respir Crit Care Med 2000;162:27–33.

50. Nahum A, Hoyt J, Schmitz L, Moody J, Shapiro R, Marini JJ. Effect of mechanical ventilation strategy on dissemination of intratracheally instilled Escherichia coli in dogs. Crit Care Med 1997;25:1733–1743.

51. van Kaam AH, Lachmann RA, Herting E, et al. Reducing atelectasis attenuates bacterial growth and translocation in experimental pneumonia. Am J Respir Crit Care Med 2004;169:1046–1053.

52. Imai Y, Parodo J, Kajikawa O, et al. Injurious mechanical ventilation and end-organ epithelial cell apoptosis and organ dysfunction in an experimental model of acute respiratory distress syndrome. JAMA 2003;289:2104–2112.

8
Prone Positioning

Nilesh M. Mehta and Martha A.Q. Curley

Introduction

The hypoxemia and undesirable respiratory mechanics in patients with acute respiratory distress syndrome (ARDS) have long been targets for intervention. Prone positioning was first proposed as a therapeutic modality for improvement of lung mechanics in 1974, when Bryan described improved oxygenation in anesthetized and muscle-relaxed patients placed in the prone position [1]. This was followed by application of prone positioning in small groups of ARDS patients with improvement in oxygenation [2,3]. Prone positioning emerged as a novel, relatively noninvasive, simple, yet logistically challenging therapeutic intervention for patients with ARDS. The past 30 years have seen increasing enthusiasm for this maneuver, which has been extensively applied to improve oxygenation and respiratory mechanics in ARDS patients.

Prone positioning is an easy, readily available treatment option for refractory hypoxemia, a characteristic feature of severe ARDS. The ultimate efficacy of prone positioning in ARDS is difficult to evaluate because of heterogeneous study populations, the variances in the application of prone positioning, and the small sample sizes used in most studies. Although there is a rationale supporting the hypothesis that prone ventilation could reduce the mortality of ARDS patients, currently there are no clinical data to support the hypothesis.

Ventilation–Perfusion Relationships: Effects of Postural Changes

In supine patients with ARDS, lung densities are predominant in the dependent dorsal regions and, in the absence of optimal positive end-expiratory pressure (PEEP), ventilation is preferentially distributed to the nondependent ventral regions. The dependent areas of the lung are more atelectatic and likely to endure collapse and inflation (atelectrauma) during mechanical ventilation at low PEEP. Meanwhile, perfusion to the lung units progressively increases from the nondependent to the dependent regions, with preferential perfusion of the dependent atelectatic lung regions [4]. Thus, in supine patients with ARDS, lung ventilation is preferentially shifted to the nondependent ventral regions, and lung perfusion is preferentially shifted to the dependent dorsal atelectatic regions. The overall effect is a mismatch between ventilation and perfusion, with a low ventilation:perfusion (V/Q) ratio, physiologic shunt, and resultant hypoxemia. This was illustrated by Pappert et al, who administered pressure-controlled ventilation in the prone position for 24 hr to 12 patients with ARDS [5]. Continuous V/Q ratios were recorded using the multiple inert gas elimination technique (MIGET). Improved oxygenation was seen in eight patients, within 30 min of prone positioning (responders), and was associated with a reduction of perfusion to the shunt regions and resultant increase in the V/Q ratio. This redirection of perfusion from nonventilated regions of the lung to those with normal V/Q ratios was thought to be caused by recruitment of previously atelectatic but healthy lung regions in the prone position. Computerized tomography (CT) scan images from patients with ARDS have shown radiographic densities predominantly located in the dependent regions (Figure 8.1).

The *transpulmonary gradient* (difference between the alveolar and pleural pressures) is higher in the ventral regions than the dorsal dependent regions of the lung and may explain increased alveolar recruitment in the ventral (nondependent) regions. This heterogeneity of alveolar ventilation distribution is largely eliminated with the application of PEEP when the previously collapsed (compression atelectasis) alveoli are recruited. Prone positioning has been associated with a more homogeneous distribution of transpulmonary pressures and hence alveolar inflation (Figure 8.2) [6].

Respiratory Mechanics

In the supine position, factors such as lung weight, cardiac mass, diaphragmatic displacement, and triangular shape of the chest are thought to influence alveolar dimensions by their effects on the transpulmonary gradient and the distribution of densities or atelectatic lung units. Computerized tomography studies have shown the vertical gradient of lung aeration in ARDS. Lung edema, on the

D.S. Wheeler et al. (eds.), The *Respiratory Tract in Pediatric Critical Illness and Injury*,
DOI 10.1007/978-1-84800-925-7_8, © Springer-Verlag London Limited 2009

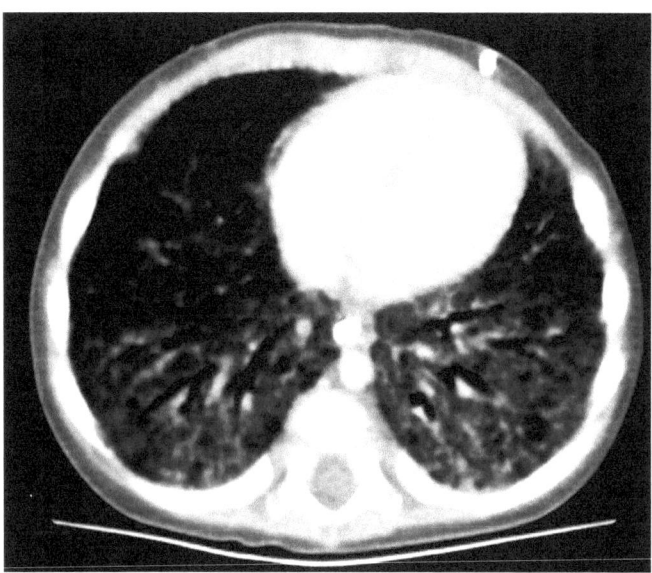

FIGURE 8.1. Computed tomography scan showing acute respiratory distress syndrome.

other hand, appears to be uniformly distributed in the lung paren-chyma. The increasing lung weight down the gravitational gradient results in deflation of alveolar units in the dependent lung regions [6]. In addition, CT imaging in patients with ARDS has shown increased cardiac dimensions, volume, and mass in this group compared with normal adults [7]. The pressure exerted by cardiac mass on underlying lung lobes was significantly higher in patients with ARDS, with a reduction in the volumes of corresponding lung regions. The cardiac mass in the thoracic cavity may also influence the pleural pressures [8]. The vertical gradient of the pleural pres-sures have been correlated with changing mass of mediastinal structures, especially the heart, in animal experiments [9,10]. However, this vertical gradient was not seen in animals in the prone position [10]. It is likely that the lung in supine position, but not in the prone position, supports the heart, and this contributes to its pleural pressure. Using a noninvasive rebreathing technique, Reutershan et al. demonstrated a continuous increase in pulmo-nary blood flow in responders when placed in the prone position [11]. The elevated pulmonary blood flow was sustained even when patients were returned to the supine position. Based on these obser-vations, suggesting beneficial cardiorespiratory profile, investiga-tors have studied the effects of prone mechanical ventilation in patients with acute respiratory failure after cardiac surgery [12].

System maturation during early childhood changes the shape, compliance, and deformability of the thorax. The horizontally extending ribs give a circular shape to the newborn thorax, and the diaphragm is horizontal. The high compliance and easy deform-ability of the newborn ribcage predisposes to sucking in of the chest wall during inspiration and reduces mechanical coupling of the diaphragm and the rib cage. Furthermore, the high ratio of the passive compliances of the chest wall to that of the lung (6.7:1) exaggerates the magnitude of the paradoxical motion between the caudal surface of the lung (driven by the diaphragm) and the remaining lung (driven by the rib cage) [13]. The efficiency of the thoracic cage and its volume is much improved with gradual caudal inclination of ribs. The adult rib cage has a smaller antero-posterior diameter, and the volume increase is achieved by the "bucket handle" or the "pump handle" effect of the elevation of ribs

during inspiration. The changes in the shape of the thorax, the effect of gravity in the upright position, the development of tho-racic muscles, and the mineralization of bone all contribute to decreased chest wall compliance and deformability. The total respi-ratory compliance progressively decreases from 5 to 16 years of age [14]. This allows opposition of the inward pull of the diaphragm on the chest wall during inspiration and improves mechanical cou-pling of the diaphragm and chest wall.

Newborns, especially preterm infants, may be more vulnerable to respiratory muscle fatigue because of the extra work imposed by the characteristics of their rib cages. The work required in distort-ing the chest wall may be 90%–96% of the work done on the lung [15]. In a cross-sectional study including children in the age range of 3 weeks to 15 years, Nicolai et al. demonstrated disproportion-ately high respiratory system compliance in infants compared with older children as an influence of chest wall configuration after adjusting for the effects of lung volume [16]. The compliant chest wall of the infant also affects the airways and impairs gas exchange. There is a reduction in the minimal outward recoil of the chest wall during end expiration in infants. This results in limited distending pressure (transpulmonary pressures are lower in infants), with a tendency to airway collapse, atelectasis, decreased functional residual capacity with consequentially impaired gas exchange, and increased work of breathing [17].

Thus, the elastance of the chest wall has a significant influence on the respiratory mechanics of the developing child. Chest wall elastance is thought to be increased in mechanically ventilated patients with acute lung injury [18]. The abdominal distension seen in acute respiratory distress patients contributes to this increased chest wall elastance [19]. In their study of 18 patients with ARDS, Ranieri et al. showed significant differences in the degree of impair-ment of respiratory system elastic properties in ARDS and also highlighted the effect of abdominal distension [20]. Some authors have described these chest wall properties to contribute to the pro-posed differences in respiratory mechanics in pulmonary and extrapulmonary ARDS [21].

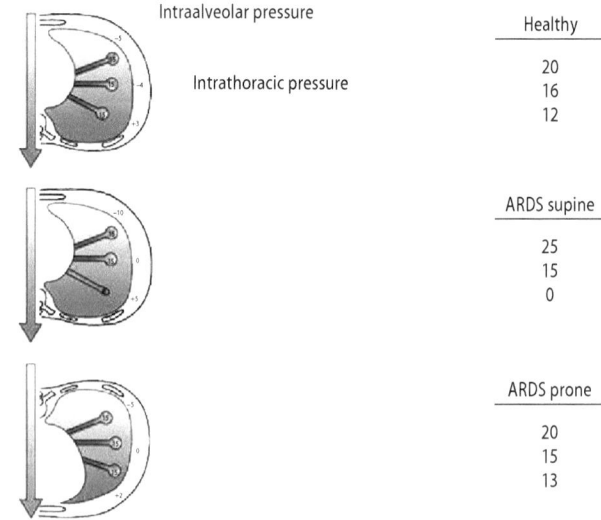

FIGURE 8.2. Transpulmonary pressure gradient in different postures. ARDS, acute respira-tory distress syndrome.

Diaphragmatic mechanics during positive pressure ventilation under anesthesia are significantly different from those during spontaneous breathing because of the differences in the distributions of the expanding forces during these two states. The pattern of volume distribution during mechanical ventilation is independent of muscle contraction and mainly determined by the relative regional elastance within the lung and chest wall. The relative contribution of the rib cage is likely to be larger in recumbent mechanically ventilated patients. Anesthesia is associated with a relative decrease in the functional residual capacity, and, at these volumes, nondependent lung appears to be preferentially ventilated [22].

In 1989, Hernandez et al. demonstrated the role of high tidal volume in ventilator-induced lung injury (VILI) [23]. In this study, white rabbits ventilated with chest wall restriction achieved by plaster cast manifested with limited pressure-induced injury compared with intact closed-chest animals that experienced larger tidal volumes. The study provided convincing evidence that volume distension (volutrauma) rather than higher peak inspiratory pressure (barotrauma) was principally responsible for producing microvascular damage in the animal lung. Susceptibility to volutrauma was thought to be inversely related to the compliance of the chest wall and static recoil forces opposing volume expansion. The highly compliant chest wall of infants is likely to suffer more damage from volutrauma than that of adults. Subsequent clinical trials have shown the benefit of low tidal volume ventilation strategy for adults with ARDS [24].

The discussion highlights the significant impact of the innate chest wall compliance in infants and the subsequent developmental changes on gas exchange in spontaneously breathing patients as well as mechanically ventilated subjects with acute lung injury. Prone positioning favorably alters chest wall compliance, and the resultant respiratory mechanics are thought to have beneficial effects in acute lung injury. Cox et al. studied 10 healthy infants undergoing clubfoot surgery and recorded the pulmonary mechanics they found in the supine and prone positions [25]. This was the first study to demonstrate the safety of prone positioning in healthy infants. Both static and dynamic compliance were significantly lower in the prone position, although this was not associated with any impairment of gas exchange. Prone positioning was reported to reduce venous admixture and improve the uniformity of ventilation distribution without affecting end-expiratory lung volume in animal models of acute lung injury [4,26].

Thus, the application of prone positioning in ARDS is based on the multiple physiologic benefits of this therapeutic maneuver on oxygenation and respiratory mechanics. These benefits include (1) improved V/Q matching, (2) homogeneous transpulmonary gradient, (3) improved recruitment of alveoli, (4) decreased chest wall and diaphragmatic asynchrony, and (5) possible prevention of VILI. Initial studies of the use of prone positioning in patients with acute lung injury showed significant variability of response. However, dramatic responses in some patients and the safety of the maneuver prompted a number of studies in which prone positioning was employed with an aim to affect physiologic outcomes such as oxygenation in ARDS.

Recruitment and Ventilator-Induced Lung Injury

Lung opacities in acute lung injury are heterogeneously distributed, with the densities seen predominantly in the most dependent regions [27]. As discussed earlier, the superimposed pressure from the lung and heart decreases the transpulmonary pressure, with a resultant progressive atelectasis along the ventrodorsal gradient. The effect of PEEP on this deflation is limited by the amount of alveolar inflation (recruitment) achieved at end inspiration. The amount of end-expiratory collapse is likely to be increased when the plateau pressure in the previous inspiration is lower [27]. The ventrodorsal gradient of transpulmonary pressures is steeper in the supine than in the prone position [28]. The results of the landmark ARDSnet trial demonstrated the beneficial effects of lower tidal volume strategy during mechanical ventilation in ARDS patients [29]. As the role of volutrauma and its effect on VILI is increasingly demonstrated, clinicians should aim to prevent VILI with the application of stress and strain within physiologic limits. Both stress (fiber tension in the lung, proportional to transpulmonary pressure) and strain (elongation of stressed fibers from resting position) are likely to be distributed more evenly in the prone position [30]. This concept was recently demonstrated by Valenza et al. in their animal model in which prone position delayed the progression of VILI [31].

The effect of the prone position on improved oxygenation is likely to be variable depending on the underlying recruitment status of individual alveolar units. Acute lung injury and ARDS are characterized by lung units with different opening pressures ranging from 45 to 70 cm H_2O [32]. Recruitment is a pan-inspiratory phenomenon and occurs along the entire volume–pressure curve, following a ventral to dorsal and cephalad to caudal distribution and progression [33]. Thus, it is conceivable that in the setting of a de-recruited lung, prone position is not likely to have benefits that would be seen in an optimally recruited lung. Lungs of patient with extrapulmonary ARDS may be more responsive to standard recruitment measures [21,34]. For these patients, it has been proposed that recruitment maneuvers (such as sustained inflation) may improve oxygenation, although these effects were not sustained in the supine position [35].

Guerin et al. studied the effects of the prone position on alveolar recruitment and oxygenation in 12 adult patients with ARDS [36]. They reported a correlation between change in oxygenation and recruited lung volume and speculated that recruitment was one of the mechanisms by which the prone position improved oxygenation [36]. Pelosi et al. also examined the effect of the prone position on enhancing the potential of recruitment maneuver (sighs) in ARDS and concluded that cyclical sighs during ventilation in the prone position may provide optimal lung recruitment [37]. Oczenski et al. showed an enhanced and persistent improvement in oxygenation after performing sustained inflation maneuvers in patients with ARDS 6 hr after placement in the prone position [38]. These observations support the hypothesis that the prone position improves the recruitment of lung units by standard recruitment maneuvers. It may be concluded that the full potential of the prone position for patients with extrapulmonary ARDS will only be achieved in an optimally recruited lung.

Pediatric Studies

Overview

Although the majority of the described work was carried out in the adult population, neonatal studies in the past and more recent pediatric studies have examined the feasibility and efficacy of the prone position in acute lung injury. Table 8.1 highlights some of the

TABLE 8.1. Studies of the prone position.

Pediatric studies

Reference	Year	Type of study	No. of Pts	Entry criteria	Time after lung injury (mean)	Frequency of PP (No. of cycles)	Percent (%) of time in PP	Duration in PP	Duration in SP	Percent (%) of responders	Adverse effects	Outcomes measured
Murdoch and Storman [63]	1994	One-center prospective case series	7	ARDS	4.5 days	1	—	0.5 hr	0.5 hr	100	—	CO, HD variables, DO_2
Numa et al. [39]	1997	One-center prospective case series	30	Intubated pts Control = 10 Obstructive = 10 Restrictive = 10	12 days	1	—	70 min	Rest of the day	NA	—	ABG, FRC, C_{RS}, R_{RS}
Curley et al. [44]	2000	One-center prospective case series	25	ALI/ARDS	<19 hr	1–12	47	20 hr/day	4 hr/day	84	Stage II skin ulcers in 24%	PaO_2:FiO_2 ratio, mortality (study, 28 days), adverse effects, COMFORT score
Kornecki et al. [45]	2001	One-center prospective case series	10	ARF OI > 12 FiO_2 > 0.5 For 12 hr		1		12 hr/day	12 hr/day	90	Facial edema in 30%	HD, OI, static C_{RS} & R_{RS}
Casado-Flores et al. [43]	2002	One-center prospective case series	23	ALI/ARDS	56 hr	2–14	36	8 hr	8 hr	78	—	PaO_2:FiO_2 ratio
Haefner et al. [61]	2003	One-center retrospective cohort	63	ECMO for respir. failure	—	15 position changes	—	—	NA	—		Adverse effects recorded
Relvas et al. [48]	2003	One-center retrospective chart review	40	ARDS	107 hr	Variable	(n = 37)	>20 hr	—	—		OI, PaO_2:FiO_2 ratio
Curley et al. [68]	2005	Randomized, multicenter study	102	ALI/ARDS	<48 hr	Up to 7	20 hr/day	20 hr/day	4 hr/day			Ventilator-free days, mortality, time to recovery from lung injury, organ failure–free days, functional outcome

Neonatal studies

Reference	Year	No. of pts	Patient population	Age at enrollment	Duration in PP	Duration in SP	Benefits of PP	Adverse effects
Wagaman et al. [64]	1979	14	34 weeks mean gestational age Recovering phase of respir. illness Vent. support (10 CPAP, 4 CMV)	5 days (2–14)	30 min with abdomen restricted; 30 min with abdomen suspended	30 min	Increased compliance and tidal volume Increased PaO_2	None reported
Lioy and Manginello [65]	1988	19	Preterm (n = 18) and full term (n = 1) 31 weeks mean gestational age RDS, requiring ventilatory support studied immediately postextubation	Mean of 5 days on ventilator before extubation	25 min	25 min	Increased PaO_2 Decreased respiratory rates and retraction scores	None reported
Mendoza et al. [66]	1991	33	27 weeks mean gestational age Mechanical vent., RDS	28 days (15–138)			Higher oxygen saturation Lower heart rate Lower pulmonary resistance	None reported
McEvoy et al. [67]	1997	55	26 weeks mean gestational age LBW (<1,000 g) RDS/CLD Mechanical ventilation (n = 17)	42 days (28–83)	60 min	60 min	Improved oxygenation Decreased periods and frequency of desaturations	None reported

Note: ABG, arterial blood gas; ALI, acute lung injury; ARDS, acute respiratory distress syndrome; ARF, acute respiratory failure; CLD, chronic lung disease; CPAP, continuous positive airway pressure; CMV, conventional mechanical ventilation; C_{RS}, compliance; ECMO, extracorporeal membrane oxygenation; FRC, functional residual capacity; HD, hemodynamic measurements; LBW, low birth weight; NA, not available; OI, oxygenation index; PP, prone position; RDS, respiratory distress syndrome; R_{RS}, resistance; SP, supine position.

salient features of the pediatric prone positioning studies. Use of prone positioning in the pediatric population has been increasingly reported in the past 10 years, although the initial reports were characterized by nonrandom assignment of this postural maneuver for varying periods of time applied to a heterogeneous population. The initial reluctance among pediatricians to employ this technique was caused by the lack of a uniform, effective, and safe guideline by which to perform the maneuver. Initial pediatric data provided limited information on the procedure, nor were its effective and safe continuation and the associated complications systematically studied. However, dramatic improvements in oxygenation were reported soon after prone positioning in children with acute lung injury. In the absence of other interventions that reduced mortality, the perceived benefits of improvement in oxygenation and the potential for reduced fractional oxygen requirement provided the impetus for continued evaluation of this intervention.

Patient Selection

Patient selection for prone positioning remains a challenging endeavor and is likely to be the key to unraveling the true potential and specific application of this intervention. Patient selection for prone positioning may be affected by feasibility of the maneuver (e.g., extreme obesity), inability to tolerate prone positioning (e.g., neurologic trauma), and associated therapies that make the postural change challenging (e.g., extracorporeal membrane oxygenation, continuous venovenous hemofiltration). Because of their size, pediatric patients appear to be easier candidates for safe prone positioning.

Numa et al. enrolled mechanically ventilated children with restrictive and obstructive lung diseases and controls and examined the influence of the prone position on functional residual capacity, oxygenation, and respiratory mechanics [39]. They demonstrated a pattern of increasing functional residual capacity in the prone position in all three subgroups, although this did not correlate with improvements in oxygenation. Patients with restrictive lung disease and controls did not demonstrate improvements in oxygenation. Moreover, in the study, patients were enrolled after relatively prolonged periods of mechanical ventilation (1–2 weeks), and the authors speculate that this may have influenced the physiologic effects of the therapeutic postural maneuver. In the absence of clear mortality benefit in the ARDS group, investigators have performed subgroup analyses to identify those select patients who might benefit most from this therapy. In the absence of a mortality benefit, prone positioning should be used as a recruitment maneuver when high settings of the ventilator are required to achieve adequate oxygenation. The improved V/Q ratio resulting from this maneuver could be desirable for this subgroup of patients, at least during the acute illness.

Responses in Pulmonary Versus Extrapulmonary Acute Respiratory Distress Syndrome

Acute lung injuries from varied etiologies do not share the same morphologic and mechanical characteristics. Literature derived from adult acute lung injury studies has long debated the distinction between pulmonary and extrapulmonary ARDS and its clinical significance [40,41]. Some investigators speculate that the two conditions have distinct pathophysiologic, biochemical, radiologic, and mechanical properties [21]. Primary ARDS and secondary ARDS may have differential responses to prone positioning, and it has been proposed that secondary ARDS (with diffuse atelectasis) may be more responsive to this intervention [6]. The altered lung elastance in pulmonary ARDS (vs. altered chest wall elastance in extrapulmonary ARDS) may not benefit from strategies such as PEEP, recruitment, and the prone position compared with patients with extrapulmonary ARDS. However, the definition of the two conditions and the clinical impact of individually tailored therapy are not known. Suntharalingam et al. showed no difference in lung function assessments, 6 months after hospital discharge, in patients with ARDS of differing etiologies [42].

Outcome Measures

Selection of clinically relevant outcome measures is crucial when evaluating therapy for complex diseases such as ARDS. The degree of oxygenation has traditionally been the main determining factor when measuring the severity of lung injury. Hypoxemia is the common denominator in ARDS, and one of the early goals of mechanical ventilatory support is optimizing oxygenation.

Indices of oxygenation have long been primary outcome measures in evaluating the role of prone positioning. Pediatric studies of prone positioning in ARDS have also used indices of oxygenation such as the oxygenation index (OI) and the PaO_2/FiO_2 (P/F) ratio as outcome measures [43–45]. In their cohort of 25 patients, Curley et al. demonstrated an immediate, cumulative improvement in oxygenation after prone positioning as measured by P/F ratios and OI at the four time points in the first 24 hr after prone positioning (Figure 8.3) [44]. A significant improvement in both indices was shown at 1 hr and up to 19 hr after prone positioning. Based on their response to prone position on day 1 as measured by the P/F ratio, patients were classified as immediate responders (n = 11, 44%) and immediate nonresponders (n = 14, 56%) (Figure 8.4). Oxygenation appears to improve early and is sustained in the immediate responders. In this subgroup of patients, the improvement in oxygenation was shown to be preserved even after returning to the supine position (persistent). The nonresponders showed a delayed improvement in oxygenation, which was not persistent. Although there is some variation in defining response to the maneuver, overall rate for responders in the pediatric age group is probably close to 80%. Casado-Flores et al. showed that the improved oxygenation in their study was not sustained after returning to the supine position [43]. Overall, authors have reported variability in the oxygenation responses to prone positioning, and responders or patients who may benefit cannot always be predicted in the immediate period after prone positioning.

To date, no studies demonstrate that improved oxygenation decreases mortality in ARDS. There is increasing evidence that survivors of ARDS may suffer from extended pulmonary morbidity (such as oxygen requirement) and nonpulmonary morbidity (such as muscle fatigue, wasting, and weakness). To assess the long-term efficacies of interventions in ARDS, it is desirable to monitor, quantify, and evaluate their effect on these functional outcomes. Herridge et al. evaluated 109 adults with ARDS 3, 6 and 9 months after intensive care unit discharge [46]. At 1 year, a significant proportion of survivors reported nonpulmonary morbidity. Future studies with pediatric ARDS patients to evaluate the role of prone positioning should incorporate clinically relevant functional outcomes to quantify long-term effects of this intervention [47].

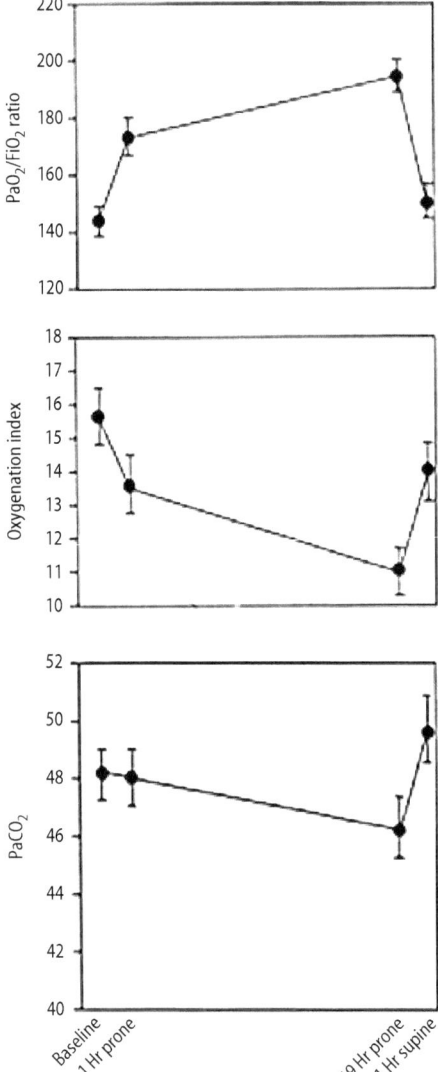

treatment values of OI with those after brief (6–10 hr) and prolonged (18–24 hr) periods in the prone position [48]. Children demonstrated a more pronounced and stable reduction in OI after prolonged periods of prone position than after brief periods. Curley et al. demonstrated the safety and feasibility of intermittent prone positioning for children admitted to the intensive care unit with respiratory failure with P/F ratios of 300 mm Hg or less who were on mechanical ventilatory support [44]. Patients ranged in age from 2 months to 17 years and were enrolled within 19 hours of meeting entry criteria. Patients were in the prone position for 20 hr each day and returned to the supine position for 4 hr. This accounted for 47% of the time of mechanical ventilation spent in the prone position.

Relvas et al. also reviewed 40 pediatric patients (aged 1 month to 18 years) over a period of 3 years who had been placed in the prone position during management of ARDS [48]. Patients in this study showed a higher benefit of decreasing OI when in the prone position for more than 12 hr compared with shorter periods of prone positioning. Kornecki et al. enrolled 10 children (8 weeks to 16 years) within the first week after acute lung injury. Patients were kept in the prone position for 12 hr, alternating between prone and supine positions [45]. Overall, the variable duration of the prone position in these studies stems from uncertainty regarding the optimal duration of this therapy. Early improvements in hypoxemia as seen in responders in the studies mentioned may be due to redistribution of ventilation and improvement of V/Q matching. However,

FIGURE 8.3. Day 1 PaO_2/FiO_2 ratio, oxygenation index (OI), and $PaCO_2$. **(Top)** The PaO_2/FiO_2 ratios among the four data collection points were significantly different ($p = 0.006$). The PaO_2/FiO_2 ratio significantly increased ($p = 0.04$) from 143 ± 10 mm Hg at baseline in the supine position to 173 ± 14 mm Hg after 1 hr in the prone position. It continued to increase significantly ($p = 0.005$) to 194 ± 15 mm Hg after 19 hr in the prone position. The PaO_2/FiO_2 ratio at hour 21 in the supine position (150 ± 11 mm Hg) was not significantly different from that at baseline. **(Middle)** The OIs among the four data collection points were significantly different ($p = 0.01$). The OI significantly decreased ($p = 0.05$) from a baseline value in the supine position from 15.7 ± 1.7 to 13.6 ± 1.6 mm Hg after 1 hr in the prone position and continued to decrease significantly ($p = 0.008$) to 10.9 ± 1.5 mm Hg after 19 hr in the prone position. The OI at hour 21 in the supine position (14 ± 1.9 mm Hg) was not significantly different from that at baseline. **(Bottom)** $PaCO_2$ values were not significantly different among the four data collection points. (From Curley et al. [44]. Copyright 2000 from the American College of Chest Physicians. Reprinted with permission.)

Duration of Prone Positioning

There is a wide variation in the duration of prone positioning used in the pediatric studies (see Table 8.1). Prospective studies have included protocols in which patients underwent repeated postural changes, spending periods ranging from 8 to 20 hr in the prone position. Relvas et al. retrospectively analyzed data from patients placed in the prone position during ARDS and compared the pre-

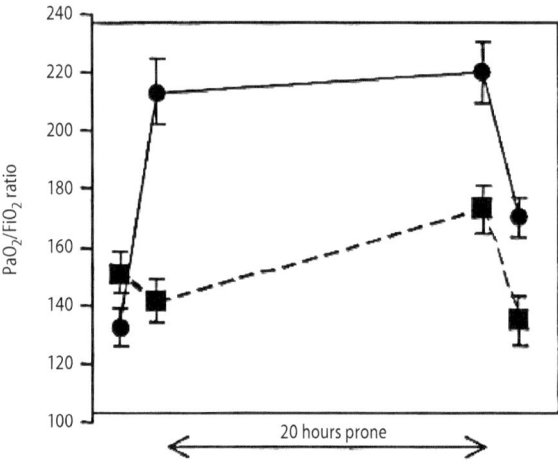

FIGURE 8.4. The PaO_2/FiO_2 ratio was significantly different between the two subgroups ($p = 0.05$) over the four data collection points ($p = 0.003$) and between the two subgroups over the four data collection points ($p = 0.03$). Immediate responder group (•): The PaO_2/FiO_2 ratio significantly increased ($p = 0.003$) from a baseline value in the supine position of 134 ± 11 to 213 ± 21 mm Hg after 1 hr in the prone position. Significant ($p = 0.02$) but not cumulative increases in oxygenation were seen after 19 hr in the prone position (220 ± 25 mm Hg). The PaO_2/FiO_2 ratio at hour 21 in the supine position (170 ± 12 mm Hg) was significantly better than that at baseline in the supine position ($p = 0.02$). Immediate nonresponder group (■): the PaO_2/FiO_2 ratio did not significantly increase from a baseline value in the supine position from 152 ± 16 to 141 ± 13 mm Hg after 1 hr in the prone position. Significant ($p = 0.02$) and cumulative increases in oxygenation were seen after 19 hr in the prone position (173 ± 15 mm Hg). The PaO_2/FiO_2 ratio at hour 21 in the supine position (135 ± 15 mm Hg) was not significantly better than that at baseline in the supine position. *Note*: with the exception of increasing the FiO_2 to keep SpO_2 at >85%, ventilator settings were held constant during the 1-hr supine-to-prone and prone-to-supine repositioning. (From Curley et al. [44]. Copyright 2000 from the American College of Chest Physicians. Reprinted with permission.)

other mechanisms have been proposed for the presumed benefits of longer periods of prone positioning.

McAuley et al. studied the effects of the prone position over a period of 18 hours in 11 patients with ARDS [49]. Respiratory parameters and extravascular lung water (EVLW) were prospectively recorded at various times during prone positioning. The study demonstrated early improvement in oxygenation followed by progressive improvement in gas exchange, pulmonary shunt, and decreased ELVW. The authors proposed that studies examining the role of prone positioning would have to offer the therapy over a prolonged period before allowing conclusions about its efficacy or benefits. It is impossible at this stage to determine the exact duration of an effective postural maneuver. The ideal duration of prone positioning may be individually variable, and it appears that patients may vary in their responses to this maneuver.

The most recent multicenter randomized controlled clinical trial, evaluating the role of prone positioning for acutely ill children with ARDS, was stopped after an interim analysis for futility. Patients (aged 2 weeks to 18 years) were enrolled from seven pediatric intensive care units within 48 hr of meeting ALI/ARDS criteria and randomized to either conventional supine management or prone positioning. The two groups were managed according to ventilator protocol, extubation readiness testing, sedation protocol, and hemodynamic, nutrition, and skin care guidelines. Thus, significant co-interventions were uniform between the groups. Patients in the treatment arm spent 20 hr/day in the prone position for a maximum of 7 days. The study was stopped after analyzing data from 102 patients (51 in the prone positioning group) when no significant differences were noted in ventilator-free days between the two groups after adjusting for age, severity of illness, and type of lung injury (direct/indirect ALI). No significant differences were observed in the secondary outcomes (mortality, time to recovery of lung function, organ failure-free days, or functional outcome) between the two groups. Overall, the study failed to show a clinically relevant outcome benefit of the prone position for pediatric ARDS/ALI patients.

Pragmatics of Prone Positioning

Since its initial description, a large number of studies have examined the effects of prone positioning in patients with a variety of respiratory illnesses. In the process, the technique has been refined with protocols, devices, and safeguards developed over the years to ensure patient safety. Patient selection, timing, and the duration of prone positioning have been discussed in the previous sections. Practical considerations for the implementation of prone positioning are discussed here.

Early investigators such as Piehl and Brown [2] used the CircOlectric bed for prone positioning without abdominal suspension. Douglas et al. [3] utilized customized foam pads, allowing space for the abdomen to prevent its restriction. Regardless of the approach, most recent investigators have made provisions for abdominal suspension during prone positioning.

As previously discussed, prone positioning is unlikely to be beneficial in the derecruited lung. Currently, clinicians rely on oxygenation and experimental methods of measuring lung dynamics to assess the response to recruitment maneuvers at bedside. Before postural change, clinicians should evaluate the patient for status of lung inflation and aim to achieve optimal recruitment. By incorporating this step as part of the prone positioning algorithm,

the chances of deriving a clinical benefit from this maneuver is maximized.

Adverse Events

The procedure of safely turning patients from a supine to prone position presents some logistical challenges. The perceived benefits of this therapeutic intervention must outweigh the potential adverse effects of this maneuver [50]. The potential complications associated with turning a patient include tissue [43] and nerve injury [51] at pressure areas, decreased venous return and edema, changes in intraocular pressure [52], difficulty in positioning and/or accessing the lines and tubes, difficult access to patients during resuscitation [53], risk of disconnection of lines and tubes [54], and delayed recognition of cardiorespiratory deterioration. With a well-designed procedural algorithm and procedurally competent personnel, the incidences of these complications can be minimized and patients safely turned even during periods of critical illness [55]. Reversible edema of the face, eyelids, conjunctiva, lips, and tongue becomes increasingly common after a few hours of prone positioning. Dependent edema may be difficult to avoid even with frequent changes in position [54,56].

Pressure ulcers were reported by Jolliet et al. [57] in 3/19 patients in their study with a 12-hr protocol and by Willems et al. [58] in one of their subjects who developed bilateral nipple ulcers after being prone for 5 days. In a 20-hr protocol for prone positioning, Fridrich et al. [54] reported some cutaneous problems but no pressure ulcers in this study where head and arm positions were changed every 2 hr. Corneal edema and ulceration have been associated with prone positioning and have the potential to cause visual loss if not detected and treated early. Stocker et al. [59] report a case of corneal ulceration, requiring corneal transplantation. Hering et al. [60] examined the effects of prone positioning on intraabdominal pressure and renal and cardiovascular function in 16 mechanically ventilated adults. The authors reported improved arterial oxygenation in their patients without alterations in hemodynamic status, renal function, and perfusion. Although no special efforts were made to suspend the abdomen in this study, intraabdominal pressure increased by only 2 to 14 mm Hg while the patients were prone with no perceived clinical effects.

Similar adverse effects of prone positioning have been reported in pediatric studies. Casado-Flores et al. [43] placed 23 children with ARDS in the prone position and then repositioned to supine every 8 hr for an average of 10 days. Pads and massage were applied to pressure points. Scars in knees (n = 2), external ear necrosis (n = 1), facial edema, and hemodynamic instability were recorded. Curley et al. [44] enrolled 25 children with ARDS/ALI and subjected them to prone positioning for a period of 20 hr each day for a median time of 4 days. In the phase one study, a prone-positioning device was used with a standardized procedure for prone positioning by a team of trained personnel. The abdomen was unrestrained from the bed and pressure-relieving material was used at patient contact areas. Stage II pressure ulcers were reported in pressure areas in 24% of patients in this study. Haefner et al. [61] reported their experience with 962 position changes in 93 patients with respiratory failure who were placed in the prone position while receiving extracorporeal membrane oxygenation (ECMO) therapy. There were no unplanned extubations, tube displacements, pressure ulcerations of skin, or corneal abrasions associated with prone positioning in this study. The incidence of bleeding from cannulae and tube insertion sites was not higher in these patients than in patients on ECMO. Prone positioning of pediatric patients has been reported to result in cephalad movement of the endotracheal tube in the trachea [62]. In this study, 15 pairs of radiographs from 14 patients were retrospectively reviewed and images before and after prone positioning were compared. Based on their observations, the authors recommend placement of the endotracheal tube tip deeper than the level of one-third tracheal length to avoid upward movement and dislodgement.

Recommendations for Safe Prone Positioning

An institutional protocol for standardizing the process of prone positioning will limit iatrogenic injury. Appendix 39.1 includes the prone positioning procedure employed in a recent pediatric multicenter clinical trial of prone positioning. The protocol includes a safety check that anticipates and makes provisions for avoiding potential problems.

A reasonable and minimum number of personnel should participate in the process of prone positioning. A respiratory therapist (RT) should be part of the repositioning team. The RT should anticipate likely changes in the pulmonary compliance and be prepared to reassess ventilatory requirements after postural changes. The need for suctioning airway secretions before prone–supine postural changes is essential. All invasive devices should be checked and re-secured if necessary before repositioning. Pressure-relieving positioning aides are used to prevent damage to the eyes, face, and skin. New protocols should be reviewed by a pediatric physical therapist. Pictorial and video training materials and reminders are helpful to maintain procedural competence. Prone-positioned patients require ongoing surveillance for pressure ulcers and corneal injury.

We have observed an important patient safety issue when placing children supported on high-frequency oscillatory ventilation (HFOV) in the prone position. Currently available HFOV ventilators do not have a safety alarm for detection of a decrease in tidal volume. Soon after placement in the prone position, the ability to monitor the efficacy of the oscillations, traditionally described as the "wiggle factor," is compromised. Any impairment in the oscillatory amplitude of HFOV could result in rapidly escalating levels of carbon dioxide. Indeed, we have observed hypercapnia in some patients with severe ARDS who were placed in the prone position during HFOV therapy. This effect should be anticipated and potentially documented with early arterial blood gases following a supine-to-prone turn. Awareness of these adverse effects will allow regular monitoring and prompt detection and intervention in the clinical setting.

Conclusion

We have reviewed what is currently known about prone positioning for pediatric patients with ALI/ARDS. The prone position has been safely applied in the pediatric population. The prone position is likely to benefit a subgroup of children with ARDS when started early after lung injury, and immediate responders may benefit from prolonged periods of prone positioning. The duration in the prone position may be restricted by the feasibility of the maneuver. There may not be much benefit in continued prone positioning of patients who do not show immediate response to this postural change.

The prone position should be used for select patients to improve lung recruitment. Improvement in oxygenation is likely to be the

Appendix 8.1. Prone Positioning Check Sheet

Preparation (prior to getting help into the room)

- ☐   • Create cushions using egg crate material (head, chest, pelvic, distal femoral, and lower limb).
- ☐ Consider transpyloric feed tube and check placement.
- ☐ Check endotracheal tube (ETT) on chest x-ray (CXR)—tip should be in the lower third of the thoracic trachea.
- ☐ Assess the security of the ETT, vascular lines, and oxyhemoglobin saturation (SpO_2) probe and reinforce as necessary.
  - • Retape the ETT to the upper lip on the side of the mouth that will end in the "up" position.
  - • Place a protective layer of plastic tape over the white adhesive tape holding the ETT.
- ☐ If cuffed ETT/trach, inflate cuff using minimal leak technique (cuff pressure under 25 mmHg).
- ☐ Protect eyes if chemically paralyzed and/or open (cleanse, lubricate, cover with plastic wrap).
- ☐ If high-frequency oscillatory ventilation (HFOV), apply plastic film dressing over anterior bony prominences to avoid friction injury.
- ☐ Move electrocardiographic electrodes to the lateral aspects of the upper arms and hips.
- ☐ Remove clothing surrounding the thorax and abdomen.
- ☐ Coil and then secure the bladder catheter to the inner thigh.
- ☐ Suction the patient's oropharynx. (If ETT suctioned, postpone turn until unit patient is returned to the presuctioning ventilator settings).
- ☐ Temporarily cap nonessential vascular lines and the patient's nasogastric tube (NGT)/nasojejunal tube (NJT).
- ☐ *Final check*—Review the start and end points of all that is left attached to the patient. Arrange the remaining vascular lines and Foley catheter tubing to prevent excessive tension.
- ☐ Premedicate with comfort medications at the discretion of the bedside nurse.

Turing (bedside nurse/respiratory therapist [RT] team)

- ☐ Call for RT and at least one other nurse.
- ☐ Preplan responsibility: RT, head/ETT; nurse 1, chest/arms; nurse 2, hips/legs.
- ☐ Review technique:
  - • *Infants/toddlers*: Levitate = levitate up, turn 45 degrees, pause/reassess, turn prone, levitate up to place cushions under the subject.
  - • *School aged/adolescents*: Mummy = using all bed linens, slide patient to the edge of the bed away from the ventilator, place new draw sheet over patient; position chest and pelvic cushions over draw sheet; place full sheet over entire patient; create a mummy effect by tucking the edges of the full sheet under patient; turn patient 45 degrees toward ventilator, pause/reassess, position patient prone on new linen and cushions/remove old linen.
- ☐ Keep head in alignment with body, avoid hyperextension, keep arms next to torso, point toes of the upper leg in the direction of turn.
- ☐ Turn toward the ventilator without disconnecting. (FiO_2 may be manipulated to maintain target SpO_2. All other ventilator settings remain constant until 1-hr post turn arterial blood gas values obtained.)
- ☐ Talk the patient through the turn.

Immediately after the turn

- ☐ Reassess the security and patency of all tubes/lines.
- ☐ Reassess SpO_2, blood pressure, cardiac rhythm, and breath sounds.
- ☐ Reassess ETT/trach leak. (May adjust cuff volume, head position, delivered tidal volume to ensure adequate ventilation.)
- ☐ Uncap/reattach capped off lines/NGT/NJT.
- ☐ Position the patient:
  - ○ Turn head to side and cushion head and ear with pressure-relieving material.
  - ○ Place an absorbent diaper under the patient's mouth.
  - ○ Avoid excessive flexion/extension of the spine, cushion the upper chest and pelvis—check that the abdomen is unrestrained. For males, check that the penis and scrotum are unrestrained. For adolescent females, check that the nipples are away from chest rolls.
  - ○ Flex arms up.
  - ○ Position knees and feet off bed using a roll under the distal femur and lower leg.
  - ○ Check that everything attached to the patient is not pressing against the skin (ETT balloon port) and that the patient's skin in not pinched in any way (periumbilical area).

Return to supine

- ☐ Precautions and techniques described above apply.
- ☐ Consider performing the patient's daily suctioning procedure
- ☐ Patients are turned away from the ventilator without disconnecting.
- ☐ Position the patient:
  - • Cushion head using pressure-relieving materials (pillow, jell pillow, or Spenco pad).
  - • Elevate the patient's heels off the bed using an appropriate sized pillow.

immediate benefit from this maneuver and will be desirable in most patients if it provides stability and minimizes potentially lung-injuring mechanical ventilatory support. With vigilance to protocol, prone positioning can be performed safely as a therapeutic maneuver to improve systemic oxygenation in the most critical of patients. Importantly, oxygenation as a single parameter has not been shown to correlate with outcomes such as mortality. Thus, the impact of the prone position on functional outcomes remains to be fully evaluated, and future studies will need to incorporate longer follow-up periods and assess quality of life, lung function, and other such functional outcomes in these children.

References

1. Bryan AC. Conference on the scientific basis of respiratory therapy. Pulmonary physiotherapy in the pediatric age group. Comments of a devil's advocate. Am Rev Respir Dis 1974;110(6 Pt 2):143–144.
2. Piehl MA, Brown RS. Use of extreme position changes in acute respiratory failure. Crit Care Med 1976;4(1):13–14.
3. Douglas WW, Rehder K, Beynen FM, Sessler AD, Marsh HM. Improved oxygenation in patients with acute respiratory failure: the prone position. Am Rev Respir Dis 1977;115(4):559–566.
4. Lamm WJ, Graham MM, Albert RK. Mechanism by which the prone position improves oxygenation in acute lung injury. Am J Respir Crit Care Med 1994;150(1):184–193.
5. Pappert D, Rossaint R, Slama K, Gruning T, Falke KJ. Influence of positioning on ventilation–perfusion relationships in severe adult respiratory distress syndrome. Chest 1994;106(5):1511–1516.
6. Pelosi P, Brazzi L, Gattinoni L. Prone position in acute respiratory distress syndrome. Eur Respir J 2002;20(4):1017–1028.
7. Malbouisson LM, Busch CJ, Puybasset L, Lu Q, Cluzel P, Rouby JJ. Role of the heart in the loss of aeration characterizing lower lobes in acute respiratory distress syndrome. CT Scan ARDS Study Group. Am J Respir Crit Care Med 2000;161(6):2005–2012.
8. Hyatt RE, Bar-Yishay E, Abel MD. Influence of the heart on the vertical gradient of transpulmonary pressure in dogs. J Appl Physiol 1985;58(1):52–57.
9. McMahon SM, Proctor DF, Permutt S. Pleural surface pressure in dogs. J Appl Physiol 1969;27(6):881–885.
10. Hubmayr RD, Walters BJ, Chevalier PA, Rodarte JR, Olson LE. Topographical distribution of regional lung volume in anesthetized dogs. J Appl Physiol 1983;54(4):1048–1056.
11. Reutershan J, Schmitt A, Dietz K, Fretschner R. Non-invasive measurement of pulmonary blood flow during prone positioning in patients with early acute respiratory distress syndrome. Clin Sci (Lond) 2004;106(1):3–10.
12. Brussel T, Hachenberg T, Roos N, Lemzem H, Konertz W, Lawin P. Mechanical ventilation in the prone position for acute respiratory failure after cardiac surgery. J Cardiothorac Vasc Anesth 1993;7(5):541–546.
13. Gerhardt T, Bancalari E. Chestwall compliance in full-term and premature infants. Acta Paediatr Scand 1980;69(3):359–364.
14. Sharp JT, Druz WS, Balagot RC, Bandelin VR, Danon J. Total respiratory compliance in infants and children. J Appl Physiol 1970;29(6):775–779.
15. Heldt GP, McIlroy MB. Distortion of chest wall and work of diaphragm in preterm infants. J Appl Physiol 1987;62(1):164–169.
16. Nicolai T, Lanteri CJ, Sly PD. Frequency dependence of elastance and resistance in ventilated children with and without the chest opened. Eur Respir J 1993;6(9):1340–1346.
17. Stocks J. Respiratory physiology during early life. Monaldi Arch Chest Dis 1999;54(4):358–364.
18. Pelosi P, Cereda M, Foti G, Giacomini M, Pesenti A. Alterations of lung and chest wall mechanics in patients with acute lung injury: effects of positive end-expiratory pressure. Am J Respir Crit Care Med 1995;152(2):531–537.
19. Mutoh T, Lamm WJ, Embree LJ, Hildebrandt J, Albert RK. Abdominal distension alters regional pleural pressures and chest wall mechanics in pigs in vivo. J Appl Physiol 1991;70(6):2611–2618.
20. Ranieri VM, Brienza N, Santostasi S, Puntillo F, Mascia L, Vitale N, et al. Impairment of lung and chest wall mechanics in patients with acute respiratory distress syndrome: role of abdominal distension. Am J Respir Crit Care Med 1997;156(4 Pt 1):1082–1091.
21. Pelosi P, D'Onofrio D, Chiumello D, Paolo S, Chiara G, Capelozzi VL, et al. Pulmonary and extrapulmonary acute respiratory distress syndrome are different. Eur Respir J Suppl 2003;42:48s–56s.
22. Milic-Emili J, Henderson JA, Dolovich MB, Trop D, Kaneko K. Regional distribution of inspired gas in the lung. J Appl Physiol 1966;21(3):749–759.
23. Hernandez LA, Peevy KJ, Moise AA, Parker JC. Chest wall restriction limits high airway pressure-induced lung injury in young rabbits. J Appl Physiol 1989;66(5):2364–2368.
24. de Durante G, del Turco M, Rustichini L, Cosimini P, Giunta F, Hudson LD, et al. ARDSnet lower tidal volume ventilatory strategy may generate intrinsic positive end-expiratory pressure in patients with acute respiratory distress syndrome. Am J Respir Crit Care Med 2002;165(9):1271–1274.
25. Cox RG, Ewen A, Bart BB. The prone position is associated with a decrease in respiratory system compliance in healthy anaesthetized infants. Paediatr Anaesth 2001;11(3):291–296.
26. Albert RK, Leasa D, Sanderson M, Robertson HT, Hlastala MP. The prone position improves arterial oxygenation and reduces shunt in oleic-acid-induced acute lung injury. Am Rev Respir Dis 1987;135(3):628–633.
27. Gattinoni L, Caironi P, Pelosi P, Goodman LR. What has computed tomography taught us about the acute respiratory distress syndrome? Am J Respir Crit Care Med 2001;164(9):1701–1711.
28. Gattinoni L, Pelosi P, Vitale G, Pesenti A, D'Andrea L, Mascheroni D. Body position changes redistribute lung computed-tomographic density in patients with acute respiratory failure. Anesthesiology 1991;74(1):15–23.
29. Ventilation with lower tidal volumes as compared with traditional tidal volumes for acute lung injury and the acute respiratory distress syndrome. The Acute Respiratory Distress Syndrome Network. N Engl J Med 2000;342(18):1301–1308.
30. Gattinoni L, Pesenti A. The concept of "baby lung." Intensive Care Med 2005.
31. Valenza F, Guglielmi M, Maffioletti M, Tedesco C, Maccagni P, Fossali T, et al. Prone position delays the progression of ventilator-induced lung injury in rats: does lung strain distribution play a role? Crit Care Med 2005;33(2):361–367.
32. Crotti S, Mascheroni D, Caironi P, Pelosi P, Ronzoni G, Mondino M, et al. Recruitment and derecruitment during acute respiratory failure: a clinical study. Am J Respir Crit Care Med 2001;164(1):131–140.
33. Puybasset L, Cluzel P, Chao N, Slutsky AS, Coriat P, Rouby JJ. A computed tomography scan assessment of regional lung volume in acute lung injury. The CT Scan ARDS Study Group. Am J Respir Crit Care Med 1998;158(5 Pt 1):1644–1655.
34. Lim CM, Jung H, Koh Y, Lee JS, Shim TS, Lee SD, et al. Effect of alveolar recruitment maneuver in early acute respiratory distress syndrome according to antiderecruitment strategy, etiological category of diffuse lung injury, and body position of the patient. Crit Care Med 2003;31(2):411–418.
35. Villagra A, Ochagavia A, Vatua S, Murias G, Del Mar Fernandez M, Lopez Aguilar J, et al. Recruitment maneuvers during lung protective ventilation in acute respiratory distress syndrome. Am J Respir Crit Care Med 2002;165(2):165–170.
36. Guerin C, Badet M, Rosselli S, Heyer L, Sab JM, Langevin B, et al. Effects of prone position on alveolar recruitment and oxygenation in acute lung injury. Intensive Care Med 1999;25(11):1222–1230.
37. Pelosi P, Bottino N, Chiumello D, Caironi P, Panigada M, Gamberoni C, et al. Sigh in supine and prone position during acute respiratory distress syndrome. Am J Respir Crit Care Med 2003;167(4):521–527.

38. Oczenski W, Hormann C, Keller C, Lorenzl N, Kepka A, Schwarz S, et al. Recruitment maneuvers during prone positioning in patients with acute respiratory distress syndrome. Crit Care Med 2005;33(1):54–62.

39. Numa AH, Hammer J, Newth CJ. Effect of prone and supine positions on functional residual capacity, oxygenation, and respiratory mechanics in ventilated infants and children. Am J Respir Crit Care Med 1997;156(4 Pt 1):1185–1189.

40. Callister ME, Evans TW. Pulmonary versus extrapulmonary acute respiratory distress syndrome: different diseases or just a useful concept? Curr Opin Crit Care 2002;8(1):21–25.

41. Pelosi P, Gattinoni L. Acute respiratory distress syndrome of pulmonary and extra-pulmonary origin: fancy or reality? Intensive Care Med 2001;27(3):457–460.

42. Suntharalingam G, Regan K, Keogh BF, Morgan CJ, Evans TW. Influence of direct and indirect etiology on acute outcome and 6-month functional recovery in acute respiratory distress syndrome. Crit Care Med 2001;29(3):562–566.

43. Casado-Flores J, Martinez de Azagra A, Ruiz-Lopez MJ, Ruiz M, Serrano A. Pediatric ARDS: effect of supine-prone postural changes on oxygenation. Intensive Care Med 2002;28(12):1792–1796.

44. Curley MA, Thompson JE, Arnold JH. The effects of early and repeated prone positioning in pediatric patients with acute lung injury. Chest 2000;118(1):156–163.

45. Kornecki A, Frndova H, Coates AL, Shemie SD. 4A randomized trial of prolonged prone positioning in children with acute respiratory failure. Chest 2001;119(1):211–218.

46. Herridge MS, Cheung AM, Tansey CM, Matte-Martyn A, Diaz-Granados N, Al-Saidi F, et al. One-year outcomes in survivors of the acute respiratory distress syndrome. N Engl J Med 2003;348(8):683–693.

47. Curley MA, Zimmerman JJ. Alternative outcome measures for pediatric clinical sepsis trials. Pediatr Crit Care Med 2005;6(3):S150–S156.

48. Relvas MS, Silver PC, Sagy M. Prone positioning of pediatric patients with ARDS results in improvement in oxygenation if maintained >12 h daily. Chest 2003;124(1):269–274.

49. McAuley DF, Giles S, Fichter H, Perkins GD, Gao F. What is the optimal duration of ventilation in the prone position in acute lung injury and acute respiratory distress syndrome? Intensive Care Med 2002;28(4):414–418.

50. Guerin C, Gaillard S, Lemasson S, Ayzac L, Girard R, Beuret P, et al. Effects of systematic prone positioning in hypoxemic acute respiratory failure: a randomized controlled trial. JAMA 2004;292(19):2379–2387.

51. Winfree CJ, Kline DG. Intraoperative positioning nerve injuries. Surg Neurol 2005;63(1):5–18.

52. Hunt K, Bajekal R, Calder I, Meacher R, Eliahoo J, Acheson JF. Changes in intraocular pressure in anesthetized prone patients. J Neurosurg Anesthesiol 2004;16(4):287–290.

53. Vollman KM. Prone positioning for the ARDS patient. Dimens Crit Care Nurs 1997;16(4):184–193.

54. Fridrich P, Krafft P, Hochleuthner H, Mauritz W. The effects of long-term prone positioning in patients with trauma-induced adult respiratory distress syndrome. Anesth Analg 1996;83(6):1206–1211.

55. Martin de la Torre Martin M, Gonzalez Priego T, Lopez Caballero T, Lopez Reusch S. [Postural technique in prone position: hemodynamic and respiratory parameters and complications]. Enferm Intensiva 2000;11(3):127–135.

56. Chatte G, Sab JM, Dubois JM, Sirodot M, Gaussorgues P, Robert D. Prone position in mechanically ventilated patients with severe acute respiratory failure. Am J Respir Crit Care Med 1997;155(2):473–478.

57. Jolliet P, Bulpa P, Chevrolet JC. Effects of the prone position on gas exchange and hemodynamics in severe acute respiratory distress syndrome. Crit Care Med 1998;26(12):1977–1985.

58. Willems MC, Voets AJ, Welten RJ. Two unusual complications of prone-dependency in severe ARDS. Intensive Care Med 1998;24(3):276–277.

59. Stocker R, Neff T, Stein S, Ecknauer E, Trentz O, Russi E. Prone positioning and low-volume pressure-limited ventilation improve survival in patients with severe ARDS. Chest 1997;111(4):1008–1017.

60. Hering R, Wrigge H, Vorwerk R, Brensing KA, Schroder S, Zinserling J, et al. The effects of prone positioning on intraabdominal pressure and cardiovascular and renal function in patients with acute lung injury. Anesth Analg 2001;92(5):1226–1231.

61. Haefner SM, Bratton SL, Annich GM, Bartlett RH, Custer JR. Complications of intermittent prone positioning in pediatric patients receiving extracorporeal membrane oxygenation for respiratory failure. Chest 2003;123(5):1589–1594.

62. Marcano BV, Silver P, Sagy M. Cephalad movement of endotracheal tubes caused by prone positioning pediatric patients with acute respiratory distress syndrome. Pediatr Crit Care Med 2003;4(2):186–189.

63. Murdoch IA, Storman MO. Improved arterial oxygenation in children with the adult respiratory distress syndrome: the prone position. Acta Paediatr 1994;83(10):1043–1046.

64. Wagaman MJ, Shutack JG, Moomjian AS, Schwartz JG, Shaffer TH, Fox WW. Improved oxygenation and lung compliance with prone positioning of neonates. J Pediatr 1979;94(5):787–791.

65. Lioy J, Manginello FP. A comparison of prone and supine positioning in the immediate postextubation period of neonates. J Pediatr 1988;112(6):982–984.

66. Mendoza JC, Roberts JL, Cook LN. Postural effects on pulmonary function and heart rate of preterm infants with lung disease. J Pediatr 1991;118(3):445–448.

67. McEvoy C, Mendoza ME, Bowling S, Hewlett V, Sardesai S, Durand M. Prone positioning decreases episodes of hypoxemia in extremely low birth weight infants (1,000 grams or less) with chronic lung disease. J Pediatr 1997;130(2):305–309.

68. Curley MA, Hibberd PL, Fineman LD, Wypij D, Shih MC, Thompson JE, et al. Effect of prone positioning on clinical outcomes in children with acute lung injury: a randomized controlled trial. JAMA 2005;294(2):229–237.

9
High-Frequency Oscillatory Ventilation

Kathleen M. Ventre and John H. Arnold

Introduction

Data supporting the feasibility of high-frequency oscillatory ventilation (HFOV) come from the observation that delivering very tidal volumes small at high frequencies can overcome the need for adequate bulk gas flow in the lung. In the early 1970s, while attempting to measure cardiac performance in large animals by assessing the myocardial response to pericardial pressure oscillations, Lunkenheimer and colleagues found that endotracheal high-frequency oscillations could produce efficient CO_2 elimination in the absence of significant chest wall excursion [1,2]. These investigators determined that CO_2 elimination was related to changes in the frequency of oscillation as well as the amplitude of the vibrations [1]. In general, CO_2 was cleared optimally at a frequency between 23–40 Hz, with smaller animals requiring higher frequencies [1]. Several years later, Butler and colleagues observed that gas exchange could be supported in humans at a frequency of 15 Hz, hypothesizing that this would enhance diffusive gas transport while minimizing dependence on bulk convective gas flow in the airways [3]. In their study, a series of patients, 9 years of age and older, were successfully ventilated with a piston pump calibrated to deliver tidal volumes in the range of 50–150 mL, and a single 2.5-kg infant was supported with a tidal volume of 7.5 mL using the same device [3].

At the moment, there are many laboratory data to suggest that repetitive cycles of pulmonary recruitment and derecruitment are associated with identifiable markers of lung injury, and experimental models of ventilatory support that reverse atelectasis, limit phasic changes in lung volume, and prevent alveolar overdistension appear to be less injurious [4–11]. There is also a growing quantity of clinical data that support these observations. A recent single-center cohort study demonstrated that among 332 patients who did not have acute lung injury (ALI) at initiation of mechanical ventilation, 80 (24%) developed it within 5 days [12]. Approximately one third of the study patients were ventilated using tidal volumes exceeding 12 mL/kg, and multivariate analysis identified large tidal volumes as the most significant risk factor for the development of ALI (odds ratio 1.3 for each 1 mL above 6 mL/kg; $p < 0.001$)[12].

Inappropriate mechanical ventilation strategies may also potentiate the dysfunction of distant organs among patients with respiratory failure. In a multicenter trial, Ranieri and colleagues randomized 37 patients to receive a strategy directed at ventilating between the upper and lower inflection points on the pressure–volume curve (Figure 9.1), versus a higher volume, lower peak end-expiratory pressure (PEEP) strategy targeted at achieving normal blood gas tensions in the control group [6]. Bronchoalveolar lavage (BAL) and blood samples showed a local and systemic inflammatory cytokine response at 36 hr among those in the control group, whereas the experimental strategy appeared to diminish this response [6]. In addition, a landmark multicenter trial has brought about the understanding that specific strategies for mechanical ventilation can have an important influence on outcomes in patients with the acute respiratory distress syndrome (ARDS). In 2000, the ARDS Network investigators demonstrated a 22% relative reduction in mortality among adult patients with ARDS on conventional mechanical ventilation who were randomized to receive relatively small tidal volumes (6 mL/kg ideal body weight) compared with those who were ventilated with larger tidal volumes (12 mL/kg ideal body weight) [13]. Collectively, these observations on the benefits of tidal volume reduction have led to the expectation that high-frequency ventilation would have an important role in the clinical arena because of its unique ability to provide adequate gas exchange using very low tidal volumes in the setting of continuous alveolar recruitment. Theoretically, high-frequency ventilation provides the ultimate *open-lung* strategy of ventilation, preserving end-expiratory lung volume, minimizing cyclic stretch, and avoiding parenchymal overdistension at end inspiration by limiting tidal volume and transpulmonary pressure (Figure 9.2) [4–7].

Modalities of High-Frequency Ventilation

The major modalities of high-frequency ventilation include high-frequency flow interruption (HFFI), high-frequency positive pressure ventilation (HFPPV), high-frequency jet ventilation (HFJV),

D.S. Wheeler et al. (eds.), The *Respiratory Tract in Pediatric Critical Illness and Injury*,
DOI 10.1007/978-1-84800-925-7_9, © Springer-Verlag London Limited 2009

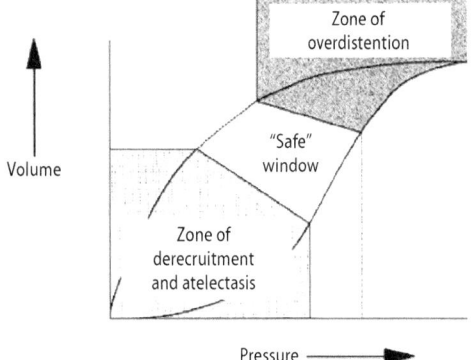

FIGURE 9.1. Pressure–volume relationships in acute lung injury. High end-expiratory pressures and small tidal volumes minimize the potential for derecruitment (lower left) and overdistension (upper right). (From Froese AB. High-frequency oscillatory ventilation for adult respiratory distress syndrome: let's get it right this time! Crit Care Med 1997;25:906–908. Copyright 1997. Reprinted with permission from Lippincott Williams & Wilkins.)

and high-frequency oscillatory ventilation (HFOV). High-frequency oscillatory ventilation is the most widely used form of high-frequency ventilation in clinical practice today. In HFOV, lung recruitment is maintained by the application of relatively high mean airway pressure, while ventilation is achieved by superimposed sinusoidal pressure oscillations that are delivered by a motor-driven piston or diaphragm at a frequency of 3–15 Hz [7,14]. High-frequency oscillatory ventilation is the only form of high-frequency ventilation in which expiration is an active process. As a result, alveolar ventilation is achieved during HFOV with the use

of tidal volumes in the range of 1–3 mL/kg, even in the most poorly compliant lungs [14].

Gas Transport and Control of Gas Exchange

A comprehensive understanding of the mechanisms of gas transport in HFOV has not emerged despite a long period of scientific investigations. Although direct bulk flow can account for ventilation of proximal alveolar units even at very low tidal volumes, it is now believed that *Pendelluft*, or mixing of gases among alveolar units with varying time constants, contributes significantly to gas exchange at high frequencies [15–17]. In addition, efficient gas mixing likely occurs along the parabolic inspiratory gas front in high-frequency oscillation, because this provides an increased area along which radial diffusion can occur [15,16]. Finally, axial asymmetry of inspiratory and expiratory gas flow profiles creates separation of fresh gas and exhaled gas so that inspiratory gas flow travels down the central axis of the airway, while expiratory flow is distributed along the airway wall [15,16].

Experimental work in healthy rabbits has shown that CO_2 elimination during HFOV is a function of frequency and the square of the tidal volume ($V_{CO2} = f \times Vt^2$) [18]. In HFOV, tidal volume is positively correlated with the amplitude of oscillation ("delta P," ΔP), and is related inversely to the frequency (Hz) [19]. Alveolar recruitment is positively correlated with the mean airway pressure (Paw) and the ratio of inspiratory time to expiratory time (I:E) [20]. Although most of the research using HFOV has focused on the use of higher frequency ranges, CO_2 elimination can probably occur at many potential combinations of f and Vt^2, with higher frequency ranges providing conditions of lowest lung impedance and, consequently,

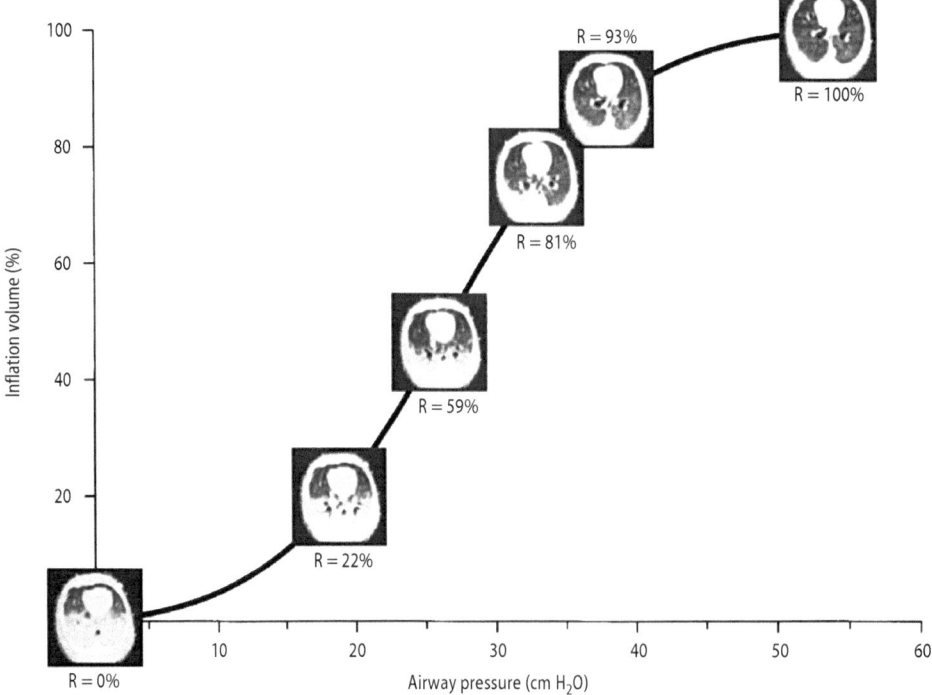

FIGURE 9.2. Open lung strategy in ARDS: alveolar recruitment along the pressure–volume curve in a large animal experimental model of ARDS, showing substantial increases in aeration of dependent lung units. R indicates percentage of total recruitment occurring at the corresponding airway pressure. At high airway pressures, nondependent regions may be vulnerable to overdistension. (From Gattinoni et al. [68]. Copyright 2001 the American Thoracic Society. Reprinted with permission.)

a lower pressure cost of ventilation [21,22]. In HFOV, Paw, ΔP, frequency, and I:E are all directly controlled by the operator.

Presently available high-frequency ventilators vary with respect to pressure waveforms, consistency of I:E ratio over a range of frequencies, and the relationship of displayed mean airway pressure to distal mean alveolar pressure [19]. Most of the experience with HFOV in the clinical arena involves the SensorMedics 3100A (SensorMedics, Yorba Linda, CA), which is approved for use in infants and children. Almost 20 years of study using this device in the laboratory have provided clinicians with a fundamental understanding of its performance characteristics. Using in vitro models as well as alveolar capsule techniques in small animals with open chests, several investigators have reported that mean airway pressure and ΔP are significantly attenuated by the tracheal tube, that alveolar pressure is inhomogeneously distributed during HFOV, and that the I:E ratio is an important determinant of alveolar pressure [20,23–25]. Specifically, early data from surfactant-deficient small animals, as well as from large animals and humans, seemed to indicate that limitation of expiratory time using an I:E ratio of 1:1 would promote alveolar gas trapping, especially at lower mean airway pressures [20,26–28]. This observation led to the suggestion that HFOV be applied in the clinical setting with an I:E ratio of no greater than 1:2.

When transitioning the patient to HFOV from conventional ventilation (Figure 9.3), the Paw on HFOV is typically set up to 5 cm H_2O above the Paw last used on the conventional ventilator in order to maintain recruitment in the face of pressure attenuation by the tracheal tube. Amplitude (ΔP) is set by adjusting the power control while observing for adequacy of chest wall vibrations, as indicated by visible vibration to the level of the groin. Frequencies of 12–15 Hz are generally used for small infants, whereas lower frequencies in the range of 3–8 Hz are typically used for larger pediatric patients and adults, with the goal of generating enough volume displacement to adequately ventilate using currently available HFOVs. If employing an *open lung* ventilation strategy, Paw is then slowly titrated upward in 1–2 cm H_2O increments, with the goal of reducing the FiO_2 to ≤0.6 with an arterial oxygen saturation of ≥90%.

Achieving acceptable oxygen saturations at this stage will often require intravascular volume expansion in order to avoid creating *zone 1* conditions [29] in the lung as pulmonary blood volume is displaced by the increasing alveolar pressure. Once adequate alveolar recruitment is achieved, it may be possible to capitalize on pulmonary hysteresis, evident in many regions of the lung early in the course of disease (see Figure 9.1) [30], by carefully adjusting the Paw downward as long as the oxygenating efficiency is preserved. Alternatively, after a brief period of aggressive volume recruitment, the Paw can be dropped to a point that is known to be above the closing pressure, with the expectation that adequate tidal volume will be preserved [30]. Adequacy of lung recruitment is verified by ensuring that both hemidiaphragms are displaced to the level of the ninth posterior rib on chest x-ray [14]. A typical sequence of steps for addressing hypercarbia once an appropriate degree of lung inflation as well as patency of the tracheal tube are verified would be (1) increasing the ΔP in increments of 3 cm H_2O until power is maximized, (2) decreasing the frequency in increments of 0.5–1 Hz, and (3) partially deflating the tracheal tube cuff, if available, to allow additional egress of CO_2 [31–33]. In the latter case, any decrement in Paw should be corrected by increasing the bias flow as necessary to maintain a stable level of distending pressure [32,33].

If employing a strategy targeted at managing active air leak, the lung is initially recruited using stepwise increases in Paw to achieve FiO_2 ≤0.6 and SaO_2 ≥90%, and then Paw and ΔP are lowered to a point just below the *leak pressure*, the value at which air is no longer seen to drain from the thoracostomy tube. If the leak pressure is relatively low, it may be necessary to tolerate an FiO_2 in excess of 0.6 with SaO_2 ≥85%, and hypercarbia if necessary, as long as pH ≥7.25, in order to provide satisfactory gas exchange while minimizing alveolar pressure [17,34–36]. As demonstrated in a small animal model of pneumothorax, higher frequencies and short inspiratory times may also minimize air leak during HFOV [36].

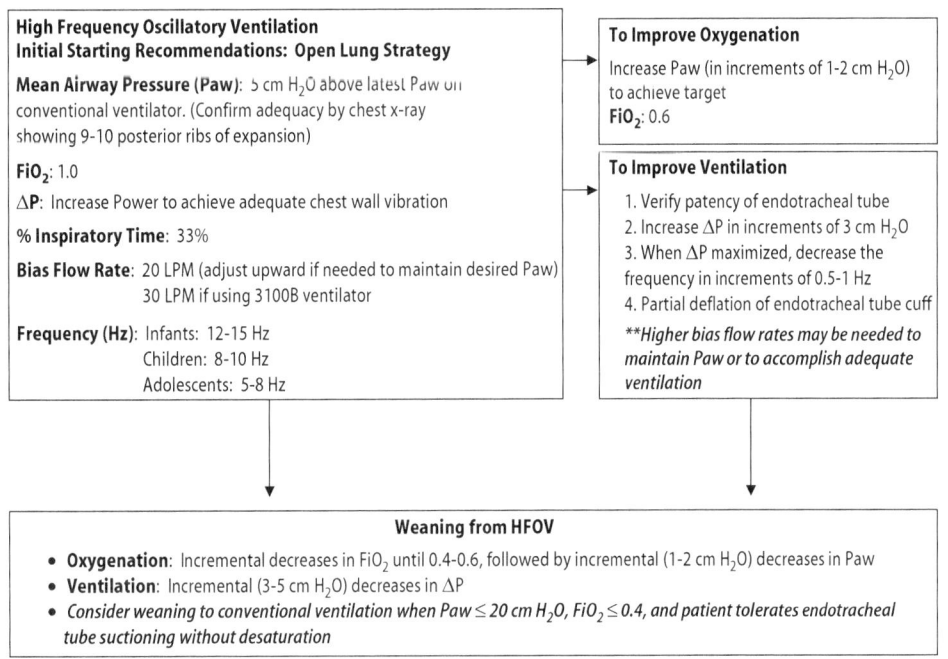

High Frequency Oscillatory Ventilation
Initial Starting Recommendations: Open Lung Strategy

Mean Airway Pressure (Paw): 5 cm H_2O above latest Paw on conventional ventilator. (Confirm adequacy by chest x-ray showing 9-10 posterior ribs of expansion)

FiO_2: 1.0

ΔP: Increase Power to achieve adequate chest wall vibration

% Inspiratory Time: 33%

Bias Flow Rate: 20 LPM (adjust upward if needed to maintain desired Paw)
30 LPM if using 3100B ventilator

Frequency (Hz): Infants: 12-15 Hz
Children: 8-10 Hz
Adolescents: 5-8 Hz

To Improve Oxygenation

Increase Paw (in increments of 1-2 cm H_2O) to achieve target
FiO_2: 0.6

To Improve Ventilation

1. Verify patency of endotracheal tube
2. Increase ΔP in increments of 3 cm H_2O
3. When ΔP maximized, decrease the frequency in increments of 0.5-1 Hz
4. Partial deflation of endotracheal tube cuff

***Higher bias flow rates may be needed to maintain Paw or to accomplish adequate ventilation**

Weaning from HFOV

- **Oxygenation**: Incremental decreases in FiO_2 until 0.4-0.6, followed by incremental (1-2 cm H_2O) decreases in Paw
- **Ventilation**: Incremental (3-5 cm H_2O) decreases in ΔP
- *Consider weaning to conventional ventilation when Paw ≤ 20 cm H_2O, FiO_2 ≤ 0.4, and patient tolerates endotracheal tube suctioning without desaturation*

FIGURE 9.3. Transitioning the critically ill child from conventional mechanical ventilatory support to high-frequency oscillatory ventilation.

High-Frequency Oscillatory Ventilation in the Neonate and Infant

Neonatal Respiratory Distress Syndrome

Surfactant deficiency, high chest wall compliance, and a dynamic functional residual capacity (FRC) that is near closing volume in the preterm infant interact to potentiate a repetitive cycle of derecruitment and reinflation that makes the neonatal lung particularly well suited to an open lung strategy of ventilation (Figure 9.4). Following laboratory investigations that demonstrated adequate gas exchange at lower intrapulmonary pressures and reduced incidence of pulmonary air leak with the use of HFOV in surfactant-deficient small animals [37,38], a substantial amount of data have accumulated on the use of HFOV in humans for the management of the neonatal respiratory distress syndrome (RDS).

The first large randomized, controlled trial with premature infants comparing high-frequency ventilation using a piston oscillator with conventional mechanical ventilation was published in the pre-surfactant era by the HIFI Study Group in 1989 [39]. The study was designed to evaluate the effect of high-frequency ventilation on the incidence of chronic lung disease of prematurity and included 673 infants weighing 750–2,000 g who had been supported less than 12 hr on conventional ventilation for respiratory failure in the first 24 hours of life. Infants randomized to receive HFOV were administered an FiO_2 and Paw equal to those administered on conventional ventilation. Infants who had not already been tracheally intubated were administered an FiO_2 equal to that received before intubation and a Paw of 8–10 cm H_2O. Hypoxemia was first addressed by increasing the FiO_2 and then by increasing the Paw [39]. Overall, the investigators did not incorporate alveolar recruitment into the HFOV strategy, and the study was unable to show a significant difference in the incidence of chronic lung disease or in 28-day mortality between the two groups. However, it did show a

significant increase in the incidence of air leak as well as high-grade intraventricular hemorrhage among the infants who were randomized to receive HFOV [39].

Two additional large multicenter trials were recently published in an effort to clarify the role of high-frequency ventilation in the management of RDS in preterm infants [40,41]. Unlike the HIFI trial and subsequent studies that produced conflicting results [42,43], these two trials were produced by centers with a great deal of experience with the use of HFOV in neonates, and each emphasized alveolar recruitment as part of the strategy for high-frequency ventilation. In a well-controlled study, Courtney and colleagues used a strategy in the conventional ventilation arm that targeted a tidal volume of 5–6 mL per kg body weight and ventilated infants in the HFOV arm at a frequency of 10–15 Hz [40]. These investigators were able to show that infants randomized to receive HFOV with the 3100A were successfully separated from mechanical ventilation earlier than those assigned to a lung-sparing strategy of conventional ventilation, and, among the infants assigned to high-frequency ventilation, there was a significant decrease in the need for supplemental oxygen at 36 weeks postmenstrual age [40]. By defining a disease threshold in the study infants, adhering to lung-protective protocols for mechanical ventilation, and extubating from the assigned ventilator according to specific criteria, this study identified a set of circumstances in which HFOV may be used with clear benefit in preterm infants with RDS [40]. In contrast, Johnson and colleagues included healthier patients, used fewer defined protocols, and used more aggressive ventilator strategies [41]. In both study arms, the investigators targeted a $PaCO_2$ of 34–53 torr, whereas Courtney and colleagues used a ventilation strategy that allowed permissive hypercapnia [40]. For those infants who were supported on HFOV, Johnson and colleagues initiated therapy at a frequency of 10 Hz, and, if maximizing amplitude (ΔP) did not achieve adequate clearance of CO_2, the frequency was subsequently reduced [41]. Finally, Johnson's group transitioned the majority of

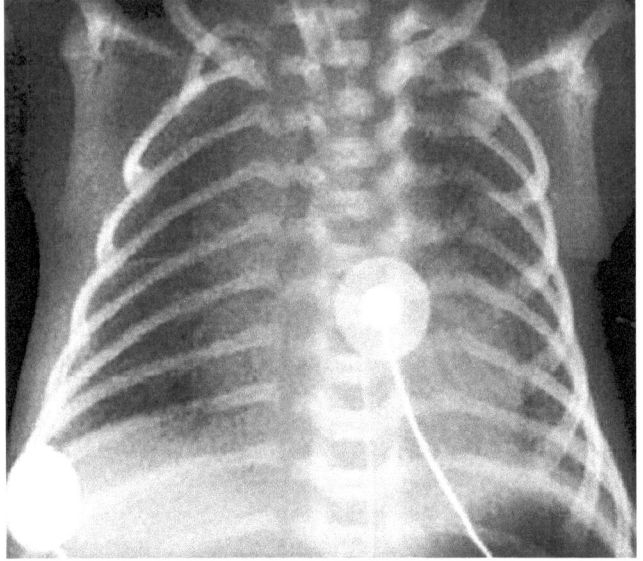

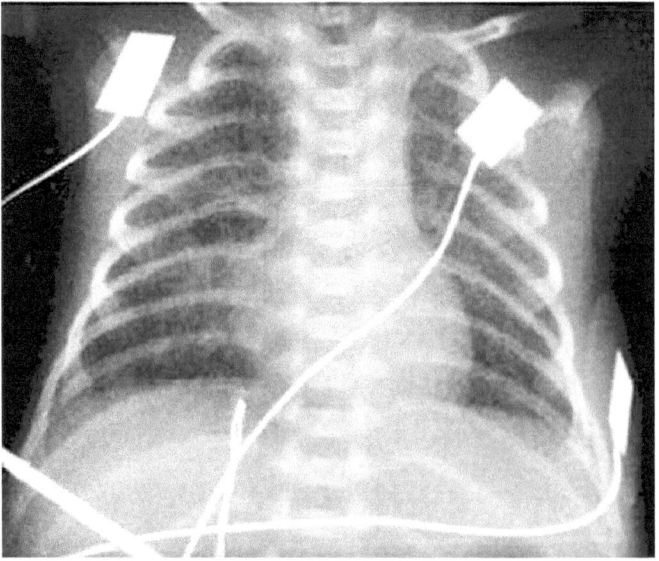

A   B

FIGURE 9.4. Conventional ventilation versus high-frequency oscillatory ventilation (HFOV) in the preterm neonate: representative chest radiographs from preterm infants with the respiratory distress syndrome assigned to receive HFOV or conventional ventilation. Each picture is taken on day 2 of mechanical ventilatory support. (A) Conventional ventilation.

(B) High-frequency oscillatory ventilation. (*Source*: Helbich TH, Popow C, Dobner M, Wunderbaldinger P, Zekert M, Herold CJ. New-born infants with severe hyaline membrane disease: radiological evaluation during high-frequency oscillatory versus conventional ventilation. Eur J Radiol 1998;28:243–249. Copyright 1998 with permission.)

study infants to conventional ventilation for weaning after a median time on HFOV of 3 days, a relatively small portion of the total duration of mechanical ventilation [41].

It is important to emphasize that neither of these studies was able to duplicate the findings of the HIFI group with respect to associating the use of HFOV with the development of high-grade intraventricular hemorrhage. However, the difference in outcomes in the two trials is striking. The rigorously controlled conditions in the Courtney study probably isolate the effect of HFOV with greater clarity, and their data suggest that only 11 infants need be supported with HFOV in order to prevent one occurrence of chronic lung disease at 36 weeks postmenstrual age [40]. Using Johnson's data, the number of infants needed to support on HFOV in order to prevent one occurrence of chronic lung disease is 50 [41]. Although the study design used by Johnson and colleagues may better represent actual practice, the outcomes indicate that exposure to aggressive conventional ventilation protocols may offset the benefits of HFOV.

Congenital Diaphragmatic Hernia

Infants with congenital diaphragmatic hernia (CDH) commonly demonstrate complex pulmonary pathophysiology that derives from alveolar and pulmonary vascular hypoplasia [44]. The discovery that ventilator-induced lung injury is evident on histopathology specimens from these patients [45,46] has continued to focus attention in recent years on applying lung-protective strategies of mechanical ventilation to infants with CDH. As a result, numerous centers have reported case series of infants with CDH in whom the application of high-frequency oscillatory ventilation has been associated with an improvement in survival [47–49]. Several retrospective studies of HFOV in infants with CDH have also reported improved survival, with dramatic reductions in $PaCO_2$ and concurrent improvements in oxygenation [48,49]. At least one center using HFOV without the use of extracorporeal membrane oxygenation (ECMO) in infants with CDH has reported an overall survival rate comparable to that of infants who were supported with conventional ventilation and ECMO, although no survival benefit specifically attributable to the use of HFOV was identified [45]. Nonetheless, some of the best survival statistics for CDH are reported in one recent single-center historical experience in which these infants were managed with conventional ventilation. This report documented a significant increase in survival from 44% to 69% among all infants with this condition during a period in which flow-triggered pressure support ventilation with permissive hypercapnia was used. Even higher survival rates were noted in those without coexisting heart disease [50].

Overall the role of HFOV in the management of infants with CDH is unclear. Despite its theoretical advantages in maintaining alveolar recruitment with minimal pressure cost, application of an open lung strategy using high-frequency ventilation in infants with CDH can lead to problems because aggressive recruitment in the setting of alveolar hypoplasia may precipitate acute increases in pulmonary vascular resistance with ensuing hemodynamic instability, air leak, or ongoing lung injury. Centers that report success with HFOV in the management of infants with CDH have found that it is important to limit Paw to ≤20 cm H_2O in order to avoid alveolar overdistension [17]. In summary, infants with CDH may suffer excess lung injury if aggressively ventilated in an attempt to manipulate pulmonary vascular resistance, and the use of high-frequency ventilation to achieve specific short-term physiologic end-points may not offset this risk.

Persistent Pulmonary Hypertension of the Newborn

Several investigators have tested the hypothesis that sustained alveolar recruitment using HFOV could enhance the delivery of therapeutic gases to patients with respiratory failure. In one large multicenter trial, therapy with HFOV was coupled with inhaled nitric oxide (iNO) in an effort to identify the relative contribution of each therapy to outcomes in patients with persistent pulmonary hypertension of the newborn (PPHN). The investigators randomized 200 neonates with severe hypoxic respiratory failure and PPHN to receive therapy with HFOV alone or conventional ventilation combined with iNO [51]. Crossover as a result of treatment failure resulted in combined therapy with HFOV and iNO. The study concluded that significant short-term improvements in PaO_2 occurred during combined treatment with HFOV and iNO among patients who failed either therapy alone [51]. This combination was particularly effective among patients with severe parenchymal disease attributable to RDS and meconium aspiration [51]. The suggestion that efficacy of iNO may depend on the adequacy of alveolar recruitment is also supported by a retrospective analysis of data from children enrolled in a multicenter randomized trial of the use of iNO in the treatment of acute hypoxic respiratory failure [52].

Air Leak Syndromes

Given the expectation that satisfactory gas exchange occurs at a relatively low Paw during HFOV, it is not surprising that this therapy has been applied with success in severe air leak syndromes. In one early case report, 27 low-birth-weight infants (mean birth weight 1.2 kg) who developed pulmonary interstitial emphysema on conventional ventilation were transitioned to HFOV. All demonstrated early improvement on HFOV, and survivors demonstrated sustained improvements in oxygenation and ventilation, allowing for lower Paw and FiO_2 and ultimate resolution of air leak. Overall survival among nonseptic patients was 80% [53].

Bronchiolitis

Despite concerns that ventilation at high frequencies may exacerbate dynamic air trapping in diseases of the lower airways, HFOV has been used in the management of bronchiolitis caused by respiratory syncytial virus [54,55]. A couple of small case series have reported the successful application of HFOV using an open lung strategy in young infants with bronchiolitis [54,55]. Applying a relatively high Paw in this clinical context derives from the observation that lower Paw may promote worsening hyperinflation by creating *choke points* that impede expiratory flow [28]. The investigators used a frequency of 10–11 Hz and an I:E of 0.33, with initial pressure amplitude (ΔP) in the 35–50 cm H_2O range. All patients survived without development of pneumothoraces attributable to HFOV and without need for ECMO [54,55].

High-Frequency Oscillatory Ventilation in the Child

Diffuse Alveolar Disease

Much of the data on the application of HFOV outside of the neonatal period comes from case series in which this therapy was applied to children with acute severe respiratory failure attributable to diffuse alveolar disease and/or air leak syndromes. In the early 1990s, two centers reported the use of HFOV in pediatric patients with these conditions who had been managed on conventional ventilation for varying periods of time [35,56]. In general, each concluded that HFOV may be applied safely as rescue therapy for pediatric patients with severe hypoxic lung injury and that its use is associated with improvement in physiologic end-points such as $PaCO_2$ and oxygenation index, OI = (Paw × FiO$_2$)/PaO$_2$) × 100. In addition, there were no reports of worsening air leak [35,56]. Each of these studies applied HFOV after recruiting the lung, but one of them [35] modified the HFOV protocol for patients with active air leak by dropping the Paw below the leak pressure following recruitment, raising the FiO$_2$ as necessary to maintain adequate oxygenation, and tolerating hypercarbia as long as the arterial pH remained above 7.25.

The first and largest multicenter randomized trial evaluating the effect of HFOV on respiratory outcomes in pediatric patients is a crossover study that enrolled patients with diffuse alveolar disease and/or air leak [34]. The investigators randomized 70 patients to receive conventional ventilation using a strategy to limit peak inspiratory pressure, or HFOV at a frequency of 5–10 Hz, using an open lung strategy in which the lung volume at which optimal oxygenation occurred was defined (SaO$_2$ ≥90% and FiO$_2$ <0.6), and, in patients with air leak, airway pressure was then limited while accepting preferential increases in FiO$_2$ to achieve saturations of ≥85% and pH ≥7.25 until it resolved [34]. The study found no difference in survival or duration of mechanical ventilatory support between the two groups, but significantly fewer patients randomized to receive HFOV remained dependent on supplemental oxygen at 30 days compared with those who were randomized to receive conventional ventilation, despite the use of significantly higher Paw in the HFOV group [34]. The OI, used often in the pediatric literature to quantify oxygenation failure, was shown in this study to discriminate between survivors and nonsurvivors after 24 hours of therapy. In addition, the time at which changes in OI were noted to occur influenced the likelihood of survival: an OI ≥42 at 24 hr predicted mortality with an odds ratio of 20.8, sensitivity of 62%, and specificity of 93% [34]. Post hoc analysis revealed that outcome benefits were not as great for those who crossed over to the HFOV arm [34], supporting the suggestion by numerous studies that HFOV may be most successful if employed early in the course of disease, using a strategy that emphasizes alveolar recruitment [9,37,56–58].

Other Conditions

Experience with the use of HFOV for treatment of lower airways disease in older pediatric patients is limited. In one interesting case report, HFOV was successfully applied to a toddler with status asthmaticus [59]. The authors achieved optimal CO$_2$ clearance using an *open lung* strategy with Paw 20 cm H$_2$O, low frequency (6 Hz), I:E 0.33, and relatively high ΔP (65–75 cm H$_2$O in the first 24 hr of therapy) without apparent air leak [59]; however, the use of HFOV in obstructive lung diseases must be considered thoughtfully.

High-Frequency Oscillatory Ventilation in the Adolescent and Adult

In recent years, the 3100B HFOV (SensorMedics, Yorba Linda, CA) has become available for use in larger pediatric patients and adult patients, addressing initial reports with large animals that adequate alveolar ventilation could not be achieved using the 3100A

model [60,61]. The 3100B differs from the 3100A model by having a higher maximal bias flow, which allows for the delivery of higher mean airway pressures. The 3100B also has a more powerful electromagnet, which produces faster acceleration to maximal oscillatory pressure (ΔP) [33].

Early experiences with the use of HFOV on adolescent and adult patients with hypoxic respiratory failure are summarized in several case series [33,62]. In each, low-frequency (maximum 5–6 Hz) HFOV with a strategy of volume recruitment was used as rescue therapy for patients with ARDS who were failing conventional ventilation. These studies included patients with severe disease, including mean values for PaO$_2$/FiO$_2$ in the 60 range at the time of enrollment [33,62]. Although neither study was powered to measure significant differences in outcomes such as mortality, the majority of patients in the two studies demonstrated an improvement in short-term physiologic variables such as FiO$_2$, PaO$_2$/FiO$_2$ ratio, and OI [33,62]. Nonsurvivors in each of these studies were exposed to significantly longer periods of conventional ventilation, suggesting once again the importance of instituting HFOV early in the course of disease.

A multicenter, prospective, randomized controlled trial designed to evaluate the safety and effectiveness of HFOV compared with conventional ventilation in the management of early ARDS (PaO$_2$/FiO$_2$ ≤200 while on PEEP 10 cm H$_2$O) in adult patients was published in 2002 [32]. Treatment strategies for both arms of the study included a volume recruitment strategy and were directed at achieving SaO$_2$ ≥88% on FiO$_2$ ≤60%. Patients in the conventional arm were managed in the pressure-control mode, targeting a delivered tidal volume of 6–10 mL/kg actual body weight, without specific attention to plateau pressures. Patients in the HFOV arm were ventilated at frequencies of 3–5 Hz and were transitioned back to conventional ventilation when FiO$_2$ ≤0.5 and Paw ≤24 cm H$_2$O with SaO$_2$ ≥88%, and conventional ventilation was reinstituted at an equivalent Paw [32]. With regard to short-term physiologic measures, these investigators also reported a significantly higher Paw among patients on HFOV and significant early increases while on HFOV in PaO$_2$/FiO$_2$ [32]. Post-study multivariate analysis also revealed that the trend in OI was the most significant post-treatment predictor of survival regardless of treatment group—survivors showed a significant improvement over the first 72 hr of the study period and nonsurvivors did not [32]. Although the OI is not a measure traditionally reported in the adult literature, it has been reported by others as predictive of mortality in adult ARDS [62].

This study was not powered to evaluate differences in mortality between the two groups, but there was a clear trend toward increased 30-day mortality among the patients randomized to receive conventional ventilation versus those who received HFOV (52% vs. 37%) [32]. At the moment, it is not known if HFOV using low frequencies is as protective as ventilating at a higher frequency range, such as what has been used with success in small animals and human infants. It is important to understand that laboratory experiments using the 3100B HFOV have demonstrated that tidal volumes approaching those used in conventional ventilation are produced under conditions of low-frequency and high-pressure amplitude (ΔP) [63].

Adjuncts: Noninvasive Assessment of Lung Volume

One of the difficulties facing intensive care clinicians is that evaluation of the adequacy of recruitment after initiating HFOV and in response to changes in ventilator settings must be guided by indirect measures such as peripheral oxygen saturations, fractional inspired oxygen concentration, blood gas tensions, anteroposterior chest radiographs, and a visual assessment of chest wall vibration. Global measures of alveolar plateau pressure, tidal volume, and pulmonary mechanics that are available from breath to breath when using conventional ventilation are not provided on the high-frequency ventilator console, and the operator must often use intuition when adjusting ventilator settings, risking sudden and clinically significant derecruitment or alveolar overdistension. In recent years, respiratory impedance plethysmography (RIP) and electrical impedance tomography (EIT) have emerged as two promising means by which pulmonary mechanics and alveolar recruitment can be assessed noninvasively at the bedside during HFOV.

Respiratory impedance plethysmography is a monitoring technique that is capable of quantifying global lung volume by relating it to measurable changes in the cross-sectional area of the chest wall and the abdominal compartment. In RIP, two elastic bands with Teflon-coated wires embedded in a zigzag distribution along their circumference are applied to the patient. One is typically placed around the chest, 3 cm above the xiphoid process, and the other is typically placed around the abdomen. Each of these two bands produces an independent signal, and the sum of the two signals is calibrated against a known volume of gas. Use of this technique in association with HFOV has been validated in animal models [64,65]. In a large animal model of acute lung injury managed with HFOV, Brazelton and colleagues have demonstrated that RIP-derived lung volumes correlated well with those that were obtained using a supersyringe ($r^2 = 0.78$) and that RIP is capable of tracking global changes in lung volume and creating a pressure–volume curve during HFOV [64]. With a newborn animal model, Weber and colleagues were able to demonstrate that RIP is capable of detecting relative changes in pulmonary compliance that were induced by saline lavage [65]. Experience with RIP in human

subjects is limited to investigations of its application in conventional phasic ventilation. One study with adult patients [66] and another with pediatric patients [67] have utilized RIP to quantify the relative degree of derecruitment that is associated with closed, in-line techniques for endotracheal tube suctioning compared with open suctioning techniques. Each study was able to demonstrate a potential role for RIP in tracking global changes in lung volume at the bedside.

Applying HFOV in a way that harmonizes with what computed tomography (CT) has revealed about the heterogeneity of parenchymal involvement in ARDS [68] will ultimately depend on developing noninvasive bedside technologies that are capable of identifying regional changes in lung volume and pulmonary mechanics. Computed tomography images of the lung in ARDS patients have demonstrated that, during a prolonged inspiratory maneuver, alveolar recruitment occurs all the way to total lung capacity, according to the specific time constants of individual lung units (Figure 9.5; see also Figure 9.2) [68,69]. Therefore, *ideal* settings on HFOV would be those that achieve ventilation above the lower inflection point on the regional pressure–volume curves for the majority of lung units, while avoiding overdistension in the most compliant alveoli. Electrical impedance tomography (EIT) is one technology that may be best suited to detecting regional heterogeneity at the bedside of the patient with diffuse alveolar disease.

In EIT, a series of electrodes is applied circumferentially to the patient's chest. The electrodes sequentially emit a small amount of electrical current that is received and processed by the other electrodes in the array. Receiving electrodes determine a local change in impedance based on the voltage differential calculated between the transmitting electrode and the receiving electrode. Well-aerated areas, which conduct current poorly, are associated with high impedance, whereas fluid and solid phases (including atelectatic or consolidated lung) would be associated with lower impedance [70].

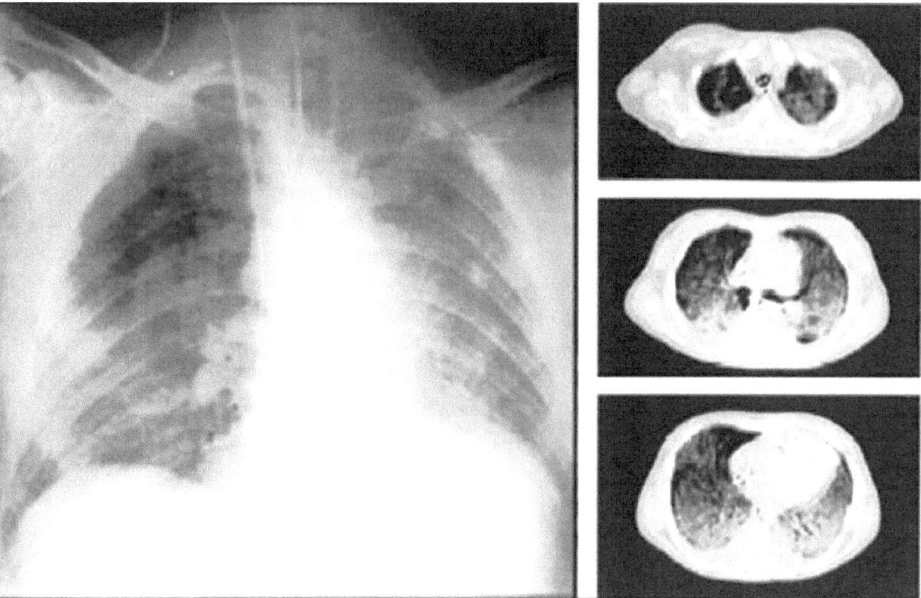

FIGURE 9.5. Heterogeneity of lung parenchymal involvement in acute respiratory distress syndrome (ARDS). Anteroposterior chest radiograph and computed tomography (CT) scans corresponding to lung apex, hilum, and base from a patient with sepsis and ARDS. Images are taken with the patient in the supine position at a positive end-expiratory pres- sure of 5 cm H_2O. The CT scans illustrate the influence of the gravitational axis on the pattern of alveolar consolidation in ARDS: nondependent regions are aerated while dependent regions remain consolidated. (From Gattinoni et al. [68]. Copyright 2001 the American Thoracic Society. Reprinted with permission.)

The impedance values that are generated are referenced to a baseline measurement and represent relative rather than absolute changes in electrical properties [69]. This process creates a tomogram that depicts the distribution of tissue electrical properties in a cross-sectional image (Figure 9.6), and the thickness of the *slice* of thorax that is represented in the image varies between approximately 15 and 20 cm, depending on the circumference of the chest [69,71]. Of the presently available EIT systems, the Goe MF II (University of Goettingen, Germany; distributed by Viasys, USA) seems to have the most favorable signal-to-noise ratio and is also capable of dynamic measurements at low lung volumes [69,72]. This system scans at a rate of 13–44 scans/sec (Hz), generating up to 44 cross-sectional images per second [69].

In the laboratory, EIT has been used in conjunction with both conventional ventilation and HFOV to describe regional lung characteristics. Investigations using conventional ventilation in large animal models of lung injury have validated EIT against supersyringe methods for the determination of regional pressure–volume (or *pressure–impedance*) curves [69,73] and have demonstrated good correlation between EIT-derived regional changes in lung impedance and CT-derived regional variations in aeration [69,74]. Using EIT to track regional lung mechanics in a large animal model of acute lung injury managed with HFOV, van Genderingen and colleagues were able to demonstrate that regional pressure–volume curves constructed using maneuvers on HFOV show less variation along the gravitational axis than pressure-volume curves that are obtained using a supersyringe method, suggesting that recruitment is more uniformly distributed between dependent and nondependent areas during HFOV [75].

Published experience with EIT in human subjects with acute lung injury or ARDS has correlated regional impedance changes induced by slow inflation maneuvers using the DAS-01P EIT system (Sheffield, UK) with regional lung density measurements obtained

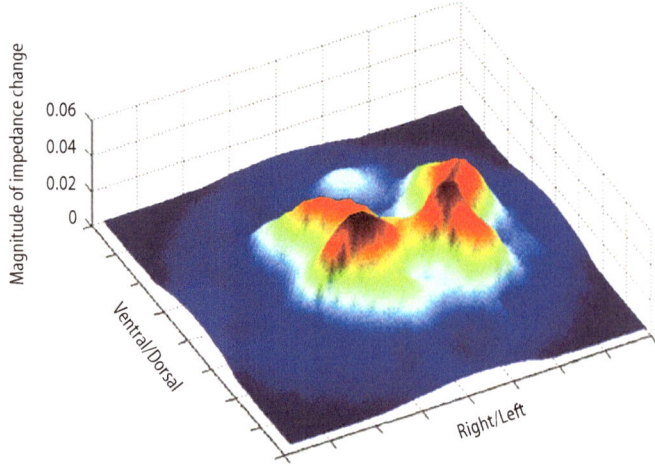

FIGURE 9.7. Three-dimensional depiction of recruitment after suctioning on high-frequency oscillatory ventilation. The standard deviation of impedance change after reconnection to the ventilator is displayed. (From Wolf and Arnold [77]. Copyright 2005. Reprinted with permission from Lippincott Williams & Wilkins.)

by CT scanning [76]. Most recently, a group of investigators at Children's Hospital Boston has utilized EIT to detect regional changes in lung volume during a standardized suctioning maneuver in children with acute lung injury or ARDS who were supported on HFOV. These data demonstrate considerable regional heterogeneity in volume changes during a derecruitment maneuver (Figure 9.7) [77].

It is tempting to expect that EIT will soon facilitate the development of strategic HFOV protocols. Theoretically, this technology can create opportunities for therapeutic intervention by dynamically tracking the regional differences in alveolar recruitment that make portions of the lung highly susceptible to ventilator-induced lung injury (VILI). However, there are important limitations to the presently available technology. For instance, substantial bias may be introduced into the EIT image because of the tendency for electrical current to follow the path of lowest impedance rather than the path of shortest distance between the transmitting and receiving electrodes [70]. This phenomenon may account in large part for the variation between EIT measures of regional lung impedance and CT measures of regional lung density [76]. In addition, because EIT measures impedance changes that are relative to baseline values, changes in baseline regional intrathoracic impedance resulting from sources other than alterations in gas volume and distribution could lead to errors in the interpretation of EIT-derived data. Despite these limitations, several investigators have reported that EIT reliably detects regional alterations in pulmonary blood flow [78] and extravascular lung water [79]. In summary, identifying a useful role for EIT as an adjunct to HFOV at the bedside will depend on additional technical modifications to make it suitable for reliably detecting very small regional tidal volumes at high frequency in the electrically hostile environment of the intensive care unit.

Weaning

Numerous studies have suggested that limiting exposure to potentially injurious strategies on conventional ventilation may enhance outcome benefits attributable to HFOV among patients with severe lung injury. Large trials in the neonatal and pediatric populations

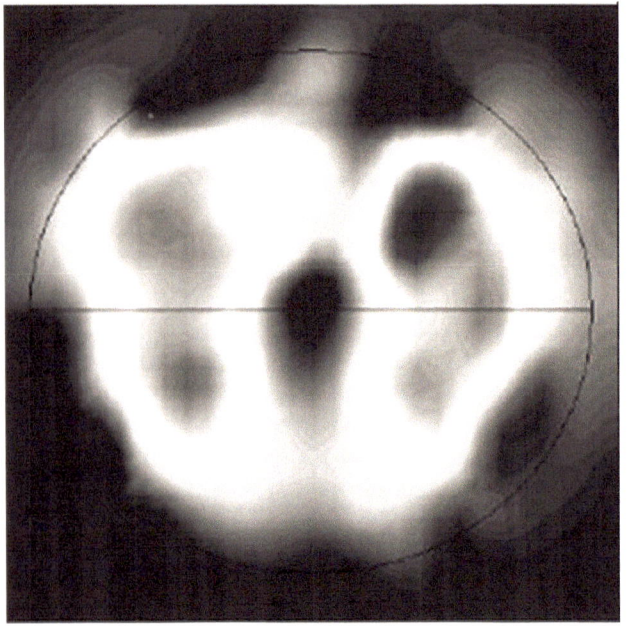

FIGURE 9.6. Electrical impedance tomography image of the lung. The orientation is the same as for a computed tomographic image. Both lung fields show equal impedance change during spontaneous breathing. (Courtesy of G.K. Wolf, MD. Children's Hospital Boston.)

have demonstrated favorable outcomes when HFOV is applied early in disease, and it seems logical to expect that timing the transition back to conventional ventilation may be of substantial importance as well.

Weaning a patient from HFOV may be considered when the clinician determines that gas exchange and pulmonary mechanics are suitable for transition to acceptable settings on conventional ventilation. Some investigators have reported successfully extubating infants directly from HFOV [40,41,57], but this is difficult to accomplish in the older pediatric and adult patient, who may be less likely to tolerate a degree of sedation that would allow spontaneous respiration while on HFOV and in whom spontaneous breathing may significantly depressurize the circuit, resulting in recurrent alveolar derecruitment. In general, when clinical improvement occurs to the point that Paw may be reduced to ≤20 cm H₂O, FiO2 is reduced to ≤0.4, and the patient tolerates endotracheal suctioning without significant desaturation, it is appropriate to undertake a more detailed evaluation of the patient's response to phasic ventilation provided by conventional means [17]. This may be done by hand ventilating (with the aid of an in-line pneumotachometer, if necessary) while noting the pressures, tidal volume, and inspiratory to expiratory time ratio necessary to sustain satisfactory oxygen saturation. It is common to find on transition to conventional ventilation that the patient will demonstrate satisfactory gas exchange on a mean airway pressure several cm H₂O below the last Paw on HFOV.

Conclusion

Despite compelling laboratory data supporting a physiologic rationale for HFOV in the treatment of diffuse alveolar disease, evidence of its superiority to conventional ventilation with regard to clinically important outcomes beyond the neonatal period is scant. The difficulty in proving significant clinical outcome benefit in pediatric and adult patients may be due in large part to the diverse potential etiologies of respiratory failure in these populations as well as a wide range of approaches to their medical management applied over a relatively long period of mechanical ventilatory support. It is also possible that low-frequency HFOV as traditionally used for larger patients may not be as protective as the higher frequency strategies that have been used with success in small animal models and human infants.

High-frequency oscillatory ventilation remains a therapeutic option in the intensive care unit that is worthy of further study because it is a safe and practical way to provide a "low stretch" form of ventilation that is less likely to produce VILI [4,6–9]. Applying this concept with greater precision in the clinical arena will depend on developing bedside technologies capable of both identifying the critical opening pressure in a majority of lung units and tracking regional changes in lung volume that follow changes in HFOV settings. Electrical impedance tomography is a promising technology that may ultimately be incorporated into the design of future trials that are powered to evaluate the benefits of specific HFOV protocols.

References

1. Lunkenheimer PP, Rafflenbeul W, Keller H, Frank I, Dickhut HH, Fuhrmann C. Application of transtracheal pressure oscillations as a modification of "diffusing respiration." Br J Anaesth 1972;44(6):627.
2. Lunkenheimer PP, Frank I, Ising H, Keller H, Dickhut HH. [Intrapulmonary gas exchange during simulated apnea due to transtracheal periodic intrathoracic pressure changes.] Anaesthesist 1973;22(5):232–238.
3. Butler WJ, Bohn DJ, Bryan AC, Froese AB. Ventilation by high-frequency oscillation in humans. Anesth Analg 1980;59(8):577–584.
4. Hernandez LA, Peevy KJ, Moise AA, Parker JC. Chest wall restriction limits high airway pressure–induced lung injury in young rabbits. J Appl Physiol 1989;66(5):2364–2368.
5. Slutsky AS, Tremblay LN. Multiple system organ failure. Is mechanical ventilation a contributing factor? Am J Respir Crit Care Med 1998;157(6 Pt 1):1721–1725.
6. Ranieri VM, Suter PM, Tortorella C, De Tullio R, Dayer JM, Brienza A, et al. Effect of mechanical ventilation on inflammatory mediators in patients with acute respiratory distress syndrome: a randomized controlled trial. JAMA 1999;282(1):54–61.
7. Doctor A, Arnold JH. Mechanical support of acute lung injury: options for strategic ventilation. New Horiz 1999;7(3):359–373.
8. McCulloch PR, Forkert PG, Froese AB. Lung volume maintenance prevents lung injury during high frequency oscillatory ventilation in surfactant-deficient rabbits. Am Rev Respir Dis 1988;137(5):1185–1192.
9. Bond DM, Froese AB. Volume recruitment maneuvers are less deleterious than persistent low lung volumes in the atelectasis-prone rabbit lung during high-frequency oscillation. Crit Care Med 1993;21(3):402–412.
10. Byford LJ, Finkler JH, Froese AB. Lung volume recruitment during high-frequency oscillation in atelectasis-prone rabbits. J Appl Physiol 1988;64(4):1607–1614.
11. Chu EK, Whitehead T, Slutsky AS. Effects of cyclic opening and closing at low- and high-volume ventilation on bronchoalveolar lavage cytokines. Crit Care Med 2004;32(1):168–174.
12. Gajic O, Dara SI, Mendez JL, Adesanya AO, Festic E, Caples SM, et al. Ventilator-associated lung injury in patients without acute lung injury at the onset of mechanical ventilation. Crit Care Med 2004;32(9):1817–1824.
13. Ventilation with lower tidal volumes as compared with traditional tidal volumes for acute lung injury and the acute respiratory distress syndrome. The Acute Respiratory Distress Syndrome Network. N Engl J Med 2000;342(18):1301–1308.
14. Priebe GP, Arnold JH. High-frequency oscillatory ventilation in pediatric patients. Respir Care Clin North Am 2001;7(4):633–645.
15. Chang HK. Mechanisms of gas transport during ventilation by high-frequency oscillation. J Appl Physiol 1984;56(3):553–563.
16. Wetzel RC, Gioia FR. High frequency ventilation. Pediatr Clin North Am 1987;34(1):15–38.
17. Arnold JH. High-frequency ventilation in the pediatric intensive care unit. Pediatr Crit Care Med 2000;1(2):93–99.
18. Boynton BR, Hammond MD, Fredberg JJ, Buckley BG, Villanueva D, Frantz ID, 3rd. Gas exchange in healthy rabbits during high-frequency oscillatory ventilation. J Appl Physiol 1989;66(3):1343–1351.
19. Hatcher D, Watanabe H, Ashbury T, Vincent S, Fisher J, Froese A. Mechanical performance of clinically available, neonatal, high-frequency, oscillatory-type ventilators. Crit Care Med 1998;26(6):1081–1088.
20. Pillow JJ, Neil H, Wilkinson MH, Ramsden CA. Effect of I/E ratio on mean alveolar pressure during high-frequency oscillatory ventilation. J Appl Physiol 1999;87(1):407–414.
21. Kolton M, McGhee I, Bryan AC. Tidal volumes required to maintain isocapnia at frequencies from 3 to 30 Hz in the dog. Anesth Analg 1987;66(6):523–528.
22. Venegas JG, Fredberg JJ. Understanding the pressure cost of ventilation: why does high-frequency ventilation work? Crit Care Med 1994;22(9 Suppl):S49–S57.
23. Gerstmann DR, Fouke JM, Winter DC, Taylor AF, deLemos RA. Proximal, tracheal, and alveolar pressures during high-frequency oscillatory ventilation in a normal rabbit model. Pediatr Res 1990;28(4):367–373.

24. Allen JL, Frantz ID, 3rd, Fredberg JJ. Heterogeneity of mean alveolar pressure during high-frequency oscillations. J Appl Physiol 1987;62(1):223–228.

25. Allen JL, Fredberg JJ, Keefe DH, Frantz ID, 3rd. Alveolar pressure magnitude and asynchrony during high-frequency oscillations of excised rabbit lungs. Am Rev Respir Dis 1985;132(2):343–349.

26. Saari AF, Rossing TH, Solway J, Drazen JM. Lung inflation during high-frequency ventilation. Am Rev Respir Dis 1984;129(2):333–336.

27. Simon BA, Weinmann GG, Mitzner W. Mean airway pressure and alveolar pressure during high-frequency ventilation. J Appl Physiol 1984;57(4):1069–1078.

28. Bryan AC, Slutsky AS. Long volume during high frequency oscillation. Am Rev Respir Dis 1986;133(5):928–930.

29. West JB. Blood flow and metabolism. In: Respiratory Physiology: The Essentials, 4th ed. Baltimore: Williams & Wilkins; 1990:41.

30. Bryan AC, Cox PN. History of high frequency oscillation. Schweiz Med Wochenschr 1999;129(43):1613–1616.

31. VandeKieft M, Dorsey D, Venticinque S, Harris A. Effects of endotracheal tube (ETT) cuff leak on gas flow patterns in a mechanical lung model during high-frequency oscillatory ventilation (HFOV) [abstract A178]. Am J Respir Crit Care Med 2003:A178.

32. Derdak S, Mehta S, Stewart TE, Smith T, Rogers M, Buchman TG, et al. High-frequency oscillatory ventilation for acute respiratory distress syndrome in adults: a randomized, controlled trial. Am J Respir Crit Care Med 2002;166(6):801–808.

33. Mehta S, Lapinsky SE, Hallett DC, Merker D, Groll RJ, Cooper AB, et al. Prospective trial of high-frequency oscillation in adults with acute respiratory distress syndrome. Crit Care Med 2001;29(7):1360–1369.

34. Arnold JH, Hanson JH, Toro-Figuero LO, Gutierrez J, Berens RJ, Anglin DL. Prospective, randomized comparison of high-frequency oscillatory ventilation and conventional mechanical ventilation in pediatric respiratory failure. Crit Care Med 1994;22(10):1530–1539.

35. Arnold JH, Truog RD, Thompson JE, Fackler JC. High-frequency oscillatory ventilation in pediatric respiratory failure. Crit Care Med 1993;21(2):272–278.

36. Ellsbury DL, Klein JM, Segar JL. Optimization of high-frequency oscillatory ventilation for the treatment of experimental pneumothorax. Crit Care Med 2002;30(5):1131–1135.

37. Meredith KS, deLemos RA, Coalson JJ, King RJ, Gerstmann DR, Kumar R, et al. Role of lung injury in the pathogenesis of hyaline membrane disease in premature baboons. J Appl Physiol 1989;66(5):2150–2158.

38. deLemos RA, Coalson JJ, deLemos JA, et al. High frequency oscillatory ventilation improves the non-uniform lung inflation of hyaline membrane disease [abstr]. Am Rev Respir Dis 1989;139:A438.

39. High-frequency oscillatory ventilation compared with conventional mechanical ventilation in the treatment of respiratory failure in preterm infants. The HIFI Study Group. N Engl J Med 1989;320(2):88–93.

40. Courtney SE, Durand DJ, Asselin JM, Hudak ML, Aschner JL, Shoemaker CT. High-frequency oscillatory ventilation versus conventional mechanical ventilation for very-low-birth-weight infants. N Engl J Med 2002;347(9):643–652.

41. Johnson AH, Peacock JL, Greenough A, Marlow N, Limb ES, Marston L, et al. High-frequency oscillatory ventilation for the prevention of chronic lung disease of prematurity. N Engl J Med 2002;347(9):633–642.

42. Clark RH, Gerstmann DR, Null DM Jr, deLemos RA. Prospective randomized comparison of high-frequency oscillatory and conventional ventilation in respiratory distress syndrome. Pediatrics 1992;89(1):5–12.

43. Ogawa Y, Miyasaka K, Kawano T, Imura S, Inukai K, Okuyama K, et al. A multicenter randomized trial of high frequency oscillatory ventilation as compared with conventional mechanical ventilation in preterm infants with respiratory failure. Early Hum Dev 1993;32(1):1–10.

44. Greenholz SK. Congenital diaphragmatic hernia: an overview. Semin Pediatr Surg 1996;5(4):216–223.

45. Azarow K, Messineo A, Pearl R, Filler R, Barker G, Bohn D. Congenital diaphragmatic hernia—a tale of two cities: the Toronto experience. J Pediatr Surg 1997;32(3):395–400.

46. Sakurai Y, Azarow K, Cutz E, Messineo A, Pearl R, Bohn D. Pulmonary barotrauma in congenital diaphragmatic hernia: a clinicopathological correlation. J Pediatr Surg 1999;34(12):1813–1817.

47. Reyes C, Chang LK, Waffarn F, Mir H, Warden MJ, Sills J. Delayed repair of congenital diaphragmatic hernia with early high-frequency oscillatory ventilation during preoperative stabilization. J Pediatr Surg 1998;33(7):1010–1016.

48. Desfrere L, Jarreau PH, Dommergues M, Brunhes A, Hubert P, Nihoul-Fekete C, et al. Impact of delayed repair and elective high-frequency oscillatory ventilation on survival of antenatally diagnosed congenital diaphragmatic hernia: first application of these strategies in the more "severe" subgroup of antenatally diagnosed newborns. Intensive Care Med 2000;26(7):934–41.

49. Cacciari A, Ruggeri G, Mordenti M, Ceccarelli PL, Baccarini E, Pigna A, et al. High-frequency oscillatory ventilation versus conventional mechanical ventilation in congenital diaphragmatic hernia. Eur J Pediatr Surg 2001;11(1):3–7.

50. Wilson JM, Lund DP, Lillehei CW, Vacanti JP. Congenital diaphragmatic hernia—a tale of two cities: the Boston experience. J Pediatr Surg 1997;32(3):401–405.

51. Kinsella JP, Truog WE, Walsh WF, Goldberg RN, Bancalari E, Mayock DE, et al. Randomized, multicenter trial of inhaled nitric oxide and high-frequency oscillatory ventilation in severe, persistent pulmonary hypertension of the newborn. J Pediatr 1997;131(1 Pt 1):55–62.

52. Dobyns EL, Anas NG, Fortenberry JD, Deshpande J, Cornfield DN, Tasker RC, et al. Interactive effects of high-frequency oscillatory ventilation and inhaled nitric oxide in acute hypoxemic respiratory failure in pediatrics. Crit Care Med 2002;30(11):2425–2429.

53. Clark RH, Gerstmann DR, Null DM, Yoder BA, Cornish JD, Glasier CM, et al. Pulmonary interstitial emphysema treated by high-frequency oscillatory ventilation. Crit Care Med 1986;14(11):926–930.

54. Medbo S, Finne PH, Hansen TW. Respiratory syncytial virus pneumonia ventilated with high-frequency oscillatory ventilation. Acta Paediatr 1997;86(7):766–768.

55. Duval EL, Leroy PL, Gemke RJ, van Vught AJ. High-frequency oscillatory ventilation in RSV bronchiolitis patients. Respir Med 1999;93(6):435–440.

56. Rosenberg RB, Broner CW, Peters KJ, Anglin DL. High-frequency ventilation for acute pediatric respiratory failure. Chest 1993;104(4):1216–1221.

57. Gerstmann DR, Minton SD, Stoddard RA, Meredith KS, Monaco F, Bertrand JM, et al. The Provo multicenter early high-frequency oscillatory ventilation trial: improved pulmonary and clinical outcome in respiratory distress syndrome. Pediatrics 1996;98(6 Pt 1):1044–1057.

58. Jackson JC, Truog WE, Standaert TA, Juul SE, Murphy JH, Chi EY, et al. Effect of high-frequency ventilation on the development of alveolar edema in premature monkeys at risk for hyaline membrane disease. Am Rev Respir Dis 1991;143(4 Pt 1):865–871.

59. Duval EL, van Vught AJ. Status asthmaticus treated by high-frequency oscillatory ventilation. Pediatr Pulmonol 2000;30(4):350–353.

60. Slutsky AS, Kamm RD, Rossing TH, Loring SH, Lehr J, Shapiro AH, et al. Effects of frequency, tidal volume, and lung volume on CO_2 elimination in dogs by high frequency (2–30 Hz), low tidal volume ventilation. J Clin Invest 1981;68(6):1475–1484.

61. Lunkenheimer PP, Redmann K, Stroh N, Gleich C, Krebs S, Scheld HH, et al. High-frequency oscillation in an adult porcine model. Crit Care Med 1994;22(9 Suppl):S37–S48.

62. Fort P, Farmer C, Westerman J, Johannigman J, Beninati W, Dolan S, et al. High-frequency oscillatory ventilation for adult respiratory distress syndrome—a pilot study [comment]. Crit Care Med 1997;25(6):937–947.

63. Sedeek KA, Takeuchi M, Suchodolski K, Kacmarek RM. Determinants of tidal volume during high-frequency oscillation. Crit Care Med 2003;31(1):227–231.

64. Brazelton TB, 3rd, Watson KF, Murphy M, Al-Khadra E, Thompson JE, Arnold JH. Identification of optimal lung volume during high-frequency oscillatory ventilation using respiratory inductive plethysmography. Crit Care Med 2001;29(12):2349–2359.

65. Weber K, Courtney SE, Pyon KH, Chang GY, Pandit PB, Habib RH. Detecting lung overdistention in newborns treated with high-frequency oscillatory ventilation. J Appl Physiol 2000;89(1):364–372.

66. Maggiore SM, Lellouche F, Pigeot J, Taille S, Deye N, Durrmeyer X, et al. Prevention of endotracheal suctioning-induced alveolar derecruitment in acute lung injury. Am J Respir Crit Care Med 2003;167(9):1215–1224.

67. Choong K, Chatrkaw P, Frndova H, Cox PN. Comparison of loss in lung volume with open versus in-line catheter endotracheal suctioning. Pediatr Crit Care Med 2003;4(1):69–73.

68. Gattinoni L, Caironi P, Pelosi P, Goodman LR. What has computed tomography taught us about the acute respiratory distress syndrome? Am J Respir Crit Care Med 2001;164(9):1701–1711.

69. Wolf GK, Arnold JH. Non-invasive assessment of lung volume: respiratory inductance plethysmography and electric impedance tomography. Yearbook of Intensive Care and Emergency Medicine, Springer-Verlag, Berlin, 2005;116–128.

70. Hedenstierna G. Using electric impedance tomography to assess regional ventilation at the bedside. Am J Respir Crit Care Med 2004; 169(7):777–778.

71. Blue RS, Isaacson D, Newell JC. Real-time three-dimensional electrical impedance imaging. Physiol Meas 2000;21(1):15–26.

72. Hahn G, Thiel F, Dudykevych T, Frerichs I, Gersing E, Schroder T, et al. Quantitative evaluation of the performance of different electrical tomography devices. Biomed Tech (Berl) 2001;46(4):91–95.

73. Kunst PW, de Vries PM, Postmus PE, Bakker J. Evaluation of electrical impedance tomography in the measurement of PEEP-induced changes in lung volume. Chest 1999;115(4):1102–1106.

74. Frerichs I, Hinz J, Herrmann P, Weisser G, Hahn G, Dudykevych T, et al. Detection of local lung air content by electrical impedance tomography compared with electron beam CT. J Appl Physiol 2002;93(2):660–666.

75. van Genderingen HR, van Vught AJ, Jansen JR. Regional lung volume during high-frequency oscillatory ventilation by electrical impedance tomography. Crit Care Med 2004;32(3):787–794.

76. Victorino JA, Borges JB, Okamoto VN, Matos GF, Tucci MR, Caramez MP, et al. Imbalances in regional lung ventilation: a validation study on electrical impedance tomography. Am J Respir Crit Care Med 2004;169(7):791–800.

77. Wolf GK, Arnold JH. Non-invasive assessment of lung volume: respiratory inductance plethysmography and electrical impedance tomography. Crit Care Med 2005;33(supl):S163–S169.

78. Kunst PW, Vonk Noordegraaf A, Hoekstra OS, Postmus PE, de Vries PM. Ventilation and perfusion imaging by electrical impedance tomography: a comparison with radionuclide scanning. Physiol Meas 1998;19(4):481–490.

79. Kunst PW, Vonk Noordegraaf A, Straver B, Aarts RA, Tesselaar CD, Postmus PE, et al. Influences of lung parenchyma density and thoracic fluid on ventilatory EIT measurements. Physiol Meas 1998;19(1):27–34.

10

Pulmonary Surfactant: Biology and Therapy

Douglas F. Willson, Patricia R. Chess, Zhengdong Wang, and Robert H. Notter

Overview of Lung Surfactant and Exogenous Surfactant Therapy

Pulmonary surfactant is the evolutionary solution to the problem of surface tension and air breathing. Without surfactant, each breath would require inordinate energy expenditure to expose the huge intrapulmonary surface (approximately the size of a badminton court) to inspired air, and life on land, at least as we know it, would be virtually impossible. One of the first insights into the existence of surface tension forces in the lungs came from the study of von Neergaard in 1929 [1]. Von Neergaard observed that it took nearly twice as much pressure to inflate excised animal lungs with air as it did with fluid. He speculated that because inflating the lungs with an aqueous solution eliminated the air–liquid interface in the alveoli, the additional work required to inflate the lungs with air must be incurred in overcoming surface tension forces at that interface. Von Neergaard's work was supported several decades later in studies by Gruenwald [2] and Mead et al. [3], which further documented the importance of surface tension forces in respiration. Moreover, additional studies indicated that surface tension forces were moderated in the normal lungs by the action of surface-active agents (i.e., surfactants). Work by Pattle [4] in 1955 suggested that the stability of bubbles in the foam expressed from the lungs was related to surfactants that acted to *abolish the tension of the alveolar surface*. Clements [5], Brown [6], and Pattle [7] subsequently confirmed the existence of surfactants in the lungs by further surface tension and biochemical studies.

The crucial physiologic importance of lung surfactant in respiration was shown by the early finding that a lack of this material in premature infants contributed to the development of hyaline membrane disease (HMD; later called the neonatal respiratory distress syndrome or RDS) [7,8]. This finding stimulated the interest of physicians, spurring further research into the function and composition of surfactant. However, clinical interest was significantly dampened by initial unsuccessful attempts by Robillard et al. [9] and Chu et al. [10,11] in the 1960s to use aerosolized dipalmitoyl phosphatidylcholine (DPPC), the major phospholipid component of pulmonary surfactant, to treat HMD in premature infants. This lack of success was misunderstood as indicating that HMD was not caused by surfactant deficiency and, consequently, that surfactant replacement was not an efficacious treatment [11]. Fifteen years of biophysical, biochemical, and animal research was required to reverse this clinical misconception and establish a firm scientific basis for exogenous surfactant therapy (see Notter [12] for detailed review). Basic science research made it clear that DPPC alone is not active lung surfactant and that the aerosolization techniques used by Robillard et al. [9] and Chu et al. [11] were ineffective for alveolar delivery. In 1980, Fujiwara et al. [13] reported the first successful use of exogenous surfactant therapy in premature infants with RDS, although it was another decade before FDA-licensed surfactant drugs were available in the United States. Exogenous surfactant therapy is now a standard of care for the treatment and prevention of RDS in premature infants, but the utility of this treatment approach in other conditions such as clinical acute lung injury (ALI) and acute respiratory distress syndrome (ARDS) is less certain and remains the subject of ongoing research as detailed later.

Pulmonary Surfactant and Its Functions

Pulmonary surfactant serves two primary functions in the lungs. It is first and foremost a *surface-active agent* that lowers and varies surface tension to reduce the work of breathing, stabilizes alveoli against collapse and overdistension, and lessens the hydrostatic driving force for edema fluid to transudate into the interstitium and alveoli. In addition, specific apoprotein components of lung surfactant have been found to play an important role in the lung's innate immune response.

Surface Tension and Surfactants

Molecules at the interface between two phases (solid, liquid, or gas) are subjected to specialized conditions that generate associated forces, which manifest as an *interfacial tension*. Surface tension is the common name given to the interfacial tension at the liquid–gas interface. In biologic systems, the most prevalent liquid–gas

D.S. Wheeler et al. (eds.), *The Respiratory Tract in Pediatric Critical Illness and Injury*,
DOI 10.1007/978-1-84800-925-7_10, © Springer-Verlag London Limited 2009

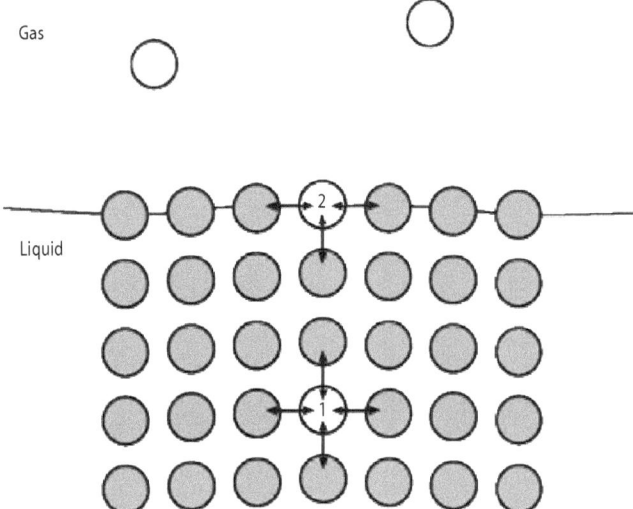

FIGURE 10.1. Molecular forces leading to surface tension at a liquid–gas interface. Attractive forces from nearest neighbors are illustrated for an idealized bulk liquid molecule (1) and an interfacial region molecule (2) contacting a gas. Because the gas is much more dilute, gas molecules exert a negligible attraction on interfacial molecules compared with the liquid. This leads to an unbalanced inward attractive force that causes the surface to minimize its area, generating surface tension. (From Notter [12], with permission from Taylor & Francis Group.)

interface involves a water-based fluid layer contacting air, as occurs in the alveoli of mammals. In the absence of lung surfactant, surface tension at the alveolar interface would be quite high—on the order of 50 dynes/cm for tissue fluid that contains nonspecific soluble proteins and other endogenous solutes [12]. The surface tension of aqueous fluids is high because water is a strongly polar substance with significant intermolecular attractive forces. Liquid (water) molecules at the interface have a strong attraction toward the bulk of the liquid with no equivalent attractive forces above the surface because molecules in the gas (air) are so dilute. These unbalanced forces cause the surface to minimize its area, giving rise to surface tension (Figure 10.1). In a construct such as a spherical bubble, surface tension forces necessitate a pressure drop to maintain the interface at equilibrium against collapse. As described by Laplace in the 18th century for a spherical bubble, this pressure drop (ΔP) is directly proportional to the surface tension (γ) and inversely proportional to the radius of curvature (R), that is, $\Delta P = 2\gamma/R$.

Surfactants are molecules that have an energetic preference for the interface. Molecules that are surface active at an air–water interface all share the characteristic of being amphipathic, that is, possessing both polar and nonpolar regions in their structure. Pulmonary surfactant is largely composed of phospholipids that are molecules with polar phosphate *head groups* and nonpolar fatty chains or *tails*. This structure gives phospholipids an energetic preference for the interface in that they can orient with the polar head group in the aqueous hypophase and the nonpolar hydrocarbon moieties in the air. Lung surfactant also contains proteins that have regions of polar and nonpolar structure, and these proteins interdigitate with phospholipid molecules in the interfacial film and in bilayers/lamellae in the aqueous phase. A surfactant film at an air–water interface acts to lower surface tension because the attractive forces between surfactant molecules and water molecules are less than those of water molecules for each other (if this

were not true, and the surfactant molecules had a stronger attraction for water, they would necessarily go into solution rather than being at the interface). The presence of a surfactant film thus reduces the net unbalanced attractive force between interfacial region and bulk liquid molecules, lowering surface tension as a function of surfactant concentration. In the lungs, the surfactant film at the alveolar interface has powerful consequences for pressure–volume (PV) mechanics and respiratory function.

Effects of Lung Surfactant on Respiratory Physiology

Pulmonary surfactant exists in the alveolar hypophase in a complex microstructure of phospholipid-rich aggregates with incorporated apoproteins. Surfactant molecules in the hypophase adsorb to the air–water interface, which is energetically preferred as described above. The resulting surface film is compressed and expanded during breathing and lowers and varies surface tension in a dynamic fashion. As alveolar size decreases during exhalation, the surfactant film is compressed and surface tension reaches very low values (<1 mN/m compared with 70 mN/m for pure water at 37°C). As alveolar size increases with inspiration, the surfactant film is expanded, and surface tension proportionately increases. This dynamic variation of surface tension with area allows alveoli of different sizes to coexist stably at fixed pressure during respiration (Figure 10.2). Small alveoli resist collapse at end expiration because their surface tension is low, and alveolar inflation is better distributed during inhalation because the ratio of surface tension to area is more uniform in different-sized alveoli. Moreover, by reducing surface tension throughout the lungs, surfactant decreases the pressures (work) needed for pulmonary inflation. There is a direct connection between the surface activity of lung surfactant and pulmonary PV mechanics. The physiologic consequences of surfactant deficiency or dysfunction are profound, as seen in the diffuse atelectasis, uneven inflation, and severe ventilation/

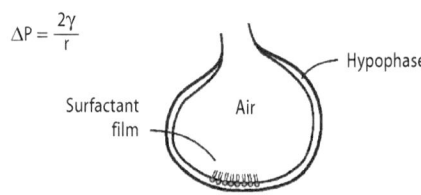

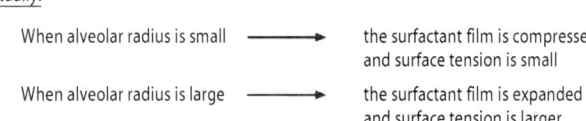

FIGURE 10.2. Schematic showing the effects of lung surfactant on pulmonary pressure–volume (P–V) behavior based on the Laplace equation. The pressure drop (ΔP) necessary to maintain alveoli at equilibrium is proportional to surface tension (γ) and inversely proportional to radius (r), i.e., $\Delta P = 2\gamma/r$ (Laplace's law for a sphere). By lowering and varying surface tension as a function of alveolar size (radius), lung surfactant acts to stabilize pulmonary P-V mechanics as shown schematically. Surfactant also greatly decreases the overall work of breathing by a generalized lowering of surface tension throughout the alveolar network. See text for discussion.

TABLE 10.1. Physiologic actions and surface properties of functional lung surfactant.

Physiologic actions of functional surfactant
    Reduces the work of breathing (increases lung compliance)
    Increases alveolar stability against collapse during expiration
    Improves alveolar inflation uniformity
    Reduces the hydrostatic driving force for edema formation
Biophysical (surface) properties of functional surfactant
    Adsorbs rapidly to the air–water interface
    Reaches very low minimum surface tensions during dynamic compression
    Varies surface tension with area during dynamic cycling
    Respreads from surface collapse phases and other film-associated structures during
        cycling

See text for discussion.
Source: Adapted from Notter [12].

tant proteins have crucial biophysical actions in facilitating the adsorption of phospholipids into the air–water interface, and SP-B and SP-C also act within the surface film itself to refine its composition, increase respreading, and optimize surface tension, lowering during dynamic cycling.

A summary of the molecular characteristics and activities of the four lung surfactant proteins is given in Table 10.3. The two small hydrophobic surfactant proteins (SP-B and SP-C) are found in approximately equal amounts in endogenous surfactant (totaling about 1.5% by weight relative to phospholipid) and are vital to surface activity. Surfactant protein B, which is the most active of the two in increasing adsorption and overall dynamic surface activity [12,14–18], is a particularly important component of functional surfactant. The presence or absence of hydrophobic

perfusion mismatching present in the lungs of preterm infants with RDS. The physiologic roles of lung surfactant, and the surface properties that generate them as described earlier, are summarized in Table 10.1.

Biophysically Functional Composition of Lung Surfactant

The surface behavior of lung surfactant results from molecular interactions between its lipid and protein components. An overall mass composition of lung surfactant is given in Table 10.2. Functional surfactant primarily contains phospholipids and three active surfactant proteins (SP), A, B, and C. A fourth apoprotein (SP-D) that does not participate in surfactant biophysics but is important in host defense (see later) also exists. Phosphatidylcholines (PCs) are the major phospholipid class in lung surfactant, including DPPC as the most prevalent single component. Dipalmitoyl phosphatidylcholine and other disaturated phospholipids form rigid, tightly packed surface films capable of reducing surface tension to very low values under dynamic compression (<1 mN/m as noted earlier). Lung surfactant also contains fluid unsaturated PCs, plus a range of other phospholipid classes with a mix of saturated and unsaturated compounds. Fluid phospholipids increase the respreading of lung surfactant films so that material ejected from the interface during compression reenters the film during expansion and remains available for subsequent respiratory cycles. Neutral lipids in lung surfactant also may help increase film respreading. Surfac-

TABLE 10.3. Molecular characteristics of lung surfactant proteins.

Surfactant protein (SP)	Selected molecular characteristics and functional activities
SP-A	Molecular weight 26–38 kD (monomer), 228 amino acids in humans
	Most abundant surfactant protein, relatively hydrophilic
	Acidic glycoprotein with multiple post-translational isoforms
	C-type lectin and member of the collectin family of host defense proteins
	Forms an active octadecamer (six triplet monomers)
	Aggregates and orders phospholipids (Ca^{2+} dependent)
	Necessary for tubular myelin formation (along with SP-B, Ca^{2+})
	Enhances ability of lung surfactant to resist biophysical inhibition
	Helps regulate reuptake/recycling in addition to aiding host defense
SP-B	Molecular weight 8.5–9 kD (monomer), 79 amino acids in humans (active peptide)
	Hydrophobic, with 2–3 amphipathic helices plus β-sheet structural regions
	Forms dimers and other oligomers of probable functional significance
	Has 10 positive Arg/Lys and 2 negative Glu/Asp residues at neutral pH
	Interacts biophysically with both head groups and chains of phospholipids
	Necessary for tubular myelin formation (along with SP-A, Ca^{2+})
	Disrupts and fuses lipid bilayers and promotes lipid insertion/mixing in surface films
	Enhances the adsorption, film spreading, and dynamic surface activity of lipids
	Most active SP in increasing overall adsorption and dynamic surface activity
SP-C	Molecular weight 4.2 kD (monomer), 35 amino acids in humans (active peptide)
	Most hydrophobic SP, with only 2 charged Arg/Lys residues
	Contains two palmitoylated cysteine residues in humans
	Can form dimers and other oligomers
	Primarily α-helical in structure, with a length that spans a lipid bilayer
	Interacts biophysically primarily with hydrophobic phospholipid chains
	Disrupts and fuses lipid bilayers
	Enhances the adsorption, film spreading, and dynamic surface activity of lipids
SP-D	Molecular weight 39–46 kD (monomer), 355 amino acids in humans
	Has significant structural similarity to SP-A
	Oligomerizes to a dodecamer (four triplet monomers)
	C-type lectin and member of the collectin family of host defense proteins
	Not implicated in lung surfactant biophysics
	Important in host defense and may also participate in surfactant metabolism

Source: Adapted from Notter [12] and Notter et al. [61].

TABLE 10.2. Average mass composition of lung surfactant lipids and proteins.

Phospholipids	85%–90%
Phosphatidylcholine (PC)	80%
Saturated PCs	55%–65%
Unsaturated PCs	45%–35%
Anionic phospholipids (PG, PI, PS)	15%
Other phospholipids	5%
Neutral lipids	4%–7%
Cholesterol, cholesterol esters, glycerides Protein*	6%–8%
SP-A, SP-B, SP-C	

Note: Tabulated values are averages in weight percent for alveolar surfactant obtained by bronchoalveolar lavage (BAL). Surfactant in BAL contains aggregates of varying sizes that can differ in specific composition (not shown). PC, phosphatidylcholine; PG, phosphatidylglycerol; PI, phosphatidylinositol; PS, phosphatidylserine.
*Only biophysically active proteins are tabulated.
Source: Notter [12], with permission from Taylor & Francis Group.

apoproteins in exogenous lung surfactants is a crucial factor in their efficacy as pharmaceutical agents as described later. Genetic deficiency of SP-B is associated with fatal respiratory distress in infancy [19–22], and mutations in SP-C have now been associated with diffuse interstitial pneumonitis and the early development of emphysema [23].

Surfactant Proteins and Innate Immune Function

Pulmonary surfactant is also important in innate (nonadaptive) pulmonary host defense. The epithelial lining of the lungs is critically positioned to participate in the neutralization and clearance of inhaled microorganisms or other particles. Two of the surfactant proteins (SP-A and SP-D) are members of a family of proteins called collectins that play a vital role in innate host defense [24–27]. Other collectins include complement, mannan binding lectin (MBL), and conglutinin. Surfactant proteins A and D are synthesized and secreted by alveolar type II cells and also by nonciliated bronchiolar cells (Clara cells) in the airways [24,25].

As a class, collectins are large multimeric proteins composed of an N-terminal cysteine-rich region, a collagen-like region, an α-helical coiled *neck* region, and a carbohydrate recognition domain (CRD) [24–26]. The basic collectin structure is a trimer of the polypeptide chain, but different collectins have different degrees of higher order oligomerization [26]. Surfactant protein A forms octadecamers (6 trimers), whereas SP-D preferentially accumulates as dodecamers (4 trimers). The C-terminal domains of SP-A and SP-D are responsible for their lectin (carbohydrate binding) activity, and trimeric clusters of the peptide chains are required for high-affinity binding to multivalent ligands. Both proteins bind to the mannose or glucose sugars present in most microbial ligands, although SP-A preferentially binds to the di-mannose repeating unit in Gram-positive capsular polysaccharides and SP-D to the glucose-containing core oligosaccharides of Gram-negative lipopolysaccharide (LPS) [24]. Both can also interact with lipids, SP-A with phospholipids and the lipid A domain of Gram-negative LPS and SP-D with the lipid and inositol moieties of phosphatidylinositol.

Surfactant proteins A and D can bind, agglutinate, and opsonize a variety of pathogens as well as induce chemotaxis, phagocytosis, and provoke killing by phagocytic cells. Table 10.4 lists organisms bound by SP-A and/or SP-D. Although no specific diseases associ-

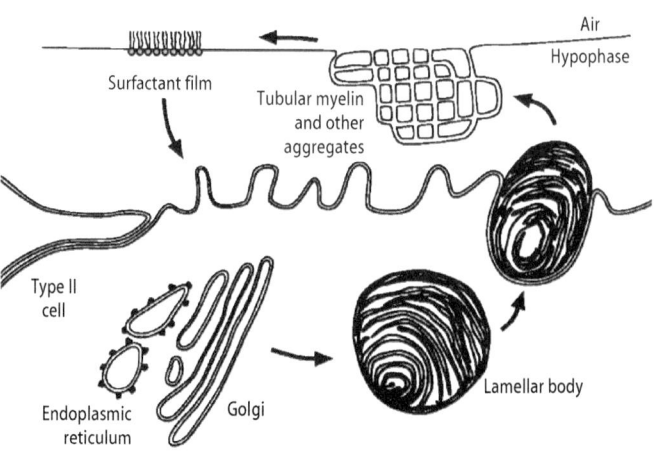

FIGURE 10.3. Schematic overview of the pulmonary surfactant system. The specific lipids and proteins that make up lung surfactant are synthesized, processed, packaged, stored, secreted, and recycled by alveolar type II cells. Surfactant is secreted from lamellar body organelles into the alveolar hypophase, where it forms heterogeneous aggregates (phospholipids plus incorporated apoproteins) that include tubular myelin plus other lamellar/vesicular structures. Surfactant absorbs from these aggregates to form a film at the air–hypophase interface, which acts to lower and vary surface tension during breathing. Over time, "spent" surface-active material in the hypophase is eventually taken up back into the type II pneumocyte for recycling. (From Notter [12], with permission from Taylor & Francis Group.)

ated with deficiencies of these proteins in humans have been described, murine knockout models have elucidated their role in host defense. Surfactant protein-A–deficient mice have normal surfactant homeostasis and respiratory function but enhanced susceptibility to a number of different bacteria, viruses, and parasites [24,28,29]. The phenotype of SP-D–deficient mice is somewhat confusing in that these animals develop a lipoproteinosis-like disease that makes effects on innate immunity difficult to separate from changes in surfactant function [30]. Nonetheless, SP-D can be shown to similarly bind, agglutinate, and opsonize a variety of pathogens [24,31,32].

Surfactant Metabolism and Recycling

A good deal of information is now available about the complex metabolism of pulmonary surfactant [e.g., 12,33–41]. Lung surfactant is synthesized, packaged, stored, secreted, and recycled in type II epithelial cells in the alveolar lining (shown schematically in Figure 10.3). The phospholipid components are synthesized in the endoplasmic reticulum and transported through the Golgi apparatus to the lamellar bodies, whereas surfactant proteins are translated in the usual fashion and then undergo extensive post-translational processing. Surfactant proteins A, B, and C [42–46], but not SP-D [47,48], are found in lamellar bodies.

Lamellar bodies are subcellular organelles, and their contents are composed of tightly packed membrane-like structures that are effectively identical in composition to surfactant obtained from the alveolar space. Lamellar bodies make their way to the cell surface where their contents are extruded into the alveolar hypophase and unwind into a lattice-like construction called *tubular myelin* [49–51] (Figure 10.4). Tubular myelin is a regularly spaced lattice of phospholipid bilayers studded with regularly spaced particles thought to be SP-A. Surfactant protein B and calcium are also

TABLE 10.4. Interactions of lung surfactant collectins with bacterial ligands.

	Bacterial ligand	Collectin
Gram-negative bacteria		
Pseudomonas aeruginosa	Lipopolysaccharide (LPS)?	SP-A
		SP-D
Klebsiella pneumoniae	LPS core (cap-phenotype)	SP-D
	Capsule (di-mannose)	SP-A
Escherichia coli	LPS core	SP-D
	Not defined	SP-A
Haemophilus influenzae, type A	P2 outer membrane protein	SP-A
Gram-positive bacteria		
Group B streptococci	Not defined	SP-A
Staphylococcus aureus		
Cowan I strain	Not defined	SP-A
Clinical isolate	Not defined	SP-A
Streptococcus pneumoniae	Not defined	SP-A

Source: Crouch and Wright [24]. Copyright 2001 the Channal Reviews.

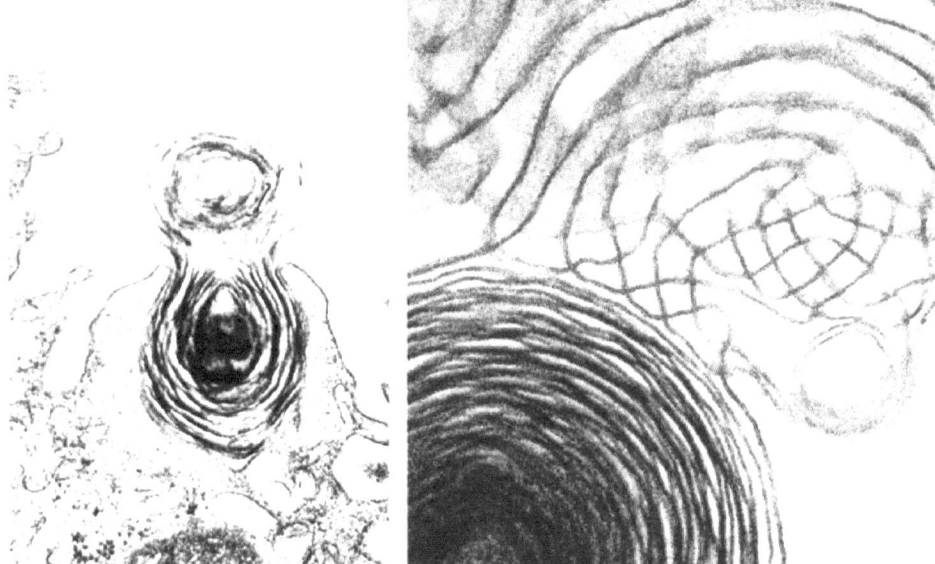

FIGURE 10.4. Lung surfactant secreted from a lamellar body and resulting tubular myelin. Lamellar body contents are extruded from a type II pneumocyte (left) and subsequently "unwind" into tubular myelin in the alveolar hypophase (right). Formation of tubular myelin requires phospholipids, SP-A, SP-B, and calcium. Alveolar surfactant also exists in a variety of large and small aggregate forms in addition to tubular myelin. (From Williams [49], with permission from Rockefeller University Press.)

required for tubular myelin formation [51,52] and are present in its lattice structure. In addition to tubular myelin, a variety of other size-distributed surfactant aggregate forms (lamellar, vesicular, and nonspecific) exist in the alveolar hypophase [12]. Lung surfactant adsorbs from tubular myelin and other active aggregates to form a complex mixed lipid–protein film at the alveolar hypophase–air interface as described earlier.

Lung surfactant has a finite life span in the alveoli and then is cleared from the alveolar space. As much as 90% of the surfactant cleared from the alveolar space is taken up and recycled by type II pneumocytes, with the highest uptake percentages found in newborn compared with adult or premature animals [12,33,53,54]. Alveolar macrophages are responsible for only about 10%–15% of surfactant clearance, and a smaller percentage (<5%) is cleared via the airways. Studies using labeled surfactant introduced into the airways have demonstrated direct uptake by type II pneumocytes, repackaging in lamellar bodies, and eventual resecretion [55]. The half-life for turnover of human surfactant is variable and has been reported to range from 1 to 24 hr in animals [12,33,53]. Surfactant protein A has been shown to enhance the uptake of surfactant phospholipids into type II pneumocytes [56–58], and SP-B/C may also influence phospholipid uptake in type II cells [59,60]. The uptake of exogenously administered surfactants as substrate is thought to be an important factor in the indirect (nonsurface-active) benefits of surfactant therapy, particularly for relatively inactive preparations with a high DPPC content such as Exosurf® and ALEC® (pharmaceutical surfactants are described in more detail later).

Acute Pulmonary Injury

The pathophysiology of acute pulmonary injury (ALI/ARDS) is multifactorial and includes inflammation, surfactant dysfunction, vascular dysfunction, edema, oxidant injury, ventilation/perfusion

mismatching, and injury to alveolar, capillary, and other pulmonary cells. A common aspect of acute pulmonary injury is damage to the cells of the alveolar–capillary membrane (type I and type II alveolar epithelial cells and capillary endothelial cells) with a loss of barrier integrity leading to interstitial and alveolar edema. Another common feature is inflammation. The innate pulmonary inflammatory response is complex, involving the recruitment and activation of circulating leukocytes as well as participation by resident lung cells. A large number of inflammatory mediators and transduction and regulatory pathways are involved in acute pulmonary inflammation and injury (for comprehensive reviews on lung injury and inflammation, see Notter et al. [61]).

In infants, although not generally labeled ALI/ARDS, common causes of respiratory failure include meconium aspiration, sepsis, and pulmonary infection. Although acute respiratory failure in preterm neonates is typically initiated by surfactant deficiency (i.e., RDS), secondary lung injury and surfactant dysfunction can arise in association with hyperoxia, mechanical ventilation, infection, edema from patent ductus arteriosus, and other factors. In addition to acute respiratory failure, ALI/ARDS can also progress to a fibroproliferative phase that leads to chronic lung injury with tissue remodeling and the initiation of fibrosis. However, surfactant dysfunction is most prominent in the acute phase of ALI/ARDS.

Surfactant Dysfunction in Acute Pulmonary Injury

In their original descriptions of ARDS, Ashbaugh, Petty, and colleagues [62,63] commented on its similarity to infantile RDS, and Petty et al. [64] subsequently reported abnormalities in surfactant function. However, respiratory failure in RDS is initiated by a quantitative deficiency in surfactant that leads to progressive atelectasis and overdistension with decreased lung compliance. Although an element of surfactant deficiency can be present in

ALI/ARDS, surfactant dysfunction (inhibition and/or inactivation) as a consequence of inflammatory injury and edema is generally much more prominent. Extensive basic research over the past two decades has identified many of the mechanisms contributing to surfactant dysfunction in lung injury (detailed reviews of lung surfactant inhibition and mechanisms of dysfunction are available [12,17,65]). Irrespective of whether the initiating event is direct injury from the alveolar side or indirect pulmonary injury from the vascular side, surfactant dysfunction may arise by multiple pathways that include the following (Table 10.5):

1. *Physicochemical interactions with inhibitory or reactive substances:* A prevalent cause of surfactant dysfunction in lung injury is through biophysical or chemical interactions with substances that gain access to the alveolar space following damage to the alveolar–capillary membrane. Albumin, hemoglobin, fibrin, fibrinogen, and other blood or serum proteins have been shown in vitro to diminish the surface tension lowering of lung surfactant by competing with the adsorption of its active components into the air-water interface, thus compromising film formation [66,67]. Other biophysical inhibitors include cell membrane lipids, lysophospholipids, or fatty acids that mix into the interfacial film itself to impair surface tension lowering during dynamic compression [67–72]. Additional biophysical inhibitors are listed in Table 10.6, which also notes chemically acting inhibitors such as phospholipases or proteases that can degrade essential surfactant lipids or proteins to impair surface activity [71–73]. Lung surfactant can also be chemically altered by interactions with reactive oxygen and nitrogen species [65]. Fortunately, although surfactant can be inhibited by these physicochemical processes, it has been well-documented, at least in vitro, that dysfunction can be overcome by increasing the concentration of active surfactant even if inhibitors are still present [12,65].

2. *Altered surfactant aggregates and metabolism:* Another pathway by which surfactant activity can be reduced during lung injury is by depletion or alteration of active large aggregates. As noted earlier, surfactant exists in the alveolar hypophase in a size-distributed microstructure of aggregates, the largest of which typically have the greatest surface activity and the highest apoprotein

TABLE 10.6. Endogenous compounds that inhibit lung surfactant activity by physical or chemical interactions.

Biophysical inhibitors
Plasma and blood proteins (e.g., albumin, hemoglobin, fibrinogen, fibrin monomer)
Cell membrane lipids
Lysophospholipids
Fluid free fatty acids
Glycolipids and sphingolipids
Meconium
Chemically acting inhibitors
Lytic enzymes (proteases, phospholipases)
Reactive oxygen and nitrogen species (ROS, RNS)

Tabulated inhibitors are examples only. See text for discussion.
Source: Adapted from Notter [12], Notter and Wang [17], and Gross [81].

content [74–81]. The percentage of large aggregates and their content of SP-A and SP-B are reduced in bronchoalveolar lavage from patients with ARDS [82–84]. Surfactant phospholipid composition can also be altered in patients with ALI/ARDS [84,85]. Animal models of ALI/ARDS show that large surfactant aggregates can be depleted or reduced in activity by interactions with inhibitors or by changes in surfactant metabolism [77,86–89]. Although large aggregates can be detrimentally affected in ALI/ARDS, information on total surfactant pools is inconsistent, with both decreased [90–92] and unchanged [85,93] amounts reported.

In assessing surfactant dysfunction in ALI/ARDS, it is important to realize that the pathology is not static. The contribution of surfactant dysfunction to ALI/ARDS is almost certainly dependent on the stage of disease, which commences with an exudative phase involving alveolar–capillary membrane damage and acute inflammation but may evolve to fibroproliferation and fibrosis. The superimposition of iatrogenic factors such as ventilator-induced lung injury and hyperoxic injury during intensive care further confounds pathology, as does the multiorgan disease that is frequently present in patients with ALI/ARDS. The multifaceted pathology of lung injury is an important issue when evaluating the potential efficacy of exogenous surfactant therapy in ALI/ARDS.

Surfactant Therapy in Acute Pulmonary Injury

The existence of surfactant dysfunction in ALI/ARDS provides a conceptional rationale for the therapeutic use of exogenous surfactant, but the use of surfactant drugs having the greatest surface activity and ability to resist inhibition is clearly required. Moreover, to be effective in ALI/ARDS, exogenous surfactant must be delivered and distributed to injured alveoli in the necessary amounts despite the presence of edema and inflammation. Similar to initial attempts to treat RDS in premature infants, the first large controlled trial of surfactant replacement in ARDS using the aerosolized protein-free synthetic surfactant Exosurf® was an unequivocal failure [94]. This failure at least partly reflects similar reasons, that is, the use of a surfactant with inadequate activity and an ineffective delivery method. However, surfactant therapy in ALI/ARDS faces more complex challenges than in the case of neonatal RDS, and this therapy remains investigational particularly for adults, as detailed next.

TABLE 10.5. Pathways and processes that can contribute to surfactant abnormalities in acute inflammatory lung injury.

Lung surfactant dysfunction/inactivation
Biophysical inactivation by inhibitory substances in edema or present as a result of inflammation
Chemical degradation by lytic enzymes or by reactive oxygen/nitrogen species
Depletion or detrimental alteration of active large aggregate surfactant subtypes
Alveolar epithelial cell damage or alteration
Type I cell injury and death leading to increased permeability of the alveolar epithelial barrier
Type II cell injury and/or hyperplasia leading to altered surfactant synthesis, secretion, recycling
Inflammation and microvascular dysfunction
Capillary endothelial injury leading to increased microvascular permeability and interstitial or alveolar edema that contains surfactant inhibitors
Multiple mediators and products produced by leukocytes and lung cells that affect the severity of injury and can directly or indirectly affect alveolar surfactant or type II cells

See text for discussion. Surfactant dysfunction and its mechanisms in ALI/ARDS are reviewed in detail by Notter [12] and Wang et al. [81].

Pharmaceutical Surfactants

Although the composition of endogenous surfactant is similar throughout mammalian species, this is not true of exogenous surfactant drugs. The degree of resemblance of pharmaceutical surfactants to native surfactant is highly variable and has direct consequences for surface and physiologic activity. Pharmaceutical surfactants can be divided into three functionally relevant groups: (1) organic solvent extracts of lavaged lung surfactant from animals, (2) organic solvent extracts of processed animal lung tissue with or without additional synthetic additives, and (3) synthetic preparations not containing surfactant material from animal lungs (Table 10.7).

Organic solvent extracts of lavaged alveolar surfactant (category I) contain all of the hydrophobic lipid and protein components of endogenous surfactant, although specific compositional details can vary depending on preparative methodology. Extracts of minced or homogenized lung tissue (category II) necessarily contain some nonsurfactant components and require more extensive processing that can further alter composition compared with native surfactant. The synthetic surfactants in category III that have been most widely studied are Exosurf® and ALEC® (artificial lung expanding compound). Exosurf is a mixture of DPPC:hexadecanol:tyloxapol (1:0.11:0.075 by weight), and ALEC is a mixture of 7:3 DPPC:egg phosphatidylglycerol (PG). These two preparations are no longer in active clinical use because they have been shown to have inferior activity compared with animal-derived surfactants [e.g., 12,95–100]. Two additional synthetic surfactants, KL4 (Surfaxin®) and recombinant SP-C surfactant (Venticute®), are currently undergoing clinical evaluation.

The compositions and activities of the exogenous surfactants listed in Table 10.7, and their efficacy in preventing or treating RDS in clinical trials in premature infants, are reviewed in detail by Notter [12]. Four exogenous surfactant preparations are currently licensed for clinical use in RDS in the United States: Infasurf®, Survanta®, Curosurf®, and Exosurf® (the latter is no longer used,

TABLE 10.7. Clinical exogenous surfactant drugs used to treat lung diseases involving surfactant deficiency/dysfunction.

I. **Organic solvent extracts of lavaged animal lung surfactant**
Infasurf® (CLSE)
bLES®
Alveofact®
II. **Supplemented or unsupplemented organic solvent extracts of processed animal lung tissue**
Survanta®
Surfactant-TA®
Curosurf®
III. **Synthetic exogenous lung surfactants**
Exosurf®
ALEC®
Surfaxin® (KL4)
Venticute® (recombinant SP-C surfactant)

Note: Infasurf® (ONY, Inc., and Forest Laboratories), Survanta® (Abbott/Ross Laboratories), and Curosurf® (Chiesi Farmaceutici and Dey Laboratories) are currently FDA approved in the United States, and Surfaxin® (KL4) is under clinical evaluation. Exosurf® (Glaxo-Wellcome) is also FDA approved but is no longer used. Details on the compositions, activities, and efficacies of these exogenous surfactants in neonatal RDS are reviewed by Notter [12], and their use in ALI/ARDS is discussed in the text.
Source: Adapted from Notter [12] and Enhorning et al. [72].

as noted earlier). Infasurf® is a direct chloroform:methanol extract of large aggregate surfactant obtained by bronchoalveolar lavage from calf lungs [12,56,101]. Survanta® is made from an extract of minced bovine lung tissue to which DPPC, tripalmitin, and palmitic acid are added [12,18]. Curosurf® is prepared from minced porcine lung tissue by a combination of washing, chloroform-methanol extraction, and liquid-gel chromatography [102]. Surfaxin®, which is under active consideration for FDA approval, contains a 21 amino acid peptide (KL4) that has repeating units of one leucine (K) and four lysine (L) residues. This peptide is combined at 3% by weight with a 3:1 mixture of DPPC and palmitoyl-oleoyl phosphatidylglycerol (POPG) plus 15% palmitic acid [12]. Venticute® contains synthetic lipids and palmitic acid plus a 34 amino acid modified human recombinant SP-C that has substitutions of phenylalanine for cysteine at two positions and isoleucine for methionine at another [12].

Relative Activity and Inhibition Resistance of Exogenous Surfactant Drugs

The relative activities and efficacies of surfactant drugs are crucial for evaluating and optimizing therapy. Differences in efficacy among pharmaceutical surfactants have been demonstrated in comparison trials in premature infants and in retrospective meta-analyses (reviewed by Notter [12]). These differences in surfactant activity can be directly linked to differences in composition. The fact that *natural* surfactants from animal lungs (categories I and II, Table 10.7) have greater efficacy than the protein-free synthetic surfactants Exosurf® and ALEC® reflects the difficulty of substituting for the highly active hydrophobic lung surfactant proteins SP-B/C in synthetic surfactants. The surface and physiologic activities of Exosurf® are significantly increased by the addition of purified bovine SP-B/SP-C, demonstrating that its synthetic components do not adequately replace these active apoproteins [95]. Animal-derived clinical surfactants also differ markedly in their surface activity and ability to resist inhibitor-induced dysfunction based on their compositions.

Biophysical research demonstrates that the surface activity, inhibition resistance, and physiologic effects of extracts of lavaged animal surfactant (category I surfactant drugs, Table 10.7) are greater than those of other clinical surfactants (Figures 10.5 to 10.7) [e.g., 18,95,96]. It has also been shown that differences in apoprotein content can help explain some of these differences in activity [14,16,18,95,103,104]. For example, the activity and inhibition resistance of Infasurf® are substantially greater than those of Survanta® in basic biophysical and animal research [18,95,96,103] (see Figures 10.5 to 10.7), and these differences correlate directly with the content of SP-B in the two preparations [18,103,105]. Survanta® contains only 0.044% SP-B by weight relative to phospholipid because of losses during processing of lung tissue [18]. In contrast, Infasurf® has a specific SP-B content of 0.9% by weight (and a total hydrophobic protein content of 1.7% by weight) equivalent to lavaged calf lung surfactant [18]. As described earlier, SP-B is the most active of the hydrophobic surfactant proteins in enhancing the adsorption and overall dynamic surface activities of phospholipids [14–16,18,106,107]. The addition of SP-B or synthetic SP-B peptides to Survanta® significantly improves its activity toward that of natural surfactant [18,103,104] (e.g., Figure 10.7), indicating that the lack of SP-B in this exogenous surfactant is functionally important. Even without SP-B, however, Survanta® still has

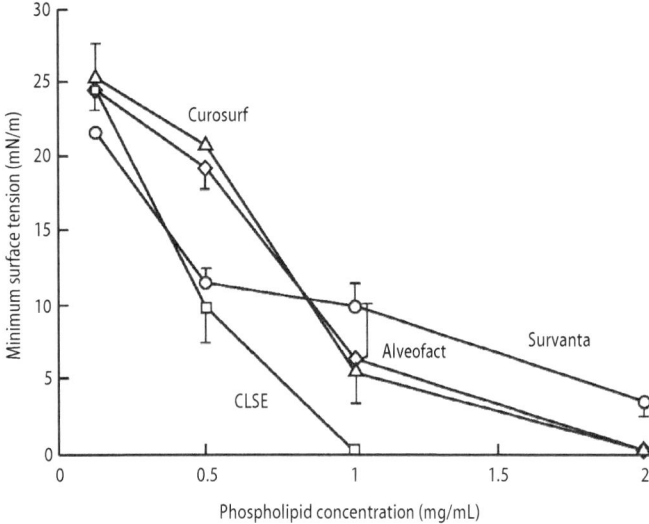

FIGURE 10.5. Overall surface tension lowering ability of clinical exogenous surfactants. Minimum surface tension after 5 min of pulsation in a bubble surfactometer (37°C, 20 cycles/min, 50% area compression) is plotted as a function of surfactant phospholipid concentration for several clinical surfactants. These surfactants vary widely in overall surface tension lowering ability, with the most active being CLSE (Infasurf®, category I, Table 10.7). (Redrawn from Seeger et al. [96].)

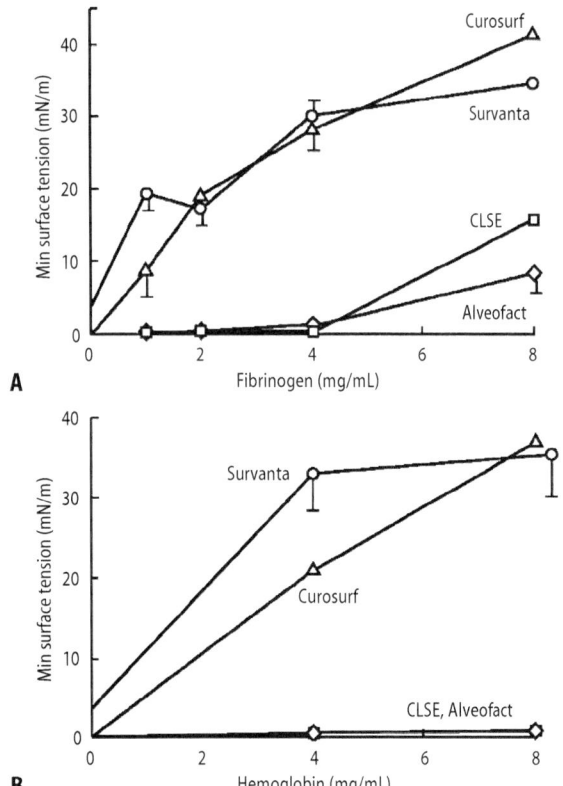

FIGURE 10.6. Resistances of clinical surfactants to inhibition by blood proteins. Minimum surface tension after 5 min of pulsation in a bubble surfactometer (37°C, 20 cycles/min, and 50% area compression) is plotted against the concentration of inhibitory blood proteins (fibrinogen **[A]** and hemoglobin **[B]**). Exogenous surfactants that most closely mimic natural surfactant (category I drugs from Table 10.7) are best able to resist inhibition and reach low surface tension despite high levels of inhibitory proteins. Surfactant phospholipid concentration was 2 mg/mL. (Redrawn from Seeger et al. [96].)

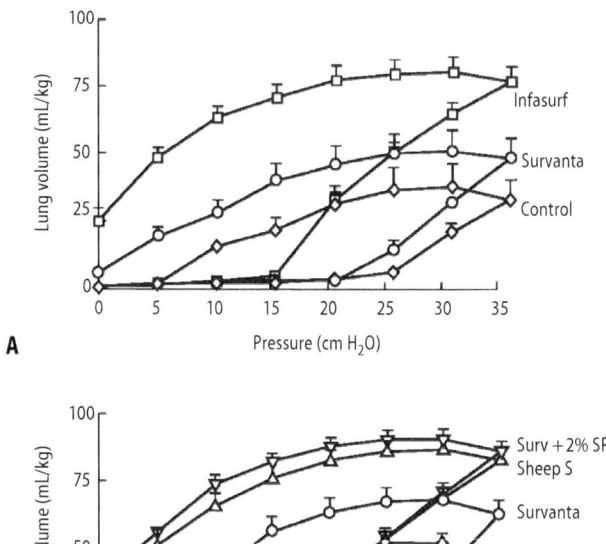

FIGURE 10.7. Effects on physiologic activity of the addition of purified SP-B to Survanta®. **(A)** Premature rabbit fetuses (27 days' gestation) treated with Survanta® or Infasurf® and untreated controls. **(B)** Premature rabbit fetuses treated with Survanta®, Survanta® + SP-B (2% by weight by ELISA), natural surfactant from adult sheep (Sheep S), or untreated controls. Infasurf® improved lung mechanics more than Survanta® (A), and the importance of SP-B in this behavior is shown by the increased activity of Survanta® + SP-B compared to Survanta® alone (B). Surfactants were instilled intratracheally at a dose of 100 mg/kg body weight, and quasistatic pressure–volume curves were measured following 15 min of mechanical ventilation. (Redrawn from Mizuno et al. [103].)

significantly better activity than protein-free surfactants like Exosurf® because of its content of SP-C and other ingredients [12].

Animal Studies of Surfactant Therapy

Animal models of ALI/ARDS in which exogenous surfactant therapy has been shown to improve respiratory function or mechanics include acid aspiration [108–110], meconium aspiration [111–114], anti-lung serum [115], bacterial or endotoxin injury [116–121], vagotomy [122], hyperoxia [123–27], in vivo lavage [104,128–132], N-nitroso-N-methylurethane (NNNMU) injury [133–135], and viral pneumonia [136,137]. In addition to demonstrating that surfactant therapy has potential benefit in ALI/ARDS, animal studies are also important in comparing surfactant activity under reproducible conditions, as well as in examining other variables of interest for clinical therapy. These variables include the method of surfactant delivery (instillation versus aerosolization), the timing of administration, the effects of different modes of ventilation, the effects of dose, and so on. For example, animal studies indicate that direct airway instillation is more effective than current aerosol techniques in delivering exogenous surfactant to the alveoli and that early therapy is preferable to later therapy in terms of distributing surfactant to injured lungs (reviewed by Notter [12]). However, despite their utility for assessing the acute effects of exogenous surfactants and comparing preparations and delivery methods, animal models offer limited insight into longer term morbidity or mortality. For this, one must ultimately turn to human studies.

Human Studies of Surfactant Replacement Therapy

Multiple clinical studies have reported benefits following the instillation of exogenous surfactants to term infants, children, or adults with ALI/ARDS or related acute respiratory failure [138–154] (Table 10.8). However, many of these are small case series or pilot studies and found improvements in only acute lung function (oxygenation). Controlled trials of surfactant therapy in patients with ALI/ARDS have met with mixed success, particularly in studies with adults [94,155]. The clinical experiences with exogenous surfactant therapy in term infants, children and adults are summarized next.

The best-studied application of surfactant therapy in term infants with acute pulmonary injury is in meconium aspiration syndrome [148–152]. Meconium obstructs and injures the lungs when aspirated and is known to cause surfactant dysfunction [156,157]. Auten et al. [148], Khammash et al. [151], and Findlay et al. [152] have all reported significant improvement from surfactant administration in infants with meconium aspiration. The randomized study of Findlay et al. [152] found reductions in the incidence of pneumothorax, duration of mechanical ventilation and oxygen therapy, time of hospitalization, and requirements for extracorporeal membrane oxygenation (ECMO) in 20 term infants treated with Survanta® compared with controls. Lotze et al. [149,150] also reported favorable results using Survanta® in a controlled trial in term infants referred for ECMO because of severe respiratory failure (meconium aspiration was a prevalent diagnosis in both studies). Twenty-eight infants treated with four doses of Survanta® (150 mg/kg) had improved pulmonary mechanics, decreased duration of ECMO treatment, and a lower incidence of complications after ECMO than control infants [149]. A subsequent multicenter controlled trial with 328 term infants also reported significant improvements in respiratory status and the need for ECMO following surfactant treatment [150]. Exogenous surfactant is now used in many institutions to treat respiratory failure in term infants with meconium aspiration or pneumonia, although fewer controlled studies are available for the latter condition. Surfactant therapy has also been studied in infants with congenital diaphragmatic hernia, but its use remains somewhat controversial in this context [158,159].

Studies of surfactant in children and adults with ALI/ARDS have followed the general pattern of initial positive case reports or series followed by more equivocal results in randomized prospective studies. The first large prospective, controlled study of surfactant therapy for adults with ARDS was definitively negative. Anzueto et al [94] administered nebulized Exosurf® versus placebo to 725 adults with ARDS secondary to sepsis and found no improvement in any measure of oxygenation and no effect on morbidity or mortality. As described earlier, Exosurf® is no longer used clinically in the United States because of its lower activity compared with animal-derived surfactants, and aerosolization is currently not as effective as airway instillation in delivering surfactant. Gregory et al. [155] reported small benefits in oxygenation in a controlled trial in adults with ARDS who received four 100 mg/kg doses of Survanta® but with no overall advantage in survival in the 43 surfactant-treated patients studied. A recent study by Spragg et al. [160] using recombinant SP-C surfactant (Venticute®) in adults with ARDS showed immediate improvements in oxygenation but no longer term improvement in duration of mechanical ventilation, lengths of stay, or mortality. Post hoc analysis did suggest, however, that the response in the subgroup of patients with ARDS caused by *direct lung injury* was quite positive, and a follow-up prospective study with this group of patients is currently underway.

Controlled studies of surfactant therapy in children with ALI/ARDS have been more encouraging. A randomized but unblinded trial by Willson et al. [143] in 42 children at eight centers with ALI/ARDS showed that those receiving Infasurf® (70 mg/kg) had immediate improvement in oxygenation and fewer ventilator days and days in intensive care. This trial followed an initial open-label trial by the same group demonstrating improved oxygenation in 29 children (0.1–16 years) treated with instilled Infasurf® [142]. Luchetti et al. [153,154] have reported two small controlled studies showing that treatment with porcine surfactant (Curosurf®, 50 mg/kg) led to improved gas exchange as well as reduced time on mechanical ventilation and in intensive care for infants with bronchiolitis. A study by Moller et al. [161] found that children with

TABLE 10.8. Clinical studies reporting benefits of exogenous surfactant therapy in acute respiratory failure (ALI/ARDS).

Study	Patients (N)	Disease or syndrome	Surfactant	Outcomes
Gunther et al. [138]	Adult (27)	ARDS	Alveofact	Improved surfactant function
Walmrath et al. [139]	Adult (10)	ARDS from sepsis	Alveofact	Improved oxygenation
Spragg et al. [140]	Adult (6)	ARDS from multiple causes	Curosurf	Improved oxygenation a and biophysical function
Wiswell et al. [141]	Adults (12)	ARDS from multiple causes	Surfaxin	Improved oxygenation
Willson et al. [142,143]	Children (29, 42)	ARDS from multiple causes	Infasurf	Improved oxygenation
Willson et al. [144]	Children (152)	ARDS from multiple causes	Infasurf	Improved survival, and improved ventilation
Lopez-Herce et al. [145]	Children (20)	ARDS + postop cardiac	Curosurf	Improved oxygenation
Hermon et al. [146]	Children (19)	ARDS + postop cardiac	Curosurf or Alveofact	Improved oxygenation
Herting et al. [147]	Children (8)	Pneumonia	Curosurf	Improved oxygenation
Auten et al. [148]	Infants (14)	Meconium aspiration or pneumonia	Infasurf (CLSE)	Improved oxygenation
Lotze et al. [149,150]	Infants (28, 328)	ECMO, multiple indications	Survanta	Improved oxygenation, decreased ECMO
Khammash et al. [151]	Infants (20)	Meconium aspiration	bLES	Improved oxygenation in 75% of patients
Findlay et al. [152]	Infants (40)	Meconium aspiration	Survanta	Improved oxygenation, decreased pneumothorax and mechanical ventilation
Luchetti et al. [153,154]	Infants (20, 40)	RSV bronchiolitis	Curosurf	Improved oxygenation

Note: Tabulated clinical studies include both controlled and noncontrolled trials as discussed in the text. ARDS, acute respiratory distress syndrome; ECMO, extracorporeal membrane oxygenation; RSV, respiratory syncytial virus.

TABLE 10.9. Clinical outcomes from a recent controlled study using exogenous surfactant (Infasurf; calfactant) in pediatric patients with ALI/ARDS.

	Calfactant (N = 77)	Placebo (N = 75)	p Value
Mortality			
Died (in hospital)	15 (19%)	27 (36%)	0.03
Died w/o extubation	12 (16%)	24 (32%)	0.02
Failed CMV*	13 (21%)	26 (42%)	0.02
ECMO	3	3	—
Use of iNO	9	10	0.80
HFOV after entry	7	15	0.07
Secondary Outcomes			
PICU LOS	15.2 ± 13.3	13.6 ± 11.6	0.85
Hospital LOS	26.8 ± 26	25.3 ± 32.2	0.91
Days O$_2$ therapy	17.3 ± 16	18.5 ± 31	0.93
Hospital charges†	$205 ± 220	$213 ± 226	0.83
Hospital charges/day†	$7.5 ± 7.6	$7.9 ± 7.5	0.74

*Some patients who failed CMV had more than one nonconventional therapy (ECMO, iNO, or HFOV);
†Costs are given in thousands of dollars.
Note: In addition to improving mortality and reducing the percentage of patients who failed CMV as reported in the table, instilled calfactant also significantly improved oxygenation index compared with placebo ($p = 0.01$, data not shown). CMV, conventional mechanical ventilation; ECMO, extracorporeal membrane oxygenation; HFOV, high-frequency oscillatory ventilation; iNO, inhaled nitric oxide.
Source: Willson et al. [144].

ARDS showed immediate improvement in oxygenation and had less need for rescue therapy following treatment with Survanta®, but it was underpowered for more definitive outcomes. Most recently, a blinded controlled study by Willson et al. [144] yielded very positive results in pediatric patients with ALI/ARDS, showing both immediate benefits with regard to oxygenation as well as a significant survival advantage for patients receiving calfactant (Infasurf®) relative to placebo (Table 10.9). None of the above studies showed any significant adverse long-term effects from surfactant administration, although transient hypoxia and some hemodynamic instability surrounding instillation appear common. Transmission of infectious agents and allergic reactions have not been reported with any of the surfactants currently licensed in the United States.

The Future of Surfactant Therapy and Related Combination Therapies

As described in preceding sections, surfactant replacement therapy is standard in the prevention and treatment of RDS in premature infants, and there is basic science and clinical evidence supporting its use in some forms of lung injury–associated respiratory failure. Clinical evidence of the efficacy of surfactant therapy for term infants with meconium aspiration is sufficiently strong that this approach is now frequently used in neonatal intensive care units (and is also being applied to other forms of neonatal respiratory failure, such as pneumonia). Controlled trials of surfactant therapy for children with ALI/ARDS also suggest significant benefits, with survival advantages shown in a recent trial [144]. It can be argued that evidence of surfactant dysfunction in ALI/ARDS, along with favorable results for surfactant treatment in animal models and evidence for efficacy in humans without significant adverse effects,

makes a strong rationale for considering surfactant therapy for any pediatric patient with pulmonary injury and ALI/ARDS. From this perspective, the major downside of the therapy is its considerable expense. However, it would be ideal if additional questions about the therapy were addressed in research before its indiscriminate adoption.

As emphasized in this chapter, some exogenous surfactants are more active and have better inhibition resistance than others, and this, along with effective delivery, will impact the success of surfactant therapy for ALI/ARDS. It is also likely that surfactant therapy is more applicable for some types of pulmonary injury than others. It is important to note that post hoc analyses in the studies of both Spragg et al. [160] and Willson et al. [144] suggested greater efficacy in direct lung injury (e.g., pneumonia, aspiration) as opposed to indirect lung injury (e.g., sepsis, systemic inflammatory response syndrome). It would obviously be helpful to focus surfactant therapy on the types of lung injury where it has maximal benefit. Also, neonatal data suggest that early surfactant administration generates improved responses compared with delayed administration [e.g., 162], possibly as a result of better intrapulmonary drug distribution coupled with minimized ventilator-induced lung injury. Intuitively, similar advantages might accompany early surfactant administration in patients with ALI/ARDS.

Finally, a major issue with regard to surfactant therapy in ALI/ARDS involves its potential use in combination with agents or interventions that target additional aspects of the complex pathophysiology of acute pulmonary injury. This kind of combination therapy approach may be particularly important for adults with ALI/ARDS, whose responses to exogenous surfactant have so far been disappointing. The use of multiple therapeutic agents or interventions based on specific rationales for potential synergy has the potential to significantly enhance patient outcomes in complex disease processes such as those involving inflammatory lung injury. The potential use of exogenous surfactant therapy in the context of specific combined-modality interventions is described in detail elsewhere [163,164]. Examples of agents that might be synergistic with exogenous surfactant in ALI/ARDS include antiinflammatory antibodies or receptor antagonists, antioxidants, and vasoactive drugs such as inhaled nitric oxide (iNO). In addition, specific ventilator modalities or ventilation strategies that reduce iatrogenic lung injury may be equally important to consider in conjunction with surfactant therapy. Given the known importance of surfactant dysfunction in inflammatory lung injury, it is likely that ongoing research will continue to identify specific populations of patients with ALI/ARDS or related acute respiratory failure who can benefit from exogenous surfactant therapy, with or without complementary agents or interventions.

References

1. von Neergaard K. Neue auffassungen uber einen grundbegriff der atemmechanik. Dieretraktionskraft der lunge, abhangig von der oberflachenspannung in den alveolen. Z Ges Exp Med 1929;66:373–394.
2. Gruenwald P. Surface tension as a factor in the resistance of neonatal lungs to aeration. Am J Obstet Gynecol 1947;53:996–1007.
3. Mead J, Whittenberger JL, Radford EP. Surface tension as a factor in pulmonary volume–pressure hysteresis. J Appl Physiol 1957;10:191–196.
4. Pattle RE. Properties, function, and origin of the alveolar lining layer. Nature 1955;175:1125–1126.
5. Clements JA. Surface tension of lung extracts. Proc Soc Exp Biol Med 1957;95:170–172.

6. Brown ES. Lung area from surface tension effects. Proc Soc Exp Biol Med 1957;95:168–170.

7. Pattle RE. Properties, function and origin of the alveolar lining layer. Proc R Soc (Lond) Ser B 1958;148:217–240.

8. Avery ME, Mead J. Surface properties in relation to atelectasis and hyaline membrane disease. Am J Dis Child 1959;97:517–523.

9. Robillard E, Alarie Y, Dagenais-Perusse P, Baril E, Guilbeault A. Microaerosol administration of synthetic b,g-dipalmitoyl-L-a-lecithin in the respiratory distress syndrome: a preliminary report. Can Med Assoc J 1964;90:55–57.

10. Chu J, Clements JA, Cotton EK, Klaus MH, Sweet AY, Thomas MA, Tooley WH. The pulmonary hypoperfusion syndrome. Pediatrics 1965;35:733–742.

11. Chu J, Clements JA, Cotton EK, Klaus MH, Sweet AY, Tooley WH. Neonatal pulmonary ischemia. Clinical and physiologic studies. Pediatrics 1967;40:709–782.

12. Notter RH. Lung Surfactants: Basic Science and Clinical Applications. New York: Marcel Dekker; 2000.

13. Fujiwara T, Maeta H, Chida S, Morita T, Watabe Y, Abe T. Artificial surfactant therapy in hyaline membrane disease. Lancet 1980;1:55–59.

14. Wang Z, Baatz JE, Holm BA, Notter RH. Content-dependent activity of lung surfactant protein B (SP-B) in mixtures with lipids. Am J Physiol 2002;283:L897–L906.

15. Wang Z, Gurel O, Baatz JE, Notter RH. Differential activity and lack of synergy of lung surfactant proteins SP-B and SP-C in surface-active interactions with phospholipids. J Lipid Res 1996;37:1749–1760.

16. Seeger W, Günther A, Thede C. Differential sensitivity to fibrinogen inhibition of SP-C- vs. SP-B-based surfactants. Am J Physiol 1992;261:L286–L291.

17. Notter RH, Wang Z. Pulmonary surfactant: physical chemistry, physiology and replacement. Rev Chem Eng 1997;13:1–118.

18. Notter RH, Wang Z, Egan EA, Holm BA. Component-specific surface and physiological activity in bovine-derived lung surfactants. Chem Phys Lipids 2002;114:21–34.

19. Whitsett JA, Nogee LM, Weaver TE, Horowitz AD. Human surfactant protein B structure, function, regulation, and genetic disease. Physiol Rev 1995;75:749–757.

20. deMello DE, Nogee LM, Heyman S, Krous HF, Hussain M, Merritt TA, Hsueh W, Haas JE, Heidelberger K, Schumacher R, Colten HR. Molecular and phenotypic variability in the congenital alveolar proteinosis syndrome associated with inherited surfactant protein B deficiency. J Pediatr 1994;125:43–50.

21. Nogee LM, Garnier G, Dietz HC, Singer L, Murphy AM, deMello DE, Colten HR. A mutation in the surfactant protein B gene responsible for fatal neonatal respiratory disease in multiple kindreds. J Clin Invest 1994;93:1860–1863.

22. Nogee LM, Wert SE, Proffit SA, Whitsett JA. Allelic heterogeneity in hereditary surfactant protein B (SP-B) deficiency. Am J Respir Crit Care Med 2000;161:973–981.

23. Nogee LM, Dunbar AE, Wert SE, Askin F, Hamvas A, Whitsett JA. A mutation in the surfactant protein C gene associated with familial interstitial lung disease. N Engl J Med 2001;344:573–579.

24. Crouch E, Wright JR. Surfactant proteins A and D and pulmonary host defense. Annu Rev Physiol 2001;63:521–554.

25. Lawson PR, Reid KBM. The roles of surfactant proteins A and D in innate immunity. Immunol Rev 2000;173:66–78.

26. Mason RJ, Greene K, Voelker DR. Surfactant protein A and surfactant protein D in health and disease. Am J Physiol 1998;275:L1–L13.

27. Wright JR. Immunomodulatory functions of surfactant. Physiol Rev 1997;77:931–962.

28. LeVine AM, Bruno MD, Huelsman KM, Ross GF, Whitsett JA. Surfactant protein A deficient mice are susceptible to group B streptococcal infection. J Immunol 1997;158:4336–4340.

29. LeVine AM, Kurak KE, Bruno MD, Stark JM, Whitsett JA, Korfhagen TA. Surfactant protein A–deficient mice are susceptible to Pseudomonas aeruginosa infection. Am J Respir Cell Mol Biol 1998;19:700–708.

30. Korfhagen TR, Sheftelyevich V, Burhans MS, Bruno MD, Ross GF, et al. Surfactant protein D regulates surfactant phospholipid homeostasis in vivo. J Biol Chem 1998;273:28438–28443.

31. Lim BL, Wang JY, Holmskov U, Hoppe HJ, Reid KB. Expression of the carbohydrate recognition domain of lung surfactant protein D and demonstration of its binding to lipopolysaccharides of Gram-negative bacteria. Biochem Biophys Res Commun 1994;202:1674–1680.

32. Ferguson JS, Voelker DR, McCormack FX, Schlesinger LS. Surfactant protein D binds Mycobacterium tuberculosis bacilli and liparabinomannan via carbohydrate-lectin interactions resulting in reduced phagocytosis of the bacteria by the macrophages. J Immunol 1999; 163:312–321.

33. Wright JR. Clearance and recycling of pulmonary surfactant. Am J Physiol 1990;259:L1–L12.

34. Batenburg JJ. Surfactant phospholipids: synthesis and storage. Am J Physiol 1992;262:L367–L385.

35. Hawgood S. Surfactant: composition, structure, and metabolism. In: Crystal RG, West JB, Weibel ER, Barnes PJ, eds. The Lung: Scientific Foundations, 2nd ed. Philadelphia: Lippincott-Raven; 1997:557–571.

36. Hawgood S, Poulain FR. The pulmonary collectins and surfactant metabolism. Annu Rev Physiol 2001;63:495–519.

37. van Golde LMG, Casals CC. Metabolism of lipids. In: Crystal RG, West JB, Weibel ER, Barnes PJ, eds. The Lung: Scientific Foundations, 2nd ed. Philadelphia: Lippincott-Raven; 1997:9–18.

38. Haagsman HP, van Golde LMG. Synthesis and assembly of lung surfactant. Annu Rev Physiol 1991;53:441–464.

39. Johansson J, Curstedt T, Robertson B. The proteins of the surfactant system. Eur Respir J 1994;7:372–391.

40. Rooney SA, Young SL, Mendelson CR. Molecular and cellular processing of lung surfactant. FASEB J 1994;8:957–967.

41. Mendelson CR, Alcorn JL, Gao E. The pulmonary surfactant protein genes and their regulation in fetal lung. Semin Perinatol 1993;17:223–232.

42. Oosterlaken-Dijksterhuis MA, van Eijk M, van Buel BLM, van Golde LMG, Haagsman HP. Surfactant protein composition of lamellar bodies isolated from rat lung. Biochem J 1991;274:115–119.

43. O'Reilly MA, Nogee L, Whitsett JA. Requirement of the collagenous domain for carbohydrate processing and secretion of a surfactant protein, SP-A. Biochim Biophys Acta 1988;969:176–184.

44. Pinto RA, Wright JR, Lesikar D, Benson BJ, Clements JA. Uptake of pulmonary surfactant protein C into adult rat lung lamellar bodies. J Appl Physiol 1993;74:1005–1011.

45. Walker SR, Williams MC, Benson B. Immunocytochemical localization of the major surfactant proteins in type II cells, Clara cells, and alveolar macrophages of rat lungs. J Histochem Cytochem 1986;34:1137–1148.

46. Weaver TE, Whitsett JA. Processing of hydrophobic pulmonary surfactant protein B in rat type II cells. Am J Physiol 1989;257:L100–L108.

47. Vorhout WF, Veenendaal T, Kuroki Y, Ogasawara Y, van Golde LMG, Geuze HJ. Immunocytochemical localization of surfactant protein D (SP-D) in type II cell, Clara cells, and alveolar macrophages of rat lung. J Histochem Cytochem 1992;40:1589–1597.

48. Crouch E, Rust K, Marienchek W, Parghi D, Chang D, Persson A. Developmental expression of pulmonary surfactant protein D (SP-D). Am J Respir Cell Mol Biol 1991;5:13–18.

49. Williams MC. Conversion of lamellar body membranes into tubular myelin in alveoli of fetal rat lungs. J Cell Biol 1977;72:260–277.

50. Williams MC. Ultrastructure of tubular myelin and lamellar bodies in fast-frozen rat lung. Exp Lung Res 1982;4:37–46.

51. Williams MC, Hawgood S, Hamilton RL. Changes in lipid structure produced by surfactant proteins SP-A, SP-B, and SP-C. Am J Respir Cell Mol Biol 1991;5:41–50.

52. Suzuki Y, Fujita Y, Kogishi K. Reconstitution of tubular myelin from synthetic lipids and proteins associated with pig lung surfactant. Am Rev Respir Dis 1989;140:75–81.

120   D.F. Willson et al.

53. Wright JR, Clements JA. Metabolism and turnover of lung surfactant. Am Rev Respir Dis 1987;135:426–444.

54. Jobe AH, Ikegami M. Surfactant metabolism. Clin Perinatol 1993;20:683–696.

55. Williams MC. Uptake of lectins by alveolar type II cells: subsequent deposition into lamellar bodies. Proc Natl Acad Sci USA 1984;81:6383–6387.

56. Wright JR, Wager RE, Hamilton RL, Huang M, Clements JA. Uptake of lung surfactant subfractions into lamellar bodies of adult rabbit lungs. J Appl Physiol 1986;60:817–825.

57. Wright JR, Wager RE, Hawgood S, Dobbs LG, Clements JA. Surfactant apoprotein Mr = 26,000–36,000 enhances uptake of liposomes by type II cells. J Biol Chem 1987;262:2888–2894.

58. Young SL, Wright JR, Clements JA. Cellular uptake and processing of surfactant lipids and apoprotein SP-A by rat lung. J Appl Physiol. 1989;66:1336–1342.

59. Claypool WD, Wang DL, Chandler A, Fisher AB. An ethanol/ether soluble apoprotein from rat lung surfactant augments liposomes uptake by isolated granular pneumocytes. J Clin Invest 1984;74:677–684.

60. Rice WR, Sarin VK, Fox JL, Baatz J, Wert S, Whitsett JA. Surfactant peptides stimulate uptake of phosphatidylcholine by isolated cells. Biochim Biophys Acta 1989;1006:237–245.

61. Notter RH, Finkelstein JN, Holm BA. Lung Injury: Mechanisms, Pathophysiology, and Therapy. Boca Raton, FL: Taylor & Francis; 2005:847.

62. Ashbaugh DG, Bigelow DB, Petty TL, Levine BE. Acute respiratory distress in adults. Lancet 1967;2:319–323.

63. Petty TL, Ashbaugh DG. The adult respiratory distress syndrome. Clinical features, factors influencing prognosis and principles of management. Chest 1971;60:233–239.

64. Petty T, Reiss O, Paul G, Silvers G, Elkins N. Characteristics of pulmonary surfactant in adult respiratory distress syndrome associated with trauma and shock. Am Rev Respir Dis 1977;115:531–536.

65. Wang Z, Holm BA, Matalon S, Notter RH. Surfactant activity and dysfunction in lung injury. In: Notter RH, Finkelstein JN, Holm BA, eds. Lung injury: Mechanisms, Pathophysiology, and Therapy. New York: Marcel Dekker; 2005:297–352.

66. Holm BA, Enhorning G, Notter RH. A biophysical mechanism by which plasma proteins inhibit lung surfactant activity. Chem Phys Lipids 1988;49:49–55.

67. Holm BA, Wang Z, Notter RH. Multiple mechanisms of lung surfactant inhibition. Pediatr Res 1999;46:85–93.

68. Holm BA, Notter RH. Effects of hemoglobin and cell membrane lipids on pulmonary surfactant activity. J Appl Physiol 1987;63:1434–1442.

69. Wang Z, Notter RH. Additivity of protein and non-protein inhibitors of lung surfactant activity. Am J Respir Crit Care Med 1998;158:28–35.

70. Hall SB, Lu ZR, Venkitaraman AR, Hyde RW, Notter RH. Inhibition of pulmonary surfactant by oleic acid: mechanisms and characteristics. J Appl Physiol 1992;72:1708–1716.

71. Pison U, Tam EK, Caughey GH, Hawgood S. Proteolytic inactivation of dog lung surfactant-associated proteins by neutrophil elastase. Biochim Biophys Acta 1989;992:251–257.

72. Enhorning G, Shumel B, Keicher L, Sokolowski J, Holm BA. Phospholipases introduced into the hypophase affect the surfactant film outlining a bubble. J Appl Physiol 1992;73:941–945.

73. Wang Z, Schwan AL, Lairson LL, O'Donnell JS, Byrne GF, Foye A, Holm BA, Notter RH. Surface activity of a synthetic lung surfactant containing a phospholipase-resistant phosphonolipid analog of dipalmitoyl phosphatidylcholine. Am J Physiol 2003;285:L550–L559.

74. Magoon MW, Wright JR, Baritussio A, Williams MC, Goerke J, Benson BJ, Hamilton RL, Clements JA. Subfractionation of lung surfactant: implications for metabolism and surface activity. Biochim Biophys Acta 1983;750:18–31.

75. Wright JR, Benson BJ, Williams MC, Goerke J, Clements JA. Protein composition of rabbit alveolar surfactant subfractions. Biochim Biophys Acta 1984;791:320–332.

76. Gross NJ, Narine KR. Surfactant subtypes in mice: characterization and quantitation. J Appl Physiol 1989;66:342–349.

77. Hall SB, Hyde RW, Notter RH. Changes in subphase surfactant aggregates in rabbits injured by free fatty acid. Am J Respir Crit Care Med 1994;149:1099–1106.

78. Putz G, Goerke J, Clements JA. Surface activity of rabbit pulmonary surfactant subfractions at different concentrations in a captive bubble. J Appl Physiol 1994;77:597–605.

79. Putman E, Creuwels LAJM, Van Golde LMG, Haagsman HP. Surface properties, morphology and protein composition of pulmonary surfactant subtypes. Biochem J 1996;320:599–605.

80. Veldhuizen RAW, Hearn SA, Lewis JF, Possmayer F. Surface-area cycling of different surfactant preparations: SP-A and SP-B are essential for large aggregate integrity. Biochem J 1994;300:519–524.

81. Gross NJ. Extracellular metabolism of pulmonary surfactant: the role of a new serine protease. Ann Rev Physiol 1995;57:135–150.

82. Günther A, Siebert C, Schmidt R, Ziegle S, Grimminger F, Yabut M, Temmesfeld B, Walmrath D, Morr H, Seeger W. Surfactant alterations in severe pneumonia, acute respiratory distress syndrome, and cardiogenic lung edema. Am J Respir Crit Care Med 1996;153:176–184.

83. Veldhuizen R, McCaig L, Akino T, Lewis J. Pulmonary surfactant subfractions in patients with the acute respiratory distress syndrome. Am J Respir Crit Care Med 1995;152:1867–1871.

84. Griese M. Pulmonary surfactant in health and human lung diseases: state of the art. Eur Respir J 1999;13:1455–1476.

85. Pison U, Seeger W, Buchhorn R, Joka T, Brand M, Obertacke U, Neuhof H, Schmit-Neuerberg K. Surfactant abnormalities in patients with respiratory failure after multiple trauma. Am Rev Respir Dis 1989;140:1033–1039.

86. Lewis JF, Ikegami M, Jobe AH. Altered surfactant function and metabolism in rabbits with acute lung injury. J Appl Physiol 1990;69:2303–2310.

87. Putman E, Boere AJ, van Bree L, van Golde LMG, Haagsman HP. Pulmonary surfactant subtype metabolism is altered after short-term ozone exposure. Toxicol Appl Pharmacol 1995;134:132–138.

88. Atochina EN, Beers MF, Scanlon ST, Preston AM, Beck JM. P. carinii induces selective alterations in component expression and biophysical activity of lung surfactant. Am J Physiol 2000;278:L599–L609.

89. Davidson BA, Knight PR, Wang Z, Chess PR, Holm BA, Russo TA, Hutson A, Notter RH. Surfactant alterations in acute inflammatory lung injury from aspiration of acid and gastric particulates. Am J Physiol Lung Cell Mol Physiol 2005;288:L699–708.

90. Seeger W, Pison U, Buchhorn R, Obestacke U, Joka T. Surfactant abnormalities and adult respiratory failure. Lung 1990;168(Suppl):891–902.

91. Gregory TJ, Longmore WJ, Moxley MA, Whitsett JA, Reed CR, Fowler AA, Hudson LD, Maunder RJ, Crim C, Hyers TM. Surfactant chemical composition and biophysical activity in acute respiratory distress syndrome. J Clin Invest 1991;88:1976–1981.

92. Pison U, Obertacke U, Brand M, et al. Altered pulmonary surfactant in uncomplicated and septicemia-complicated courses of acute respiratory failure. J Trauma 1990;30:19–26.

93. Hallman M, Spragg R, Harrell JH, Moser KM, Gluck L. Evidence of lung surfactant abnormality in respiratory failure. J Clin Invest 1982;70:673–683.

94. Anzueto A, Baughman RP, Guntupalli KK, Weg JG, Wiedemann HP, Raventos AA, Lemaire F, Long W, Zaccardelli DS, Pattishall EN, Exosurf ARDS Sepsis Study Group. Aerosolized surfactant in adults with sepsis-induced acute respiratory distress syndrome. N Engl J Med 1996;334:1417–1421.

95. Hall SB, Venkitaraman AR, Whitsett JA, Holm BA, Notter RH. Importance of hydrophobic apoproteins as constituents of clinical exogenous surfactants. Am Rev Respir Dis 1992;145:24–30.

96. Seeger W, Grube C, Günther A, Schmidt R. Surfactant inhibition by plasma proteins: differential sensitivity of various surfactant preparations. Eur Respir J 1993;6:971–977.

97. Hudak ML, Farrell EE, Rosenberg AA, Jung AL, Auten RL, Durand DJ, Horgan MJ, Buckwald S, Belcastro MR, Donohue PK, Carrion V, Maniscalco WM, Balsan MJ, Torres BA, Miller RR, Jansen RD, Graeber JE, Laskay KM, Matteson EJ, Egan EA, Brody AS, Martin DJ, Riddlesberger MM, Montogomery P, 21 Center Group. A multicenter randomized masked comparison of natural vs synthetic surfactant for the treatment of respiratory distress syndrome. J Pediatr 1996;128: 396–406.

98. Hudak ML, Martin DJ, Egan EA, Matteson EJ, Cummings J, Jung AL, Kimberlin LV, Auten RL, Rosenberg AA, Asselin JM, Belcastro MR, Donahue PK, Hamm CR, Jansen RD, Brody AS, Riddlesberger MM, Montgomery P, 10 Center Group. A multicenter randomized masked comparison trial of synthetic surfactant versus calf lung surfactant extract in the prevention of neonatal respiratory distress syndrome. Pediatrics 1997;100:39–50.

99. Vermont-Oxford Neonatal Network. A multicenter randomized trial comparing synthetic surfactant with modified bovine surfactant extract in the treatment of neonatal respiratory distress syndrome. Pediatrics 1996;97:1–6.

100. Horbar JD, Wright LL, Soll RF, Wright EC, Fanaroff AA, Korones SB, Shankaran S, Oh W, Fletcher BD, Bauer CR, NIH NICHHD Neonatal Research Network. A multicenter randomized trial comparing two surfactants for the treatment of neonatal respiratory distress syndrome. J Pediatr 1993;123:757–766.

101. Willson DF. Calfactant. Expert Opin Pharmacother 2001;2:1479–1493.

102. Wiseman LR, Bryson HM. Porcine-Derived Lung Surfactant. A review of the therapeutic efficacy and clinical tolerability of a natural surfactant preparation (Curosurf) in neonatal respiratory distress syndrome. Drugs 1994;48:387–400.

103. Mizuno K, Ikegami M, Chen C-M, Ueda T, Jobe AH. Surfactant protein-B supplementation improves in vivo function of a modified natural surfactant. Pediatr Res 1995;37:271–276.

104. Walther FJ, Hernandez-Juviel J, Bruni R, Waring A. Spiking Survanta with synthetic surfactant peptides improves oxygenation in surfactant-deficient rats. Am J Respir Crit Care Med 1997;156:855–861.

105. Hamvas A, Cole FS, deMello DE, Moxley M, Whitsett JA, Colten HR, Nogee LM. Surfactant protein B deficiency: antenatal diagnosis and prospective treatment with surfactant replacement. J Pediatr 1994;125:356–361.

106. Yu SH, Possmayer F. Comparative studies on the biophysical activities of the low-molecular-weight hydrophobic proteins purified from bovine pulmonary surfactant. Biochim Biophys Acta 1988;961:337–350.

107. Oosterlaken-Dijksterhuis MA, van Eijk M, van Golde LMG, Haagsman HP. Lipid mixing is mediated by the hydrophobic surfactant protein SP-B but not by SP-C. Biochim Biophys Acta 1992;1110:45–50.

108. Kobayashi T, Ganzuka M, Taniguchi J, Nitta K, Murakami S. Lung lavage and surfactant replacement for hydrochloric acid aspiration in rabbits. Acta Anaesthesiol Scand 1990;34:216–221.

109. Zucker A, Holm BA, Wood LDH, Crawford G, Ridge K, Sznajder IA. Exogenous surfactant with PEEP reduces pulmonary edema and improves lung function in canine aspiration pneumonitis. J Appl Physiol 1992;73:679–686.

110. Schlag G, Strohmaier W. Experimental aspiration trauma: comparison of steroid treatment versus exogenous natural surfactant. Exp Lung Res 1993;19:397–405.

111. Al-Mateen KB, Dailey K, Grimes MM, Gutcher GR. Improved oxygenation with exogenous surfactant administration in experimental meconium aspiration syndrome. Pediatr Pulmonol 1994;17:75–80.

112. Sun B, Curstedt T, Robertson B. Exogenous surfactant improves ventilation efficiency and alveolar expansion in rats with meconium aspiration. Am J Respir Crit Care Med 1996;154:764–770.

113. Cochrane CG, Revak SD, Merritt TA, Schraufstatter U, Hoch RC, Henderson C, Andersson S, Takamori H, Oades ZG. Bronchoalveolar lavage with KL4-surfactant in models of meconium aspiration syndrome. Pediatr Res 1998;44:705–715.

114. Sun B, Curstedt T, Song GW, Robertson B. Surfactant improves lung function and morphology in newborn rabbits with meconium aspiration. Biol Neonate 1993;63:96–104.

115. Lachmann B, Hallman M, Bergman K-C. Respiratory failure following anti-lung serum: study on mechanisms associated with surfactant system damage. Exp Lung Res 1987;12:163–180.

116. Nieman G, Gatto L, Paskanik A, Yang B, Fluck R, Picone A. Surfactant replacement in the treatment of sepsis-induced adult respiratory distress syndrome in pigs. Crit Care Med 1996;24:1025–1033.

117. Lutz C, Carney D, Finck C, Picone A, Gatto L, Paskanik A, Langenbeck E, Nieman G. Aerosolized surfactant improves pulmonary function in endotoxin-induced lung injury. Am J Respir Crit Care Med 1998;158: 840–845.

118. Lutz CJ, Picone A, Gatto LA, Paskanik A, Landas S, Nieman G. Exogenous surfactant and positive end-expiratory pressure in the treatment of endotoxin-induced lung injury. Crit Care Med 1998;26:1379–1389.

119. Tashiro K, Li W-Z, Yamada K, Matsumoto Y, Kobayashi T. Surfactant replacement reverses respiratory failure induced by intratracheal endotoxin in rats. Crit Care Med 1995;23:149–156.

120. Eijking EP, van Daal GJ, Tenbrinck R, Luyenduijk A, Sluiters JF, Hannappel E, Lachmann B. Effect of surfactant replacement on Pneumocystis carinii pneumonia in rats. Intensive Care Med 1990;17:475–478.

121. Sherman MP, Campbell LA, Merritt TA, Long WA, Gunkel JH, Curstedt T, Robertson B. Effect of different surfactants on pulmonary group B streptococcal infection in premature rabbits. J Pediatr 1994;125:939–947.

122. Berry D, Ikegami M, Jobe A. Respiratory distress and surfactant inhibition following vagotomy in rabbits. J Appl Physiol. 1986;61:1741–1748.

123. Matalon S, Holm BA, Notter RH. Mitigation of pulmonary hyperoxic injury by administration of exogenous surfactant. J Appl Physiol 1987;62:756–761.

124. Loewen GM, Holm BA, Milanowski L, Wild LM, Notter RH, Matalon S. Alveolar hyperoxic injury in rabbits receiving exogenous surfactant. J Appl Physiol 1989;66:1987–1992.

125. Engstrom PC, Holm BA, Matalon S. Surfactant replacement attenuates the increase in alveolar permeability in hyperoxia. J Appl Physiol 1989;67:688–693.

126. Matalon S, Holm BA, Loewen GM, Baker RR, Notter RH. Sublethal hyperoxic injury to the alveolar epithelium and the pulmonary surfactant system. Exp Lung Res 1988;14:1021–1033.

127. Novotny WE, Hudak BB, Matalon S, Holm BA. Hyperoxic lung injury reduces exogenous surfactant clearance in vitro. Am J Respir Crit Care Med 1995;151:1843–1847.

128. Lachmann B, Fujiwara T, Chida S, Morita T, Konishi M, Nakamura K, Maeta H. Surfactant replacement therapy in experimental adult respiratory distress syndrome (ARDS). In: Cosmi EV, Scarpelli EM, eds. Pulmonary Surfactant System. Amsterdam: Elsevier; 1983:221–235.

129. Kobayashi T, Kataoka H, Ueda T, Murakami S, Takada Y, Kobuko M. Effect of surfactant supplementation and end expiratory pressure in lung-lavaged rabbits. J Appl Physiol 1984;57:995–1001.

130. Berggren P, Lachmann B, Curstedt T, Grossmann G, Robertson B. Gas exchange and lung morphology after surfactant replacement in experimental adult respiratory distress induced by repeated lung lavage. Acta Anaesthesiol Scand 1986;30:321–328.

131. Lewis JF, Goffin J, Yue P, McCaig LA, Bjarneson D, Veldhuizen RAW. Evaluation of exogenous surfactant treatment strategies in an adult model of acute lung injury. J Appl Physiol 1996;80:1156–1164.

132. Walther F, Hernandez-Juviel J, Bruni R, Waring AJ. Protein composition of synthetic surfactant affects gas exchange in surfactant-deficient rats. Pediatr Res 1998;43:666–673.

133. Harris JD, Jackson F, Moxley MA, Longmore WJ. Effect of exogenous surfactant instillation on experimental acute lung injury. J Appl Physiol 1989;66:1846–1851.

134. Lewis JF, Ikegami M, Jobe AH. Metabolism of exogenously administered surfactant in the acutely injured lungs of adult rabbits. Am Rev Respir Dis 1992;145:19–23.

135. Lewis J, Ikegami M, Higuchi R, Jobe A, Absolom D. Nebulized vs. instilled exogenous surfactant in an adult lung injury model. J Appl Physiol 1991;71:1270–1276.

136. van Daal GJ, So KL, Gommers D, Eijking EP, Fievez RB, Sprenger MJ, van Dam DW, Lachmann B. Intratracheal surfactant administration restores gas exchange in experimental adult respiratory distress syndrome associated with viral pneumonia. Anesth Analg 1991;72:589–595.

137. van Daal GJ, Bos JAH, Eijking EP, Gommers D, Hannappel E, Lachmann B. Surfactant replacement therapy improves pulmonary mechanics in end-stage influenza A pneumonia in mice. Am Rev Respir Dis 1992;145:859–863.

138. Gunther A, Schmidt R, Harodt J, Schmehl T, et al. Bronchoscopic administration of bovine natural surfactant in ARDS and septic shock: impact on biophysical and biochemical surfactant properties. Eur Respir J 2002;10:797–804.

139. Walmrath D, Gunther A, Ghofrani HA, Schermuly R, Schnedier T, Grimminger F, Seeger W. Bronchoscopic surfactant administration in patients with severe adult respiratory distress syndrome and sepsis. Am J Respir Crit Care Med 1996;154:57–62.

140. Spragg RG, Gilliard N, Richman P, et al. Acute effects of a single dose of porcine surfactant on patients with acute respiratory distress syndrome. Chest. 1995;105:195–202.

141. Wiswell TE, Smith RM, Katz LB, Mastroianni L, Wong DY, Willms D, Heard S, Wilson M, Hite RD, Anzueto A, Revak SD, Cochrane CG. Bronchopulmonary segmental lavage with Surfaxin (KL(4)—surfactant) for acute respiratory distress syndrome. Am J Respir Crit Care Med 1999;160:1188–1195.

142. Willson DF, Jiao JH, Bauman LA, Zaritsky A, Craft H, Dockery K, Conrad D, Dalton H. Calf lung surfactant extract in acute hypoxemic respiratory failure in children. Crit Care Med 1996;24:1316–1322.

143. Willson DF, Bauman LA, Zaritsky A, Dockery K, James RL, Stat M, Conrad D, Craft H, Novotny WE, Egan EA, Dalton H. Instillation of calf lung surfactant extract (calfactant) is beneficial in pediatric acute hypoxemic respiratory failure. Crit Care Med 1999;27:188–195.

144. Willson DF, Thomas NJ, Markovitz BP, Bauman LA, DiCarlo JV, Pon S, Jacobs BR, Jefferson LS, Conaway MR, Egan EA, Pediatric Acute Lung Injury and Sepsis Investigators. Effect of exogenous surfactant (calfactant) in pediatric acute lung injury: a randomized controlled trial. JAMA 2005;293:470–476.

145. Lopez-Herce J, de Lucas N, Carrillo A, Bustinza A, Moral R. Surfactant treatment for acute respiratory distress syndrome. Arch Dis Child 1999;80:248–252.

146. Hermon MM, Golej J, Burda H, et al. Surfactant therapy in infants and children: three years experience in a pediatric intensive care unit. Shock 2002;17:247–251.

147. Herting E, Moller O, Schiffman JH, Robertson B. Surfactant improves oxygenation in infants and children with pneumonia and acute respiratory distress syndrome. Acta Paediatr 2002;91:1174–1178.

148. Auten RL, Notter RH, Kendig JW, Davis JM, Shapiro DL. Surfactant treatment of full-term newborns with respiratory failure. Pediatrics 1991;87:101–107.

149. Lotze A, Knight GR, Martin GR, Bulas DI, Hull WM, O'Donnell RM, Whitsett JA, Short BL. Improved pulmonary outcome after exogenous surfactant therapy for respiratory failure in term infants requiring extracorporeal membrane oxygenation. J Pediatr 1993;122:261–268.

150. Lotze A, Mitchell BR, Bulas DI, Zola EM, Shalwitz RA, Gunkel JH. Multicenter study of surfactant (beractant) use in the treatment of term infants with severe respiratory failure. J Pediatr 1998;132: 40–47.

151. Khammash H, Perlman M, Wojtulewicz J, Dunn M. Surfactant therapy in full-term neonates with severe respiratory failure. Pediatrics 1993;92:135–139.

152. Findlay RD, Taeusch HW, Walther FJ. Surfactant replacement therapy for meconium aspiration syndrome. Pediatrics 1996;97:48–52.

153. Luchetti M, Casiraghi G, Valsecchi R, Galassini E, Marraro G. Porcine-derived surfactant treatment of severe bronchiolitis. Acta Anaesthesiol Scand 1998;42:805–810.

154. Luchetti M, Ferrero F, Gallini C, Natale A, Pigna A, Tortorolo L, Marraro G. Multicenter, randomized, controlled study of porcine surfactant in severe respiratory syncytial virus–induced respiratory failure. Pediatr Crit Care Med 2002;3:261–268.

155. Gregory TJ, Steinberg KP, Spragg R, Gadek JE, Hyers TM, Longmere WJ, Moxley MA, Guang-Zuan CAI, Hite RD, Smith RM, Hudson LD, Crim C, Newton P, Mitchell BR, Gold AJ. Bovine surfactant therapy for patients with acute respiratory distress syndrome. Am J Respir Crit Care Med 1997;155:109–131.

156. Clark DA, Nieman GF, Thompson JE, Paskanik AM, Rokhar JE, Bredenberg CE. Surfactant displacement by meconium free fatty acids: an alternative explanation for atelectasis in meconium aspiration syndrome. J Pediatr 1987;110:765–770.

157. Moses D, Holm BA, Spitale P, Liu M, Enhorning G. Inhibition of pulmonary surfactant function by meconium. Am J Obstet Gynecol 1991;164:477–481.

158. Ivascu FA, Hirschl RB. New approaches to managing congenital diaphragmatic hernia. Semin Perinatol 2004;28:185–198.

159. Van Meurs K, The Congenital Diaphragmatic Hernia Study Group. Is surfactant therapy beneficial in the treatment of the term newborn infants with congenital diaphragmatic hernia? J Pediatr 2004;145: 312–316.

160. Spragg RG, Lewis JF, Wurst W, Hafner D, Baughman RP, Wewers MD, Marsh JJ. Treatment of acute respiratory distress syndrome with recombinant surfactant protein C surfactant. Am J Respir Crit Care Med 2003;167:1562–1566.

161. Moller JC, Schaible T, Roll C, et al. with the Surfactant ARDS Study Group. Treatment with bovine surfactant in severe acute respiratory distress syndrome in children: a randomized multicenter study. Intensive Care Med 2003;29:437–446.

162. Kendig JW, Notter RH, Cox C, Reubens LJ, Davis JM, Maniscalco WM, Sinkin RA, Bartoletti A, Dweck HS, Horgan MJ, Risemberg H, Phelps DL, Shapiro DL. A comparison of surfactant as immediate prophylaxis and as rescue therapy in newborns of less than 30 weeks gestation. N Engl J Med 1991;324:865–871.

163. Notter RH, Apostolakos M, Holm BA, Willson D, Wang Z, Finkelstein JN, Hyde RW. Surfactant therapy and its potential use with other agents in term infants, children and adults with acute lung injury. Perspect Neonatol 2000;1(4):4–20.

164. Pryhuber G, D'angio C, Finkelstein JN, Notter RH. Combination therapies for lung injury. In: Notter RH, Finkelstein JN, Holm BA, eds. Lung Injury: Mechanisms, Pathophysiology, and Therapy. Boca Raton, FL: Taylor & Francis; 2005:779–838.

11
Nitric Oxide

Emily L. Dobyns and Eva N. Grayck

Introduction

The discovery that nitric oxide (NO) is produced in living systems and participates in diverse biologic processes generated tremendous excitement in the scientific community and stimulated extensive research on NO biology. These investigations continue to provide new insight into the pathophysiology of numerous disease processes and open new opportunities for therapeutic interventions. To understand the rationale and limitations of inhaled NO and other therapies that modulate NO bioactivity in neonatal and pediatric lung diseases, it is useful to highlight the production, chemistry, and biologic functions of NO in the lung.

Nitric oxide (NO) and other higher nitrogen oxides were first identified as atmospheric pollutants long before it was recognized that NO could be produced endogenously. A pivotal study by Furchgott and Zawadzki in 1980 demonstrated that aortic endothelial cells released a factor responsible for vasorelaxation by acetylcholine [1]. Subsequently, two research groups lead by Ignarro and Moncada simultaneously determined that the endothelium-derived relaxing factor was NO, an extraordinary discovery leading to the Nobel Prize in Medicine [2,3]. In the diverse fields of immunology and neurobiology, researchers also found inducible release of NO by macrophages during inflammation and constitutive production of NO by neuronal cells [4,5]. Parallel studies in neurons, macrophages, and endothelial cells lead to the identification of three distinct isoforms of the enzyme nitric oxide synthase (NOS) that are responsible for the production of NO.

Nitric Oxide Synthase: Structure and Regulation

The three NOS isoforms, NOS I (nNOS), NOS II (iNOS), and NOS III (eNOS), which share more than 50% amino acid sequence homology, release NO during the oxygen-dependent five-electron oxidation of L-arginine to L-citrulline [6]. A mitochondrial NOS has been identified, although it is still unclear if this is a distinct isoform or, more likely, a post-translational modification of NOS I [7,8]. The structure of NOS is complex, containing a reductase domain and oxygenase domain separated by a calmodulin-binding motif [9]. The COOH-terminal reductase domain contains binding sites for nicotine adenine dinucleotide phosphate (NADPH), which serves as the source of electrons, as well as flavin mononucleotide (FMN) and flavin adenine dinucleotide (FAD), which transfer electrons to the oxygenase domain [10]. The NH_2-terminal oxygenase domain contains a cytochrome P450–like heme site and binding site for the essential cofactor tetrahydrobiopterin (BH_4). Binding of Ca^{2+}/calmodulin enables the flow of electrons from the reductase to the oxygenase domain with the resultant oxidation of L-arginine to L-citrulline and release of NO. Nitric oxide synthases I and III contain a region that destabilizes calmodulin-binding and inhibits electron transfer from FMN at low Ca^{2+} levels and accounts for the Ca^{2+} dependence of these NOS isoforms. In contrast, NOS II is less responsive to changes in intracellular Ca^{2+} because of tight calmodulin binding.

Although originally described as constitutive (NOSs 1 and III) or inducible (NOS II) and attributed to specific cell types, it is now recognized that constitutive production of NO may be further induced, NOS II may release NO constitutively, and isoforms are not confined to specific organs or cell types. The regulation of NOS expression and activity is essential for normal cellular functioning under physiologic conditions and alterations in NOS contribute to disease states. In the lung, for example, each isoform is present in multiple cell types. In the perinatal lung, NOS expression increases to prepare the high resistance fetal pulmonary circulation to release NO at birth to facilitate the transition to the low resistance adult pulmonary circulation. Decreased NOS activity and NO production can lead to persistent pulmonary hypertension of the newborn. Conversely, in septic shock, increased production of NO by NOS II leads to nitrosative stress and systemic hypotension.

The expression and activity of the NOS isoforms are regulated at the level of transcription and translation and through posttranslational modifications and protein–protein interactions. A detailed review of the regulation of the NOS isoforms is beyond the scope of this chapter, but the reader is referred to recent reviews [9–11]. A variety of stimuli can increase NOS transcription, including cytokines, estrogen, growth factors, oxidative stress, and

D.S. Wheeler et al. (eds.), The *Respiratory Tract in Pediatric Critical Illness and Injury*,
DOI 10.1007/978-1-84800-925-7_11, © Springer-Verlag London Limited 2009

glucocorticoids. These stimuli mediate their effects by increasing a variety of transcription factors that can bind to specific consensus sequences within the promoter region of the NOS genes. The three NOS genes contain binding sites for many transcription factors, including nuclear factor-κB (NFκB), activating proteins 1 and 2 (AP-1 and AP-2), a shear stress response element, and cAMP response element binding protein (CREB). In addition, regulation of mRNA stability has also been shown to modulate translation of the NOS isoforms.

Nitric oxide synthase protein activity is regulated by many factors, including substrate availability, dimerization, and post-translational modifications such as myristoylation, palmitoylation, phosphorylation, and nitrosylation. In vitro, conditions that limit substrate availability, including L-arginine or BH_4 deficiency, or compounds that uncouple the two enzymatic domains, such as the heat shock protein 90 (HSP-90) inhibitor geldanamycin, promote NADPH oxidation without NO formation, leading to release of superoxide anion [12]. This is very interesting given that superoxide can, in turn, inactivate NO bioactivity. The in vivo conditions that determine whether NOS will produce NO or superoxide are not well understood at this time. In both plasma and cells, naturally occurring L-arginine inhibitors including dimethyl arginine (ADMA) are present that decrease NO release and may contribute to NOS-dependent production of superoxide [13]. Myristoylation and palmitoylation of NOS III targets the protein to the membrane calveolae, whereas phosphorylation and nitrosylation regulate NOS III activity [12]. Post-translational modifications and inactivation of NOS III by NO contributes to the rebound pulmonary hypertensive effects that can be observed when inhaled NO therapy is discontinued.

One additional important property of NOS, which influences its localization, activity, and function, is its ability to form numerous protein–protein interactions [14]. Nitric oxide synthase can bind to activators such as calmodulin, the chaperone protein, HSP-90, as well as isoform-specific inhibitors to regulate enzyme activity. Nitric oxide synthase can also bind to scaffolding proteins such as the calveolin proteins to direct its subcellular localization. Nitric oxide synthase also interacts with G protein–coupled receptors, transporters, kinases, and GTPases, which influences both activity and function. Binding of NOS III to the arginine transporter (cationic amino acid transporter-1) may serve to transport L-arginine directly to NOS to facilitate NO production. Bradykinin triggers NOS III phosphorylation via the kinase Akt, which increases NOS activity. Interestingly, NOS III binds to both the bradykinin G protein–coupled receptor and Akt.

A unique feature of NOS I is its PDZ domain, which determines a number of specific protein interactions [10]. For example, the PDZ domain enables NOS I to bind to scaffolding proteins in skeletal muscle and directs it to the sarcolemma to influence blood flow in contracting muscle. In the brain, the PDZ domain associates NOS I to the N-methyl-D-aspartate (NMDA) receptor and links glutamate-stimulated Ca^{2+} influx with NO release. The extensive research on NOS structure, regulation, and protein–protein interactions provide further insight into the diverse signaling pathways by NO. It is important to note that NO production does not depend entirely on the activities of constitutive and inducible NOS. Other sources of NO include exogenous nitrogen oxides (NO_x), such as nitrite (NO_2^-) from food or bacterial flora, or stores of endogenous NO bound to transitional metals or existing as low-mass S-nitrosothiols (SNOs).

Nitric Oxide: Reactions and Targets

Nitric oxide is a free radical that exists in the aqueous environment as a number of NO-related molecules, such as multiple NO_x species including peroxynitrite ($OONO^-$), metal–NO complexes, and SNOs. In the gaseous state, NO reacts rapidly with oxygen to form the toxic species nitrogen dioxide, which is an important consideration when delivering NO as an inhaled gas. The reactions of NO are part of a broad redox-based signaling system that mediates diverse physiologic processes. In the vasculature, NO not only functions as a vasodilator but also has antiproliferative, antiinflammatory, antiatherogenic, and metabolic effects.

Early studies demonstrated that NO can mediate its biologic effects through cGMP-dependent signaling pathways. Nitric oxide binds to the heme in guanylate cyclase to increase cGMP and relax vascular smooth muscle. One important cGMP-dependent mechanism to regulate vascular tone is through the inactivation of the Rho A/Rho kinase pathway by protein kinase G to activate myosin light chain phosphatase, decrease phosphorylation of myosin light chain, and produce vasorelaxation [15]. Nitric oxide can also be released following activation of specific subtypes of the serotonin and endothelin G protein receptors to mediate cGMP-dependent vasodilation.

Nitric oxide can also transduce cellular signals through cGMP-independent mechanisms. One pathway is through peroxynitrite ($OONO^-$), which is formed by rapid reaction of superoxide with NO and has been characterized as a highly reactive nitrating species [16]. Peroxynitrite can inactivate proteins, and its footprint, nitrotyrosine, is detectable in multiple animal models and in human tissues in diseases associated with nitrosative stress, including acute respiratory distress syndrome (ARDS).

Another important cGMP-independent pathway for NO to mediate its biologic effects is via S-nitrosylation. The reaction of NO with thiols, or S-nitrosylation, is now recognized as an important post-translational modification that can regulate the function of numerous enzymes, transcription factors, ion channels, and receptors [17–20]. S-nitrosothiols, including S-nitrosoglutathione and S-nitrosoalbumin, form a stable reservoir of NO that can participate in transfer of NO to other protein thiols through transnitrosylation. One novel role for SNO in the circulation is the contribution of SNO-hemoglobin (Hg) in hypoxic vasodilation. SNO-Hg forms in the high oxygen environment of the lung microvasculature. When the blood reaches the peripheral tissues, the low oxygen tension induces a conformational change in Hg to enable the release of NO to promote vasodilation and facilitate oxygen delivery [21,22]. S-nitrosothiol levels are decreased in a number of disease states, including asthma, cystic fibrosis, and hypoxic lung diseases [23,24]. A role overall for an imbalance in reactive oxygen and nitrogen species has important implications for disease processes encountered in the pediatric intensive care unit.

In the intensive care setting, excessive NO production may augment hypotension and cellular injury in septic shock and systemic inflammatory conditions, whereas endothelial dysfunction and loss of endothelium-derived vascular NO may contribute to pulmonary hypertension. This chapter reviews the current therapeutic tools, including inhaled NO, pharmacologic NO donors, and phosphodiesterase inhibitors (to protect the downstream mediator cGMP), that are utilized to augment NO-mediated pulmonary vasodilation and improve right ventricular function and ventilation/perfusion matching.

Exogenous Nitric Oxide

Nitric oxide exists not only as an endogenous molecule but also as a gas that can be inhaled. The ability to deliver NO as an inhaled gas directly to ventilated regions of the lung makes NO a unique and selective pulmonary vasodilator [25,26]. When inhaled, NO diffuses from the ventilated areas of the lung, across the alveolar capillary membrane, to the smooth muscle cells of the adjacent pulmonary vessels. Once in the vascular smooth muscle cell, NO selectively binds to soluble guanylate cyclase to activate cyclic GMP, resulting in pulmonary vasodilation. The NO that diffuses into the blood stream is rapidly bound to hemoglobin and inactivated. The rapid inactivation of NO by hemoglobin limits its effects to the lung and avoids dilating systemic blood vessels. This distinguishes NO from systemic (intravenous) vasodilators that can result in systemic hypotension because these agents nonselectively dilate both the systemic and the pulmonary vasculatures. The systemic administration of vasodilators can also increase pulmonary shunt and worsen oxygenation by dilating both ventilated and nonventilated lung units. Inhaled NO has been used in a variety of diseases to improve oxygenation and lower pulmonary vascular resistance [27].

Clinical Applications of Inhaled Nitric Oxide

Persistent Pulmonary Hypertension of the Newborn

The onset of ventilation during the normal transition at birth results in a decrease in pulmonary vascular resistance and an increase in pulmonary blood flow, and the failure to make this transition results in persistent pulmonary hypertension of the newborn (PPHN). A variety of insults may result in PPHN, but common to each is the presence of extrapulmonary right-to-left shunting of blood across a patent ductus arteriosus or foramen ovale because of high pulmonary vascular resistance, leading to hypoxemia and a high morbidity and mortality. Low-dose inhaled NO was shown to cause pulmonary vasodilation and increase pulmonary blood flow in near-term fetal lambs during perinatal transition [28,29]. Roberts et al. demonstrated that 30 min of inhalation of 80 ppm NO improved oxygenation in infants with PPHN [29]. At the same time, Kinsella et al. demonstrated improved oxygenation in infants with severe PPHN treated with lower doses (6–20 ppm) of inhaled NO and that continuous inhalation of NO caused a sustained improvement in oxygenation [28]. These early studies showed that treatment with inhaled NO resulted in improved oxygenation in neonates with PPHN, but that oxygenation rapidly decreased after discontinuing NO, and that additional therapies were then needed.

Pilot studies of continuous inhalation of NO in neonates with echocardiographic evidence of high pulmonary vascular resistance with right-to-left shunting showed a sustained improvement in oxygenation without the need for additional therapies [30]. Several multicenter randomized trials, based on these early results, were conducted to determine the efficacy of inhaled NO in term neonates with PPHN [31,32]. The largest of these trials (the Neonatal Inhaled NO Study—NINOS) randomized 235 neonates to treatment with inhaled NO or placebo gas [31]. The hypothesis of this trial was that treatment with inhaled NO would decrease mortality and the need for extracorporeal membrane oxygenation (ECMO).

Infants treated with inhaled NO showed an acute improvement in oxygenation and a significant reduction in the need for ECMO compared with the placebo-treated group. There was no difference in mortality between the two groups. The toxicities associated with NO, including methemoglobinemia, high exhaled nitrogen dioxide concentrations, or intracranial hemorrhage, were rare, and study gas was not stopped in any patient because of toxicity. Based on the findings of these trials, the U.S. Food and Drug Administration approved the use of inhaled NO for the treatment of term or near-term neonates with clinical or echocardiographic evidence of PPHN.

Respiratory Distress Syndrome

The role of inhaled NO in premature newborns with hypoxemic respiratory failure is another area of investigation. As stated earlier, NO may have direct effects on lung inflammation and vascular permeability and a potential protective effect on surfactant function in addition to its effects on vascular tone and reactivity. Preliminary studies of low-dose inhaled NO in premature neonates with severe hypoxemic respiratory failure have demonstrated an improvement in oxygenation without additional adverse events. Randomized controlled trials of low-dose inhaled NO in premature neonates are currently underway.

Acute Respiratory Distress Syndrome

The role of inhaled NO in the treatment of ARDS in adults or pediatric patients is less well defined. The predominant mechanism for hypoxemia in ARDS is intrapulmonary shunting caused by lung parenchymal disease (edema, inflammation). Rossaint et al. compared intravenous infusion of prostacyclin to short-term inhalation of two doses (18 and 36 ppm) of NO in adults with severe ARDS [33]. They found that both agents decreased pulmonary artery pressure but that only inhaled NO decreased intrapulmonary shunting and resulted in an improvement in oxygenation [33]. Prostacyclin caused systemic hypotension and decreased oxygen saturation. Seven patients were then treated with continuous inhalation (3–53 days) of NO [33]. The investigators observed a sustained decrease in pulmonary pressure and improved oxygenation, and neither significant toxicities nor tachyphylaxis was seen. Subsequent multicenter placebo controlled trials of inhaled NO in adult patients with ARDS have demonstrated acute but transient improvement in oxygenation [34,35]. No difference in either mortality or days alive off of mechanical ventilation has been shown in these trials. Dellinger et al. enrolled 231 adults with ARDS; 54 were randomized to placebo, and 177 were randomized to five different concentrations (1.25, 5, 20, 40, or 80 ppm) of inhaled NO [35]. In this study, a higher percentage of patients treated with 5 ppm inhaled NO than with placebo were alive and off of mechanical ventilation at 28 days in a post hoc subgroup analysis [35]. Pediatric patients with acute hypoxemic respiratory failure treated with inhaled NO have also shown a similar transient acute improvement in oxygenation [36,37]. Because the mortality seen in ARDS is most often associated with multiorgan failure, additional studies are needed to determine whether these acute/transient improvements in oxygenation are important in the long-term management of patients with ARDS.

Pulmonary Hypertension and Right Ventricular Failure

The development of acute pulmonary hypertension with resultant right-sided heart failure and death is a significant cause of morbidity and mortality following surgical repair of congenital cardiac lesions and cardiac death [38,39]. One possible precipitating mechanism may be endothelial dysfunction resulting in decreased NO production [40]. Postoperative inhalation of NO has been shown in several small studies [41,42] to selectively reduce pulmonary vascular resistance and improve right ventricular function and stroke volume. A randomized trial of inhaled NO following congenital heart surgery demonstrated a reduction in pulmonary hypertensive crises and earlier extubation in the group treated with inhaled NO compared with the placebo group [43].

Post-Lung Transplantation

Ischemia–reperfusion is a major cause of graft failure in lung transplantation. In animal models of ischemia–reperfusion injury, inhaled NO has been shown to reduce leukocyte adhesion and distal microvascular constriction [44]. Several clinical trials have also shown a reduction in ischemia–reperfusion injury in lung transplantation [45,46]. Based on this rationale, adults undergoing lung transplantation were randomized to inhaled NO initiated 10 min after reperfusion of the lung or to placebo [47]. There was no effect on outcome of these patients following lung transplantation.

Inhaled Nitric Oxide as a Diagnostic Tool

Inhaled NO is also used as a diagnostic tool in pediatric and adult patients with pulmonary hypertension from cardiac or pulmonary etiologies. Inhaled NO is used during cardiac catheterization to measure pulmonary vasoreactivity and to assess the severity and reversibility of pulmonary hypertension [48]. A reduction in pulmonary artery pressure or pulmonary vascular resistance of 20% or more in these patients in response to vasodilating agents predicts a favorable response to oral vasodilators and an improved long-term clinical outcome [49]. The rapidity of action of inhaled NO and its lack of systemic effects have allowed inhaled NO to be used safely to assess pulmonary vasoreactivity in pediatric and adult patients with pulmonary hypertension. This contrasts with the systemic administration of vasodilators such as calcium channel blockers or prostacyclin, which can result in systemic hypotension, increased intrapulmonary right-to-left shunting, and even death during diagnostic cardiac catheterization [50]. Pulsed delivery of low-dose inhaled NO via nasal cannula has been used in the chronic treatment of pulmonary hypertension [51].

In summary, numerous clinical applications for inhaled NO exist; however, it remains to be determined whether its use will be associated with clinically important benefits in these various indications. Although long-term follow-up studies of neurodevelopment and lung function are ongoing, current data appear to favor the use of inhaled NO for neonatal patients [52,53].

Toxicities and Monitoring

Methemoglobinemia is a rare complication that occurs after exposure to high concentrations ($\geq$80 ppm) of inhaled NO. Methemoglobinemia has not been reported at doses less than 20 ppm inhaled NO. Because methemoglobin reductase deficiency may occur unpredictably, measurement of methemoglobin levels by co-oximetry 4 hr after starting inhaled NO and every 24 hr of therapy could be considered.

Formation of nitrogen dioxide from NO can occur in gas mixtures of high oxygen concentrations. Breathing concentrations of $\geq$5 ppm of nitrogen dioxide have been shown to cause diffuse inflammation and hyperreactivity. Levels of nitrogen dioxide remain low when inhaled NO is delivered within the recommended doses. Early monitoring of both nitrogen dioxide and NO were done with chemiluminescence devices. These were cumbersome and expensive. Electrochemical sensors are used now but are relatively slow and are not accurate when measurements of acute change in concentrations are needed.

Dosing and Rebound

A wide range of doses for inhaled NO have been used in both preclinical and clinical trials. All doses of inhaled NO (5, 20, or 80 ppm) studied in a randomized, controlled, dose–response trial in neonates with hypoxemic respiratory failure improved oxygenation when compared to placebo [31]. The highest dose tested, 80 ppm, was no more effective than the other doses, but it was more often associated with the adverse effects of increased methemoglobinemia and high exhaled nitrogen dioxide concentrations. Increasing the dose to 40 ppm generally does not improve oxygenation in patients who did not respond to a dose of 20 ppm inhaled NO [32]. As stated above, the inhalation of 5 ppm NO by adults with ARDS in the Dellinger et al. trial showed better outcomes in post hoc subgroup analysis than the placebo group [35]. Doses between 5 and 20 ppm NO, depending on the patient population and underlying pathophysiology, would be supported by these data.

There can be variability in the clinical response to inhaled NO. Inadequate lung inflation appears to be the most frequent etiology associated with a poor response to inhaled NO [54,55]. Improper dosing, abnormal pulmonary vascular function or structure, unsuspected anatomic cardiac disease, or myocardial dysfunction can also contribute to a lack of response to inhaled NO.

Abrupt discontinuation of inhaled NO may result in a "rebound response" that is characterized by decreases in oxygenation and elevation of pulmonary vascular resistance [56,57]. Generally, these responses are mild and respond to a brief increase in FiO$_2$. Postoperative cardiac patients with high pulmonary artery pressures at the time of NO withdrawal appear to be most at risk for developing this rebound response. The mechanisms that contribute to this *rebound response* are unclear, but the factors that may be active include the following. Exogenous (inhaled) NO may downregulate endogenous NO production by inhibiting NOS production and has also been associated with increased expression of the potent vasoconstrictor endothelin-1 [58]. Alterations in other components of the NO–cGMP pathway may decrease vascular sensitivity to NO and contribute to vasospasm after withdrawal of inhaled NO [57]. The rise in pulmonary vascular resistance and drop in oxygenation after stopping inhaled NO may represent the presence of more severe underlying pulmonary vascular disease. Several recent anecdotal reports and preclinical studies have suggested that a slower weaning of the inhaled NO dose to discontinuation, addition of a phosphodiesterase inhibitor (e.g., milrinone) at a low dose, or addition of sildenafil before inhaled NO discontinuation may prevent a clinically compromising rebound effect.

Phosphodiesterase Inhibitors

Nitric oxide activates soluble guanylate cyclase, converting guanosine triphosphate to cGMP and resulting in relaxation of the vascular smooth muscle. Hydrolysis of cGMP by cyclic nucleotide phosphodiesterases (PDEs) limits the action of cGMP [59]. The isozyme PDE-5 has a high affinity for cGMP and is the most active cGMP-hydrolyzing PDE in vascular smooth muscle. Selective inhibition of this isoform with PDE-5 inhibitors such as sildenafil and zaprinast is being used to prolong the effects of endogenous NO [60–62]. Early studies of diseases with increased pulmonary arterial pressure suggest that oral dosing of sildenafil to inhibit PDE-5 lowers pulmonary artery pressure and may be effective in a synergistic manner when combined with inhaled NO.

Although inhaled NO has been shown to be an important therapeutic tool for newborn infants with PPHN, it is unclear whether it will be beneficial in other lung diseases, particularly in those characterized by inflammation and increased NO production. New studies are investigating the potential benefit of repletion of SNOs in diseases associated with increased NO production but depletion of SNO. In a pilot study with nine adult patients with cystic fibrosis, treatment with aerosolized nitrosoglutathione acutely raised oxygen saturations [63]. In a study of seven neonates with PPHN, treatment with an S-nitrosoglutathione donor, O-nitrosoethanol, also improved oxygenation [64]. Understanding the role of NO in the pathogenesis of pediatric lung disease will lead to the optimal use of current treatment strategies and development of new therapeutic approaches to improve the outcome of these critically ill patients.

References

1. Furchgott RF, Zawadzki JV. The obligatory role of endothelial cells in the relaxation of arterial smooth muscle by acetylcholine. Nature 1980;288(5789):373–376.
2. Palmer RM, Ferrige AG, Moncada S. Nitric oxide release accounts for the biological activity of endothelium-derived relaxing factor. Nature 1987;327(6122):524–526.
3. Ignarro LJ, Buga GM, Wood KS, Byrns RE, Chaudhuri G. Endothelium-derived relaxing factor produced and released from artery and vein is nitric oxide. Proc Natl Acad Sci USA 1987;84(24):9265–9269.
4. Stuehr DJ, Gross SS, Sakuma I, Levi R, Nathan CF. Activated murine macrophages secrete a metabolite of arginine with the bioactivity of endothelium-derived relaxing factor and the chemical reactivity of nitric oxide. J Exp Med 1989;169(3):1011–1020.
5. Snyder SH. Nitric oxide: first in a new class of neurotransmitters. Science 1992;257(5069):494–496.
6. Bruckdorfer R. The basics about nitric oxide. Mol Aspects Med 2005;26(1–2):3–31.
7. Tatoyan A, Giulivi C. Purification and characterization of a nitric-oxide synthase from rat liver mitochondria. J Biol Chem 1998;273(18):11044–11048.
8. Schild L, Reinheckel T, Reiser M, Horn TF, Wolf G, Augustin W. Nitric oxide produced in rat liver mitochondria causes oxidative stress and impairment of respiration after transient hypoxia. FASEB J 2003;17(15):2194–2201.
9. Kone BC. Nitric oxide synthesis in the kidney: isoforms, biosynthesis, and functions in health. Semin Nephrol 2004;24(4):299–315.
10. Alderton WK, Cooper CE, Knowles RG. Nitric oxide synthases: structure, function and inhibition. Biochem J 2001;357(Pt 3):593–615.
11. Kone BC, Kuncewicz T, Zhang W, Yu ZY. Protein interactions with nitric oxide synthases: controlling the right time, the right place, and the right amount of nitric oxide. Am J Physiol Renal Physiol 2003;285(2):F178–F190.
12. Pritchard KA Jr, Ackerman AW, Gross ER, Stepp DW, Shi Y, Fontana JT, et al. Heat shock protein 90 mediates the balance of nitric oxide and superoxide anion from endothelial nitric-oxide synthase. J Biol Chem 2001;276(21):1762–1764.
13. Leiper J, Vallance P. Biological significance of endogenous methylarginines that inhibit nitric oxide synthases. Cardiovasc Res 1999;43(3):542–548.
14. Kone BC. Protein-protein interactions controlling nitric oxide synthases. Acta Physiol Scand 2000;168(1):27–31.
15. Fagan KA, Oka M, Bauer NR, Gebb SA, Ivy DD, Morris KG, et al. Attenuation of acute hypoxic pulmonary vasoconstriction and hypoxic pulmonary hypertension in mice by inhibition of Rho-kinase. Am J Physiol Lung Cell Mol Physiol 2004;287(4):L656–L664.
16. Greenacre SA, Ischiropoulos H. Tyrosine nitration: localisation, quantification, consequences for protein function and signal transduction. Free Radic Res 2001;34(6):541–581.
17. Hess DT, Matsumoto A, Kim SO, Marshall HE, Stamler JS. Protein S-nitrosylation: purview and parameters. Nat Rev Mol Cell Biol 2005;6(2):150–166.
18. Foster MW, McMahon TJ, Stamler JS. S-nitrosylation in health and disease. Trends Mol Med 2003;9(4):160–168.
19. Hare JM, Stamler JS. NO/redox disequilibrium in the failing heart and cardiovascular system. J Clin Invest 2005;115(3):509–517.
20. Gaston BM, Carver J, Doctor A, Palmer LA. S-nitrosylation signaling in cell biology. Mol Intervent 2003;3(5):253–263.
21. McMahon TJ, Moon RE, Luschinger BP, Carraway MS, Stone AE, Stolp BW, et al. Nitric oxide in the human respiratory cycle. Nat Med 2002;8(7):711–717.
22. Stamler JS. S-nitrosothiols in the blood: roles, amounts, and methods of analysis. Circ Res 2004;94(4):414–417.
23. Gaston B, Sears S, Woods J, Hunt J, Ponaman M, McMahon T, et al. Bronchodilator S-nitrosothiol deficiency in asthmatic respiratory failure. Lancet 1998;351(9112):1317–1319.
24. Grasemann H, Gaston B, Fang K, Paul K, Ratjen F. Decreased levels of nitrosothiols in the lower airways of patients with cystic fibrosis and normal pulmonary function. J Pediatr 1999;135(6):770–772.
25. Frostell C, Fratacci MD, Wain JC, Jones R, Zapol WM. Inhaled nitric oxide. A selective pulmonary vasodilator reversing hypoxic pulmonary vasoconstriction. Circulation 1991;83(6):2038–2047.
26. Pepke-Zaba J, Higenbottam TW, Dinh-Xuan AT, Stone D, Wallwork J. Inhaled nitric oxide as a cause of selective pulmonary vasodilatation in pulmonary hypertension. Lancet 1991;338(8776):1173–1174.
27. Ichinose F, Roberts JD Jr, Zapol WM. Inhaled nitric oxide: a selective pulmonary vasodilator: current uses and therapeutic potential. Circulation 2004;109(25):3106–3111.
28. Kinsella JP, Neish SR, Shaffer E, Abman SH. Low-dose inhalation nitric oxide in persistent pulmonary hypertension of the newborn. Lancet 1992;340(8823):819–820.
29. Roberts JD, Polaner DM, Lang P, Zapol WM. Inhaled nitric oxide in persistent pulmonary hypertension of the newborn. Lancet 1992;340(8823):818–819.
30. Kinsella JP, Neish SR, Ivy DD, Shaffer E, Abman SH. Clinical responses to prolonged treatment of persistent pulmonary hypertension of the newborn with low doses of inhaled nitric oxide. J Pediatr 1993;123(1):103–108.
31. Inhaled nitric oxide in full-term and nearly full-term infants with hypoxic respiratory failure. The Neonatal Inhaled Nitric Oxide Study Group. N Engl J Med 1997;336(9):597–604.
32. Kinsella JP, Truog WE, Walsh WF, Goldberg RN, Bancalari E, Mayock DE, et al. Randomized, multicenter trial of inhaled nitric oxide and high-frequency oscillatory ventilation in severe, persistent pulmonary hypertension of the newborn. J Pediatr 1997;131(1 Pt 1):55–62.
33. Rossaint R, Falke KJ, Lopez F, Slama K, Pison U, Zapol WM. Inhaled nitric oxide for the adult respiratory distress syndrome. N Engl J Med 1993;328(6):399–405.
34. Lundin S, Mang H, Smithies M, Stenqvist O, Frostell C. Inhalation of nitric oxide in acute lung injury: results of a European multicentre

study. The European Study Group of Inhaled Nitric Oxide. Intensive Care Med 1999;25(9):911–919.

35. Dellinger RP, Zimmerman JL, Taylor RW, Straube RC, Hauser DL, Criner GJ, et al. Effects of inhaled nitric oxide in patients with acute respiratory distress syndrome: results of a randomized phase II trial. Inhaled Nitric Oxide in ARDS Study Group. Crit Care Med 1998;26(1): 15–23.

36. Abman SH, Griebel JL, Parker DK, Schmidt JM, Swanton D, Kinsella JP. Acute effects of inhaled nitric oxide in children with severe hypoxemic respiratory failure. J Pediatr 1994;124(6):881–888.

37. Dobyns EL, Cornfield DN, Anas NG, Fortenberry JD, Tasker RC, Lynch A, et al. Multicenter randomized controlled trial of the effects of inhaled nitric oxide therapy on gas exchange in children with acute hypoxemic respiratory failure. J Pediatr 1999;134(4):406–412.

38. Ardehali A, Hughes K, Sadeghi A, Esmailian F, Marelli D, Moriguchi J, et al. Inhaled nitric oxide for pulmonary hypertension after heart transplantation. Transplantation 2001;72(4):638–641.

39. Humbert M, Sitbon O, Simonneau G. Treatment of pulmonary arterial hypertension. N Engl J Med 2004;351(14):1425–1436.

40. Celermajer DS, Cullen S, Deanfield JE. Impairment of endothelium-dependent pulmonary artery relaxation in children with congenital heart disease and abnormal pulmonary hemodynamics. Circulation 1993;87(2):440–446.

41. Roberts JD, Jr., Lang P, Bigatello LM, Vlahakes GJ, Zapol WM. Inhaled nitric oxide in congenital heart disease. Circulation 1993;87(2):447–453.

42. Goldman AP, Delius RE, Deanfield JE, Miller OI, de Leval MR, Sigston PE, et al. Pharmacological control of pulmonary blood flow with inhaled nitric oxide after the fenestrated Fontan operation. Circulation 1996;94(9 Suppl):II44–II48.

43. Miller OI, Tang SF, Keech A, Pigott NB, Beller E, Celermajer DS. Inhaled nitric oxide and prevention of pulmonary hypertension after congenital heart surgery: a randomised double-blind study. Lancet 2000; 356(9240):1464–1469.

44. Fox-Robichaud A, Payne D, Hasan SU, Ostrovsky L, Fairhead T, Reinhardt P, et al. Inhaled NO as a viable antiadhesive therapy for ischemia/reperfusion injury of distal microvascular beds. J Clin Invest 1998;101(11):2497–2505.

45. Date H, Triantafillou AN, Trulock EP, Pohl MS, Cooper JD, Patterson GA. Inhaled nitric oxide reduces human lung allograft dysfunction. J Thorac Cardiovasc Surg 1996;111(5):913–919.

46. Ardehali A, Laks H, Levine M, Shpiner R, Ross D, Watson LD, et al. A prospective trial of inhaled nitric oxide in clinical lung transplantation. Transplantation 2001;72(1):112–115.

47. Meade MO, Granton JT, Matte-Martyn A, McRae K, Weaver B, Cripps P, et al. A randomized trial of inhaled nitric oxide to prevent ischemia-reperfusion injury after lung transplantation. Am J Respir Crit Care Med 2003;167(11):1483–1489.

48. Ricciardi MJ, Knight BP, Martinez FJ, Rubenfire M. Inhaled nitric oxide in primary pulmonary hypertension: a safe and effective agent for predicting response to nifedipine. J Am Coll Cardiol 1998;32(4):1068–1073.

49. Balzer DT, Kort HW, Day RW, Corneli HM, Kovalchin JP, Cannon BC, et al. Inhaled nitric oxide as a preoperative test (INOP Test I): the INOP Test Study Group. Circulation 2002;106(12 Suppl 1):I76–I81.

50. Sitbon O, Humbert M, Jagot JL, Taravella O, Fartoukh M, Parent F, et al. Inhaled nitric oxide as a screening agent for safely identifying responders to oral calcium-channel blockers in primary pulmonary hypertension. Eur Respir J 1998;12(2):265–270.

51. Ivy DD, Parker D, Doran A, Kinsella JP, Abman SH. Acute hemodynamic effects and home therapy using a novel pulsed nasal nitric oxide delivery system in children and young adults with pulmonary hypertension. Am J Cardiol 2003;92(7):886–890.

52. Dobyns EL, Griebel J, Kinsella JP, Abman SH, Accurso FJ. Infant lung function after inhaled nitric oxide therapy for persistent pulmonary hypertension of the newborn. Pediatr Pulmonol 1999;28(1): 24–30.

53. Rosenberg AA, Kennaugh JM, Moreland SG, Fashaw LM, Hale KA, Torielli FM, et al. Longitudinal follow-up of a cohort of newborn infants treated with inhaled nitric oxide for persistent pulmonary hypertension. J Pediatr 1997;131(1 Pt 1):70–75.

54. Dobyns EL, Anas NG, Fortenberry JD, Deshpande J, Cornfield DN, Tasker RC, et al. Interactive effects of high-frequency oscillatory ventilation and inhaled nitric oxide in acute hypoxemic respiratory failure in pediatrics. Crit Care Med 2002;30(11):2425–2429.

55. Kinsella JP, Abman SH. High-frequency oscillatory ventilation augments the response to inhaled nitric oxide in persistent pulmonary hypertension of the newborn: Nitric Oxide Study Group. Chest 1998; 114(1 Suppl):100S.

56. Davidson D, Barefield ES, Kattwinkel J, Dudell G, Damask M, Straube R, et al. Safety of withdrawing inhaled nitric oxide therapy in persistent pulmonary hypertension of the newborn. Pediatrics 1999;104 (2 Pt 1):231–236.

57. Ivy DD, Kinsella JP, Ziegler JW, Abman SH. Dipyridamole attenuates rebound pulmonary hypertension after inhaled nitric oxide withdrawal in postoperative congenital heart disease. J Thorac Cardiovasc Surg 1998;115(4):875–882.

58. Oka M, Ohnishi M, Takahashi H, Soma S, Hasunuma K, Sato K, et al. Altered vasoreactivity in lungs isolated from rats exposed to nitric oxide gas. Am J Physiol 1996;271(3 Pt 1):L419–L424.

59. Reffelmann T, Kloner RA. Therapeutic potential of phosphodiesterase 5 inhibition for cardiovascular disease. Circulation 2003;108(2):239–244.

60. Ghofrani HA, Wiedemann R, Rose F, Schermuly RT, Olschewski H, Weissmann N, et al. Sildenafil for treatment of lung fibrosis and pulmonary hypertension: a randomised controlled trial. Lancet 2002; 360(9337):895–900.

61. Michelakis E, Tymchak W, Lien D, Webster L, Hashimoto K, Archer S. Oral sildenafil is an effective and specific pulmonary vasodilator in patients with pulmonary arterial hypertension: comparison with inhaled nitric oxide. Circulation 2002;105(20):2398–2403.

62. Prasad S, Wilkinson J, Gatzoulis MA. Sildenafil in primary pulmonary hypertension. N Engl J Med 2000;343(18):1342.

63. Synder AH, McPherson ME, Hunt JF, Johnson M, Stanker JS, Gaston B. Acute effects of aerosolized S-nitrosogluathione in cystic fibrosis. Am J Respir Crit Care Med 2002:165(7):922–926.

64. Moya MP, Gow AJ, Califf RM, Goldberg RN, Stamler JS. Inhaled ethyl nitrite gas for persistent pulmonary hypertension of the newborn. Lancet 2002:360(9327):141–143.

12
Extracorporeal Life Support for Children with Acute Respiratory Failure

Heidi J. Dalton and Angela T. Wratney

Introduction

Extracorporeal life support has been used for over 30 years for more than 30,000 infants, children, and adults. This chapter focuses on the use of extracorporeal membrane oxygenation (ECMO), or extracorporeal life support (ECLS), as it is also known, for children predominately with acute respiratory failure. The overall survival rate for patients is shown in Table 12.1. Neonates with severe respiratory failure have historically been the predominate recipients of ECMO support. Most of these infants suffer from a combination of pulmonary parenchymal and vascular dysfunction that leads to impaired gas exchange [1].

As alternative support methods, such as high-frequency oscillatory ventilation, surfactant, and inhaled nitric oxide, have been developed and become accepted for the neonatal population, the need for ECMO support has declined [2]. Annual neonatal ECMO cases now number around 800 per year, down from the peak of 1,500 cases in the early 1990s. Survival has also decreased in the neonatal population over the past few years. This is speculated to be related to delays in institution of ECMO while other, less-invasive therapies are attempted. Infants who fail all other therapies and require ECMO may thus be sicker than in years past when ECMO was the only "rescue" therapy available. Although this explanation seems logical, in an evaluation of the Extracorporeal Life Support Organization (ELSO) registry data, there was no difference in outcomes among infants who received treatment with inhaled nitric oxide, with high-frequency ventilation, or with both prior to ECMO and those who did not [3]. Similarly, there were no statistical differences in measures of respiratory severity, such as alveolar-arterial oxygen gradient (AaDO$_2$) or oxygenation index

(OI), in the past few years. An alternative explanation is that use of ECMO has expanded from neonates with only respiratory failure to include neonates with a variety of comorbidities that may also influence survival

Approximately 200 to 300 non-neonatal pediatric patients receive ECMO each year for severe respiratory failure, with an overall survival rate of 53% (Table 12.2) [4]. Most patients suffer from severe hypoxia, hypercapnia, or intractable air leaks. Pulmonary dysfunction resulting from bacterial or viral pneumonia, aspiration syndromes, intrapulmonary hemorrhage, acute respiratory distress syndrome, and other poorly defined disorders have been successfully treated with ECMO. The uncertainties accompanying the use of ECMO for neonates, who compose a homogeneous group relative to other age groups, are compounded for older children. The enormously heterogeneous older pediatric population spans nearly two decades of physiologic development, and cardiorespiratory failure develops from a multitude of disorders. Furthermore, many patients have varying degrees of multiple-organ failure along with respiratory failure at the time ECMO is instituted. Resolution of both lung disease and secondary organ dysfunction must occur to achieve survival. These factors result in lower survival rates for older patients treated with ECMO than that achieved with the neonatal patient population [5].

Despite attempts to define predictive models that identify optimal candidates for the institution of ECMO, none have proved universally applicable. The clinician still most often relies on clinical judgment at the bedside as to when conventional medical therapy has failed. Perhaps the largest change in non-neonatal ECMO in the past few years is the variety of patients to whom it has been applied. Patients with recent trauma, tracheal injury requiring reconstruction, burns, smoke inhalation, severe sepsis, compromised immune systems, and toxic ingestions with cardiopulmonary collapse are but a few of the types of patients who may have been excluded from ECMO support in the past but have now been successfully supported with ECMO therapy [6–9]. The multiple exclusion criteria used in the early days of ECMO have now been fairly well eliminated, and potential patients are often considered on a case-by-case basis. Even patients with known bleeding disorders such as hemophilia have received ECMO support [10].

Perhaps one group for whom ECMO is still cautiously avoided or rarely applied is patients with malignancy and transplanted bone marrow. The continued high mortality rate for these patients when respiratory failure develops, however, has recently caused several

D.S. Wheeler et al. (eds.), The *Respiratory Tract in Pediatric Critical Illness and Injury*,
DOI 10.1007/978-1-84800-925-7_12, © Springer-Verlag London Limited 2009

TABLE 12.1. Total numbers of extracorporeal life support patients.

Group	Total cases	Survive to DC or transfer	
Neonatal			
Respiratory	19,463	14,942	77%
Cardiac	2,344	896	38%
ECPR	174	72	41%
Pediatric			
Respiratory	2,883	1,608	56%
Cardiac	3,059	1,312	43%
ECPR	322	124	39%
Adult			
Respiratory	1,025	542	53%
Cardiac	499	159	32%
ECPR	139	51	37%
Total	29,908	19,706	66%

Note: ECPR, extracorporeal cardiopulmonary resuscitation; DC, discharge.
Source: Adapted with permission from ELSO International Summary, January 2005.

clinicians to advocate application of ECMO at an early time in disease for such patients to see if outcome can be improved. A recent review of the use of ECMO in 30 cancer patients from 58 centers noted an overall survival rate of 37%. Of seven patients who underwent bone marrow transplantation and received ECMO, two (29%) patients survived [11].

In addition to respiratory support, ECMO can readily be combined with hemofiltration to augment renal function, provide stable hemodynamics to allow use of plasmapheresis or plasma exchange, allow use of hepatic support devices, or be coupled with a variety of these adjunct therapies. As a consequence, ECMO may benefit patients with established multiorgan dysfunction. Implementation of ECMO during multiple-organ dysfunction syndrome (MODS) now occurs under a variety of conditions, with resolution of organ dysfunction and good outcome for some patients [12]. Furthermore, because it avoids the circulatory derangements that often result from extreme forms of mechanical ventilation and provides systemic perfusion without the need for high doses of inotropic agents, ECMO may also prevent damage to other systems.

A smaller number of adult patients have also received ECMO support (Table 12.3). Several attempts at randomized trials of ECMO use for adults did not show benefit of ECMO, and this has precluded the consideration of ECMO for adults in many clinicians' eyes [13]. All these studies, however, had design and procedural flaws that may have affected results. Multiple case reports and

TABLE 12.2. Extracorporeal life support for pediatric respiratory failure.

Primary diagnosis	Total No.	No. surviving	% Surviving
Bacterial pneumonia	309	171	55
Viral pneumonia	747	471	63
Aspiration pneumonia	170	111	65
ARDS	358	193	54
ARF, non-ARDS	608	288	47
Other	720	386	54
Total	2,912	1,720	59

Note: ARF, acute respiratory failure; ARDS, acute respiratory distress syndrome.
Source: Adapted with permission from ELSO International Summary, January 2005.

TABLE 12.3. Extracorporeal life support for adult respiratory failure.

Primary diagnosis	No. cases	No. surviving	% Surviving
Bacterial pneumonia	191	100	52
Viral pneumonia	88	55	63
Aspiration pneumonia	32	18	56
ARDS, postop/trauma	136	70	51
ARDS, not postop/trauma	200	101	51
ARF, non-ARDS	59	37	63
Other	352	172	49
Total	1,058	553	52

Note: ARF, acute respiratory failure; ARDS, acute respiratory distress syndrome.
Source: Adapted with permission from ELSO International Summary, January 2005.

series of successful use of ECMO for adults exist [14,15]. In a recent report of ECMO for 255 adults with severe respiratory failure, 68% of patients were weaned off ECMO support and 53% survived to discharge. Multivariate analysis noted that age, gender, pH < 7.10, pre-ECMO ventilator days, and pre-ECMO PaO_2/FiO_2 ratio were associated with outcome [16]. Other reports of the successful use of ECMO for adult patients with burns, trauma, myocardial infarct with arrest, and a variety of other disease processes exist in the literature. The large size of adult patients makes them ideal for venovenous ECMO support, which may be important for older patients. The need to use the carotid artery for ECMO support in older patients has been another reason why clinicians have avoided ECMO in this age group. Recent advances in ECMO technology and a newly funded study by the NIH to develop large double-lumen single cannulae that can be used in adult-sized patients may make ECMO a more attractive and accepted modality for this population. The lack of adult ECMO centers and poor awareness of the technique and potential benefits among adult clinicians are major obstacles to acceptance of ECMO for adults. Currently, many pediatric ECMO centers (including the authors') are opening their ECMO programs to adults and trying to teach adult caregivers about the potential benefits of ECMO for selected patients. Alternative support techniques such as the implantable artificial lung are also close to clinical application and may also provide rescue modalities for adults in respiratory failure [17–19].

Methods of Support

Several modes of ECLS have been developed that differ according to cannulation site and minor physiologic principles. However, the basic circuit is similar for all modes (Figure 12.1). Blood is drained from the body via venous access, circulated through tubing to a membrane oxygenator by either a roller head or a centrifugal pump, and returned to the body. More specific details regarding cannulation, circuit design, and types of pumping devices are provided elsewhere (1,2,4,5).

Patient Selection

Various mortality prediction criteria have been put forth as indicators of when ECMO rescue is best applied, although many of these criteria have been derived from small series of historical data for respiratory failure patients or extrapolated from neonatal

FIGURE 12.1. Common components of an extracorporeal membrane oxygenation circuit.

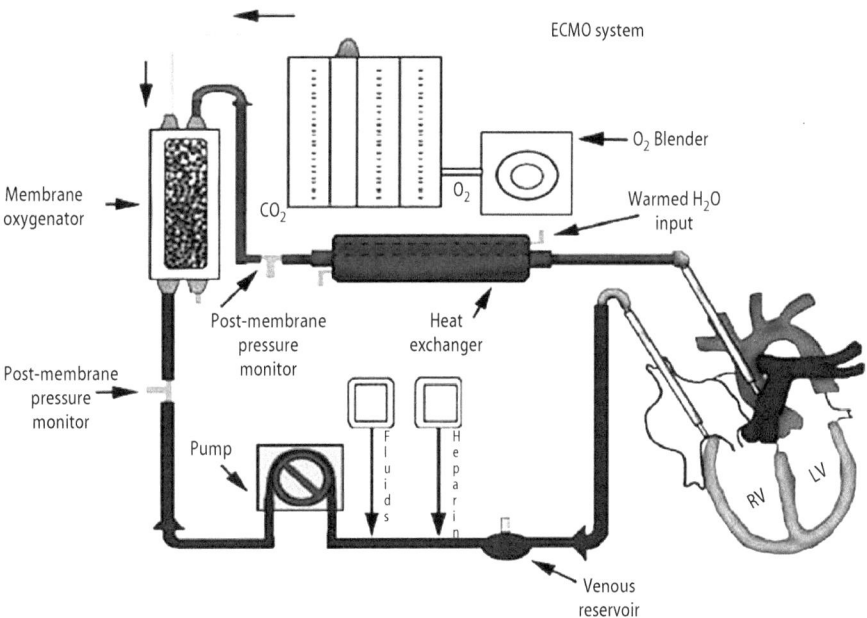

respiratory failure data [20–24]. Attempts to provide universally accepted criteria for institution of ECMO have proved difficult. The predominant listed criterion for placing a pediatric patient on ECMO remains *failure to respond*. Over 50% of pediatric ECMO patients reported to the ELSO registry have *failure to respond* as the major criterion for initiation of ECMO. Although no strict definition of what *failure to respond* entails exists, the basic premise may be interpreted as the clinician caring for the patient determining that current support is insufficient and death is imminent without ECMO rescue. The majority of patients who are placed on ECMO have failed less invasive methods of respiratory support. Such methods of support often include conventional mechanical ventilation in pressure-controlled or pressure-regulated volume control (PRVC) modes, high positive end-expiratory pressure (PEEP), high-frequency oscillatory ventilation (HFOV), surfactant, and/or inhaled nitric oxide (iNO). An evaluation of the ELSO registry noted that for pediatric patients who received ECMO, use of both iNO and HFOV before ECMO was associated with poorer outcome than for patients who received neither or only one of these modalities before ECMO [25], although it is unknown whether this simply reflects disease severity.

There has been concern that respiratory severity indices reported in the past are not applicable to today's respiratory failure patients, although there are few recent reports comparing past severity indices to outcome in the current era. One recent report examined the current utility of respiratory severity indices used in the past for potential ECMO eligibility for 118 children with acute hypoxemic respiratory failure [25]. Indices examined included the $AaDO_2$, OI, PaO_2/FiO_2, ventilation index (VI), mean airway pressure (Paw), as well as individual ventilator settings and arterial blood gas values. When risk of mortality predictions based on respiratory severity indices were compared to the observed mortality of the 118 children, survival was much better than would have been predicted based on historical data [26]. As an example, in the past, an OI > 40 had been associated with > 80% risk of death. Although only 15 patients reached an OI > 40 in this study, the positive predictive risk of mortality in these patients was only 40%, signifi-

cantly lower than predicted by past reports. An $AaDO_2$ > 450 for 24 hr, Paw > 23, or $AaDO_2$ > 420 had positive predictive value for mortality of 32%–40%. Using logistic regression, no respiratory parameter ($AaDO_2$, OI, Paw, ventilator settings, or blood gas values) was independently correlated with death. All deaths were associated with multiorgan system failure, coincident pathology, or perceived treatment futility leading to limitation or withdrawal of care. The overall mortality rate for these 118 children was 22%, with no previously healthy child expiring from respiratory failure. Nonconventional therapies applied included high-frequency ventilation in 25/119 (21%, survival 64%), surfactant administration in 15/119 (13%, survival 73%), iNO in 38/119 (32%, survival 69%), and ECMO in 4/119 (3%, survival 75%) of patients. In contrast, a more recent prospective clinical study of 131 pediatric patients, age range 1 month to 18 years, with acute hypoxemic respiratory failure found the OI measured during any time point during mechanical ventilation to be an independent predictor of mortality [27]. No threshold value of OI, however, was identified that could accurately predict mortality. As a result, precise criteria for initiating ECMO support for any single patient do not exist, leaving the decision up to the clinical team caring for any given patient.

Gas Exchange and Oxygen Delivery

Oxygenation

The difference between the partial pressure of oxygen (PO_2) in the gas supplied to the oxygenator and that in the patient's systemic venous blood provides the "driving pressure" across the membrane lung. As an example, 30% oxygen blended into the gas entering the oxygenator will result in an estimated PAO_2 of 228 torr at sea level. The PO_2 of venous blood entering the oxygenator depends on the difference between oxygen delivery and consumption in the patient but is usually about 40 torr. The driving pressure for oxygen diffusion into the blood would thus be approximately 188 torr (228 torr − 40 torr = 188 torr), which is usually adequate to achieve 100%

saturation of hemoglobin. Higher oxygen concentrations in the gas phase may be necessary to compensate for loss of membrane surface area over time to maintain hemoglobin saturation. Once the oxy-hemoglobin saturation exceeds 95%, higher oxygen concentration in the sweep gas results in a higher PO_2 in postoxygenator blood without a significant increment in overall oxygen content. For this reason, oxygen concentration in sweep gas is usually adjusted to maintain an oxygen saturation of approximately 95% in postoxygenator blood.

Carbon Dioxide Exchange (Ventilation)

The pressure gradient for carbon dioxide between blood and gas is less than that for oxygen. The partial pressure of carbon dioxide in the body is usually low (the venous partial pressure of carbon dioxide, $PvCO_2$, is 45–55 torr) so that the pressure difference between the blood and gas phase in the oxygenator is much less than with oxygen. Despite the small pressure difference, the membrane's high diffusion coefficient for carbon dioxide (at least six times that for oxygen) allows excellent carbon dioxide removal, even at low flow rates. To eliminate more carbon dioxide, the gas flow in the membrane must be increased, much as alveolar ventilation must increase to eliminate carbon dioxide from the body under physiologic conditions. Carbon dioxide removal is also limited by the surface area across which gas exchange can occur. Thus, increased carbon dioxide clearance may be obtained by using larger oxygenators or using more than one oxygenator in parallel in the circuit. Conversely, to prevent excessive carbon dioxide removal and hypocapnia in small infants and neonates, carbon dioxide may be blended into the gas mixture to further reduce the partial pressure difference between blood and gas and maintain normocarbia.

Oxygen Delivery

During venoarterial ECMO, both increasing oxygen delivery and increasing the patient's PaO_2 and arterial saturation can be accomplished by increasing the ECMO flow rate. This diverts more of the systemic venous return into the ECMO circuit for oxygenation while at the same time proportionally decreasing the amount of venous blood that enters the diseased pulmonary circuit. The result of increasing ECMO flow, then, will be an increase in oxygen delivery provided by the circuit and an elevation in measured systemic arterial saturation and PaO_2. Another means to change the proportion of native blood flow to that from the ECMO circuit is to decrease the overall blood volume in the patient. During cardiopulmonary bypass, filling pressures and overall blood volume can be adjusted by removal of blood volume into the bypass circuit. Circulating volume is also frequently decreased by modified ultra-filtration. During ECMO, these same principles can be followed: excessively high filling pressures can be lowered by simple removal of blood volume from the circuit, and diuretics and renal replacement strategies can be used to control fluid balance. Care must be taken, however, to avoid decreasing circulating volume excessively, as this may in turn cause tissue hypoperfusion or an increase in oxygen extraction.

Systemic oxygen delivery is defined as the product of cardiac output and arterial oxygen content [28]. By altering the amount of cardiac output diverted from the patient to the ECMO circuit, venoarterial ECMO can be viewed as either *complete* or *partial*. In the patient on *complete* venoarterial ECMO, the cardiopulmonary circuit is almost totally bypassed, and oxygen delivery is determined by the product of pump flow and the oxygen content of blood leaving the oxygenator. Most centers use partial venoarterial ECMO because adequate systemic oxygenation can be achieved by diverting less than 100% of cardiac output to the ECMO circuit. Studies have suggested that complete bypass of the pulmonary circuit may lead to pulmonary alkalosis or ischemia and cause direct damage of the pulmonary capillary bed [29]. Furthermore, microsphere studies have shown that the majority of coronary artery perfusion comes from native left heart ejection during ECMO, which is another important reason to avoid total bypass [30]. Monitoring of adequate oxygen delivery is aided by following venous saturation [31]. Most ECMO circuits contain a sensor along the venous return line that continuously measures and displays venous saturation. Other centers use an indwelling blood gas monitor for the same purpose. Low venous saturation and other markers such as elevated lactate, poor perfusion, decreased urine output, and mental status changes may indicate need for improved oxygen delivery. If ECMO flow cannot be increased to provide adequate support, an additional drainage cannula to improve ECMO flow may be needed.

For patients cannulated via the venovenous route, reduced systemic oxygenation caused by either less bypass obtained in this mode or the effect of recirculation may be observed compared with patients supported with venoarterial ECMO. Recirculation is the phenomenon where too proximal a juxtaposition between the venous drainage lumen and the oxygenated blood return lumen results in blood being recirculated through the cannulae and circuit and not delivered to the patient (Figure 12.2). This can result in an artificially high venous saturation while other markers of inadequate oxygen delivery (elevated lactate, poor perfusion, decreased urine output) are present. Persistent signs of inadequate oxygen delivery or continued hemodynamic instability with venovenous ECMO may require conversion to venoarterial ECMO. Patients with venovenous ECMO support or who have a left atrial communication to the ECMO circuit may have artificially high measured venous saturations due to mixing of well-oxygenated blood with systemic venous return. Following venous saturations from another site in the body may be helpful to monitor adequacy of support in this circumstance.

One novel means to improve oxygenation to the head and upper body in patients cannulated through bilateral femoral veins is to add an additional venous cannula via the right internal jugular vein to the right atrium. Connecting this cannula into the inflow return side of the ECMO circuit will thus increase the amount of oxygenated bypass directly returning to the right heart. This may improve overall oxygen delivery to the patient while still avoiding the need for arterial vessel cannulation.

Loose occlusion of the roller heads against the raceway tubing can also lead to less blood being propelled forward through the ECMO circuit and reduce systemic oxygen delivery. Although this is an uncommon problem, failure to recognize it can be harmful to the patient. Finally, persistent vasodilation, which can occur with sepsis, may require the administration of low levels of vasoconstricting agents to maintain adequate central venous pressures and adequate pump return without massive fluid administration.

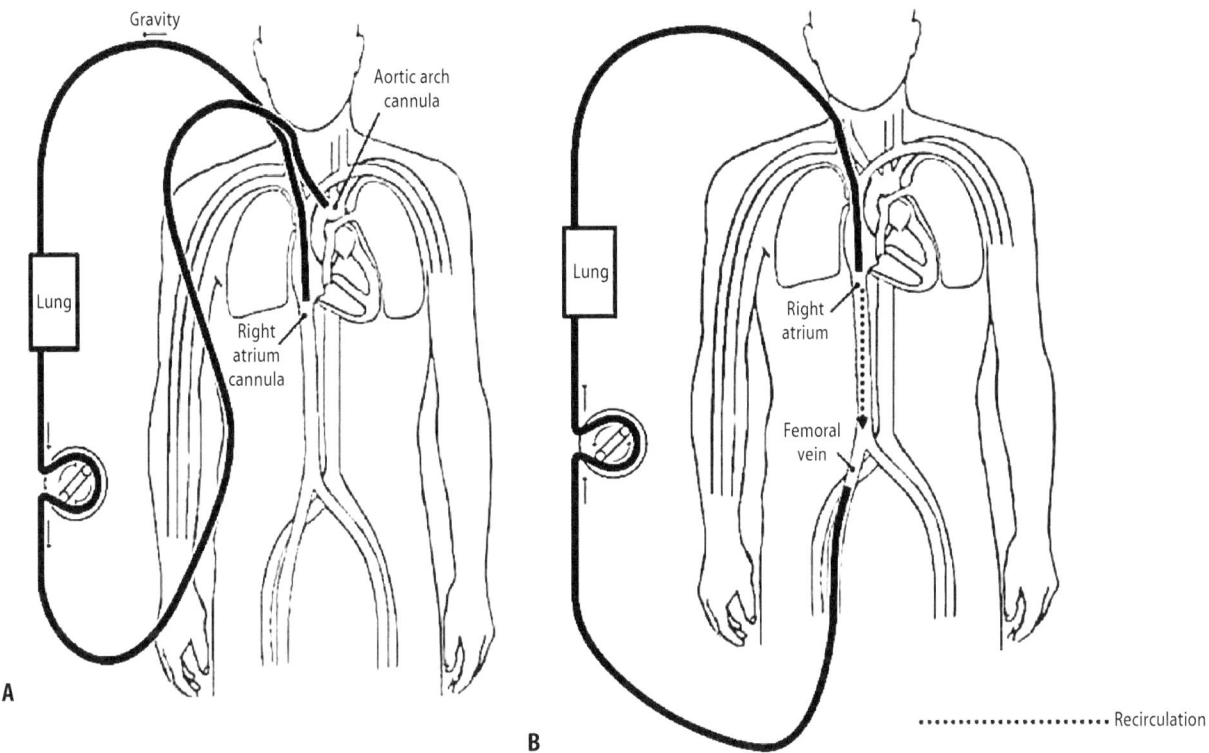

Figure 12.2. Schema of venoarterial (**A**) versus venovenous (**B**) support.

Patient Management

Screening

Infants who are candidates for ECMO undergo routine cranial ultrasonography to identify existing intracranial hemorrhage [32,33]. The presence of hemorrhage greater than that confined to the germinal matrix (grade I) is a contraindication to ECMO because heparinization may cause additional bleeding. Older patients may also have evaluation of intracranial bleeding by ultrasound if an open fontanelle is present. Computed tomography can be useful if the patient is stable enough to undergo such an examination. Frequently, however, older patients are not stable enough to undergo computed tomography, and clinical neurologic evaluation may be hampered by sedation or neuromuscular blockade before ECMO. The decision to place a patient on ECMO is thus made on best assessment of neurologic function. For infants, echocardiography is usually performed before ECMO to determine if hypoxia is caused by structural defects in the heart that may be better served by surgical repair than by ECMO support. Echocardiography is also used to detect the presence and direction of central shunts and to assess myocardial function [34,35].

Cannulation and Initiation of Extracorporeal Life Support

A guideline for selection of cannula size and circuit components based on patient weight is shown in Table 12.4A (cardiac patients) and Table 12.4B (respiratory failure patients). Cannulation is usually performed at the bedside, with the patient receiving a combination of local anesthetics and intravenous analgesics, sedatives, and neuromuscular blocking drugs. An initial bolus of heparin (usually 50–200 units/kg) and continued heparin infusion ensures systemic anticoagulation for the duration of ECMO. Activated clotting time (ACT) is measured at the bedside and provides a gauge for adjusting the heparin dose to avoid either catastrophic clotting in the circuit or bleeding complications [36]. The ECMO flow is initially begun at 50 mL/kg/min and increased in 50–100 mL/kg/min increments. For infants, a rate of 100–200 mL/kg/min usually provides adequate perfusion and oxygenation, although patients in a state of high cardiac output, such as sepsis, may require more. Some centers use high-flow ECMO in patients cannulated with single ventricle physiology, especially those patients with a systemic-to-pulmonary artery shunt, to provide adequate circulation for both systemic and pulmonary organs [37]. Pediatric patients usually require about 90 mL/kg/min of flow to maintain adequate oxygen delivery, and adult patients require rates of 70 mL/kg/min. Estimates of flow needs can also be predicted by using cardiac index data based on body surface area. One caution in estimating ECMO flow in this manner is that patients with sepsis or MODS may require flow rates that are much higher than that predicted. These factors must be taken into account when selecting cannula size, as larger cannulas than predicted by body surface area may be required. In venoarterial ECMO, the arterial waveform provides a rough estimation of the degree of bypass provided by the ECMO circuit. Because ECMO flow is nonpulsatile, increasing flow and decreasing left ventricular output will result in a flattening of the arterial wave contour. Severe myocardial dysfunction may also cause a flattened wave contour. This effect must be kept in mind when waveform contour is used to monitor the extent of bypass.

TABLE 12.4A. Sample components for cardiac extracorporeal life support based on patient weight.

	Weight (kg)					
	2.5–6	6–12	12–25	25–40	40–70	70+
Tubing pack	$\frac{1}{4}''$	$\frac{1}{4}''$	$\frac{3}{8}''$	$\frac{3}{8}''$	$\frac{1}{2}''$	$\frac{1}{2}''$
Raceway	$\frac{1}{4}''\ \frac{3}{8}''$	$\frac{3}{8}''$	$\frac{3}{8}''\ \frac{1}{2}''$	$\frac{1}{2}''$	$\frac{1}{2}''$	$\frac{1}{2}''$
Oxygenator model	0800	1500	I-2500	I-3500	I-4500	I-4500 × 2
Venous cannula (French)	10–15	14–19	17–19	19–21	19–23	19–29
Chest venous cannula (French)	16	20	22	24–28	28–32	32–36
Arterial cannula (French)	8–12	12–15	14–17	17–21	17–21	19–23
Blood prime(units of PRBCs)*	1	1–2	2–3	3–4	4	4–5

Note: These are guidelines only. Individual variables must be considered! Estimates are for a roller head pump with silicone membrane oxygenator. All cannula references are for Biomedicus. PRBCs, packed red blood cells.
*Consider adding albumin 25% 200 cc after crystalloid priming. Also may add fresh-frozen plasma 50 cc/unit PRBCs
Source: Data provided by University of Michigan, Ann Arbor, MI, and Children's National Medical Center, Washington, DC.

Priming

Priming of the ECMO circuit before initiation is accomplished with a crystalloid solution that is then replaced with blood. Because required blood usually has been citrated and stored, it may be calcium depleted, have a high potassium level, and possess a low pH. Addition of calcium (usually as calcium chloride), bicarbonate, or THAM (tromethamine) and heparin is performed during the priming procedure. Electrolytes should be measured in the priming blood before bypass is begun, as disturbances of cardiac rhythm or frank cardiac arrest can occur on initiation of ECMO [38]. Hyperkalemia exists almost universally in the ECMO primed circuit despite buffering by calcium and bicarbonate. The potassium level rarely causes systemic effects once the ECMO prime is diluted with the patient's intrinsic blood volume. As an example, if a neonatal patient with a blood volume similar to that of the ECMO circuit has a potassium level of 3 and the ECMO prime has a potassium level of 7, the circulating potassium level may be around 5 on ECMO initiation. This is unlikely to cause systemic or cardiac effects. Larger patients with blood volumes proportionally much less than that of the ECMO circuit will have less risk of hyperkalemia or hypocalcemia. Use of the freshest blood available may also lessen the degree of hyperkalemia in the primed circuit. Rarely, hyperkalemia may be of such concern that blood must be washed before ECMO use or the primed ECMO circuit cannot be used until the potassium level is reduced. In this circumstance, replacement of blood in the circuit with fresh-frozen plasma or albumin can be done to lower the circulating potassium concentration in the prime.

Patient Management

Hypovolemia causes low central venous pressures and results in decreased venous return to the circuit. This can be easily corrected with fluid administration. Increased oxygen delivery also can be accomplished by increasing the pump flow rate, which increases blood diverted into the ECMO circuit for oxygenation. Anemia can be corrected with transfusion of blood products. Maintenance of hematocrit at 30%–33% is usually sufficient to sustain adequate oxygen content [39,40]. Intermittent administration of packed red blood cells to maintain adequate blood volume and hematocrit will be required [41–43]. Fresh-frozen plasma may also be given intermittently to provide adequate clotting factors and help prevent excessive bleeding [44]. Platelet sequestration in the ECMO circuit is a constant problem. Historically, platelet counts of 80,000–100,000/mm^3 have been maintained routinely on ECMO to deter bleeding, but there are now multiple examples of patients placed on ECMO with thrombocytopenia of 30,000/mm^3 or lower and in whom massive bleeding was not a problem [15,16]. Although patients often require frequent platelet transfusions, the capacity of transfusions to increase platelet counts to high levels may be limited in patients such as those with cancer. For these patients, lower platelet counts may be allowed and a careful watch for bleeding maintained.

TABLE 12.4B. Sample components for respiratory failure extracorporeal life support based on patient weight.

	Weight (kg)					
	2.5–6	6–12	12–25	25–40	40–70	70+
Tubing pack	$\frac{1}{4}''$	$\frac{1}{4}''$	$\frac{3}{8}''$	$\frac{3}{8}''$	$\frac{1}{2}''$	$\frac{1}{2}''$
Raceway	$\frac{1}{4}''$	$\frac{1}{4}''\ \frac{3}{8}''$	$\frac{3}{8}''$	$\frac{1}{2}''$	$\frac{1}{2}''$	$\frac{1}{2}''$
Oxygenator model	0800	1500	I-2500	I-3500	I-4500	I-4500 × 2
Venous cannula (French)	10–15*	14–18*	15–19	19–21	19–23	19–29
Arterial cannula (French)	8–12	12–1	14–17	17–21	17–21	19–23
Blood prime (units of PRBCs)†	1	1–2	2–3	3–4	4	4–5

Note: These are guidelines only. Individual variables must be considered! Estimates are for a roller head pump with silicone membrane oxygenator. All cannula references are for Biomedicus, the shortest cannulas available in specified sizes except the dual-lumen cannulas as indicated. PRBCs, packed red blood cells.
*Venovenous double-lumen cannula available in 12, 15, 18 French by Origen and 14 French by Kendall.
Consider adding albumin 25% 200 cc after crystalloid priming. Also may add fresh-frozen plasma 50 cc/unit PRBCs.
Source: Data provided by University of Michigan, Ann Arbor, MI, and Children's National Medical Center, Washington, DC.

Another recently identified problem with ECMO, especially during prolonged runs, is heparin-induced thrombocytopenia (HIT) [45,46]. Heparin-induced thrombocytopenia should be suspected in any patient receiving heparin who develops a drop in platelet count that is unresponsive to platelet transfusion or continues to fall without an identified reason. Although HIT usually develops 5–15 days after initial exposure to heparin, it can occur immediately in patients with previous exposure to heparin, such as cardiac surgical patients. Heparin-induced thrombocytopenia associated with immune response to heparin can result in severe thrombocytopenia and thrombotic complications.

The only *cure* is to remove heparin exposure from the patient. During ECMO, this necessitates the use of other anticoagulation methods. Currently, lepirudin and Argatroban are the two alternatives which have been commented on in ECMO, although neither is widely used in the pediatric population in general [47–49]. Lepirudin is a derivative of the leech anticoagulant hirudin. Two reports of its use during ECMO noted no bleeding or clotting complications. It is rapidly active, has a relatively short half life (1.3 hr), and is dosed by weight of the patient. One pediatric report used 0.1 mg/kg bolus dosing followed by an infusion of 0.12 mg/kg/hr and monitored to maintain the activated partial thromboplastin time at two times the control level. It is relatively contraindicated in renal failure. Argatroban is also a direct thrombin inhibitor approved for use in HIT. It is metabolized predominantly by the liver but excreted normally even in severe renal failure. One report of two infants with CDH and HIT treated with Argatroban at a dose of 0.5–10 μg/kg/min to maintain an activated clotting time of ~200 sec had no associated bleeding or thrombotic complications. Another report of thrombin production in ECMO circuits comparing heparin-prepared circuits with Argatroban-primed circuits found that those circuits with Argatroban had less thrombin generation [50]. Thrombocytopenia caused by platelet antibodies has also been described.

Adequate nutrition is essential for healing and can be provided as total parenteral nutrition, enteral feeding, or a combination of both in patients on ECMO. The prior concern of lipids potentially causing either platelet malfunction (bleeding) or increased lung damage from metabolism of arachidonic acid has not been substantiated. Anecdotally, lipids have been associated with the development of cracks in stopcocks used to connect the lipid infusion line to the ECMO circuit [51]. Use of lipids may also be associated with shortened life span of hollow-fiber oxygenators. Enteral feeding has been shown to be safe and effective during ECMO and may limit the need for total parenteral nutrition with its associated complications [52,53].

It is currently popular to maintain a strict fluid balance in critically ill patients, and patients supported with ECMO are no exception. Diuretic use to promote urine excretion, concentrating fluids to balance intake and output, and the use of hemofiltration in patients with renal insufficiency are all important considerations with ECMO [54,55]. Concomitant use of continuous renal replacement therapy during ECMO has become commonplace as a means to maintain fluid balance, support failing kidneys, and potentially clear pathogenic mediators/cytokines from the blood. One recent abstract noted that continuous renal replacement therapy (in the form of continuous venous-venous hemofiltration [CVVH]) was used in 27/84 (32%) of pediatric ECMO patients usually for fluid overload. Overall survival rate was 75% for respiratory failure patients. Of these 84 patients, 27 were matched for age, diagnosis, and PRISM III score with ECMO patients who did not receive CVVH. Improved fluid balance over time, less diuretic use, and faster time to reach caloric-intake goals were noted in patients receiving renal replacement, although there was no difference in survival (67% CVVH, 82% non-CVVH, $p = 0.352$), duration of ventilation post-ECMO, or need for potassium supplementation between groups [56]. Data from the ELSO registry show that about 30% of pediatric and adult ECMO patients receive renal replacement therapy either by hemofiltration or dialysis, although elevations of creatinine >1.5 were reported in only 15% of pediatric patients. Other adjunct extracorporeal therapies such as plasmapheresis and liver support systems have also been used successfully during ECMO.

The optimal ventilatory management for patients on ECMO is not known, and each center may have its own preference for how to treat the lungs during ECMO. Minimizing further barotrauma or oxygen toxicity and providing an environment that promotes lung healing are basic tenets. For neonatal patients on venoarterial ECMO, most centers use ventilator settings with low peak inspiratory pressure (PIP; 25 to 30 cm H_2O), PEEP (5 cm H_2O), intermittent mandatory ventilation rates (6–12 breaths per minute), and fraction of inspired oxygen (FiO$_2$, 0.21). Lung volume decreases dramatically with such settings in most ECMO patients, often resulting in generalized opacification on the chest radiograph. Maintaining lung expansion and functional residual capacity with higher levels of PEEP (10–15 cm H_2O) were associated with shorter ECMO duration in one neonatal study, and this approach is also used frequently at many centers [57]. Given the recent evidence supporting the role of atelectasis in ongoing cytokine production, maintaining some lung distention with PEEP even during ECMO seems prudent. For older patients, use of PEEP with reduced peak airway pressures, low ventilator rates, and low concentrations of inspired oxygen are also the predominant method of support. Common settings reported in the pediatric and adult ECMO literature include PEEP levels in the range of 5–15 cm H_2O, PIP less than 30 cm H_2O, and respiratory rates of 10–12 with FIO$_2$ between 0.3 and 0.4.

Patients with barotrauma and persistent air leaks even at low distending airway pressures on ECMO may benefit from a period of total apnea to allow the lungs to rest [58]. Allowing airway pressure to equilibrate with atmospheric pressure has been used successfully to promote healing of ruptured parenchyma within 48 to 72 hours. Reinflation is accomplished by lavage to remove accumulated secretions, gentle hand ventilation to begin recruiting collapsed alveoli, and then resumption of mechanical ventilation to complete alveolar reexpansion. Use of HFOV to improve lung recruitment, bronchoscopy to remove inspissated secretions, and prone positioning to improve lung mechanics have all been successful in ECMO patients.

At high flow rates in venoarterial ECMO, there is minimal blood entering the pulmonary circuit. Therefore, manipulating ventilator settings, especially in diseased lungs with impaired gas exchange, generally has little effect on blood gas tensions. Oxygenation and carbon dioxide elimination depend on the function of the ECMO circuit. With venovenous cannulation, less overall bypass is obtained, and the systemic oxygenation provided by ECLS is less than with venoarterial bypass. Systemic arterial oxygen saturations are thus lower with venovenous support. Although the majority of patients do well with saturations in the 80s, monitoring of adequate oxygen delivery by following lactate, venous saturation, urine output, metabolic acid–base balance, and mental status is recommended with patients supported with venovenous ECMO.

Increasing oxygenation over time may herald recovery of native pulmonary function. As the lungs heal, compliance and tidal volume increase [59]. The radiograph of the lung fields gradually improves from atelectatic opacification to increasing lung aeration. Increasing concentration and absolute volume of expired carbon dioxide also heralds improved alveolar–capillary gas exchange. These changes along with evidence of decreasing pulmonary artery pressure (indicating resolution of right-to-left intracardiac shunting) may signal that the patient is ready to be weaned from ECMO [60].

Maintaining patient comfort during ECMO can be a challenge, especially during prolonged ECMO runs. Sedation and analgesia are provided by routine medications such as morphine, fentanyl, midazolam, lorazepam, and other agents. If lorazepam infusions are used, intermittent osmolality and osmol gap should be calculated to prevent propylene glycol toxicity [61]. Medications may be absorbed by the membrane oxygenator, and patients can become tolerant to them over time [62]. The extraordinary amount of medications some patients require has led some centers to use anesthesia gas in the membrane oxygenator, although a protocol for appropriate scavenging of these gases must be developed for use. European centers are facile in maintaining patients in a "normal" awake status in which they can play games, read books, and even eat during their ECMO course. Nursing and family support play a major role in the success of providing ECMO with little sedation.

Weaning

The most common mode of weaning from ECMO involves reducing the flow rate in increments every 1–2 hr provided that arterial and mixed venous oxygen saturations remain adequate. Once ECMO flow is reduced to provide only about two-thirds of cardiac output, ventilator support is increased (PIP 20–30 cm H_2O; intermittent mandatory ventilation of 20–30 breaths per minute; PEEP 5 cm H_2O; and FiO_2 0.30–0.40). Weaning continues until an ECMO flow rate of 50–100 mL/min in infants or an estimated 10% of cardiac output is reached. If the patient remains physiologically stable with acceptable blood gas tensions at this low flow, the ECMO cannulas are clamped, and the infant is observed off ECMO support for a short time. If respiration and circulation remain stable during the trial, the cannulas are removed and the patient is returned to conventional therapy. Quicker weaning methods involve decreasing ECMO flow in larger increments over shorter periods of time, similar to what is performed during cardiopulmonary bypass in the operating room [63].

Complications

Complications that occur during ECMO can be mechanical or patient related. The most common adverse events that are reported to the ELSO registry are shown in Table 12.5 (respiratory failure patients).

Bleeding

Bleeding from systemic heparinization is the major complication associated with ECMO [64]. Although bleeding occurs predominately from cannulation or surgical sites, intracranial hemorrhage

TABLE 12.5. Mechanical and patient-related complications for respiratory failure patients.

Complication	Neonatal	Pediatric	Adult
Mechanical			
Oxygenator failure	5.7 (55)	13.7 (45)	18.0 (42)
Tubing rupture	0.7 (74)	3.8 (47)	3.9 (29)
Pump malfunction	1.8 (68)	3.0 (48)	4.1 (35)
Cannula problems	11.2 (69)	13.9 (49)	10.8 (40)
Patient related			
Gastrointestinal hemorrhage	1.7 (46)	4.0 (25)	4.3 (24)
Cannula site bleeding	6.2 (68)	9.4 (61)	12.2 (45)
Surgical site bleeding	6.1 (46)	15.6 (47)	22.2 (35)
Hemolysis	12.0 (67)	8.8 (42)	5.2 (27)
Brain death	1.0 (0)	6.0 (0)	3.8 (0)
Seizures: clinically determined	10.7 (62)	7.2 (34)	1.9 (45)

Note: Data are percent reported (percent survival).
Source: Adapted with permission from ELSO International Summary, January 2005.

is the most dreaded site for bleeding to occur. Intracranial bleeding occurs in approximately 11% of patients overall, with the rate highest in the neonatal population and lowest in the adult population. Bleeding that occurs outside the head that cannot be controlled with medical means requires surgical investigation. Although there are obvious risks of surgical intervention in a bleeding patient who is systemically anticoagulated, many operative repairs have been accomplished during ECMO support [65].

Initial attempts to control bleeding focus on decreasing the rate of heparin infusion and lowering activated clotting time levels. Limitation of heparin may put the circuit at risk for increased clotting, especially at lower flow levels that must be balanced against the bleeding risk. Medications to help prevent clot breakdown in the patient are also used. Aminocaproic acid, also known by the trade name Amicar, has historically been the predominant medication used during ECMO [66]. Amicar functions as an antifibrinolytic amino acid by displacing plasminogen from fibrin and inhibiting clot breakdown. Although a recent survey found a wide range of doses used, we have commonly followed a dosage scheme of 100 mg/kg as a loading dose followed by an infusion of 25–50 mg/kg/hr. Although Amicar has been used in ECMO centers for many years, a recent randomized controlled trial of Amicar versus placebo in neonates found no difference between groups in need for transfusion or need for circuit changes caused by thrombosis.

More recently, aprotinin has become the favored agent in many centers [67]. Aprotinin is a serine protease inhibitor that is antifibrinolytic by inhibiting protein C and factors Va and VIIIa in the extrinsic coagulation pathway and inhibiting the intrinsic pathway as well. It also preserves platelet function, reduces vascular permeability, and has been suggested to decrease the inflammatory response to cardiopulmonary bypass. It has not been compared in a randomized fashion to Amicar or placebo during ECMO, but many centers now use it as their first agent for bleeding patients. Aprotinin is administered as a loading dose of 10,000 units/kg and continued at an infusion rate of 10,000 units/kg/hr. Circuit thromboses may be noted with use of Amicar or aprotinin. Several recent reports of intractable bleeding on ECMO have commented on the benefits of factor VIIa, although the data with this medication are still too sparse to recommend it without further investigation [68]. Discontinuation of heparin to help control intractable bleeding can also be beneficial and has been used for variable periods of time up to 36 hr or more without significant clotting in the ECMO circuit [69]. Larger patients with faster ECMO flow rates are more likely to tolerate discontinuation of heparin without significant clotting. It is wise, however, to have a backup circuit readily available if clotting does occur and the ECMO system requires an emergent replacement.

Infection

Infection is another potential complication of ECMO [70]. Colonization of indwelling catheters, selective adherence of bacteria to polyurethane surfaces, sequestration of bacteria from the body's normal antibody and phagocytic defense mechanisms, and the patient's prior debilitated state are all factors that may increase the risk of infection [71,72]. Successful therapy may be difficult without eliminating invasive equipment, most significantly the ECMO catheters. Viral infection from blood transfusions also may occur. The risk may be limited by minimizing the exposure to blood products from multiple donors by using multiple aliquots sequentially dispensed from a single unit of packed red blood cells. Although sepsis, either preexisting or developing on ECMO, was once seen as a reason to exclude patients from ECMO support, several recent reports have demonstrated that sepsis can be cleared and septic patients may be successfully treated with ECMO. In fact, the most recent guidelines for hemodynamic support of pediatric patients with septic shock note that ECMO should be considered for patients with refractory catecholamine-resistant shock [73]. There is still some debate over whether patients in high-cardiac output shock will obtain any benefit from augmenting cardiac output further with ECMO, but such patients have been treated successfully with ECMO support.

Troubleshooting

Use of an extracorporeal device such as an ECMO circuit is fraught with potential complications that the intensivist should be familiar with in order to compliment the expertise commonly provided by the ECMO technician/perfusionist manning the circuit. Common scenarios include the following: (1) Air might enter the circuit. In this instance the arterial and venous lines should be clamped and the pump turned off while emergent ventilatory and circulatory support is provided the patient. Potential locations of air entry are identified and air removed using the three-way stopcock most proximal to the site of entry. Extracorporeal life support is then restarted. (2) The power might fail. In this setting either emergent ventilatory and circulatory support is provided to the patient, or, if practical, hand-cranking of the pump can be maintained. (3) Increase in negative pump inlet pressure and/or bladder "chirping" can indicate diminished blood return to the circuit, a change in the venous cannula position, or hypovolemia. This can be addressed in a number of ways, including decreasing the pump flow if measures of oxygen delivery are adequate, changing the patient position, raising the patient higher, or administering volume. (4) Decreased oxygenation or evidence of increasing $PaCO_2$ in the patient can be a reflection of a number of problems, but membrane failure particularly as the circuit ages during long runs must be excluded. Assessment of a postoxygenator blood gas will often reveal decreased gas exchange function of the membrane. This can often be overcome simply by increasing the flow of the sweep gases and/or increasing the FiO_2, but failure to improve may eventually require changing the membrane oxygenator, which can usually be done in under a minute off bypass support. Other common causes of low saturations include inadequate pump flow, anemia, inadequate ventilatory support for the percentage of native pulmonary blood flow, sweep gas disconnection, and pneumothorax. Increasing experience with this modality in the setting of available technical expertise is the optimal way to gain an enhanced ability to identify either patient- or circuit-related problems in order to effectively and expeditiously remedy them without unintended injury to the patient while using this life-saving technology.

Long-Term Outcome

Patients undergoing ECMO are at risk of neurologic damage from hypoxia, acidosis, hypotension, induced alkalosis before ECMO, hemorrhage or ischemia related to systemic heparinization, and alterations in cerebral blood flow following ligation of the carotid artery and internal jugular vein [74–79]. Nevertheless, two thirds of the neonatal survivors appear to have a normal neurodevelopmental outcome. The remaining one third suffer from mild to severe deficits in motor or cognitive function. Sensorineural hearing loss has been noted in 23% of patients, an incidence comparable to that in infants with persistent pulmonary hypertension treated conventionally. The long-term effects of carotid artery and jugular vein ligation remain unknown.

Severe chronic respiratory disease in patients treated with ECMO is uncommon [80]. Most reports relate an incidence of bronchopulmonary dysplasia (defined as the need for oxygen beyond the first month of life) from 4% to 27%. Most cases occurred in patients who had required extreme ventilator settings for more than 7 days before ECMO rescue. A follow-up report of neonates treated with ECMO and evaluated at 10–15 years post-ECMO found that, although patients had some diminished lung function by pulmonary function testing, they had similar aerobic capacity and were able to reach anaerobic exercise goals similar to those of age-matched healthy controls [81].

Of 2,800 pediatric respiratory ECMO patients listed in the ELSO registry through January 2005, 6% of patients had intracranial infarct or hemorrhage found on computed tomography examination. Brain death occurred in 6% of the patients, and 7% of patients had reported seizures. Long-term neurologic outcome data are sorely missing in the pediatric population. Few centers maintain regular follow-up clinics, and patients are often referred for ECMO from distant sites, making follow-up studies difficult. In one report of 15 pediatric and 4 adult patients, 58% survived to discharge. Patients were evaluated by use of the Pediatric Cerebral Performance Category (PCPC; which measures cognitive impairment) and the Pediatric Overall Performance Category (POPC; which measures functional morbidity). Overall, 64% of survivors had normal PCPC scores, 27% had mild disabilities, and 9% had moderate cognitive disability. Functional outcome was normal in 27%, while 45% had mild disability, 18% moderate disability, and 9% severe disability [82]. In another small series of 26 patients studied 1–3 years after ECMO, 38% of pre-school-aged children were described as normal, and 31% had observed abnormalities. Four patients (31%) who had prior neurologic dysfunction remained at baseline following ECMO. Among children who were school-aged, 77% were described as normal by parental report [83]. More specific neurologic follow-up studies of the pediatric age groups are needed.

The Future

The current extension of ECLS systems to older pediatric and adult patients in a variety of clinical settings highlights the changes that have occurred in the ECLS environment. Progress in renal replacement, liver support, and plasmapheresis and the development of new cardiac support devices applicable to pediatrics may also expand the use of ECMO or related techniques. Additionally, the development of small, portable systems for cardiopulmonary resuscitation may herald a new age of extracorporeal support. Technical advances in extracorporeal life support equipment continue to make such support safer and more efficient. Venovenous ECMO techniques have been refined and used successfully in a wide age range of patients: neonatal to adults. Single-cannula, double-lumen catheters for venovenous ECMO may obviate the risks of arterial cannulation and offer the benefit of requiring only one surgical site for venous access. Heparin- or novel anticoagulant-bonded circuits may decrease the need for systemic anticoagulation and the risk of hemorrhagic complications. Until the day when medical science may make the need for ECLS obsolete, research into ways to make it safer and more efficient should continue.

References

1. Dalton HJ, Heulitt MJ. Extracorporeal membrane oxygenation. Invited review. Respir Care 1998;43:966–977.
2. Tulenko DR. An update on ECMO. Neonatal Netw 2004;23(4):11–18.
3. Dalton HJ, Rycus P. Unpublished data. Extracorporeal Life Support Organization, Ann Arbor, MI, 2002.
4. ECMO Registry of the Extracorporeal Life Support Organization, Ann Arbor, MI, January 2005.
5. O'Rourke PP, Crone RK. Pediatric applications of extracorporeal membrane oxygenation. J Pediatr 1990;116(3):393.
6. Fortenberry JD, Meier AH, Pettignano R, Heard M, Chambliss CR, Wulkan M. Extracorporeal life support for posttraumatic acute respiratory distress syndrome at a children's medical center. J Pediatr Surg 2003;38:1221–1226.
7. Szocik J. Rudich S, Csete M. ECMO resuscitation after massive pulmonary embolism during liver transplantation. Anesthesiology 2002;97:763–764.
8. Sheridan RL, Schnitzer JJ. Management of the high risk pediatric burn patient. J Pediatr Surg 2001;36:1308–1312.
9. Linden V, Karlen J, Olsson M, Palmer K, Ehren H, Henter JI, Kalin M. Successful extracorporeal membrane oxygenation in four children with malignant disease and severe *Pneumocystis carinii* pneumonia. Med Pediatr Oncol 1999;32(1):25–31.
10. Thiagarajan RR, Roth SJ, Margossian S, Mackie AS, Neufeld EJ, Laussen PC, Forbess JM, Blume ED. Extracorporeal membrane oxygenation as a bridge to cardiac transplantation in a patient with cardiomyopathy and hemophilia A. Intensive Care Med 2003;29(6):985–988.
11. Gow KW, Heard ML, Heiss KF, KAtzenstein HM, Wulkan ML, Fortenberry JD. Extracorporeal membrane oxygenation (ECMO) in children with malignancy. 20th Annual CNMC Symposium on ECMO and Advanced Respiratory Therapies, A23. Keystone, CO, 2004.
12. MacLaren G, Pellegrino V, Butt W, Preovolos A, Salamonsen R. Successful use of ECMO in adults with life-threatening infections. Anaesth Intensive Care 2004;32(5):707–710.
13. Zapol WM, Snider MT, Hill JD, Fallat RJ, Bartlett RH, Edmunds LH, Morris AH, Peirce EC 2nd, Thomas AN, Proctor HJ, Drinker PA, Pratt PC, Bagniewski A, Miller RG Jr. Extracorporeal membrane oxygenation in severe acute respiratory failure. A randomized prospective study. JAMA 1979;242(20):2193–2196.
14. Gattinoni L, Kolobow T, Tomlinson T, et al. Low frequency positive pressure ventilation with extracorporeal carbon dioxide removal (LFPPV-ECCO₂R): an experimental study. Anesth Analg 1978;57:470.
15. Kolla S, Awad SS, Rich PB, Schreiner RJ, Hirschl RB, Bartlett RH. Extracorporeal life support for 100 adult patients with severe respiratory failure. Ann Surg 1997;226(4):544–564.
16. Hemmila MR, Rowe SA, Boules TN, Miskulin J, McGillicuddy JW, Schuerer DJ, Haft JW, Swaniker F, Arbabi S, Hirschl RB, Bartlett RH. Extracorporeal life support for severe acute respiratory distress syndrome in adults. Ann Surg 2004;240(4):595–605.
17. Kolobow T. An update on adult extracorporeal membrane oxygenation: extracorporeal CO₂ removal. Trans Am Soc Artif Intern Organs 1988;4:1004.
18. Alpard SK, Zwischenberger JB, Tao W, Deyo DJ, Bidani A. Reduced ventilator pressure and improved P/F ratio during percutaneous arteriovenous carbon dioxide removal for severe respiratory failure. Ann Surg 1999;230(2):215–224.
19. Kolobow T. The artificial lung: the past. A personal retrospective. ASAIO J 2004;50(6):xliii–xlviii.
20. Morris MC, Wernovsky G, Nadkarni VM. Survival outcomes after extracorporeal cardiopulmonary resuscitation instituted during active chest compressions following refractory in-hospital pediatric cardiac arrest. Pediatr Crit Care Med 2004;5(5):440–446.
21. Marsh TD, Wilkerson SA, Cook LN. Extracorporeal membrane oxygenation selection criteria: partial pressure of arterial oxygen versus alveolar-arterial oxygen gradient. Pediatrics 1988;82:162.
22. Beck R, Anderson KD, Pearson GD, et al. Criteria for extracorporeal membrane oxygenation in a population of infants with persistent pulmonary hypertension of the newborn. J Pediatr Surg 1986;21:297.
23. Ortiz RM, Cilley RE, Bartlett RH. Extracorporeal membrane oxygenation in pediatric respiratory failure. Pediatr Clin North Am 1987;34:39.
24. Nading JH. Historical controls for extracorporeal membrane oxygenation in neonates. Crit Care Med 1989;17:423.
25. Dalton HJ, Rycus P. Unpublished data. Extracorporeal Life Support Organization Registry, Ann Arbor, MI, 2004.
26. Peters MJ, Tasker RC, Kiff KM, Yates R, Hatch DJ. Acute hypoxemic respiratory failure in children: case mix and the utility of respiratory severity indices. Intensive Care Med 1998;24:699–705.
27. Traschel D, McCrindle BW, Nakagawa S, Bohn D. Oxygenation index predicts outcome in children with acute hypoxemic respiratory failure. Am J Respir Crit Care Med 2005;172:206–211.
28. Gilbert EM, Haupt MT, Mandanas RY, et al. The effect of fluid loading, blood transfusion and catecholamine infusion on oxygen delivery and consumption in patients with sepsis. Am Rev Respir Dis 134:873, 1986.
29. Kolobow T, Spragg RG, Pierce JE. Massive pulmonary infarction during total cardiopulmonary bypass in unanesthetized spontaneously breathing lambs. Int J Artif Organs 1981;4(2):76.
30. Secker-Walker JS, Edmonds JF, Spratt EH, Conn AW. The source of coronary perfusion during partial bypass for extracorporeal membrane oxygenation (ECMO). Ann Thorac Surg 1976;21:138–143.
31. Mims BC: Physiologic monitoring of SO₂ monitoring. Crit Care Nurs Clin North Am 1989;1(3):619.
32. Babcock DS, Han BK, Weiss RG, Ryckman FC Brain abnormalities in infants on extracorporeal membrane oxygenation: sonographic and CT findings. Am J Roentgenol 1989;153(3):571.
33. Taylor GA, Fitz CR, Kapur S, Short BL. Cerebrovascular accidents in neonates treated with extracorporeal membrane oxygenation: sonographic-pathologic correlation. Am J Roentgenol 1989;153(2):355.
34. Kimball TR, Weiss RG, Meyer RA, et al. Color flow mapping to document normal pulmonary venous return in neonates with persistent pulmonary hypertension being considered for extracorporeal membrane oxygenation. J Pediatr 1989;114(3):433.
35. Martin GR, Short BL. Doppler echocardiographic evaluation of cardiac performance in infants on prolonged extracorporeal membrane oxygenation. Am J Cardiol 1988;62:929.

36. Green TP, Isham-Schopf B, Steinhorn RH, et al. Whole blood activated clotting time in infants during extracorporeal membrane oxygenation. Crit Care Med 1990;18(5):494.

37. Jaggers JJ, Forbes JM, Shah AS, Meliones JN, Kirshbom PM, Miller CE, Ungerleider RM. Extracorporeal membrane oxygenation for infant postcardiotomy support: significance of shunt management. Ann Thorac Surg 2000;69(5):1476–1483.

38. Meliones JN, Moler FW, Custer JR, Dekeon MK, Chapman RA, Bartlett RH. Normalization of priming solution ionized calcium concentration improves hemodynamic stability of neonates receiving venovenous ECMO. ASAIO J 1995;41(4):884–888.

39. Mink RB, Pollack MM. Effect of blood transfusion on oxygen consumption in pediatric septic shock. Crit Care Med 1990;18(10):1087.

40. Gilbert EM, Haupt MT, Mandanas RY, et al. The effect of fluid loading, blood transfusion and catecholamine infusion on oxygen delivery and consumption in patients with sepsis. Am Rev Respir Dis 1986;134: 873.

41. Bjerke HS, Kelly RE Jr, Foglia RP, Barcliff L, Petz L. Decreasing transfusion exposure risk during extracorporeal membrane oxygenation (ECMO). Transfus Med 1992;2(1):43–49.

42. Zavadil DP, Stammers AH, Willett LD, et al. Hematological abnormalities in neonatal patients treated with extracorporeal membrane oxygenation. J Extra Corpor Technol 1998;30:83–90.

43. McCoy-Pardington D, Judd WJ, Knafl P, Abruzzo LV, Coombes KR, Butch SH, Oberman HA. Blood use during extracorporeal membrane oxygenation. Transfusion 1990;30(4):307–309.

44. Plotz F. Extracorporeal membrane oxygenation and clotting revisited. J Pediatr 1997;130:847–848.

45. Alsoufi B, Boshkov LK, Kirby A, Ibsen L, et al. Heparin-induced thrombocytopenia (HIT) in pediatric cardiac surgery: and emerging cause of morbidity and mortality. Semin Thorac Cardiovasc Surg Pediatr Card Surg Annu 2004;7:155–171.

46. Klenner AF, Lubenow N, Raschke R, Greinacher A. Heparin-induced thrombocytopenia in children: 12 new cases and review of the literature. Thromb Haemost 2004;91:719–724.

47. Dager WE, Gosselin RC, Yoshikawa R, Owings JT. Lepirudin in heparin-induced thrombocytopenia and extracorporeal membranous oxygenation. Ann Pharmacother 2004;38(4):598–601.

48. Deitcher SR, Topoulos AP, Bartholomew JR, Kichuk-Chrisant MR. Lepirudin anticoagulation for heparin-induced thrombocytopenia. J Pediatr 2002;140(2):264–266.

49. Mejak B, Giacomuzzi C, Heller E, You X, Ungerleider R, Shen I, Boshkov L. Argatroban usage for anticoagulation for ECMO on a post-cardiac patient with heparin-induced thrombocytopenia. J Extra Corpor Technol 2004;36(2):178–181.

50. Young G, Yonekawa KE, Nakagawa P, Nugent DJ. Argatroban as an alternative to heparin in extracorporeal membrane oxygenation circuits. Perfusion 2004;19(5):283–288.

51. Buck ML, Ksenich RA, Wooldridge P. Effect of infusing fat emulsion into extracorporeal membrane oxygenation circuits. Pharmacotherapy 1997;17(6):1292–1295.

52. Scott LK, Boudreaux K, Thaljeh F, Grier LR, Conrad SA. Early enteral feedings in adults receiving venovenous extracorporeal membrane oxygenation. J Parenter Enteral Nutr 2004;28(5):295–300.

53. Piena M, Albers MJ, Van Haard PM, Gischler S, Tibboel D. Introduction of enteral feeding in neonates on extracorporeal membrane oxygenation after evaluation of intestinal permeability changes. J Pediatr Surg 1998;33(1):30–34.

54. Lochan S, Adeniyi-Jones S, Assadi F. Coadministration of theophylline enhances diuretic response to furosemide in infants during extracorporeal membrane oxygenation: a randomized controlled pilot study. J Pediatr 1998;133:86–89.

55. Foland JA, Fortenberry JD, Warshaw BL, Pettignano R, Merritt RK, Heard ML, Rogers K, Reid C, Tanner AJ, Easley KA. Fluid overload before continuous hemofiltration and survival in critically ill children: a retrospective analysis. Crit Care Med 2004;32(8):1771–1776.

56. Hoover NG, Fortenberry JD, Heard M, Wagoner S, Tanner A, Foland J. Continuous venovenous hemofiltration use in pediatric respiratory failure patients on ECMO: a case–control study. 20th Annual CNMC Symposium on ECMO and Advanced Respiratory Therapies, A24. Keystone, CO, 2004.

57. Keszler M, Subramanian KN, Smith YA. Pulmonary management during extracorporeal membrane oxygenation. Crit Care Med 1989;17:495–500.

58. Frattalone J, Fuhrman BP, Thompson AE. Treatment of air leak during extracorporeal membrane oxygenation: total apneic lung rest. Clin Res 1987;35:912A.

59. Kugelman A, Saiki K, Platzker AC, Garg M. Measurement of lung volumes and pulmonary mechanics during weaning of newborn infants with intractable respiratory failure from extracorporeal membrane oxygenation. Pediatr Pulmonol 1995;20(3):145–151.

60. Tanke R, Daniels O, Van Heyst A, Van Lier H, Festen C The influence of ductal left-to-right shunting during extracorporeal membrane oxygenation. J Pediatr Surg 2002;37(8):1165–1168.

61. Yaucher NE, Fish JT, Smith HW, Wells JA. Propylene glycol–associated renal toxicity from lorazepam infusion. Pharmacotherapy 2003;23(9):1094–1099.

62. Arnold JH, Truog RD, Orav DJ. Tolerance and dependence in neonates sedated with fentanyl during extracorporeal membrane oxygenation. Anesthesiology 1990;73:1136–1140.

63. Cronin J. Cycling: an alternative method for weaning ECMO. CNMC National ECMO Symposium, Breckenridge, CO, 1990:69.

64. Sell LL, Cullen ML, Whittlesey GC, et al. Hemorrhagic complications during extracorporeal membrane oxygenation: prevention and treatment. J Pediatr Surg 1986;21:1087.

65. Fortenberry JD, Meier AH, Pettignano R, Heard M, Chambliss CR, Wulkan M. Extracorporeal life support for posttraumatic acute respiratory distress syndrome at a children's medical center. J Pediatr Surg 2003;38(8):1221–1226.

66. Downard CD, Betit P, Chang RW, Garza JJ, Arnold JH, Wilson JM. Impact of AMICAR on hemorrhagic complications of ECMO: a ten-year review. Pediatr Surg 2003;38(8):1212–1216.

67. Jamieson WR, Dryden PJ, O'Connor JP, Sadeghi H, Ansley DM, Merrick PM. Beneficial effect of both tranexamic acid and aprotinin on blood loss reduction in reoperative valve replacement surgery. Circulation 1997;96(9 Suppl):II-96–II-100.

68. Verrijckt A, Proulx F, Morneau S, Vobecky S. Activated recombinant factor VII for refractory bleeding during extracorporeal membrane oxygenation. J Thorac Cardiovasc Surg 2004;127(6):1812–1813.

69. Shanley CJ, Hultquist KA, Rosenberg DM, et al. Prolonged extracorporeal membrane circulation without heparin. Evaluation of the Medtronic Minimax oxygenator. ASAIO J 1992;38:M311-M3116.

70. Schutze GE, Heulitt MJ. Infections during extracorporeal life support. J Pediatr Surg 1995;30:809–812.

71. Brody J. Altered lymphocyte subsets during cardiopulmonary bypass. Am J Clin Pathol 1987;87:626–628.

72. Zach TL. Leukopenia associated with extracorporeal membrane oxygenation in newborn infants. J Pediatr 1990;116:440–444.

73. Carcillo JA, Fields AI, American College of Critical Care Medicine Task Force Committee Members. Clinical practice parameters for hemodynamic support of pediatric and neonatal patients in septic shock. Crit Care Med 2002;30(6):1365–1378.

74. Adolph V, Ekelund C, Smith C, et al. Developmental outcome of neonates treated with extracorporeal membrane oxygenation. J Pediatr Surg 1990;25:38.

75. Matamoros A, Anderson JC, McConnell J, et al. Neurosonographic findings in infants treated by extracorporeal membrane oxygenation (ECMO). J Child Neurol 4(Suppl):S52, 1989.

76. Krummel TM, Greenfield LJ, Kirkpatrick BV, et al. The early evaluation of survivors after extracorporeal membrane oxygenation for neonatal pulmonary failure. J Pediatr Surg 1984;19:585.

77. Towne BH, Lott IT, Hicks DA, et al. Long-term follow-up of infants and children treated with extracorporeal membrane oxygenation (ECMO): a preliminary report. J Pediatr Surg 1985;20:410.

78. Lott IT, McPherson D, Towne B, et al. Long-term neurophysiologic outcome after neonatal extracorporeal membrane oxygenation. J Pediatr 1990;116:343.

79. Hofkosh D, Clouse H, Smith-Jones J, et al. Ten years of ECMO: neurodevelopmental outcome among survivors. Pediatr Res 1990;27:246A.

80. Koumbourlis AC, Motoyama EK, Mutich RL. Lung mechanics during and after extracorporeal membrane oxygenation for meconium aspiration syndrome. Crit Care Med 1992;20:751–756.

81. Boykin AR, Quivers ES, Wagenhoffer KL, Sable CA, Chaney HR, Glass P, Bahrami KR, Short BL. Cardiopulmonary outcome of neonatal extracorporeal membrane oxygenation at ages 10–15 years. Crit Care Med 2003;31(9):2380–2384.

82. Heulitt MJ, Moss MM, Walker WM. Morbidity and mortality in pediatric patients with respiratory failure. Extracorporeal Life Support Meeting, 1993:41.

83. Fajardo EM. Outcome and follow-up of children following extracorporeal life support in ECMO: extracorporeal cardiopulmonary support in critical care. In: Zwischenberger JB, Barlett RH eds. Extracorporeal Cardiopulmonary Support in Critical Care. Ann Arbor, MI: Extracorporeal Life Support Organization; 1975;373–381.

13
Diseases of the Upper Respiratory Tract

Renuka Mehta, Suriyanarayana P. Hariprakash, Peter N. Cox, and Derek S. Wheeler

Developmental Anatomy

Prenatal development of the upper airway is divided into the embryonic phase (0–8 weeks of gestation) and the fetal phase (8–40 weeks of gestation). The embryonic phase is characterized by organogenesis, whereas the fetal phase is characterized by organ maturation. The human embryo develops at the interface between two sacs, a dorsal, ectodermal sac and a ventral, endodermal yolk sac. The part of the yolk sac incorporated into the arching head fold forms the foregut. One outgrowth of the foregut into the dorsally aligned mesodermal beds is termed the *laryngotracheal groove*, the primordium of the tracheal and pulmonary diverticula. Laterally, the foregut is limited by a thick wall of mesoderm in which the branchial or pharyngeal arches develop. These paired arches are intimately involved in the ultimate formation of the mouth, nasal cavities, pharynx, and larynx. The ear and mandible share the first and second arch derivation. The laryngotracheal groove develops furrows along its lateral aspect, which deepen and eventually unite, separating the laryngotracheal tube from the esophagus. The anterior portion of the cranial end of the laryngotracheal tube forms the laryngeal slit, covered by an epithelial lamina. Caudally it progresses to form lung buds. On either side of the slit, two lateral swellings appear that ultimately become the arytenoids. The epiglottis forms from an anteriorly sited, central elevation of the primitive larynx, and the lateral arms develop into the aryepiglottic folds.

The thyroid, cricoid, and corniculate cartilages are first recognizable in the seventh week of gestation as condensations of mesenchyme paralleled by the appearance of the laryngeal muscles. By 10–11 weeks, the major structures of the larynx have developed and the cartilages are chondrifying. At this stage, the epithelial lamina dissolutes and the glottic aperture appears. By the end of second trimester the laryngeal development enters the differentiation phase during which it attains the inverted cone shape. The cunei-

form cartilages are the last to develop, late in the seventh month, within the aryepiglottic folds.

The respiratory tract begins with the nasal and oral cavities, which together comprise the pharynx. The pharynx is connected to the esophagus and the larynx. The larynx and its unique anatomy continue into the chest in the form of a cylindrical structure called the *trachea*, which divides into the right and left main bronchi. The bronchi continue dividing approximately 23 more times until the terminal bronchioles and the accompanying alveoli are reached. The larynx is a unique structure whose primary functions are in speech production and protection of the airway. It is formed by cartilaginous, bony, and connective tissue structures. The glottis is the area around the vocal cords. The subglottis is the area directly below the vocal cords leading into the trachea. The cords are closed during the end of the expiratory phase and rest, and they open at the beginning of the inspiratory phase. The narrowest part of the adult airway is the vocal cords, but, in children, the narrowest part is the cricoid cartilage located in the subglottic area of the larynx. The trachea is a cylindrical structure formed by 16–20 U-shaped cartilaginous rings and a muscular/cartilaginous part that completes the tube. The airway is divided into the upper airway, which begins with the nose and lips and extends down to the glottis, and the lower airway, which is the airway below the glottis.

Although basic principles in the management of the airway in children are the same as in adults, there are important developmental characteristics that distinguish the pediatric airway from the adult airway (Table 13.1). These affect both mask ventilation and tracheal intubation. In the neonate and infant, important anatomic differences include a proportionately larger head and tongue, narrower nasal passages, an anterior and cephalad larynx, long epiglottis, and a short trachea and neck. These factors contribute to making infants "obligate" nasal breathers. The cricoid cartilage is the narrowest point of the airway in children younger than 10 years of age as opposed to the glottis in the adult. Even minimal edema will have a proportionately greater effect in children because of their smaller tracheal diameters. In older children, prominent adenoidal and tonsillar tissue can obstruct visualization of the larynx. Also, there are specific congenital anatomic airway anomalies that occur in children that make management of these airways even more complex. As the child becomes older the airway becomes more comparable to the adult anatomy, and by 8 or 9 years of age the airway is considered similar to the adult airway, with the exception of size.

TABLE 13.1. Major anatomic differences between the airways of infants and adults.

	Infant	Adult
Head	Large, prominent occiput	Flat occiput
Tongue	Relatively larger	Relatively smaller
Larynx	Cephalad position Opposite to C2–C3	Opposite to C4–C6
Epiglottis	Omega-shaped and soft	Flat and flexible
Vocal cords	Short and concave	Horizontal
Narrowest portion	Cricoid ring, below cords	Vocal cords
Cartilage	Soft	Firm
Lower airways	Smaller, less developed	Larger, more cartilage

All parts of the pediatric airway are very small and fragile. Even trauma that occurs during tracheal intubation can cause significant edema and obstruction of the upper airway. For example, 1 mm of circumferential edema can result in a 16-fold increase in resistance in a 4-mm infant airway (Figure 13.1). The narrowness of the airway results in greater baseline resistance. Any process that narrows the airway further will cause an exponential rise in airway resistance and a secondary increase in the work of breathing. When the child perceives distress, the resultant increase in respiratory effort will further augment turbulence and raise resistance.

Because the neonate is primarily a nasal breather, any degree of obstruction of the nasopharynx may result in a significant increase in the work of breathing and present clinically as retractions. The tongue of infants and small children dominates the overall capacitance of the oropharynx, so any pediatric patient who presents with altered mental status will be at risk for the development of upper airway obstruction secondary to loss of muscle tone affecting the tongue. Occlusion of the oropharynx by the tongue is not uncommon in this setting, but tilting of the head, lifting the chin, or insertion of an oral airway may correct this obstruction.

Older children have tonsillar and adenoidal tissues that are large in proportion to available airways. Although these rarely cause an upper airway catastrophe, they are vulnerable to traumatization and bleeding during clinical interventions such as insertion of an oral or a nasal airway. The pediatric trachea is easily distensible and compressible because of incomplete closure of semiformed cartilaginous rings. Any maneuver that overextends the neck will contribute to compression of this structure and secondary upper airway obstruction. As the cricoid ring represents the narrowest portion of the upper airway in children, it is often the site of occlusion in tracheobronchial foreign body aspiration.

The lower airway tract consists of all structures below the level of the midtrachea, including the bronchi, bronchioles, and alveoli. Developmental immaturity of these structures in infancy is reflected by a decreased number of subunits necessary for appropriate oxygenation and ventilation. In addition, the pediatric patient possesses a diminished pulmonary vascular bed. The relatively small caliber of the pediatric lower airway predisposes it to occlusion. Even partial occlusion will result in an increased degree of airway resistance. Immaturity of musculoskeletal and central nervous systems of the pediatric patient also contributes to the development of respiratory failure. In infancy, the diaphragm remains the primary muscle of respiration, with only minor contributions provided by the intercostal musculature. Any degree of abdominal distension will provide significant interference to diaphragmatic function and secondary ventilatory insufficiency. The infantile diaphragm possesses muscle fibers that are more prone to fatigue than their adult counterparts. In addition, the chest wall of the pediatric patient is quite compliant, preventing adequate stabilization during periods of increased respiratory distress. Also, infants are less responsive to hypoxemia because of immature development of central respiratory control, placing them at risk for insufficient respiratory responses to disease states.

Congenital Anomalies of the Upper Airway

Congenital anomalies of the upper airway are relatively common and typically present with signs and symptoms of upper airway obstruction [1–5]. As these disorders are discussed in length in Chapter 17, they are only briefly mentioned here.

Supralaryngeal Anomalies

Syndromes Associated With Upper Airway Obstruction

Several malformation syndromes are commonly associated with upper airway obstruction. The Pierre-Robin sequence [6–10] is a pattern of malformations that arise from a single primary defect in early morphogenesis—in this case, mandibular hypoplasia—which include micrognathia, cleft palate, and glossoptosis. Mandibular hypoplasia forces the tongue posteriorly, keeping it high in the oral cavity and causing a cleft in the palate by preventing the closure of the palatal shelves. This leads to the classic inverted U-shaped cleft and the absence of an associated cleft lip common in these children. The tongue is not actually larger than normal, but, because of the small mandible, the tongue is large relative to the airway and therefore causes obstruction. Although the Pierre-Robin sequence is associated with multiple malformation syndromes, Stickler syndrome, deletion 22q11.2 spectrum, and Treacher-Collins syndrome account for the vast majority [6–10]. Trisomy 21 (Down syndrome),

	Normal	Edema	Δ diameter	Δ resistance
Infant	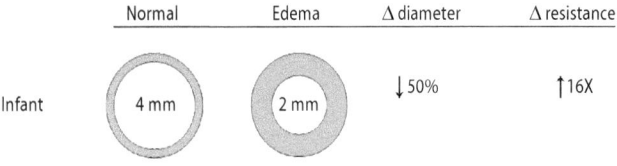 4 mm	2 mm	↓50%	↑16X
Adult	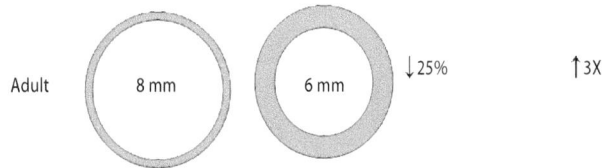 8 mm	6 mm	↓25%	↑3X

FIGURE 13.1. Age-dependent effects of a reduction in airway caliber on the airway resistance and air flow. Normal airways are represented on the left (top, infants; bottom, adults), and edematous airways are represented on the right. According to Poiseuille's law, airway resistance is inversely proportional to the radius of the airway to the *fourth power* when there is laminar flow and to the *fifth power* when there is turbulent flow. One millimeter of circumferential edema will reduce the diameter of the airway by 2 mm, resulting in a 16-fold increase in airway resistance in the pediatric airway versus a 3-fold increase in the adult (cross-sectional area reduced by 75% in the pediatric airway versus a 44% decrease in the adult airway). Note that turbulent air flow (such as occurs during crying) in the child would increase the resistance by 32-fold.

Crouzon disease, Beckwith-Wiedemann syndrome, and Goldenhar syndrome are also commonly associated with upper airway obstruction.

Choanal Atresia

Choanal atresia occurs in approximately 1:8,000 live births and may be unilateral or bilateral. Cases of unilateral and bilateral choanal atresia appear to be evenly distributed (i.e., 50% of cases are unilateral and 50% are bilateral) [1,11,12]. The majority of cases (71%) are of the *mixed* type (bony and membranous), while the remaining cases (29%) are primarily of the *bony* type. The *membranous* type is exceedingly rare [1,11,12]. Because infants are *obligate* nasal breathers, most children with this condition present with respiratory distress and poor feeding in early infancy.

Affected infants have episodes of respiratory distress with cyanosis that is relieved with crying (paradoxical cyanosis). Bilateral choanal atresia always produces symptoms during the neonatal period, although the degree and severity of airway obstruction are variable. Unilateral choanal atresia often presents with unilateral rhinorrhea and persistent obstruction between the ages of 2 and 5 years. Rarely an infant with unilateral choanal atresia may present early because of contralateral obstruction such as a deviated septum. Diagnosis is confirmed at the bedside by the inability to pass a soft catheter through the nose. Radiologic evaluation of the nose and nasopharynx by computed tomography (CT) scanning is helpful in establishing the diagnosis as well as the extent of disease. Flexible fiberoptic examination after topical decongestion usually confirms the presence of atresia, but axial CT is necessary to assess the thickness of the atresia plate, the degree of lateral pterygoid plate and vomerine involvement, and the plan for surgical intervention. Associated anomalies are common and occur in 20%–50% of infants with choanal atresia. The CHARGE association includes coloboma or other ophthalmic anomalies, heart disease, choanal atresia, growth retardation, genital hypoplasia, and ear anomalies associated with hearing loss. Definitive management is surgical and includes either transnasal or transpalatal repair [1,11–13].

Intranasal Tumors

Significant airway obstruction secondary to intranasal tumors (e.g., dermoids, gliomas, encephaloceles, or teratomas) usually present in the neonatal period. Encephaloceles contain herniated brain tissue, dura, and cerebrospinal fluid, and early surgical resection is recommended (regardless of the degree of airway obstruction) in order to alleviate the risk of meningitis [1,11].

Tongue Cysts

Cysts at the base of the tongue are rare but potentially life-threatening causes of upper airway obstruction during infancy [1,11,14,15]. These include thyroglossal duct cysts, dermoid cysts, and vallecular cysts. Vallecular cysts [16–18] are a rare but well-recognized cause of stridor and respiratory distress in infants and have been associated with sudden airway obstruction resulting in death. Vallecular cysts are also called *mucous retention cysts, epiglottic cysts, base-of-the-tongue cysts*, and *ductal cysts* [18]. Infants typically present with inspiratory stridor and respiratory distress in the first weeks of life. Feeding difficulties and failure to thrive are also common manifestations. Vallecular cysts consist of a unilocular, cystic mass that arises from the lingual surface of the epi-

glottis. Diagnosis is usually made by direct laryngoscopy, and surgery is curative.

Laryngeal Anomalies

Laryngomalacia

Laryngomalacia is the most common cause of stridor in infants, accounting for 60% of cases with congenital anomalies [1–3,19–21]. Boys appear to be affected twice as often as girls. Although severe cases can produce obstructive apnea, cor pulmonale, and failure to thrive, most cases are self-limited. The etiology of this disorder is not known, but gastroesophageal reflux may play a contributing role.

Children with laryngomalacia most commonly present with noisy respirations, often since the first few weeks of life, which are accentuated by the supine position, feeding, and agitation. Feeding difficulties may also occasionally occur, although failure to thrive, respiratory distress, and cyanosis are rare. The stridor of laryngomalacia is inspiratory in character and is typically milder in the prone position or when the neck is extended. The severity of stridor typically worsens with growth and increasing oxygen demands and then slowly resolves between 6 and 18 months of age. Central nervous system disorders associated with neuromuscular coordination difficulties are likely to exacerbate laryngomalacia in affected infants. The diagnosis is made based on a classic history and physical examination and is confirmed by endoscopy. During awake, flexible laryngoscopy, the epiglottis may be omega shaped and appear to fold posteriorly with inspiration. The arytenoids are bulky and prolapse into the glottis with inspiration (Figure 13.2). Radiologic evaluation will show downward and inferior displacement and bowing of the aryepiglottic folds [22,23]. The majority of cases can be managed with observation alone, and symptoms generally resolve by 18–24 months of age. Gastroesophageal reflux should be treated if present, as it is known to exacerbate symptoms. Surgical management is rarely required, but, when indicated, supraglottoplasty is the procedure of choice [1–3,19–21].

Vocal Cord Paralysis

Vocal cord paralysis is the second most common congenital anomaly of the larynx, accounting for nearly 10% of all cases [1–3,19–21,24–26]. Vocal cord paralysis may be unilateral or bilateral. Most cases of unilateral vocal cord paralysis are idiopathic but may also occur secondary to peripheral nerve injury (e.g., injury to the recurrent laryngeal nerve following Norwood stage I palliation for hypoplastic left heart syndrome, during repair of tracheoesophageal fistula, or resulting from birth trauma). Unilateral vocal cord paralysis is usually well tolerated and is suggested by the presence of a weak cry and occasional stridor in the right historical context. Congenital anomalies of the cardiovascular system frequently are associated with unilateral vocal cord paralysis. The left vocal cord is more commonly affected than the right because of its longer course and closer proximity to the heart, placing it at greater risk for injury during surgery for congenital heart disease. Bilateral vocal cord paralysis, on the other hand, usually results from central nervous system (CNS) injury or disease (hemorrhage, hypoxia/ischemia, Arnold-Chiari malformation, spina bifida, etc.) [1,25]. Central nervous system involvement is almost always the result of brain stem pathology. Supranuclear etiologies are rare causes of bilateral vocal cord paralysis caused by the extensive interhemispheric connections of laryngeal efferent neural pathways. The

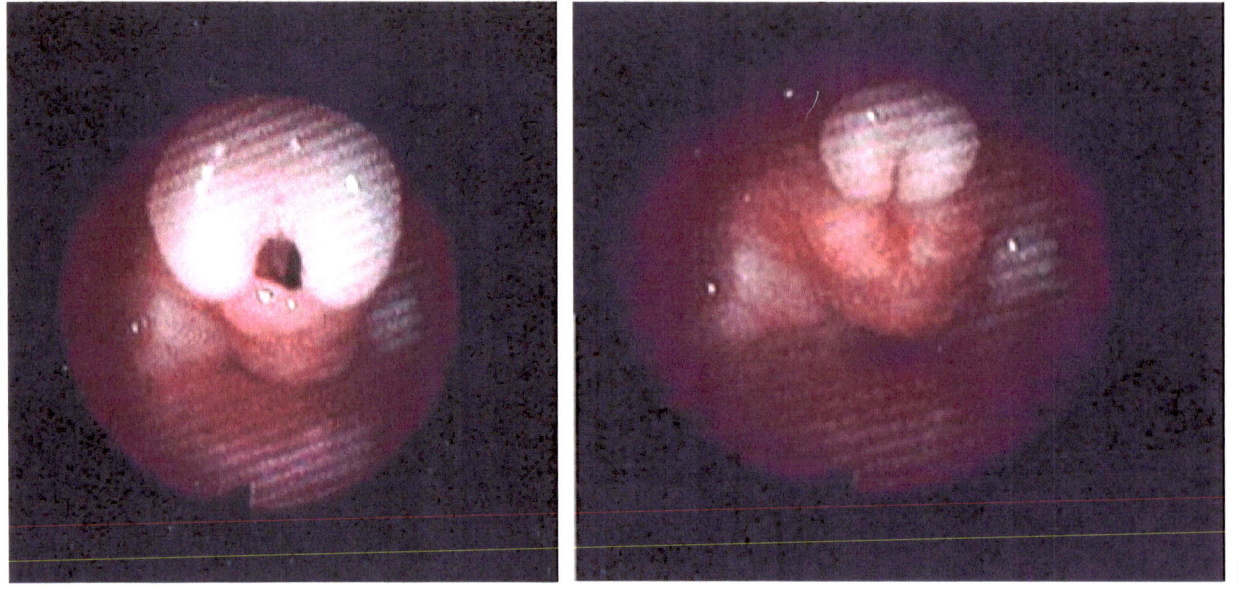

FIGURE 13.2. Endoscopic appearance, laryngomalacia. (**A**) Severe laryngomalacia during expiration. (**B**) Same patient during inspiration with total collapse of the airway. (Courtesy of Mitchell B. Austin, MD, Department of Otolaryngology, Medical College of Georgia.)

Arnold-Chiari malformation is the most common cause of bilateral vocal cord paralysis, which probably results from brain stem compression and stretching of vagal nerve rootlets due to caudal displacement of the brain stem or cerebellum into the foramen magnum [1–3,19–21,24–26].

Infants with bilateral vocal cord paralysis present with marked inspiratory stridor and respiratory distress, although the cry is often normal. Aspiration leading to recurrent pneumonia is common. The diagnosis of vocal cord paralysis is suggested by the history and physical examination and confirmed by endoscopy. Radiologic evaluation is important to evaluate for potential etiologies (e.g., head CT for bilateral vocal cord paralysis). Most cases of unilateral vocal cord paralysis can be managed with observation alone. Upright positioning may be required to alleviate feeding difficulties and minimize the risk of aspiration. However, children with bilateral vocal cord paralysis often require urgent management of the airway. A tracheotomy is generally necessary and should remain in place for 2 years to allow for potential recovery of function. If spontaneous recovery does not occur, further operative procedures (e.g., arytenoidectomy) may be attempted in an effort to decannulate the patient [1–3,19–21,24–26].

Congenital Subglottic Stenosis

Congenital subglottic stenosis is the third most common laryngeal anomaly, accounting for nearly 15% of all cases [1–3,19–21,21,27,28]. Males are affected twice as commonly as females. Congenital subglottic stenosis can be classified into a membranous subtype and a cartilaginous subtype. The membranous subtype results from circumferential submucosal hypertrophy with excess fibrous connective tissue and mucous glands and is the most common and milder form of congenital subglottic stenosis. The cartilaginous subtype

results from an abnormal shape of the cricoid cartilage. Infants with congenital subglottic stenosis usually present within the first 2–3 months of life with biphasic stridor, often following an upper respiratory tract infection or *croup-like illness*. Even the slightest degree of inflammation and edema can precipitate partial to complete airway obstruction in these infants. Milder cases often present as recurrent croup.

Diagnosis is made with a suggestive history and endoscopy. The severity of stenosis is assessed by the ability to pass a tracheal tube through the airway using the rigid bronchoscope. Congenital subglottic stenosis is diagnosed when the lumen diameter is less than 4 mm in a term infant or less than 3 mm in a preterm infant. Although the majority of cases of congenital subglottic stenosis resolve spontaneously with normal growth, laryngotracheoplasty may be required in severe cases [1–3,19–21,21,27,28].

Subglottic Hemangiomas

Subglottic hemangiomas are seldom present at birth and usually present before 6 months of age with worsening respiratory distress. Females appear to be affected twice as often as males. Initially, children present with signs and symptoms similar to croup. Inspiratory stridor is exacerbated by agitation and crying. As the lesion grows, symptoms worsen, and affected infants develop biphasic stridor. Approximately one-half of children will also have cutaneous hemangiomas on the head and neck. Diagnosis is made by identification of the lesion by rigid bronchoscopy. Management is usually conservative, as most hemangiomas will regress spontaneously, usually disappearing by 2 years of age. Larger lesions may require surgical intervention via one of several options, including carbon dioxide laser ablation, cryosurgery, intralesional interferon or sclerosing agent injection, and systemic steroids. Tracheotomy is only rarely necessary [1–3,19–21,27,28–31].

Congenital Laryngeal Webs and Atresia

Congenital laryngeal webs are rare and arise from defects in recannulation of the embryonic larynx during the third month of gestation, with laryngeal atresia representing the extreme end of the spectrum of these disorders [1–3,19–21,27,28,32–34]. Laryngeal webs are often noted at birth, presenting with upper airway obstruction, a weak or feeble cry, and occasionally aphonia. Complete obstruction of the airway may occur and requires immediate recognition and definitive management. Nearly 75% of webs are located at the level of the glottis and are usually anterior in position. Supraglottic and subglottic webs comprise the remaining 25% of children. Nearly one third of children will also have associated anomalies of the respiratory tract, most commonly congenital subglottic stenosis. Diagnosis is easily made with rigid bronchoscopy. Management includes close observation when the web is small to emergent tracheotomy when the web is large. Laryngeal atresia, also known as *congenital high airway obstruction syndrome* (CHAOS) is fortunately an extremely rare anomaly [32,33]. It presents with immediate airway obstruction upon clamping of the umbilical cord unless there is a concomitant tracheoesophageal fistula (TEF) that is sufficiently large to sustain adequate ventilation. Physical examination reveals a newborn with markedly severe respiratory distress associated with strong respiratory efforts and inability to inhale air or cry. Emergent tracheotomy must be performed; otherwise, death is imminent. If a TEF is present, mask ventilation and esophageal intubation may be sufficient to stabilize the infant before tracheotomy. Successful treatment with the ex utero intrapartum treatment (EXIT) procedure has been encouraging [32,33,35–38].

Laryngeal Clefts

Laryngotracheoesophageal clefts are extremely rare, accounting for 0.3%–0.5% of all laryngeal malformations [1–3,19–21,27,28,32–34,39,40]. They result from a failure of the tracheoesophageal septum to fuse at approximately 35 days of gestation and, if complete, are associated with 90% mortality. The clinical presentation depends on the severity of the cleft. Infants typically present with recurrent aspiration and respiratory distress following a feeding. Coughing, choking, and stridor are commonly observed, and there is a history of maternal polyhydramnios in more than 30% of cases. Diagnosis is made by endoscopy, although radiographic studies are typically helpful during the initial evaluation of a suspected laryngeal cleft. Chest radiography often shows aspiration pneumonia, while lateral radiographs of the neck frequently show a posteriorly displaced tracheal tube or an anteriorly displaced nasal or oral gastric tube. Minor clefts can usually be treated medically (positioning, antireflux medications, etc.) with close observation. Surgical management is required for more severe cases.

Bifid Epiglottis

Congenital bifid epiglottis is a rare anomaly that usually presents with a constellation of signs and symptoms similar to laryngomalacia [1–3,19–21,27,28,41]. The midline defect in the epiglottis often renders it incompetent in protecting the airway during feeding, and aspiration is common in affected infants. Surgical management is often required in severe cases.

Laryngoceles and Laryngeal Cysts

Laryngoceles are sac-like, air-filled structures corresponding to a remnant of the lateral laryngeal air sac of the higher anthropoid apes. They may be internal (i.e., remaining within the laryngeal cartilage) or external (i.e., extending through the thyrohyoid membrane). Laryngeal cysts are saccular cysts that are similar in their embryologic development to laryngoceles. However, in contrast to the air-filled laryngocele, saccular cysts are fluid filled. Both laryngoceles and laryngeal cysts may present with stridor and respiratory distress in severe cases. Surgery is indicated when airway obstruction is severe [1–3,19–21,27,28,42–44].

Tracheal Anomalies

As a group, tracheal anomalies are much less common than laryngeal anomalies [1–3,19–21,27,28,45–49]. Because of the normal compliance of the trachea and its position within the thorax, the trachea dilates somewhat with inspiration and narrows with expiration, reflecting the difference between intrathoracic and intraluminal pressures. This phenomenon is accentuated whenever intrathoracic pressure is substantially greater than intraluminal pressure, as during forced expiration, cough, and the Valsalva maneuver or if there is any degree of anatomic obstruction in the trachea. Therefore, tracheal anomalies typically present with expiratory stridor, although the stridor may also have an inspiratory component if there is a fixed obstruction. Feeding difficulties are also common, as the bolus of food passing through the esophagus may compress the trachea and exacerbate the severity of obstruction.

Tracheomalacia

Tracheomalacia [45–49] is a relatively uncommon anomaly that results from an intrinsic weakness in the cartilaginous support of the trachea such that it is prone to collapse, especially during expiration. If the main bronchi are also affected (which they are commonly), the term *tracheobronchomalacia* is used. Although much less common than laryngomalacia, tracheomalacia is the most common congenital anomaly of the trachea. Primary (or congenital) and secondary (acquired) forms exist. The secondary or acquired form of tracheomalacia is perhaps more common than the congenital form and is frequently associated with prematurity and extrinsic vascular compression of the trachea. Several conditions are commonly associated with tracheomalacia, including tracheoesophageal fistula (see below), congenital heart disease, and gastroesophageal reflux [1–3,19–21,27,28,45–49].

Tracheomalacia commonly presents with expiratory stridor (in contrast to inspiratory stridor) and a croup-like cough. Tracheomalacia is frequently misdiagnosed as asthma. Most of these infants have impaired clearance of secretions as a result of luminal closure during cough and are therefore prone to aspiration pneumonia. Feeding difficulties are also common. Diagnosis is made by a relevant history and endoscopic examination of the trachea (Figure 13.3). Tracheomalacia is self-limiting in the majority of cases and rarely requires surgical intervention. Most infants outgrow the symptoms by age 18–24 months. However, when severe, tracheomalacia is potentially life-threatening. Historically, tracheotomy and long-term mechanical ventilatory support have been the mainstays of treatment. Recent technological improvements in noninvasive positive pressure ventilation (NIPPV) will likely improve the outcomes of children with this

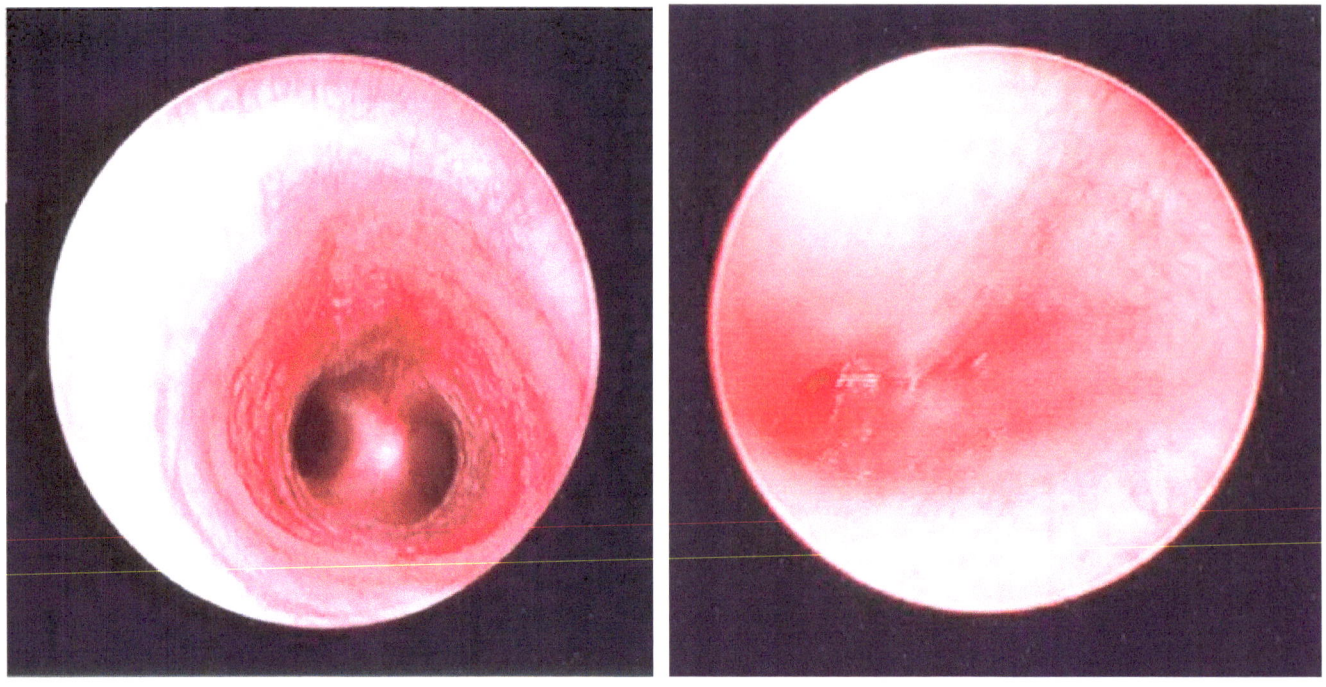

A   B

FIGURE 13.3. Endoscopic appearance, tracheomalacia. **(A)** Normal trachea. **(B)** Child with severe tracheomalacia demonstrating total collapse of the airway during expiration. The child required tracheotomy. (Courtesy of Mitchell B. Austin, MD, Department of Otolaryngology, Medical College of Georgia.)

disease. Aortopexy is now widely considered the surgical procedure of choice, although this is by no means a panacea because of a small, but significant, failure rate and potential for complications [1–3,19–21,27,28,45–49].

Tracheal Stenosis

Tracheal stenosis is also rare with a variable clinical presentation depending on its severity [1–3,19–21,27,28,45–50). It is best viewed in the context of laryngeal stenosis, as the two entities frequently coexist; hence use of the term *laryngotracheal stenosis* is preferred. Isolated tracheal stenosis is most commonly a result of a complete, circumferential tracheal ring. Associated anomalies are common and include tracheoesophageal fistula, pulmonary hypoplasia, and skeletal abnormalities. These infants typically present with biphasic stridor, although the expiratory phase is usually more pronounced. Failure to thrive because of feeding difficulties is also common. Diagnosis is made by endoscopy, although CT or magnetic resonance imaging (MRI) of the trachea may be helpful. Surgical options for severe cases include endoscopic dilation, resection of the stenotic segment with end-to-end reanastomosis, laryngotracheoplasty with either costal cartilage interposition or a pericardial patch, and slide tracheoplasty. If the stenotic segment is short, resection and end-to-end anastomosis is generally preferred. Slide tracheoplasty, frequently performed under cardiopulmonary bypass, is rapidly becoming the preferred technique for long segment stenosis [51–55].

Tracheoesophageal Fistula

Tracheoesophageal fistula results from an incomplete development of the tracheoesophageal septum and is usually associated with esophageal atresia [56]. Infants with TEF typically present soon after birth with recurrent pneumonia, choking or coughing during feeding, stridor, and retention of secretions. Direct visualization of the fistulous tract on rigid bronchoscopy is diagnostic, although a barium swallow is helpful as well. Surgical treatment is curative. As discussed earlier, children with TEF frequently have tracheomalacia and/or stenosis.

Vascular Compression on the Trachea

Nonvascular causes of extrinsic compression of the trachea include thoracic masses such as mediastinal tumors and cystic hygromas. The three most common vascular causes of extrinsic compression of the trachea and airways include (1) double aortic arch, in which the trachea and esophagus are completely encircled by bilateral aortic arches (derived from the embryonic paired fourth aortic arches); (2) pulmonary artery sling, in which an aberrant left pulmonary artery arises abnormally from the right pulmonary artery; and (3) aberrant innominate artery, which causes compression of the anterior trachea [57–59]. Affected children typically present with stridor, wheezing, lobar atelectasis, and recurrent pneumonia. As mentioned earlier, tracheomalacia at the site of the extrinsic compression is common. Surgical correction is required in severe cases.

Infectious Disorders of the Pediatric Airway

The clinical spectrum of infectious causes of upper airway obstruction has changed dramatically in the past few decades, especially following the introduction of vaccines against diphtheria and *Haemophilus influenzae*. Many of the infectious causes of upper airway obstruction pose less of a threat today as a result of advances in

TABLE 13.2. Common causes of upper airway obstruction in children.

Anatomic
    Altered level of consciousness (airway muscle laxity)
    Postextubation airway obstruction
    Tonsillar hypertrophy
    Subglottic stenosis (acquired or congenital)
    Macroglossia
    Vocal cord paralysis
External or internal compression
    Tumor
    Hemangioma
    Hematoma
    Cyst
    Papilloma
    Vascular rings and slings
Infectious
    Laryngotracheobronchitis (croup)
    Peritonsillar abscess
    Retropharyngeal abscess
    Bacterial tracheitis
    Supraglottitis (epiglottitis)
    Infectious mononucleosis
Miscellaneous
    Postextubation airway obstruction
    Angioedema
    Foreign body aspiration
    Airway trauma

prevention, early diagnosis, and treatment. Nevertheless, infectious causes of upper airway obstruction remain an important source of morbidity and potential mortality in the pediatric age group (Tables 13.2 and 13.3) [60–63].

Viral Laryngotracheobronchitis

Viral laryngotracheobronchitis, or croup, is the most common infectious cause of upper airway obstruction in children, with an annual incidence of 18 per 1,000 children in the United States [61–64]. Croup primarily affects children between the ages of 6 months

and 4 years, with a peak incidence between 1 and 2 years of age. Although sporadic cases may occur throughout the year, the peak incidence is during late fall and winter. Males are affected slightly more commonly than females [60,61–64]. Croup is caused by an inflammation affecting the subglottic tissues, occasionally affecting the tracheobronchial tree as well, usually because of a viral infection. Croup is most commonly caused by parainfluenza virus type 1, although parainfluenza virus types 2 and 3, influenzas A and B, respiratory syncytial virus (RSV), adenovirus, and *Mycoplasma pneumoniae* are commonly implicated as well [65–68].

Most children with croup can be managed in the outpatient setting, although between 1% and 30% of children require hospitalization, and 2% of hospitalized children require tracheal intubation and mechanical ventilatory support [69,70]. Children with croup typically present with several days of viral prodromal symptoms (cough, coryza, rhinorrhea, low-grade fever) with progressively worsening hoarseness, the classic "seal-like" or barky cough, and stridor (most commonly inspiratory in nature, although biphasic stridor is indicative of a more severe degree of airway obstruction). Conversely, children with high fevers and/or a toxic appearance are more likely to have a more serious infection, such as bacterial tracheitis, retropharyngeal abscess, or supraglottitis. The classic harsh cough or bark may progress to inspiratory stridor and frank dyspnea in severe cases, and various scales have been devised to quantify the severity of stridor and document the progression of the illness and subsequent response to therapy [71–74].

Although radiographic examination is useful to rule out other important causes of airway obstruction (e.g., supraglottitis, foreign body, retropharyngeal abscess), the classic *steeple sign* (Figure 13.4) may be absent in as many as half of children with croup [65,75,76]. When visible, the subglottic narrowing is dynamic and is more accentuated during inspiration because of the more negative intraluminal airway pressure during inspiration [77]. Children with a long-standing history of stridor or those under 4 months of age should be carefully evaluated for anatomic airway obstruction, such as laryngeal cyst or papillomatosis, vocal cord paralysis

TABLE 13.3. Infectious causes of upper airway obstruction.

	Croup	Epiglottitis	Bacterial tracheitis	Retropharyngeal abscess
Onset	Gradual Viral prodrome 1–7 days	Rapid onset 6–12 hr	Viral prodrome followed by rapid deterioration	Viral prodrome followed by rapid deterioration
Typical age at onset	6 months to 4 years	2–8 years	6 months to 8 years	<5 years
Seasonal occurrence	Late fall to winter	Throughout the year	Fall to winter	Throughout the year
Causative agents	Parainfluenza, respiratory syncytial virus, influenza A	*Haemophilus influenzae* type b (classically), *Streptococcus pneumoniae*, GABHS	*Staphylococcus aureus* (classically), GABHS, *Streptococcus pneumoniae*	Anaerobic bacteria, GABHS, *Staphylococcus aureus*
Pathology	Subglottic edema	Inflammatory edema of supraglottis	Thick, mucopurulent, membranou stracheal secretions	Abscess formation in the deep cervical fascia
Fever	Low-grade	High fever	High fever	High fever
Cough	"Barking" or "seal-like"	None	Usually absent	Usually absent
Sore throat	None	Severe	None	Severe
Drooling	None	Frequent	None	Frequent
Posture	Any position	Sitting forward, mouth open, neck extended ("tripod position")	Any position	Sitting forward, mouth open, neck extended ("tripod position")
Voice	Normal or hoarse	Muffled	Normal or hoarse	Muffled
Appearance	Nontoxic	Toxic	Toxic	Toxic

Note: GABHS, group A β-hemolytic *Streptococcus*.

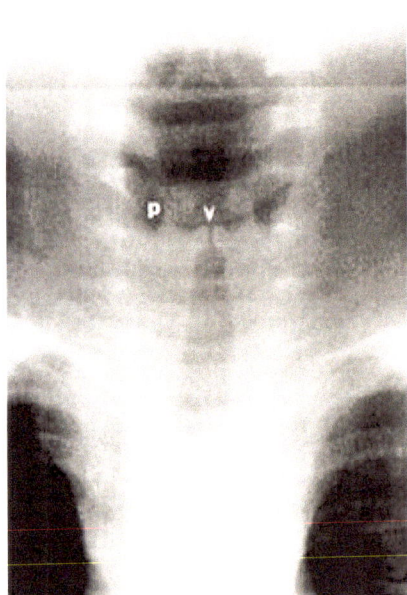 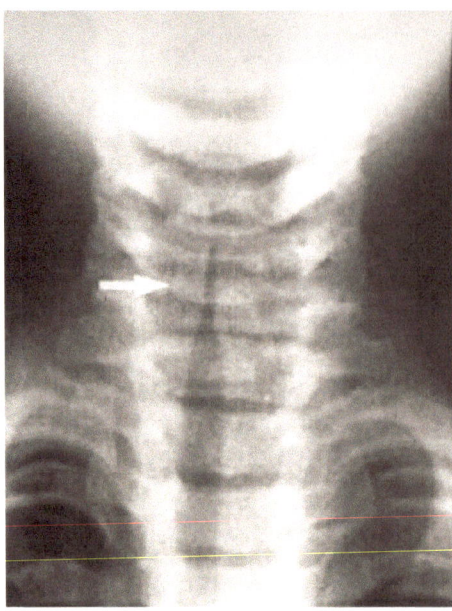

FIGURE 13.4. Typical radiographic appearance of croup demonstrating symmetric narrowing of the subglottic region ("steeple sign"). (**A**) Normal anatomy (v, vestibule; p, pyriform sinuses). (**B**) Subglottic narrowing (arrow) consistent with croup.

A

B

extrinsic airway compression (e.g., vascular ring), or laryngotracheal stenosis.

Croup is generally self-limited and frequently requires only supportive care. Humidification with continuous cool mist has been the standard accepted treatment for many years [75,77–79]. The mechanism by which humidified cool mist improves symptomatology is not well understood and probably reflects a placebo effect [78–80]. Nebulized racemic epinephrine rapidly reduces airway edema and improves symptoms, although the effect is transient and disappears within 2–3 hr of administration [81–86]. Both the racemic and L-isomer forms of epinephrine appear to be safe and effective; however, racemic epinephrine has not been shown to decrease the need for either tracheal intubation or tracheotomy in children with croup [83,85,86]. Rebound or worsening of airway obstruction after the drug effect wears off may occur with the use of racemic epinephrine, and for this reason treated patients should be observed for 4–6 hr after administration [87].

Several recent studies have shown substantial improvement in symptoms following administration of corticosteroids. Administration of corticosteroids appears to improve symptomatology, shorten the duration of hospital stay, and reduce the need for racemic epinephrine [69,88]. A single dose of dexamethasone is usually adequate for mild to moderate croup. The dose of dexamethasone ranges from 0.15 mg/kg of oral preparation to 0.6 mg/kg of parenteral preparation. Children with severe croup who are managed in the pediatric intensive care unit setting may require a more prolonged course of corticosteroids. Although few adequately controlled, randomized studies exist to suggest any benefit to prolonged administration of corticosteroids in critically ill children with acute respiratory failure secondary to croup, the wealth of anecdotal experience would suggest this to be a reasonable practice. Corticosteroids appear to be advantageous in relieving upper airway obstruction regardless of the route of administration [89–92]. Although the precise mechanism of action of corticosteroids in croup is not readily known, the rapid response observed following corticosteroid administration suggests that decreased capillary permeability and peripheral vasoconstriction plays an important role [93]. The antiinflammatory effects of corticosteroids (via inhi-

bition of proinflammatory gene expression) require 6–12 hr for maximal effect [94–96].

The use of helium–oxygen mixtures may be beneficial for some children with croup. Laminar flow is determined by the Reynolds number (Re):

$$Re = 2 V r \rho / \eta$$

where V is the velocity of the air flow, ρ is the density of the air, r is the radius of the airway, and η is the viscosity of the air. When Re is <2,000, laminar flow is present. Conversely, when Re is >4,000, turbulent flow is present. Airway resistance is inversely proportional to the airway radius to the fifth power (r^5) under conditions of turbulent air flow (versus airway radius to the fourth power when laminar flow is present). Helium is a colorless, odorless gas with the lowest density of any gas except hydrogen. As such, helium will reduce Re and change a turbulent flow pattern to a laminar flow pattern, resulting in lower airway resistance and improved bulk flow [97]. Helium–oxygen gas (heliox) mixtures have been shown to improve the work of breathing and gas exchange in children with croup [98–104]. Heliox has few side effects and is easy to administer by face mask, hood, or tracheal tube in children on mechanical ventilatory support [104]. To minimize the risk of asphyxia secondary to administration of 100% helium, heliox mixtures should only be administered from premixed helium–oxygen cylinders. Currently, 80:20, 70:30, and 60:40 helium:oxygen mixtures are available. Therefore, children with a high oxygen requirement are unlikely to benefit (and may actually worsen) from heliox administration. The beneficial effects of helium are reduced with lower ratios of helium to oxygen, although it appears likely that helium will have at least some therapeutic value even at low concentrations [97,105]. Heliox may also be an effective alternative for those children in whom the administration of corticosteroids or racemic epinephrine is contraindicated. Additionally, heliox may help to prevent the need for tracheal intubation in those children with impending respiratory failure [98–104].

Until the airway inflammation resolves, severe upper airway obstruction may develop and occasionally necessitate tracheal intubation. Before the introduction of corticosteroid therapy, tracheal intubation was required in approximately 2% of children hospitalized with croup [60–63]. Tracheal intubation is now commonly limited to those children who either have preexisting airway abnormalities or who have been tracheally intubated in an outside facility before transfer. Generally, tracheal intubation with a tube smaller than what would be normally predicted for age and weight should be used in the minority of children requiring tracheal intubation and mechanical ventilatory support. Extubation can usually be accomplished within 2–3 days once an air leak has developed around the tracheal tube. Bronchoscopy is reserved for children who fail to develop an air leak after 7 days or who are less than 6 months of age, who have a high likelihood of congenital malformations of the airway [60–63]. Although the etiologies of many infections of upper respiratory tract are viral, there may be bacterial superinfection or injury to the respiratory mucosa that may invite bacterial infection. Uncomplicated croup is viral in origin and should not be treated with antibiotics. Antibiotic therapy may be considered for those children who fail to improve or who require tracheal intubation.

Supraglottis (Epiglottitis)

Epiglottitis is a true emergency, although the term is somewhat misleading as the supraglottic structures are most severely affected. Supraglottitis is perhaps a more appropriate term for this reason. It classically affects children between the ages of 2 and 8 years [60–63]. Historically, supraglottitis was most commonly caused by *Haemophilus influenzae* type B (HIB). *Streptococcus pneumoniae*, group A β-hemolytic *Streptococcus* (GABHS), and *Staphylococcus aureus* are reported more commonly in the post-HIB vaccination era [106–111]. Since the development and widespread use of the conjugated HIB vaccine, there has been a significant decrease in the incidence of supraglottitis. The incidence of supraglottitis in children <5 years of age has decreased from 41 cases per 100,000 in 1987 to 1.3 cases per 100,000 in 1997 [112]. The incidence of supraglottitis appears to have stabilized at around 1.3 cases per 100,000 children, primarily because of low or incomplete vaccination coverage in localized populations, as well as cases of supraglottitis caused by microorganisms other than HIB [113].

Supraglottitis requires a high index of suspicion, especially now in the post-HIB vaccination era when many physicians have never seen a child with true supraglottitis. In addition, especially now in the post-HIB vaccination era, epiglottitis may present with atypical features, especially in children under 2 years of age [107,114,115]. Children classically present with rapidly progressive signs and symptoms, including high fever, irritability, drooling, and respiratory distress (the "4 Ds" include drooling, dysphagia, dyspnea, and dysphonia). These children are toxic in appearance and prefer to rest in the tripod position. Stridor is relatively late and ominous. There is usually no viral prodrome. By the time that affected children present for medical attention, they are generally toxic and have inspiratory stridor [60–63]. The voice tends to be muffled rather than hoarse as in children with croup. Affected children assume a characteristic sniffing position in an attempt to maintain optimal airway patency. These children are usually anxious, which is a strong indication that their airway is significantly compromised.

When supraglottitis is suspected, intraoral examination and lateral neck radiograph should be deferred and only performed if equipment and personnel are available to secure the airway immediately. Excessive manipulation of the child and his or her airway should be avoided to minimize the risk of acute exacerbation of airway obstruction. The appearance on a lateral neck radiograph obtained with hyperextension of the neck is classic (Figure 13.5), although diagnosis is usually confirmed by direct inspection of the airway in the operating room. When a diagnosis of supraglottitis is entertained based on initial history and physical examination, the child should be accompanied by a physician skilled in airway management to the operating room. The child should be allowed to remain in his or her "position of comfort" and all anxiety-provoking procedures (e.g., phlebotomy, oral examination) should be deferred.

Direct laryngoscopy under anesthesia should be performed while maintaining spontaneous breathing [60–63,116–119]. Cultures of the supraglottic region should be obtained, and the trachea should be intubated. Treatment with broad-spectrum antibiotics effective against β-lactamase–producing microorganisms (e.g., a

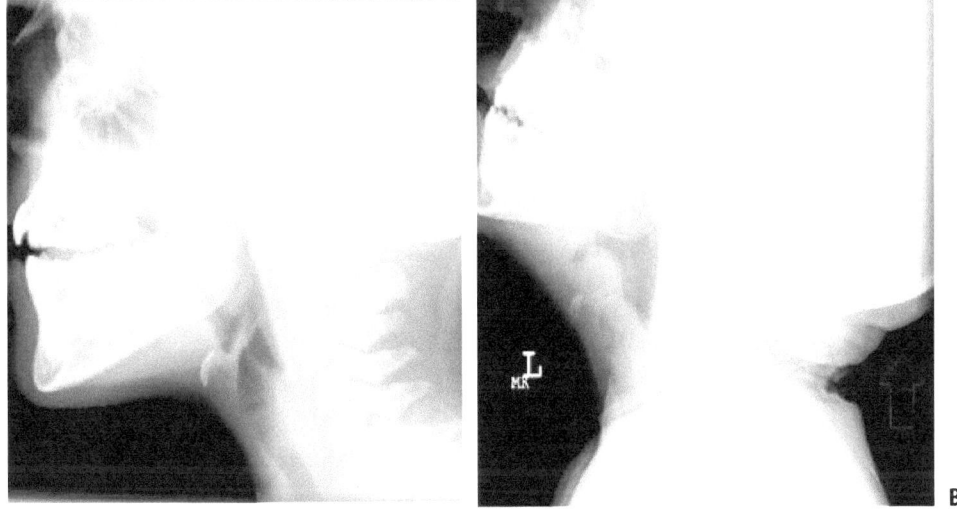

FIGURE 13.5. Typical radiographic appearance of supraglottitis. **(A)** Normal lateral neck x-ray showing normal epiglottis. **(B)** Lateral neck x-ray showing the classic appearance of supraglottitis: loss of cervical lordosis; thick, rounded epiglottis ("thumb sign"); loss of the vallecular air space; and thickening of the aryepiglottic folds.

second- or third-generation cephalosporin such as cefuroxime or ceftriaxone or, alternatively, ampicllin/sulbactam) is initiated once cultures have been obtained [60–63,120,121]. Antibiotic therapy should be tailored to the pathogenic organism, and the duration of antibiotic therapy is determined by the clinical response. Generally, symptomatic improvement and the development of an audible air leak around the tracheal tube occur within 24–48 hr [122]. Despite the virtual elimination of invasive HIB infection, it is important for pediatric intensivists to understand the management issues surrounding patients with supraglottitis to avoid disastrous outcomes.

Bacterial Tracheitis

Bacterial tracheitis, also known as *pseudomembranous croup*, is a relatively uncommon, but potentially life-threatening cause of infectious upper airway obstruction in children [60–63]. It is characterized by thick, mucopurulent, membranous tracheal secretions that do not clear with cough, which have the potential to occlude the airway. Bacterial tracheitis is more insidious than supraglottitis and affects children between the ages of 6 months and 8 years, with a peak incidence during fall and winter [60–63,123–125]. Children frequently present with a viral prodrome of several days' duration, accompanied by low-grade fever, cough, and stridor (similar to croup). The viral prodrome is followed by rapid clinical deterioration characterized by a high fever and upper airway obstruction. Affected children are more toxic in appearance than children with croup. Radiographic examination often is indistinguishable from that of croup (*steeple sign*), and, in fact, the noted similarities between these two disorders have led some authors to suggest that bacterial tracheitis represents a bacterial superinfection of croup.

Historically, bacterial tracheitis is most commonly secondary to *Staph. aureus*, although *Strep. pneumoniae*, GABHS, *H. influenzae*, *Moraxella catarrhalis*, anaerobic bacteria, and viruses have been implicated as well ([23–127]. Infection with the parainfluenza virus has been implicated as the prodromal infection in many cases, further lending credence to the suggestion that bacterial tracheitis represents a bacterial superinfection of croup. Children with bacterial tracheitis are managed using the epiglottis management algorithm described earlier [128]. Direct inspection of the airway under anesthesia should be performed in the operating room and usually reveals subglottic edema with ulcerations, erythema, and pseudomembrane formation in the trachea. Removal of pseudomembranes and dead tissue from the airway at diagnosis, tracheal intubation, and administration of broad-spectrum antibiotics directed against staphylococcal and streptococcal species are the cornerstone of treatment. Empiric therapy should be broadly directed against both Gram-positive and Gram-negative organisms until culture results are available. *Staph. aureus* is treated with a penicillinase-resistant drug, such as methicillin or nafcillin, that has been effective against resistant staphylococci. Anaerobic organisms may be treated with clindamycin. Extubation may be attempted following clinical improvement and the development of an air leak around the tracheal tube, usually within 3–5 days [60–63,128].

Retropharyngeal Abscess

Retropharyngeal abscess has been called "the epiglottitis of the new millennium" [129]. The retropharyngeal space is composed of a loose network of connective tissue and lymph nodes that drain the nasopharynx, paranasal sinuses, middle ear, teeth, and facial bones. Infection and abscess formation in this area generally result from lymphatic spread of infection or direct spread from the nasopharynx, paranasal sinuses, or middle ear. These lymph nodes atrophy during early childhood, thereby decreasing the risk of disease in older children and adolescents [60–63,130–132]. For this reason, trauma (e.g., from placing a pencil or stick in the mouth) and foreign body ingestion account for the majority of cases in older children and adolescents. Most cases of retropharyngeal abscess occur in children less than 5 years of age, so there is a significant overlap in the affected age range compared with supraglottitis and bacterial tracheitis [60–63].

Children with retropharyngeal abscess present with a nonspecific constellation of symptoms that progress to high fever, sore throat, and neck stiffness. Fever, sore throat, dysphagia, drooling, muffled voice, and limited neck movement or torticollis are the most common presenting symptoms. Airway symptoms include stridor or stretor and difficulty in breathing. Symptoms often mimic those of supraglottitis. However, in contrast to supraglottitis, children with retropharyngeal abscess normally have a sore throat and cough for several days before showing symptoms of fever and respiratory distress. The neck stiffness may mimic that seen in children with meningitis such that these children are often evaluated for meningitis. Physical examination may reveal the presence of a bulging unilateral neck mass. Additional physical findings commonly include diffuse erythema, tonsillar exudates, and swelling or bulging of the involved tonsillar region. Cervical adenopathy appears to be greatest on the side of the neck where deep infection is most involved [60–63,133–135].

The diagnosis of retropharyngeal abscess is confirmed by the presence of an abnormally increased prevertebral space on lateral neck radiographs (Figure 13.6). Additional radiographic findings include the presence of gas or air–fluid levels in the retropharyngeal space and the loss of the normal cervical lordosis. Computed tomography with contrast confirms the presence of abscess, determines its extent, and identifies its relationship to the airway [135–137]. Although blood cultures are generally negative, culture of the abscess often yields anaerobic microorganisms such as *Prevotella*, *Porphyromonas, Fusobacterium*, and *Peptostreptococcus* spp., as well as *Staph. aureus*, GABHS, and *H. influenzae* [138].

Treatment with broad-spectrum antibiotics and close observation are highly effective, with drainage of the abscess recommended in children refractory to antibiotic therapy. Complications are rare with early recognition and appropriate treatment, although complications include spontaneous rupture into the pharynx leading to aspiration or spread of the infection laterally to the side of the neck or dissection into the posterior mediastinum through the facial planes and the prevertebral space. Although rare, death can occur from aspiration, upper airway obstruction, erosion into major blood vessels, or extension into the mediastinum with mediastinitis. Tracheal intubation is often necessary to protect the patient from aspiration of the purulent content [60–63,135].

Peritonsillar Abscess ("Quinsy" Tonsillitis)

Peritonsillar abscess (PTA) rarely requires admission to the pediatric intensive care unit, but can lead to significant airway obstruction and respiratory compromise if not recognized and therefore left untreated [139]. Peritonsillar abscess, also known as *quinsy tonsillitis*, is the most common deep space head and neck infection in children and is thought to result from the direct contiguous

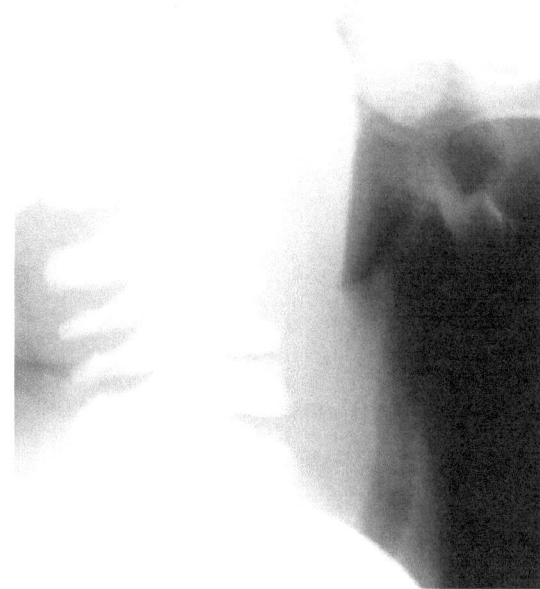

FIGURE 13.6. Typical radiographic appearance of a retropharyngeal abscess (RPA). A retropharyngeal space measured from the most anterior aspect of C2 to the soft tissues of the posterior pharyngeal wall >7 mm (normal 3–6 mm) or a retrotracheal space >14 mm is suggestive of RPA. Normal prevertebral spaces are as follows: anterior to C2, less than or equal to 7 mm; anterior to C3–C4, less than 5 mm or less than 40% of the anteroposterior diameter of the C3 and C4 vertebral bodies. A good rule of thumb to remember is that the upper prevertebral soft tissue should be no wider than one vertebral body width. *Note:* Adequate hyperextension of the head and neck is necessary in order to properly interpret the film. If the head and neck are not properly positioned, the prevertebral space will appear widened. In addition, crying can cause rapid changes in the size of the retropharyngeal space. If there is any doubt, repeated radiographic examination with more hyperextension of the neck, fluoroscopy, or computed tomography imaging is indicated.

spread of infection from the tonsils. Older children and adolescents appear to be most commonly affected, with no seasonal predilection. Children with PTA present with sore throat, neck pain, odynophagia or dysphagia, and fever. Physical examination typically reveals enlargement of the cervical lymph nodes, uvular deviation, and a muffled voice. Treatment options include broad-spectrum antibiotics, needle aspiration of the abscess, incision and drainage, and tonsillectomy. Complications include extension of the infection, acute upper airway obstruction (rare), and rupture of the abscess with aspiration of purulent material and subsequent pneumonia [139,140].

Recurrent Respiratory Papillomatosis

Recurrent respiratory papillomatosis (RRP) is the most common benign laryngeal neoplasm in children and is usually caused by perinatal transmission of human papilloma virus (HPV) 6 or HPV-11. Recurrent respiratory papillomatosis is characterized by the proliferation of squamous epithelial cells in the upper respiratory tract, which occasionally form lesions that cause severe to life-threatening airway obstruction. Affected children are usually between the ages of 2 and 5 years and typically present with stridor and voice changes. The classic triad consists of a first-born child delivered vaginally to an adolescent mother. The diagnosis of RRP is based on endoscopic observation of characteristic lesions. Because any region of the upper aerodigestive tract is involved,

laryngoscopy, bronchoscopy, and careful inspection of the oropharynx and nasopharynx should be performed [61,63,141].

The primary goal of treatment is to prevent airway obstruction while the lesions are in the proliferative phase and minimize any complications of therapy. The mainstay of treatment for RRP is surgical debulking of the lesions in the operating room by one of several methods, including physical debridement with forceps and/or CO_2 laser vaporization, as often as weekly to ensure a safe airway. Adjuvant medical therapies to control aggressive papillomatosis include topical chemotherapy, corticosteroids, podophyllin, tetracycline, autogenous vaccine, immune stimulators, acyclovir, isotretinoin, and interferon. Recently successful treatment of respiratory papillomatosis with adjunctive intralesional injection of cidofovir has been reported [142]. Cidofovir suppresses cytomegalovirus replication by selective inhibition of viral DNA synthesis. Specifically, cidofovir diphosphate, the active intracellular metabolite of cidofovir, inhibits the activity of cytomegalovirus DNA polymerase. Tracheotomy should be avoided if at all possible, although tracheotomy is occasionally required because of acquired tracheal stenosis [61,63,141].

Infectious Mononucleosis

Acute airway obstruction secondary to enlargement of the tonsils and adenoids is a well-recognized complication of infectious mononucleosis [143–146]. Fortunately, this complication is exceedingly rare and appears to occur primarily in younger children. Parenteral corticosteroids are recommended, based primarily on case reports and retrospective series [143–147]. Tracheal intubation may be required if airway obstruction is severe, and in such cases tonsillectomy is generally recommended [148,149].

Noninfectious Disorders of the Pediatric Airway

Obesity

The prevalence of childhood obesity has increased dramatically in recent years. Obesity is associated with decreased upper airway patency, principally related to increased fat deposition in the lateral walls of the pharynx [150] and is a common cause of obstructive sleep apnea syndrome (OSAS) in children [151,152]. Adenotonsillectomy is a commonly performed surgical procedure in this population, and children with OSAS secondary to obesity occasionally require postoperative monitoring and care in the pediatric intensive care unit [153,154].

Angioedema

Angioedema is an immunologically mediated, nonpitting edema that frequently results in acute airway obstruction. It is caused by a kinin- and complement-mediated increase in capillary permeability that leads to edema, usually affecting the head and neck, face, lips, tongue, and larynx. Angioedema is most often caused by ingestion (either food or medication), upper respiratory tract infection, and insect envenomation [62].

Angioedema represents a type 1 anaphylactic reaction and results from immunoglobulin E (IgE)–mediated activation of mast cells leading to the release of histamine and other mediators. Signs and symptoms typically occur approximately 15 min after exposure to an allergen and may lead to respiratory and circulatory collapse. Early symptoms include itching of the eyes, nose, and throat associated with facial flushing and a tightening sensation in the throat. Tachycardia, bronchospasm, urticaria, and a "feeling of impending doom" are other features suggestive of an anaphylactic reaction. Respiratory distress is secondary to edema of the larynx, trachea, and even hypopharynx. The type 1 reaction may also lead to a "late" allergic response causing airway obstruction that appears several hours after exposure to the allergen, such as food or medications. Children with angioedema rapidly improve with intravenous corticosteroids, antihistamines, and subcutaneous epinephrine, which are the mainstay of treatment. The airway should be secured in any child demonstrating signs and symptoms of acute airway obstruction, such as stridor and respiratory distress [62].

Adenotonsillar Hypertrophy

Adenotonsillar hypertrophy is usually the result of infection. The majority of the children with adenotonsillar hypertrophy present with symptoms of chronic airway obstruction, especially at night time; however, a small group will present suddenly during an acute viral upper respiratory tract infection that causes additional swelling. Infectious mononucleosis commonly causes enlargement of lymphoid tissue and may precipitate acute obstruction in rare situations (see preceding paragraphs). Children with underlying craniofacial abnormalities such as Down syndrome [155,156] and children with hypotonia are more susceptible to acute episodes of obstruction from adenotonsillar swelling. Careful questioning of caregivers will often elicit a history of preceding chronic airway obstruction, especially at night time with loud snoring, obstructed and irregular breathing, and even brief periods of apnea. During an acute infection, these symptoms become more severe. Severe, long-standing airway obstruction may progress to cor pulmonale and right heart failure. Therefore, failure to respond to medical therapy is usually an indication for tonsillectomy and adenoidectomy.

Acquired Subglottic Stenosis

A history of previous tracheal intubation dramatically increases the incidence of subglottic injury [157–160]. Subglottic stenosis may be congenital (see preceding paragraphs) or acquired. Before 1965 and before the advent of neonatal intensive care, acquired subglottic stenosis more commonly affected older children and adults following either trauma or infection (particularly supraglottitis, diphtheria, and tuberculosis). Acquired subglottic stenosis in these cases was frequently observed as a complication following tracheotomy and not prolonged tracheal intubation. Significant advances in pediatric critical care medicine, vaccination, and antimicrobial therapy have decreased the incidence of tracheotomy in this age group [157–160], and since 1965 the majority of cases of acquired subglottic stenosis involve children who develop subglottic stenosis following prolonged tracheal intubation because of preterm delivery. Acquired subglottic stenosis occurs in 1.8% of infants less than 1,500 g and in 1 in 678 of infants more than 1,500 g [158].

Affected children generally present with feeding difficulty, changes in voice, stridor (usually biphasic), and respiratory distress. The feeding problems are so severe that failure to thrive is common. Occasionally affected children will present with recurrent croup or asthma that is refractory to medical therapy. The mainstay for diagnosis of subglottic stenosis is rigid bronchoscopy under general anesthesia. Flexible broncoscopy may help to identify the level of airway collapse. Computed tomography or MRI scan may be necessary to rule out the possibility of extrinsic vascular compression. Finally, affected children should undergo a thorough evaluation for swallowing dysfunction, gastroesophageal reflux, and pulmonary function before surgical correction. Surgical options include an anterior cricoid spilt, tracheotomy, and laryngotracheoplasty [157,159,161–164].

Laryngeal Neoplasms and Mediastinal Masses

With the exception of laryngeal papillomatosis, laryngeal tumors are rare in children. Some of the rapidly developing malignant mediastinal masses (e.g., lymphomas, certain types of acute leukemias) may impinge on the intrathoracic trachea and lead to severe respiratory compromise. Aggressive medical therapy should be commenced immediately to decrease the size of tumor mass. Tracheal intubation should only be considered for severe respiratory compromise, as these masses may also impinge on the bronchial tree distal to the tip of the endotracheal tube and will not improve with positive-pressure ventilation [165–168].

Airway Trauma

Damage to the upper airway can occur from multiple causes, including foreign body aspiration, thermal or chemical injury, and direct trauma to the airway itself, either blunt or penetrating.

Postextubation Stridor

Tracheal intubation, although vital to facilitate mechanical ventilation in the intensive care and operating room setting, is associated with the potential development of glottic or subglottic edema (Figure 13.7), resulting in stridor on extubation [169]. Postextubation stridor is an inspiratory stridor that occurs within 24 hr of extubation and is associated with tachypnea, increased work of breathing, and occasionally the need for reintubation. Postextubation stridor is a relatively common problem and occurs in as may as 37% of critically ill children [170]. Postextubation stridor may prolong length of stay in the intensive care unit, particularly if airway obstruction is severe and reintubation proves necessary. Reactive edema develops in the glottic or subglottic mucosa because of pressure necrosis and often worsens upon removal of the tracheal tube [169–171].

Historically, cuffed tracheal tubes have not been generally recommended for children less than 8 years of age. Using an uncuffed tracheal tube, for example, does allow a tube of larger internal diameter to be used, minimizing resistance to air flow and the work of breathing in the spontaneously breathing child. A prolonged period of tracheal intubation and a poorly fitted tracheal tube are significant risk factors for damage to the tracheal mucosa regardless of whether the tracheal tube is cuffed or uncuffed. Cuffed tracheal tubes may have significant advantages over uncuffed tracheal tubes, including better control of air leakage and decreased risk of aspiration and infection in mechanically ventilated children. Therefore, cuffed tracheal tubes are being used with greater frequency in this age group [172,173], especially when high inflation pressures are required to provide adequate oxygenation and ventilation in the setting of severe acute lung disease. The available data suggest that there is no difference in the incidence of

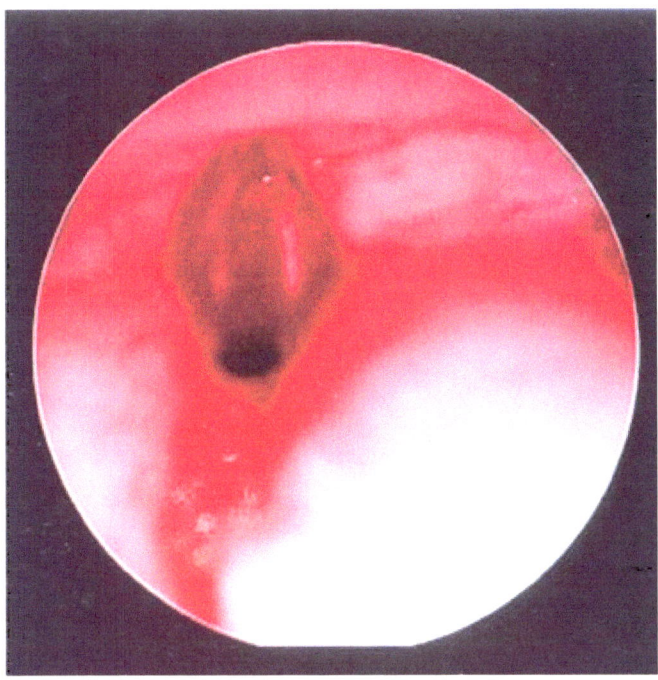

Figure 13.7. Endoscopic appearance, subglottic edema from prolonged tracheal intubation. (Courtesy of Mitchell B. Austin, MD, Department of Otolaryngology, Medical College of Georgia.)

postextubation stridor in children who were tracheally intubated with cuffed tubes compared with those who received uncuffed tubes [174–176].

There are several factors associated with postextubation stridor, including age, size of tracheal tube, and type of injury [170,171,177]. Patients suffering from burn and trauma appear to be at particularly significant risk [170]. Children with trisomy 21 are also at significant risk of developing postextubation stridor [155,156]. Children with trisomy 21 have smaller airways than other children because of an overall decrease in the diameter of the tracheal lumen. Tracheal intubation should therefore be performed with a tracheal tube at least two sizes smaller than would be used in a child of the same age without trisomy 21 in order to avert potential trauma to the airway [178].

The *air-leak test* before extubation is a poor predictor of extubation success, although it may predict the presence of postextubation stridor with some degree of accuracy [179,180]. Several treatment options for postextubation stridor exist, although none has been shown to prevent subsequent reintubation in severe cases. The vasoconstrictive properties of racemic epinephrine and its proven efficacy in the treatment of croup have led to its routine use immediately following extubation in many neonatal and pediatric intensive care units [81–86,181]. The use of corticosteroids in the prevention and/or treatment of postextubation stridor are advocated by many pediatric intensivists, although there is very little evidence to support the universal use of corticosteroids at this time. Dexamethasone at a dose of 1 to 1.5 mg/kg/day every 6–8 hr (maximum daily dose 40 mg/day) has also been administered in an attempt to interrupt the progressive cycle of inflammation that results in edema of injured tissue following extubation. Again, the evidence that this therapy prevents reintubation is limited [182–186], although a recent meta-analysis suggested a possible benefit

[186]. Regardless, in a recent national survey of pediatric critical care fellowship program directors, 66% of those surveyed continue to rely on the air-leak test and use corticosteroids to prevent postextubation stridor and extubation failure. Furthermore, the majority stated that they would delay extubation and administer corticosteroids in the presence an air leak of ≥30 cm H_2O [187]. Finally, helium–oxygen mixtures (see preceding discussion) have also been used in several studies [188–191]. Heliox should be viewed only as a temporizing measure until either the aforementioned therapies become effective or the disease process naturally resolves. In the majority of cases, postextubation stridor is self-limited, although reintubation is occasionally required. Unfortunately, reintubation further exacerbates the reactive airway edema. Ideally, a smaller tracheal tube (generally one size smaller) than previously used should be placed with the hope of causing less airway injury. The new tracheal tube is generally left in place until air leak is observed 24–48 hr later. Anatomic airway problems such as subglottic stenosis and tracheal compression should be considered if postextubation stridor persists following the second attempt at extubation.

Foreign Body Aspiration

Foreign body aspiration is an important cause of accidental death in infants and young children compounded by the fact that infants seem to place almost any object in their mouths [192]. Although most foreign bodies pass through the vocal cords and lodge in the lower airways, laryngeal foreign bodies are not uncommon and are immediately life threatening. The clinical presentation depends on the location of the foreign body as well as the degree of obstruction. Importantly, the actual aspiration event is not always identified, and a high index of suspicion is required. Foreign bodies that are lodged in the glottic or subglottic airway (extrathoracic obstruction) often produce symptoms that mimic croup such as sudden onset of stridor and respiratory distress. In contrast, foreign bodies lodged in the distal trachea (intrathoracic obstruction) tend to produce coughing and wheezing, mimicking asthma or bronchiolitis.

The most commonly aspirated foreign bodies include vegetable matter such as peanuts (Figure 13.8), grapes, and popcorn [192]. Large objects that are lodged in the proximal esophagus and apply pressure to the posterior larynx may also produce stridor and signs of upper airway obstruction. Coins are the most common foreign bodies ingested (Figure 13.9) [193,194]. Coins are radiopaque and usually easy to remove via rigid esophagoscopy. Children with a history of choking and respiratory distress should undergo immediate rigid bronchoscopy, which is both diagnostic and therapeutic. Radiographs may be helpful if the child is otherwise stable. Most distal tracheal or bronchial foreign objects can often be identified on inspiratory/expiratory films, lateral decubitus films, or chest fluoroscopy. Lateral neck radiographs are helpful if the foreign body is radiopaque (see Figure 13.9). However, most aspirated foreign bodies are not radiopaque and lodge in the bronchi. The presence of atelectasis (i.e., distal to a bronchus that is completely occluded by a foreign body) or air trapping and hyperinflation (i.e., distal to a partially obstructing foreign body), which are viewed best on expiratory films, are findings that are highly suggestive of foreign body aspiration (Figure 13.10) [195,196]. Basic life support maneuvers (Figures 13.11–13.13) should be initiated in the field whenever possible. Rigid bronchoscopy is the gold standard for diagnosis of foreign body aspiration and is the treatment of choice [192]. Occasionally, tracheotomy is required. If bronchoscopic

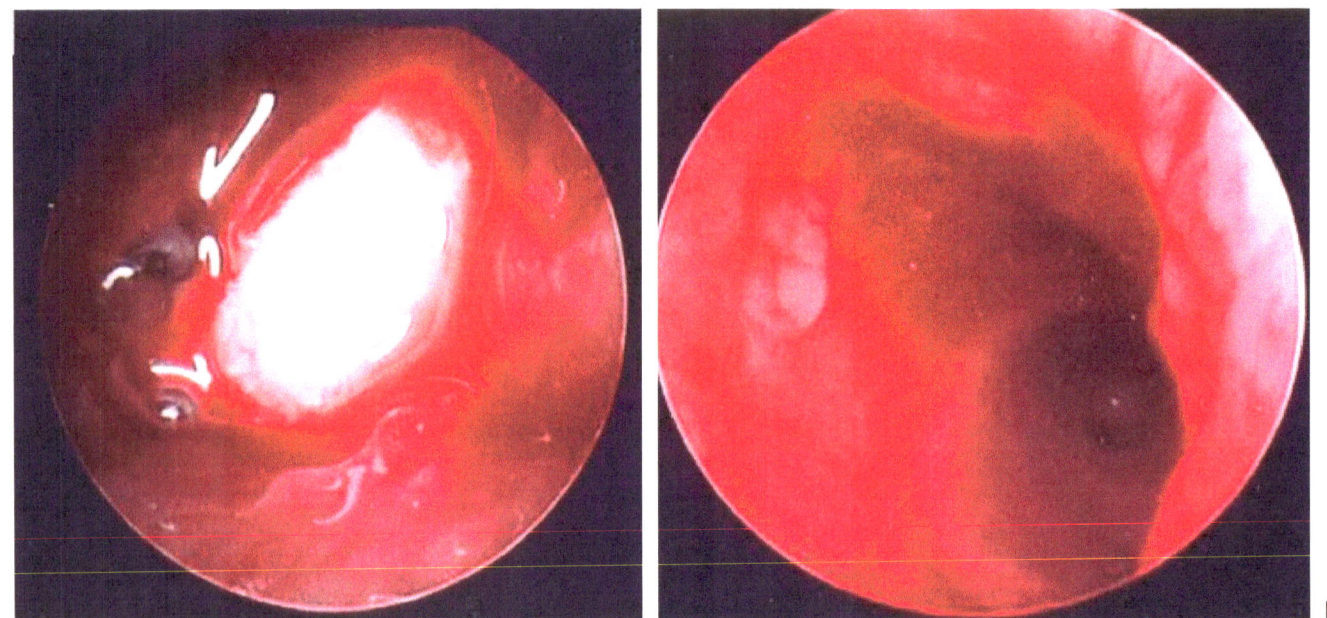

Figure 13.8. Endoscopic appearance, foreign body aspiration (in this case, a peanut is lodged in the right main bronchus) before **(A)** and after **(B)** removal. Note the resultant tissue reaction and formation of granulation tissue. (Courtesy of Mitchell B. Austin, MD, Department of Otolaryngology, Medical College of Georgia.)

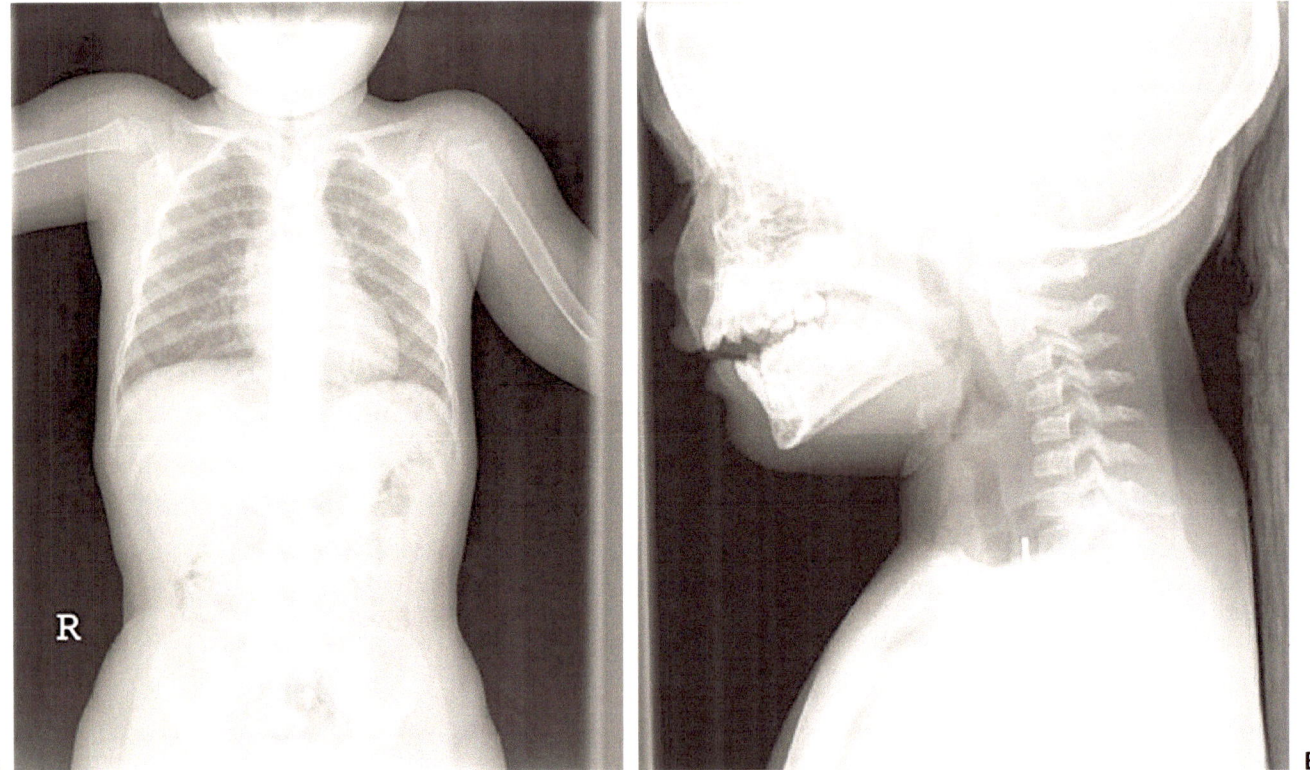

Figure 13.9. Radiopaque foreign body (coin) in the esophagus. **(A)** Anteroposterior chest view. **(B)** Lateral neck view.

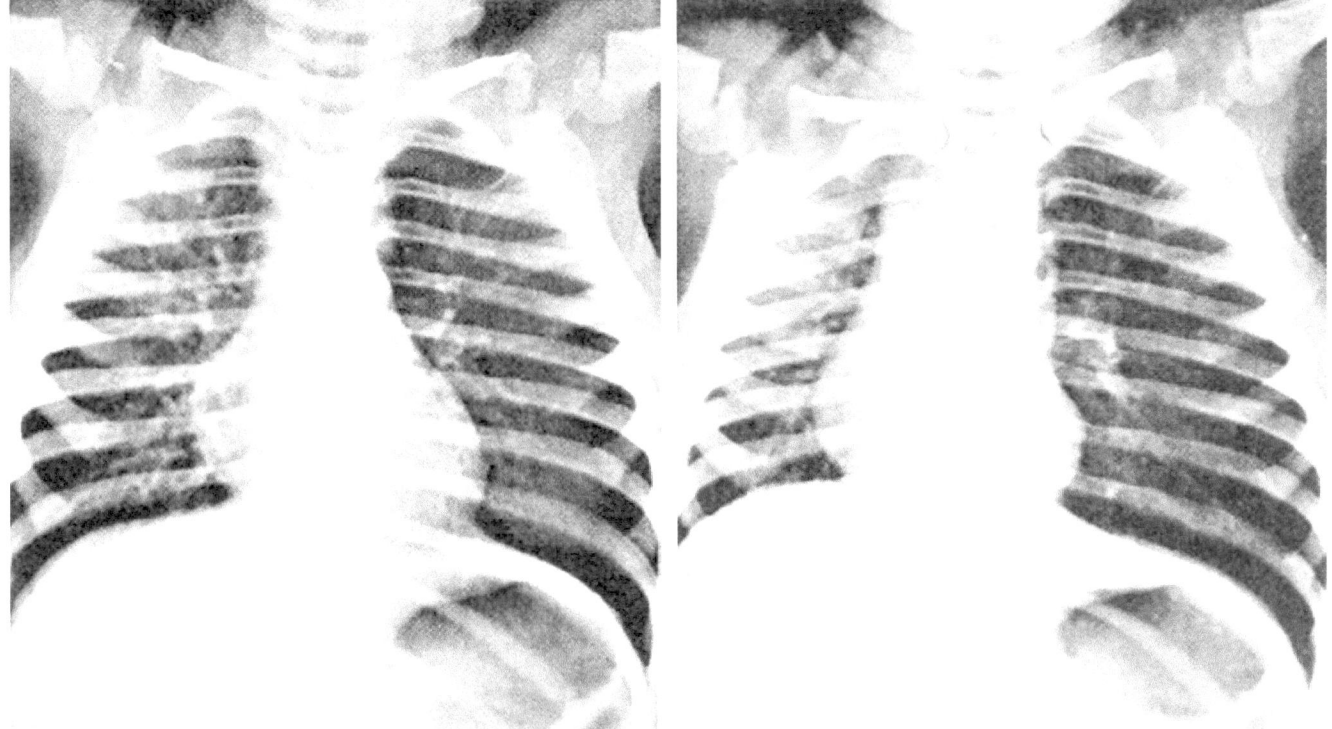

A   **B**

FIGURE 13.10. Foreign body aspiration. Inspiratory and expiratory chest radiographs demonstrate hyperinflation caused by a peanut fragment in the left main stem bronchus. (A) The inspiratory film appears relatively normal except for a slight mediastinal shift to the right. (B) In expiration, the left lung remains overaerated (i.e., ball-valve mechanism), and the mediastinum moves far to the right.

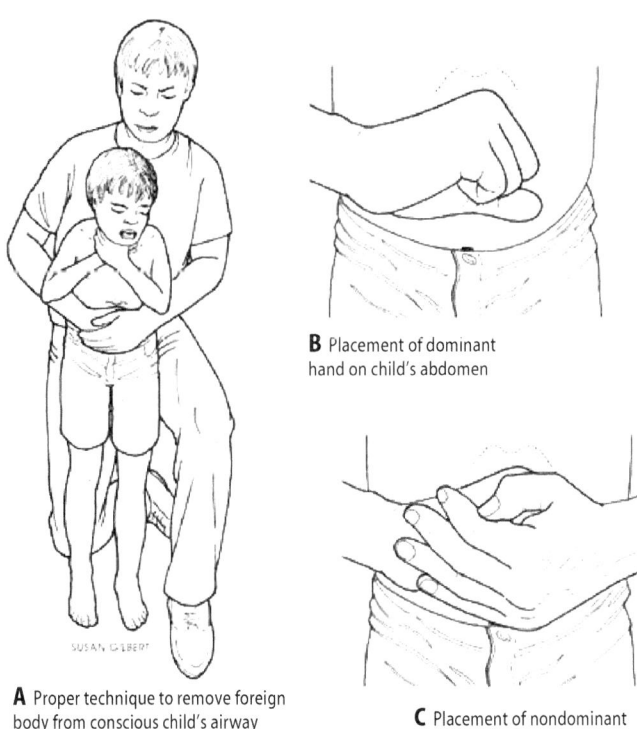

B Placement of dominant hand on child's abdomen

A Proper technique to remove foreign body from conscious child's airway

C Placement of nondominant hand on child's abdomen

FIGURE 13.11. Basic life support—removal of foreign body in the airway in a conscious child. (Reprinted from Foltin GL, Tunik MG, Cooper A, Markenson D, Treiber M, Phillips R, Karpeles T. Teaching Resource for Instructors in Prehospital Pediatrics. New York: Center for Pediatric Emergency Medicine; 1998.)

extraction is unsuccessful, pulmonary lobectomy may be necessary. Foreign bodies often elicit a local inflammatory response, which is generally self-limited. Racemic epinephrine and systemic corticosteroids may be beneficial in this scenario.

Inhalational Injury

Life-threatening airway obstruction may develop as a result of inhalational injury, laryngeal burns, or caustic ingestions. Any child with a scald injury to the face or neck should be evaluated for potential inhalational injury. Inhalational injury should also be suspected in children with any of the following signs or symptoms: evidence of soot in sputum or vomitus, burns of the face, singed nasal hairs, lip burns, wheezing, stridor, or the presence of severe burns. An aggressive approach with early endoscopic evaluation in the operating room suite and management of the airway with either tracheal intubation or tracheotomy is recommended.

Direct Trauma

Although direct trauma resulting in serious injury to the craniofacial skeleton and larynx is relatively uncommon, the types of injuries sustained are likely to be significant and potentially life threatening. The anatomic features of the pediatric airway (e.g., cephalad position of the larynx) may explain the relative infrequency of airway injuries in children versus adults. However, although the pediatric larynx is soft, pliable, and less likely to fracture, the ligamentous and soft tissue support is less well-developed such that laryngotracheal separation is not uncommon [197–203].

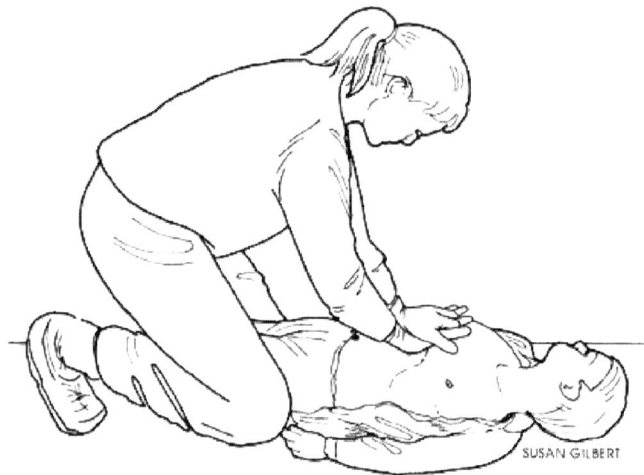

Proper technique to remove foreign body from unconscious child's airway

FIGURE 13.12. Basic life support—removal of foreign body in the airway in an unconscious child. (Reprinted from Foltin GL, Tunik MG, Cooper A, Markenson D, Treiber M, Phillips R, Karpeles T. Teaching Resource for Instructors in Prehospital Pediatrics. New York: Center for Pediatric Emergency Medicine; 1998.)

Blunt trauma to the airway appears to be more common in children than is penetrating trauma and is more common in the adolescent age group [197–203]. The most frequent causes of injury are motor vehicle accidents or direct blows to the larynx. Edema and hematoma formation frequently lead to acute upper airway obstruction. Although less common than in adults, laryngeal fractures occasionally occur. Laryngotracheal separation, although relatively uncommon, is potentially life-threatening. The severity of airway obstruction dictates the extent of the initial evaluation and management. An unstable airway should be immediately secured using the flexible bronchoscope. Tracheal intubation without endoscopic evaluation is best avoided. If immediate surgical intervention is required, tracheotomy is preferable to cricothyrotomy. If the airway is stable, radiographic evaluation should include chest radiograph (to look for associated injuries, such as pneumothorax, pneumomediastinum, or subcutaneous emphysema), lateral neck radiograph (to evaluate the cervical spine), and CT. A barium swallow may be helpful to rule out the possibility of esophageal tear or laceration [197–203].

Tracheotomy

The indications for performing tracheotomy in children have changed significantly in the past 30 years [204–207]. Historically, the most common indication for tracheotomy was infectious upper airway obstruction secondary to epiglottitis, diphtheria, or viral laryngotracheobronchitis. The advent of vaccines against *Corynebacterium diphtheriae* and *H. influenzae* as well as the increased use of tracheal intubation has almost eliminated the need for tracheotomy in these children. Common indications now include prolonged tracheal intubation (e.g., prematurity), neurologic impairment (e.g., cerebral palsy, Werdnig-Hoffman syndrome, hypoxic–ischemic encephalopathy), congenital airway malformations (discussed below), craniofacial syndromes (e.g., Pierre-Robin

sequence, CHARGE association), and vocal cord paralysis [204–207]. A recent national study showed that pediatric tracheotomies are relatively infrequent, occurring at a rate of 6.6 children per 100,000 child-years. However, children who received tracheotomies accounted for an average of nearly $200,000 in health care costs and a mean length of hospital stay of 50 days, reflecting the inherent complexity of care for these children [205]. Potential complications in the immediate postoperative period, before the first tracheostomy tube change, are well described and include tube occlusion, accidental decannulation, and false passage. Serious, potentially life-threatening complications, such as pneumomediastinum, pneumothorax, and innominate artery erosion are infrequent. Late complications include laryngeal stenosis, tracheal stenosis, stomal

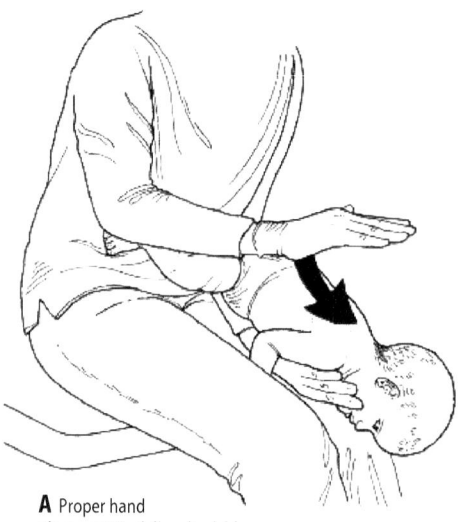

A Proper hand placement to deliver back blows

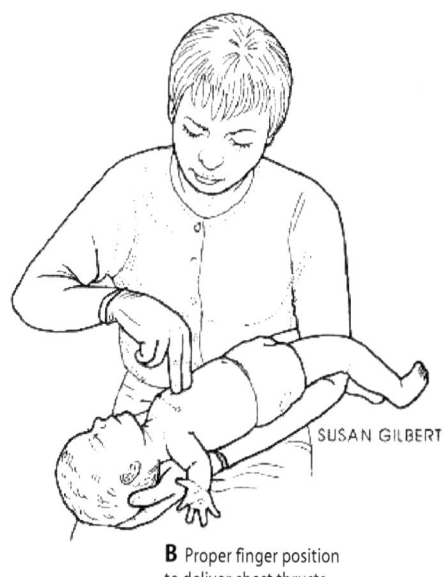

B Proper finger position to deliver chest thrusts

FIGURE 13.13. Basic life support—removal of foreign body in the airway in an infant. (Reprinted from Foltin GL, Tunik MG, Cooper A, Markenson D, Treiber M, Phillips R, Karpeles T. Teaching Resource for Instructors in Prehospital Pediatrics. New York: Center for Pediatric Emergency Medicine; 1998.)

granuloma formation, stomal bleeding, tube occlusion, and lower respiratory tract infection [204–208].

The decision to perform an elective tracheotomy is complex and depends on several factors. The decision-making process should be multidisciplinary in nature and at a minimum include the child's parent(s) or other primary caregiver, the child's primary care physician, the pediatric intensive care team, and the otolaryngologist. Tracheotomy is more commonly performed in the critically ill adult population and is frequently performed at the bedside [209–211]. In contrast, children appear to tolerate prolonged tracheal intubation without significant laryngeal complications and may remain safely tracheally intubated even for several months before tracheotomy is considered [212–219]. Currently there are no studies of early tracheostomy in critically ill children on which to base additional recommendations, although the wealth of evidence obtained from retrospective studies in critically ill children with Guillain-Barré syndrome, tetanus, botulism, and so forth would suggest that prolonged tracheal intubation with meticulous care is relatively safe.

References

1. Richardson MA, Cotton RT. Anatomic abnormalities of the pediatric airway. Pediatr Clin North Am 1984;31:821–834.
2. Altman KW, Wetmore RF, Marsh RR. Congenital airway abnormalities in patients requiring hospitalization. Arch Otolaryngol Head Neck Surg 1999 May;125:525–528.
3. Ward RF, April MM. Congenital malformations of the nose, nasopharynx, and sinuses. In: Westmore RF, Muntz HR, McGill TJI, eds. Pediatric Otolaryngology. Principles and Practice Pathways. New York: Thieme Medical Publishers; 2000:775–786.
4. Infosino A. Pediatric upper airway and congenital anomalies. Anesthesiol Clin North Am 2002;20:747–766.
5. Dinwiddie R. Congenital upper airway obstruction. Paediatr Respir Rev 2004;5:17–24.
6. Dennison WM. The Pierre Robin syndrome. Pediatrics 1965;36:336–341.
7. Lyons Jones K. Robin sequence. In: Lyons Jones K, ed. Smith's Recognizable Patterns of Human Malformation. Philadelphia: WB Saunders; 1997:234–235.
8. Caouette-Laberge L, Bayet B, Larocque Y. The Pierre Robin sequence: review of 125 cases and evolution of treatment modalities. Plast Reconstruct Surg 1994;93:934–941.
9. St-Hilaire H, Buchbinder D. Maxillofacial pathology and management of Pierre Robin sequence. Otolaryngol Clin North Am 2000;33:1241–1256.
10. van den Elzen AP, Semmekrot BA, Bongers EM, Huygen PL, Marres HA. Diagnosis and treatment of the Pierre Robin sequence: results of a retrospective clinical study and review of the literature. Eur J Pediatr 2001;160:47–53.
11. Brown OE, Pownell P, Manning SC. Choanal atresia: a new anatomic classification and clinical management applications. Laryngoscope 1996;106:97–101.
12. Keller JL, Kacker A. Choanal atresia, CHARGE association, and congenital nasal stenosis. Otolaryngol Clin North Am 2000;33:1343–1351.
13. Samadi DS, Shah UK, Handler SD. Choanal atresia: a twenty-year review of medical comorbidities and surgical outcomes. Laryngoscope 2003;113:254–258.
14. Canty TG, Hendren WH. Upper airway obstruction from foregut cysts of the hypopharynx. J Pediatr Surg 1975;10:807–812.
15. Kuint J, Horowitz Z, Kugel C, Toper L, Birenbaum E, Linder N. Laryngeal obstruction caused by lingual thyroglossal duct cyst presenting at birth. Am J Perinatol 1997;14:353–356.
16. Myer CH. Vallecular cyst in the newborn. Ear Nose Throat J 1988;67:122–124.
17. Gutiérrez JP, Berkowitz RG, Robertson CF. Vallecular cysts in newborn and young infants. Pediatr Pulmonol 1999;27:282–285.
18. Ahrens B, Lammert I, Schmitt M, Wahn U, Paul K, Niggemann B. Life-threatening vallecular cyst in a 3-month-old infant: Case report and literature review. Clin Pediatr (Phila) 2004;43:287–290.
19. Zalzal GH. Pediatric stridor and airway management. International Congress Series 2003;1240:803–808.
20. Hollinger ID. Etiology of stridor in the neonate, infant, and child. Ann Otol Rhinol Laryngol 1980;89:397–400.
21. Hughes CA, Dunham ME. Congenital anomalies of the larynx and trachea. In: Westmore RF, Muntz HR, McGill TJI, eds. Pediatric Otolaryngology. Principles and Practice Pathways. New York: Thieme Medical Publishers; 2000:775–786.
22. Jasin ME, Osguthrope JD. The radiographic evaluation of infants with stridor. Otolaryngol Head Neck Surg 1982;90:736–739.
23. Zawin JK. Radiologic evaluation of the upper airway. In: Westmore RF, Muntz HR, McGill TJI, eds. Pediatric Otolaryngology. Principles and Practice Pathways. New York: Thieme Medical Publishers; 2000:689–736.
24. Parnell FW, Brandenberg JH. Vocal cord paralysis: a review of 100 cases. Laryngoscope 1970;80:1036–1045.
25. Holinger LD, Holiner PC, Holinger PH. Etiology of bilateral vocal cord paralysis: a review of 389 cases. Ann Otol Rhinol Laryngol 1976;85:428–436.
26. deJonge AL, Friedman EM. Vocal cord paralysis. In: Westmore RF, Muntz HR, McGill TJI, eds. Pediatric Otolaryngology. Principles and Practice Pathways. New York: Thieme Medical Publishers; 2000:787–798.
27. Holinger PH, Kutnick SL, Schild JA, Holinger LD. Subglottic stenosis in infants and children. Ann Otol Rhinol Laryngol 1976;85:591–599.
28. Sichel JY, Dangoor E, Eliashar R, Halperin D. Management of congenital laryngeal malformations. Am J Otolaryngol 2000;21:22–30.
29. Chatrath P, Black M, Jani P, Albert DM, Bailey CM. A review of the current management of infantile subglottic haemangioma, including a comparison of CO(2) laser therapy versus tracheostomy. Int J Pediatr Otorhinolaryngol 2002;64:143–157.
30. Rahbar R, Nicollas R, Roger G, Triglia JM, Garabedian EN, McGill TJ, Healy GB. The biology and management of subglottic hemangioma: past, present, future. Laryngoscope 2004;114:1880–1891.
31. Bitar MA, Moukarbel RV, Zalzal GH. Management of congenital subglottic hemangioma: trends and success over the past 17 years. Otolaryngol Head Neck Surg 2005;132:226–231.
32. Hartnick CJ, Rutter M, Lang F, Willging JP, Cotton RT. Congenital high airway obstruction syndrome and airway reconstruction: an evolving paradigm. Arch Otolaryngol Head Neck Surg 2002;128:567–570.
33. Lim FY, Crombleholme TM, Hedrick HL, Flake AW, Johnson MP, Howell LJ, Adzick NS. Congenital high airway obstruction syndrome: natural history and management. J Pediatr Surg 2003;38:940–945.
34. Wyatt ME, Hartley BE. Laryngotracheal reconstruction in congenital laryngeal webs and atresias. Otolaryngol Head Neck Surg 2005;132:232–238.
35. DeCou JM, Jones DC, Jacobs HD, Touloukian RJ. Successful ex utero intrapartum treatment (EXIT) procedure for congenital high airway obstruction syndrome (CHAOS) owing to laryngeal atresia. J Pediatr Surg 1998;33:1563–1565.
36. Crombleholme TM, Sylvester K, Flake AW, Adzick NS. Salvage of a fetus with congenital high airway obstruction syndrome by ex utero intrapartum treatment (EXIT) procedure. Fetal Diagn Ther 2000;15:280–282.
37. Bui TH, Grunewald C, Frenckner B, Kuylensierna R, Dahlgren G, Edner A, Granstrom L, Sellden H. Successful EXIT (ex utero intrapartum treatment) procedure in a fetus diagnosed prenatally with congenital high-airway obstruction syndrome due to laryngeal atresia. Eur J Pediatr Surg 2000;10:328–333.

38. Bouchard S, Johnson MP, Flake AW, Howell LJ, Myers LB, Adzick NS, Crombleholme TM. The EXIT procedure: experience and outcome in 31 cases. J Pediatr Surg 2002;37:418–426.

39. Evans KL, Courteney-Harris R, Bailey CM, Evans JN, Parsons DS. Management of posterior laryngeal and laryngotracheoesophageal clefts. Arch Otolaryngol Head Neck Surg 1995;121:1380–1385.

40. Chitkara AE, Tadros M, Kim HJ, Harley EH. Complete laryngotracheoesophageal cleft: complicated management issues. Laryngoscope 2003;113:1314–1320.

41. Goldenberg JD, Holinger LD, Bressler FJ, Hutchinson LR. Bifid epiglottis. Ann Otol Rhinol Laryngol 1996;105:155–157.

42. Civantos FJ, Holinger LD. Laryngoceles and saccular cysts in infants and children. Arch Otolaryngol Head Neck Surg 1992;118:296–300.

43. Sniezek JC, Johnson RE, Ramirez SG, Hayes DK. Laryngoceles and saccular cysts. South Med J 1996;89:427–430.

44. Forte V, Fuoco G, James A. A new classification system for congenital laryngeal cysts. Laryngoscope 2004;114:1123–1127.

45. Austin J, Ali T. Tracheomalacia and bronchomalacia in children: pathophysiology, assessment, treatment, and anaesthesia management. Paediatr Anaesth 2003;13:3–11.

46. Berrocal T, Madrid C, Novo S, Gutierrez J, Arjonilla A, Gomez-Leon N. Congenital anomalies of the tracheobronchial tree, lung, and mediastinum: embryology, radiology, and pathology. Radiographics 2004;24:e17.

47. McNamara VM, Crabbe DC. Tracheomalacia. Paediatr Respir Rev 2004;5:147–154.

48. Carden KA, Boiselle PM, Waltz DA, Ernst A. Tracheomalacia and tracheobronchomalacia in children and adults: an in-depth review. Chest 2005;127:984–1005.

49. Bluestone CD. Humans are born too soon: impact on pediatric otolaryngology. Int J Pediatr Otorhinolaryngol 2005;69:1–8.

50. Messineo A, Filler RM. Tracheomalacia. Semin Pediatr Surg 1994;3:253–258.

51. Elliot M, Roebuck D, Noctor C, McLaren C, Hartley B, Mok Q, Dunne C, Pigott N, Patel C, Patel A, Wallis C. The management of congenital tracheal stenosis. Int J Pediatr Otorhinolaryngol 2003;67(Suppl 1):S183–S192.

52. Nicolai T. Therapeutic concepts in upper airway obstruction. Paediatr Respir Rev 2004;5:34–39.

53. Wright CD, Grillo HC, Wain JC, Wong DR, Donahue DM, Gaissert HA, Mathisen DJ. Anastomotic complications after tracheal resection: prognostic factors and management. J Thorac Cardiovasc Surg 2004;128:731–739.

54. Kocyildirim E, Kanani M, Roebuck D, Wallis C, McLaren C, Noctor C, Pigott N, Mok Q, Hartley B, Dunne C, Uppal S, Elliott MJ. Long-segment tracheal stenosis: slide tracheoplasty and a multidisciplinary approach improve outcomes and reduce costs. J Thorac Cardiovasc Surg 2004;128:876–882.

55. Airway Reconstruction Team. Recent challenges in the management of congenital tracheal stenosis: an individualized approach. J Pediatr Surg 2005;40:774–780.

56. Merei JM, Hutson JM. Embryogenesis of tracheo-esophageal anomalies: a review. Pediatr Surg Int 2002;18:319–326.

57. Bove T, Demanet H, Casimir G, Viart P, Goldstein JP, Deuvaert FE. Tracheobronchial compression of vascular origin. Review of experience in infants and children. J Cardiovasc Surg (Torino) 2001;42:663–666.

58. Yilmaz M, Ozkan M, Dogan R, Demircin M, Ersoy U, Boke E, Pasaoglu I. Vascular anomalies causing tracheobronchial compression: a 20-year experience in diagnosis and management. Heart Surg Forum 2003;6:149–152.

59. Kussman BD, Geva T, McGowan FX. Cardiovascular causes of airway compression. Paediatr Anaesth 2004;14:60–74.

60. Rotta AT, Wiryawan B. Respiratory emergencies in children. Respir Care 2003;48:248–258.

61. Sie KCY. Infectious and inflammatory disorders of the larynx and trachea. In: Westmore RF, Muntz HR, McGill TJI, eds. Pediatric Otolaryngology. Principles and Practice Pathways. New York: Thieme Medical Publishers; 2000:811–825.

62. Hammer J. Acquired upper airway obstruction. Paediatr Respir Rev 2004;5:25–33.

63. Myer CM. Inflammatory diseases of the pediatric airway. In: Cotton RT, Myer CM, eds. Practical Pediatric Otolaryngology. Philadelphia: Lippincott-Raven; 1999:547–559.

64. Leung AK, Kellner JD, Johnson DW. Viral croup: a current perspective. J Pediatr Health Care 2004;18:297–301.

65. Cunningham MJ. The old and new of acute laryngotracheal infections. Clin Pediatr (Phila) 1992;31:56–64.

66. Denny FW, Murphy TF, Clyde WA Jr, Collier AM, Henderson FW. Croup: an 11-year study in a pediatric practice. Pediatrics 1983;71:871–876.

67. Yang TY, Lu CY, Kao CL, Chen RT, Ho YH, Yang SC, Lee PI, Chen JM, Lee CY, Huang LM. Clinical manifestations of parainfluenza infection in children. J Microbiol Immunol Infect 2003;36:270–274.

68. Crowe JE Jr. Human metapneumovirus as a major cause of human respiratory tract disease. Pediatr Infect Dis J 2004;23:S215–S21.

69. Kairys SW, Olmstead EM, O'Connor GT. Steroid treatment of laryngotracheitis: A meta-analysis of the evidence from randomized trials. Pediatrics 1989;83:683–693.

70. Durward AD, Nicoll SJ, Oliver J, Tibby SM, Murdoch IA. The outcome of patients with upper airway obstruction transported to a regional paediatric intensive care unit. Eur J Pediatr 1998;157:907–911.

71. Chin R, Browne GJ, Lam LT, McCaskill ME, Fasher B, Hort J. Effectiveness of a croup clinical pathway in the management of children with croup presenting to an emergency department. J Paediatr Child Health 2002;38:382–387.

72. Fitzgerald DA, Mellis CM, Johnson M, Allen H, Cooper P, Van Asperen P. Nebulized budesonide is as effective as nebulized adrenaline in moderately severe croup. Pediatrics 1996;97:722–725.

73. Westley CR, Cotton EK, Brooks JG. Nebulized racemic epinephrine by IPPB for the treatment of croup: a double-blind study. Am J Dis Child 1978;132:484–487.

74. Husby S, Agertoft L, Mortensen S, Pedersen S. Treatment of croup with nebulized steroid (budesonide): a double blind, placebo controlled study. Arch Dis Child 1993;68:352–355.

75. Skolnik NS. Treatment of croup: a critical review. Am J Dis Child 1989;36:1389–1402.

76. Dawson KP, Steinberg A, Capaldi N. The lateral radiograph of neck in laryngo-tracheo-bronchitis (croup). J Qual Clin Pract 1994;14:39–43.

77. Swishchuk LE. Upper airway, nasal passages, sinuses, and mastoids. In: Swishchuk LE, ed. Emergency Radiology of the Acutely Ill and Injured Child, 2nd ed. Baltimore: Williams & Wilkins; 1986:127–140.

78. Bourchier D, Dawson KP, Fergusson DM. Humidification in viral croup: a controlled trial. Aust Paediatr J 1984;20:289–291.

79. Lenney W, Milner AD. Treatment of acute viral croup. Arch Dis Child 1978;53:704–706.

80. Neto GM, Kentab O, Klassen TP, Osmond MH. A randomized controlled trial of mist in the acute treatment of moderate croup. Acad Emerg Med 2002;9:873–879.

81. Westley CR, Cotton EK, Brooks JG. Nebulized racemic epinephrine by IPPB for the treatment of croup: a double-blind study. Am J Dis Child 1978;132:484–487.

82. Kelley PB, Simon JE. Racemic epinephrine use in croup and disposition. Am J Emerg Med 1992;10:181–183.

83. Waisman Y, Klein BL, Boenning DA, et al. Prospective randomised double-blind study comparing L-epinephrine and racemic epinephrine aerosols in the treatment of laryngotracheitis (croup). Pediatrics 1992;89:302–306.

84. Prendergast M, Jones JS, Hartman D. Racemic epinephrine in the treatment of laryngotracheitis: can we identify children for outpatient therapy? Am J Emerg Med 1994;12:613–616.

85. Gardner HG, Powell KR, Roden VJ, Cherry JD. The evaluation of racemic epinephrine in the treatment of infectious croup. Pediatrics 1973;52:52–55.

86. Kristjansson S, Berg-Kelly K, Winso E. Inhalation of racemic adrenaline in the treatment of mild and moderately severe croup: clinical symptom score and oxygen saturation measurements for evaluation of treatment effects. Acta Paediatr 1994;83:1156–1160.

87. Rizos JD, DiGravio BE, Sehl MJ, Tallon JM. The disposition of children with croup treated with racemic epinephrine and dexamethasone in the emergency department. J Emerg Med 1998;16:535–539.

88. Ausejo M, Saenz A, Pham B, Kellner JD, Johnson DW, Moher D, Klassen TP. The effectiveness of glucocorticoids in treating croup: meta-analysis. BMJ 1999;319:595–600.

89. Geelhoed GC, Macdonald WB. Oral and inhaled steroids in croup: a randomized, placebo-controlled trial. Pediatr Pulmonol 1995;20:355–361.

90. Johnson DW, Jacobson S, Edney PC, Hadfield P, Mundy ME, Schuh S. A comparison of nebulized budesonide, intramuscular dexamethasone, and placebo for moderately severe croup. N Engl J Med 1998;339:498–503.

91. Klassen TP, Craig WR, Moher D, Osmond MH, Pasterkamp H, Sutcliffe T, et al. Nebulized budesonide and oral dexamethasone for treatment of croup: a randomized, controlled trial. JAMA 1998;279:1629–1632.

92. Donaldson D, Poleski D, Knipple E, Filips K, Reetz L, Pascual RG, Jackson RE. Intramuscular versus oral dexamethasone for the treatment of moderate-to-severe croup: a randomized, double-blind trial. Acad Emerg Med 2003;10:16–21.

93. Falkenstein E, Wehling M. Nongenomically initiated steroid actions. Eur J Clin Invest 2000;30:51–54.

94. Klaustermeyer WB, Hale FC. The physiologic effect of an intravenous glucocorticoid in bronchial asthma. Ann Allergy 1976;37:80–86.

95. Wolfson DH, Nypaver MM, Blaser M, Hogan A, Evans RI, Davis AT. A controlled trial of methylprednisolone in the early emergency department treatment of acute asthma in children. Pediatr Emerg Care 1994;10:335–338.

96. Rodrigo C, Rodrigo G. Early administration of hydrocortisone in the emergency room treatment of acute asthma: a controlled clinical trial. Respir Med 1994;88:755–761.

97. Gupta VK, Cheifetz IM. Heliox administration in the pediatric intensive care unit: an evidence-based review. Pediatr Crit Care Med 2005;6:204–211.

98. Duncan PG. Efficacy of helium–oxygen mixtures in the management of severe viral and post-intubation croup. Can Anaesth Soc J 1979;26:206–212.

99. Skrinskas GJ, Hyland RH, Hutcheon MA. Using helium oxygen mixtures in the management of acute airway obstruction. Can Med Assoc J 1983;128:555–558.

100. Mizrahi S, Yaari Y, Lugassy G, Cotev S. Major airway obstruction relieved by helium/oxygen breathing. Crit Care Med 1986;14:986–987.

101. Terregino CA, Nairn SJ, Chansky ME, Kass JE. The effect of heliox on croup: a pilot study. Acad Emerg Med 1998;5:1130–1133.

102. Grosz AH, Jacobs IN, Cho C, Schears GJ. Use of helium–oxygen mixtures to relieve upper airway obstruction in a pediatric population. Laryngoscope 2001;111:1512–1514.

103. Weber JE, Chudnofsky CR, Younger JG, Larkin GL, Boczar M, Wilkerson MD, Zuriekat GY, Nolan B, Eicke DM. A randomized comparison of helium–oxygen mixture (heliox) and racemic epinephrine for the treatment of moderate to severe croup. Pediatrics 2001;107:E96.

104. DiCecco RJ, Rega PP. The application of heliox in the management of croup by an air ambulance service. Air Med J 2004;23:33–35.

105. Ho AM-H, Dion PW, Karmakar MK, Chung DC, Tay BA. Use of heliox in critical upper airway obstruction. Physical and physiologic considerations in choosing the optimal helium:oxygen mix. Resuscitation 2002;52:297–300.

106. Glenn GM, Schofield T, Krober M. Group A streptococcal supraglottitis. Clin Pediatr (Phila) 1990;29:674–676.

107. Senior BA, Radkowski D, MacArthur C, Sprecher RC, Jones D. Changing patterns in pediatric supraglottitis: a multi-institutional review, 1980 to 1992. Laryngoscope 1994;104:1314–1322.

108. Gorelick MH, Baker MD. Epiglottitis in children, 1979 through 1992. Effects of Haemophilus influenzae type b immunization. Arch Pediatr Adolesc Med 1994;148:47–50.

109. Gonzalez Valdepena H, Wald ER, Rose E, Ungkanont K, Casselbrant ML. Epiglottitis and Haemophilus influenzae immunization: the Pittsburgh experience-a five-year review. Pediatrics 1995;96:424–427.

110. McEwab J, Giridharan W, Clarke RW, Shears P. Paediatric acute epiglottitis: not a disappearing entity. Int J Pediatr Otorhinolaryngol 2003;67:317–321.

111. Shah RK, Roberson DW, Jones DT. Epiglottitis in the Hemophilus influenzae type B vaccine era: a changing trends. Laryngoscope 2004;114:557–560.

112. Talan DA, Moran GJ, Pinner RW. Progress toward eliminating Haemophilus influenzae type b disease among infants and children—United States, 1987–1997. Ann Emerg Med 1999;34:109–111.

113. Centers for Disease Control and Prevention. Progress toward elimination of Haemophilus influenzae type b invasive disease among infants and children—United States, 1998–2000. JAMA 2002;287:2206–2207.

114. Brilli RJ, Benzing G 3rd, Cotcamp DH. Epiglottitis in infants less than 2 years of age. Pediatr Emerg Care 1989;5:16–21.

115. Losek JD, Dewitz-Zink BA, Melzer-Lange M, Havens PL. Epiglottitis: comparison of signs and symptoms in children less than 2 years of age and older. Ann Emerg Med 1990;19:55–58.

116. Kimmons HC Jr, Peterson BM. Management of acute epiglottitis in pediatric patients. Crit Care Med 1986;14:278–279.

117. Crockett DM, Healy GB, McGill TJ, Friedman EM. Airway management of acute supraglottitis at the Children's Hospital, Boston: 1980–1985. Ann Otol Rhinol Laryngol 1988;97:114–119.

118. Crysdale WS, Sendi K. Evolution in the management of acute epiglottitis: a 10-year experience with 242 children. Int Anesthesiol Clin 1988;26:32–38.

119. Damm M, Eckel HE, Jungehulsing M, Roth B. Airway endoscopy in the interdisciplinary management of acute epiglottitis. Int J Pediatr Otorhinolaryngol 1996;38:41–51.

120. Wald E, Reilly JS, Bluestone CD, Chiponis D. Sulbactam/ampicillin in the treatment of acute epiglottitis in children. Rev Infect Dis 1986;5:S617–S619.

121. Sawyer SM, Johnson PD, Hogg GG, Robertson CF, Oppedisano F, MacIness SJ, Gilbert GL. Successful treatment of epiglottitis with two doses of ceftriaxone. Arch Dis Child 1994;70:129–132.

122. Gonzalez C, Reilly JS, Kenna MA, Thompson AE. Duration of intubation in children with acute epiglottitis. Otolaryngol Head Neck Surg 1986;95:477–481.

123. Jones R, Santos JI, Overall JC Jr. Bacterial tracheitis. JAMA 1979;242:721–726.

124. Liston SL, Gehrz RC, Siegel LG, Tilelli J. Bacterial tracheitis. Am J Dis Child 1983;137:764–767.

125. Donaldson JD, Maltby CC. Bacterial tracheitis in children. J Otolaryngol 1989;18:101–104.

126. Bernstein T, Brilli R, Jacobs B. Is bacterial tracheitis changing? A 14-month experience in a pediatric intensive care unit. Clin Infect Dis 1998;27:458–462.

127. Salamone FN, Bobbitt DB, Myer CM, Rutter MJ, Greinwald JH Jr. Bacterial tracheitis reexamined: is there a less severe manifestation? Otolaryngol Head Neck Surg 2004;131:871–876.

128. Stroud RH, Friedman NR. An update on inflammatory disorders of the pediatric airway: epiglottitis, croup, and tracheitis. Am J Otolaryngol 2001;22:268–275.

129. Lee SS, Schwartz RH, Bahadori RS. Retropharyngeal abscess: epiglottitis of the new millennium. J Pediatr 2001;138:435–437.

130. Yeoh LH, Singh SD, Rogers JH. Retropharyngeal abscesses in a children's hospital. J Laryngol Otol 1985;99:555–566.

131. Coutlhard M, Isaacs D. Retropharyngeal abscess. Arch Dis Child 1991;66:1227–1230.

132. Broughton RA. Nonsurgical management of deep neck infections in children. Pediatr Infect Dis J 1992;11:14–18.

133. Thompson JW, Cohen SR, Reddix P. Retropharyngeal abscess in children: a retrospective and historical analysis. Laryngoscope 1988;98:589–592.

134. Morrison JE Jr, Pashley NR. Retropharyngeal abscesses in children: a 10-year review. Pediatr Emerg Care 1988;4:9–11.

135. Craig FW, Schunk JE. Retropharyngeal abscess in children: clinical presentation, utility of imaging, and current management. Pediatrics 2003;111:1394–1398.

136. Coticchia JM, Getnick GS, Yun RD, Arnold JE. Age-, site-, and time-specific differences in pediatric deep neck abscesses. Arch Otolaryngol Head Neck Surg 2004;130:201–207.

137. Vural C, Gungor A, Comerci S. Accuracy of computerized tomography in deep neck infections in the pediatric population. Am J Otolaryngol 2003;24:143–148.

138. Asmar BI. Bacteriology of retropharyngeal abscess in children. Pediatr Infect Dis J 1990;9:595–597.

139. Brook I. Microbiology and management of peritonsillar, retropharyngeal, and parapharyngeal abscesses. J Oral Maxillofac Surg 2004;62:1545–1550.

140. Schraff S, McGinn JD, Derkay CS. Peritonsillar abscess in children: a 10-year review of diagnosis and management. Int J Pediatr Otorhinolaryngol 2001;57:213–218.

141. Kashima HK, Mounts P, Shah K. Recurrent respiratory papillomatosis. Obstet Gynecol Clin North Am 1996;23:699–706.

142. Peyton Shirley W, Wiatrak B. Is cidofovir a useful adjunctive therapy for recurrent respiratory papillomatosis in children? Int J Pediatr Otorhinolaryngol 2004;64:413–418.

143. Boglioli LR, Taff ML. Sudden asphyxial death complicating infectious mononucleosis. Am J Forensic Med Pathol 1998;19:174–177.

144. Burstin PP, Marshall CL. Infectious mononucleosis and bilateral peritonsillar abscesses resulting in airway obstruction. J Laryngol Otol 1998;112:1186–1188.

145. Irving JA, Cameron BR, Ludemann JP, Taylor G. Florid infectious mononucleosis: clinicopathological correlation in acute tonsillectomy. Int J Pediatr Otorhinolaryngol 2002;66:87–92.

146. Lobo S, Williams H, Singh V. Massive retropharyngeal lymphadenopathy in an infant: an unusual presentation of infectious mononucleosis. J Laryngol Otol 2004;118:983–984.

147. Ganzel TM, Goldman JL, Padhya TA. Otolaryngologic clinical patterns in pediatric infectious mononucleosis. Am J Otolaryngol 1996;17:397–400.

148. Stevenson DS, Webster G, Stewart IA. Acute tonsillectomy in the management of infectious mononucleosis. J Laryngol Otol 1992;106:989–991.

149. Wohl DL, Isaacson JE. Airway obstruction in children with infectious mononucleosis. Ear Nose Throat J 1995;74:630–638.

150. Pierce RJ, Worsnop CJ. Upper airway function and dysfunction in respiration. Clin Exp Pharmacol Physiol 1999;26:1–10.

151. Arens R, Marcus CL. Pathophysiology of upper airway obstruction: a developmental perspective. Sleep 2004;27:997–1019.

152. Erler T, Paditz E. Obstructive sleep apnea syndrome in children: a state-of-the-art review. Treat Respir Med 2004;3:107–122.

153. Spector A, Scheid S, Hassink S, Deutsch ES, Reilly JS, Cook SP. Adenotonsillectomy in the morbidly obsess child. Int J Pediatr Otorhinolaryngol 2003;67:359–364.

154. Mitchell RB, Kelly J. Adenotonsillectomy for obstructive sleep apnea in obese children. Otolaryngol Head Neck Surg 2004;131:104–108.

155. Jacobs IN, Gray RF, Todd NW. Upper airway obstruction in children with Down syndrome. Arch Otolaryngol Head Neck Surg 1996;122:945–950.

156. de Jong AL, Sulek M, Nihill M, Duncan NO, Friedman EM. Tenuous airway in children with trisomy 21. Laryngoscope 1997;107:345–350.

157. McMurray JS, Myer III CM. Management of chronic airway obstruction. In: Westmore RF, Muntz HR, McGill TJI, eds. Pediatric Otolaryngology. Principles and Practice Pathways. New York: Thieme Medical Publishers; 2000:863–881.

158. Ratner I, Whitfield J. Acquired subglottic stenosis in the very-low-birth-weight infant. Am J Dis Child 1983;137:40–43.

159. da Silva OP. Factors influencing acquired upper airway obstruction in newborn infants receiving assisted ventilation because of respiratory failure: an overview. J Perinatol 1996;16:272–275.

160. Wiel E, Vilette B, Darras JA, Scherpereel P, Leclerc F. Laryngotracheal stenosis in children after intubation. Report of five cases. Paediatr Anaesth 1997;7:415–419.

161. Cotton RT, Myer CM 3rd. Contemporary surgical management of laryngeal stenosis in children. Am J Otolaryngol 1984;5:360–368.

162. Cotton RT. Pediatric laryngotracheal stenosis. J Pediatr Surg 1984;19:699–704.

163. Cotton RT, Myer CM 3rd, Bratcher GO, Fitton CM. Anterior cricoid split, 1977–1987. Evolution of a technique. Arch Otolaryngol Head Neck Surg 1988;114:1300–1302.

164. Cotton RT. Management of subglottic stenosis. Otolaryngol Clin North Am 2000;33:111–130.

165. Robie DK, Gursoy MH, Pokorny WJ. Mediastinal tumors-airway obstruction and management. Semin Pediatr Surg 1994;3:259–266.

166. Goh MH, Liu XY, Goh YS. Anterior mediastinal masses: an anaesthetic challenge. Anaesthesia 1999;54:670–674.

167. Dilworth K, Thomas J. Anaesthetic consequences for a child with complex multilevel airway obstruction—recommendations for avoiding life-threatening sequelae. Paediatr Anaesth 2003;13:620–623.

168. Lam JC, Chui CH, Jacobsen AS, Tan AM, Joseph VT. When is a mediastinal mass critical in a child? An analysis of 29 patients. Pediatr Surg Int 2004;20:180–184.

169. Koka BV, Jeon IS, Andre JM, MacKay I, Smith RM. Postintubation croup in children. Anesth Analg 1977;56:501–505.

170. Kemper KJ, Benson MS, Bishop MJ. Predictors of postextubation stridor in pediatric trauma patients. Crit Care Med 1991;19:352–355.

171. Gomes Cordeiro AM, Fernandes JC, Troster EJ. Possible risk factors associated with moderate or severe airway injuries in children who underwent endotracheal intubation. Pediatr Crit Care Med 2004;5:364–368.

172. Newth CJ, Rachman B, Patel N, Hammer J. The use of cuffed versus uncuffed endotracheal tubes in pediatric intensive care. J Pediatr 2004;144(3):333–337.

173. Silver GM, Freiburg C, Halerz M, Tojong J, Supple K, Gamelli RL. A survey of airway and ventilator management strategies in North American pediatric burn units. J Burn Care Rehabil 2004;25:435–440.

174. Deakers TW, Reynolds G, Stretton M, Newth CJ. Cuffed endotracheal tubes in pediatric intensive care. J Pediatr 1994;125(1):57–62.

175. Khine HH, Corddry DH, Kettrick RG, Martin TM, McCloskey JJ, Rose JB, et al. Comparison of cuffed and uncuffed endotracheal tubes in young children during general anesthesia. Anesthesiology 1997;86(3):627–631.

176. Fine GF, Borland LM. The future of the cuffed endotracheal tube. Paediatr Anaesth 2004;14(1):38–42.

177. Kurachek SC, Newth CJ, Quasney MW, Rice T, Sachdeva RC, Patel NR, Takano J, et al. Extubation failure in pediatric intensive care: a multiple-center study of risk factors and outcomes. Crit Care Med 2003;31:2657–2664.

178. Shott SR. Down syndrome: analysis of airway size and a guide for appropriate intubation. Laryngoscope 2000;110:585–592.

179. Maury E, Guglielminotti J, Alzieu M, Qureshi T, Guidet B, Offenstadt G. How to identify patients with no risk for postextubation stridor? Crit Care Med 2004;19:23–28.

180. Mhanna MJ, Zamel YB, Tichy CM, Super DM. The "air leak" test around the endotracheal tube, as a predictor of postextubation stridor, is age dependent in children. Crit Care Med 2002;30:2639–2643.

181. Nutman J, Brooks LJ, Deakins KM, Baldesare KK, Witte MK, Reed MD. Racemic versus l-epinephrine aerosol in the treatment of postextubation laryngeal edema: results from a prospective, randomized, double-blind study. Crit Care Med 1994;22:1591–1594.

182. Tellez DW, Galvis AG, Storgion SA, Amer HN, Hoseyni M, Deakers TW. Dexamethasone in the prevention of postextubation stridor in children. J Pediatr 1991;118:289–294.

183. Couser RJ, Ferrara TB, Falde B, Johnson K, Schilling CG, Hoekstra RE. Effectiveness of dexamethasone in preventing extubation failure in preterm infants at increased risk for airway edema. J Pediatr 1992;121:591–596.

184. Anene O, Meert KL, Uy H, Simpson P, Sarnaik AP. Dexamethasone for the prevention of postextubation airway obstruction: a prospective, randomized, double-blind, placebo-controlled trial. Crit Care Med 1996;24:1666–1669.

185. Meade MO, Guyatt GH, Cook DJ, Sinuff T, Butler R. Trials of corticosteroids to prevent postextubation airway complications. *Chest* 2001;120(Suppl):464S–468S.

186. Markovitz BP, Randolph AG. Corticosteroids for the prevention of reintubation and postextubation stridor in pediatric patients: a meta-analysis. Pediatr Crit Care Med 2002;3:223–226.

187. Foland JA, Super DM, Dahdah NS, Mhanna MJ. The use of the air leak test and corticosteroids in intubated children: a survey of pediatric critical care fellowship directors. Respir Care 2002;47:662–666.

188. Kemper KJ, Izenberg S, Marvin JA, Heimbach DM. Treatment of postextubation stridor in a pediatric patient with burns: the role of heliox. J Burn Care Rehabil 1990;11:337–339.

189. Kemper KJ, Ritz RH, Benson MS, Bishop MS. Helium-oxygen mixture in the treatment of postextubation stridor in pediatric trauma patients. Crit Care Med 1991;19:356–359.

190. Jaber S, Carlucci A, Boussarsar M, Fodil R, Pigeot J, Maggiore S, Harf A, Isabey D, Brochard L. Helium–oxygen in the postextubation period decreases inspiratory effort. *Am J Respir Crit Care Med* 2001;164:633–637.

191. Berkenbosch JW, Grueber RE, Graff GR, Tobias JD. Patterns of helium-oxygen (heliox) usage in the critical care environment. J Intensive Care Med 2004;19:335–344.

192. Lima JA, Fischer GB. Foreign body aspiration in children. Paediatr Respir Rev 2002;3:303–307.

193. Wai Pak M, Chung Lee W, Kwok Fung H, van Hasselt CA. A prospective study of foreign-body ingestion in 311 children. Int J Pediatr Otorhinolaryngol 2001;58:37–45.

194. Arana A, Hauser B, Hachimi-Idrissi S, Vandeplas Y. Management of ingested foreign bodies in childhood and review of the literature. Eur J Pediatr 2001;160:468–472.

195. Donnelly LF, Frush DP, Bisset GS III. The multiple presentations of foreign bodies in children. AJR 1998;170:471–477.

196. Girardi G, Contador AM, Castro-Rodriguez JA. Two new radiological findings to improve the diagnosis of bronchial foreign-body aspiration in children. Pediatr Pulmonol 2004;38:261–264.

197. Ford HR, Gardner MJ, Lynch JM. Laryngotracheal disruption from blunt pediatric neck injuries: impact of early recognition and intervention on outcome. J Pediatr Surg 1995;30:331–335.

198. Gold SM, Gerber ME, Shott SR, Myer CM 3rd. Blunt laryngotracheal trauma in children. Arch Otolaryngol Head Neck Surg 1997;123:83–87.

199. Grant WJ, Meyers RL, Jaffe RL, Johnson DG. Tracheobronchial injuries after blunt chest trauma in children—hidden pathology. J Pediatr Surg 1998;33:1707–1711.

200. Cay A, Imamoglu M, Sarihan H, Kosucu P, Bektas D. Tracheobronchial rupture due to blunt trauma in children: report of two cases. Eur J Pediatr Surg 2002;12:419–422.

201. Lichenstein R, Gillette DL. An unusual presentation of stridor: blunt pediatric laryngotracheal trauma. J Emerg Med 2002;22:375–378.

202. Corsten G, Berkowitz RG. Membranous tracheal rupture in children following minor blunt cervical trauma. Ann Otol Rhinol Laryngol 2002;111:197–199.

203. Myer CM 3rd. Trauma of the larynx and craniofacial structures: airway implications. Paediatr Anaesth. 2004;14:103–106.

204. Ward RF, Jones J, Carew JF. Current trends in pediatric tracheotomy. Int J Pediatr Otorhinolaryngol 1995;32:233–239.

205. Lewis CW, Carron JD, Perkins JA, Sie KCY, Feudtner C. Tracheotomy in pediatric patients: a national perspective. Arch Otolaryngol Head Neck Surg 2003;129:523–529.

206. Carron JD, Derkay CS, Strope GL, Nosonchuk JE, Darrow DH. Pediatric tracheotomies: changing indications and outcomes. Laryngoscope 2000;110:1099–1104.

207. Lee W, Koltai P, Harrison AM, Appachi E, Bourdakos D, Davis S, et al. Indications for tracheotomy in the pediatric intensive care unit population: a pilot study. Arch Otolaryngol Head Neck Surg 2002;128:1249–1252.

208. Carr MM, Poje CP, Kingston L, Kielma D, Heard C. Complications in pediatric tracheostomies. Laryngoscope 2001;111:1925–1928.

209. Plummer AL, Gracey DR. Consensus conference on artificial airways in patients receiving mechanical ventilation. Chest 1989;96:178–180.

210. Heffner JE. Tracheotomy application and timing. Clin Chest Med 2003;24:389–398.

211. Maziak DE, Meade MO, Todd TR. The timing of tracheotomy: a systematic review. Chest 1998;114:605–609.

212. Mattila MA, Suutarinen T, Sulamaa M. Prolonged endotracheal intubation or tracheostomy in infants and children. J Pediatr Surg 1969;4:674–682.

213. Battersby EF, Hatch DJ, Towney RM. The effects of prolonged naso-endotracheal intubation in children. A study in infants and young children after cardiopulmonary bypass. Anaesthesia 1977;32:154–157.

214. Cantrell RW, Bell RA, Morioka WT. Acute epiglottitis: intubation versus tracheostomy. Laryngoscope 1978;88:994–1005.

215. Pather M, Hariparsad D, Wesley AG. Nasotracheal intubation versus tracheostomy for intermittent positive pressure ventilation in neonatal tetanus. Intensive Care Med 1985;11:30–32.

216. Wohl D, Tucker JA. Infant botulism: considerations for airway management. Laryngoscope 1992;102:1251–1254.

217. Anderson TD, Shah UK, Schreiner MS, Jacobs IN. Airway complications of infant botulism: ten-year experience with 60 cases. Otolaryngol Head Neck Surg 2002;126:234–239.

218. Shann FA, Duncan AW, Brandstater B. Prolonged per-laryngeal endotracheal intubation in children: 40 years on. Anaesth Intensive Care 2003;31:664–666.

219. Kadilak PR, Vanasse S, Sheridan RL. Favorable short- and long-term outcomes of prolonged translaryngeal intubation in critically ill children. J Burn Care Rehabil 2004;25:262–265.

14
Congenital Airway and Respiratory Tract Anomalies

Michael J. Rutter

Introduction

Airway management in the pediatric intensive care unit (PICU) environment carries the inherent potential of becoming problematic. For children with underlying congenital anomalies of the airway, this potential may be greatly compounded. Congenital anomalies of the airway frequently have predictable patterns by which the airway is compromised. If anticipated, these patterns may be either prevented or ameliorated. Management of the pediatric patient in the PICU with a congenitally abnormal airway may significantly influence surgical options and patient outcomes both pre- and postoperatively. This chapter presents an overview of airway management in critically ill infants and children, with particular emphasis on infants and children with anatomic airway abnormalities.

General Considerations

Prevention of Complications

Although prolonged tracheal intubation may be tolerated for weeks or even months by neonates, this tolerance decreases with age. The longer the period of tracheal intubation, the greater the relative risk of developing subglottic stenosis or posterior glottic stenosis. A variety of factors may act synergistically to increase the risk of laryngeal scar formation secondary to tracheal intubation. These factors include the composition of the tracheal tube, the length of time intubated, patient agitation while intubated, and factors that predispose patients to mucosal damage, such as extraesophageal reflux and airway burns. The most potent predisposing factor to laryngeal damage is the size of the tracheal tube. Ideally, the size of the tracheal tube selected should be *child appropriate* more so than *age appropriate*.

An ideal tracheal tube should be large enough to allow adequate ventilation but small enough to permit a leak of air through the subglottis at a subglottic pressure of less than 20 cm H_2O. Although the average 4 year old should accommodate a 5.0-mm tracheal tube, a 4 year old with an asymptomatic, mild congenital subglottic stenosis may require a 3.0-mm tracheal tube. In some children, the size of the tracheal tube ideal for the larynx may not allow adequate pulmonary ventilation and toilet. In such cases, a larger tracheal tube without a leak may be tolerated for a period of time— a calculated risk, as the true risk of developing subglottic stenosis is still small.

To minimize the risk of developing subglottic stenosis in this situation, consideration should be given to early tracheotomy. A similar problem may occur with poor pulmonary compliance, whereby a leak pressure of less than 20 cm H_2O may not allow adequate ventilation. One possible solution is the use of a low-pressure cuffed tracheal tube that permits higher pressure ventilation while still minimizing laryngeal trauma. For some children, the risks associated with tracheal intubation may be circumvented by the use of alternatives to intubation, such as continuous positive airway pressure (CPAP), bilevel positive airway pressure (BiPAP), high-flow nasal cannula, or even tracheotomy.

Difficult Intubation

In some children tracheal intubation is difficult, while in others tracheal intubation may carry undue risks. In some cases, problems with tracheal intubation are predictable; in other cases, such problems cannot be anticipated. As such, it is prudent to have a cascade of options to secure an airway should difficulties be encountered. Maintaining spontaneous ventilation during attempts to intubate is recommended, as children who are not paralyzed may be able to at least partly maintain their own airway should problems be encountered during attempts at tracheal intubation.

Anatomic anomalies of the mandible present a predictable challenge, especially in the neonate. The retrognathic child, particularly infants with Pierre-Robin sequence, may be extraordinarily difficult to intubate; furthermore, the degree of difficulty may not necessarily be reflected by the clinical degree of retrognathia or the severity of obstruction. Children with microsomia, temporomandibular fixation, macroglossia, and maxillofacial trauma may be similarly challenging to intubate.

Standard tracheal intubation techniques also may be challenging in children in whom neck extension should be avoided. The child with an unstable cervical spine is the best example of this. The risk may be known, such as in a child with Down syndrome or atlanto-occipital instability, or unknown, such as in an unconscious child

D.S. Wheeler et al. (eds.), The *Respiratory Tract in Pediatric Critical Illness and Injury*,
DOI 10.1007/978-1-84800-925-7_14, © Springer-Verlag London Limited 2009

with a head injury and possibly a cervical injury. If intubation is elective, flexion extension views of the cervical spine of children at risk of cervical instability are prudent. Children with Down syndrome, mucopolysaccharide storage disorders, and any major chromosomal anomalies are most at risk. Intubation without neck extension may still be safely performed in most cases.

Even in children who are difficult to intubate, it is usually possible to intubate in a standard fashion, with an anesthetic laryngoscope blade (larger is usually better), a styleted tracheal tube (with the tip of the stylet being angled anteriorly 30°–45° in a retrognathic child), and with laryngeal pressure applied. If this is unsuccessful, options include transnasal fiberoptic intubation, intubation with a rigid ventilating bronchoscope, intubation with a tracheal tube threaded over a Hopkins rod telescope, or placement of a laryngeal mask airway. It should be emphasized that even in children who are difficult to intubate, a bag and mask with an oral airway may be sufficient to temporarily stabilize the airway until a more definitive solution can be arranged. For children in whom intubation is very difficult, either elective or emergent tracheotomy is generally required. It is desirable to place a tracheotomy with the airway already secured with a tracheal tube whenever possible.

The Child With a Tracheotomy

In the PICU setting, the airway of a child with a tracheotomy tube should be easily managed, as the child may be conveniently ventilated and usually does not require sedation. However, a tracheotomy is not without risk, and tube blockage or displacement may result in abrupt airway obstruction. Tracheotomy tube complications may be divided into those related to a fresh tracheotomy tract and those related to tube obstruction. With a fresh tracheotomy, the risk is that of tube displacement and subsequent difficulty with tube replacement. Precautions to prevent displacement include maturing the stoma (the skin is sewn directly to the tracheal cartilage) and placing stay sutures. These precautions are taken so that if the tracheotomy is displaced, traction on the stay sutures will open the tracheotomy and aid in replacement of the tube. Ensuring that the tip of the tracheotomy tube is well distal to the tracheotomy site is also prudent, as this lessens the risk of displacement. Flexible bronchoscopy at the time of tracheotomy is a simple method of ensuring that the tracheotomy tube is in sufficiently and that it is not too close to the carina or down a bronchus.

Obstructive symptoms may be due to either obstruction within the tube or obstruction distal to the tube. Regular suctioning to the tip of the tube, but not beyond, will usually prevent tube obstruction, and, whenever the tube appears obstructed, suctioning is the first intervention. If this does not rapidly resolve the problem, the tube should be replaced. If obstruction persists, obstruction distal to the tube should be suspected. Ideally, flexible bronchoscopy down the tracheotomy tube will confirm the site of obstruction, and a longer tube may be all that is required to bypass the obstruction (usually granulation tissue or tracheomalacia). Positive pressure will alleviate obstruction caused by tracheomalacia or bronchomalacia. In an emergency situation, a longer tracheotomy tube or even a tracheal tube placed through the stoma will usually bypass the obstruction.

Single-Stage Airway Reconstruction

Airway surgery is frequently performed without retaining a tracheotomy tube, but rather relying on a tracheal tube to both act as a temporary stent and to maintain the airway; this is referred to as *single-stage reconstruction*. The tracheal tube may be required for only a few hours or may be placed for up to 2 weeks. In general, the more complex the surgery, the longer the period of tracheal intubation required. A prerequisite for successful single-stage surgery is a capable PICU staff that can manage a child who may be tracheally intubated for a prolonged period and minimize the risk of accidental extubation, as reintubation may potentially compromise the reconstruction. Ideally, paralytic agents should be avoided, for, should an accidental extubation occur, nonparalyzed children may be able to manage their own airway for a time that is sufficient to arrange reintubation under controlled conditions.

Many children requiring airway surgery have a history of prolonged tracheal intubation and sedation before tracheotomy placement. These children may be quite tolerant to a range of sedatives. Most children younger than 3 years of age require sedation, while most neurologically normal children older than age 3 do not. Despite tracheal intubation, neurologically normal children older than 3 years of age may be able to ambulate and even eat. For children who require sedation, the amount of sedation required may be remarkable, resulting in a need for ventilation and inotropic support. This may also present problems of oversedation upon extubation. As such, conversion to a rapidly metabolized agent such as propofol or dexmedetomidine for the 12 hr before extubation is useful. The child should be as awake as possible before extubation.

A bronchoscopic evaluation of the airway the day before extubation is very useful to (1) assess whether it is prudent to attempt extubation, (2) remove excessive glottic granulation tissue, and (3) place a smaller tracheal tube that allows resolution of some of the laryngeal edema. Once a child is extubated, glottic or subglottic edema is common, and stridor and retractions are to be expected. Laryngeal edema typically worsens for the first 24–36 hr and then subsides. Every effort should be made to avoid reintubation during this period. Useful adjunctive measures include the use of racemic epinephrine, heliox, CPAP, high-flow nasal cannula, corticosteroids (dexamethasone, 0.5 mg/kg daily), and chest physiotherapy. If a child requires reintubation, it is usually worth reattempting extubation after an additional 48 hr. If a child has failed a trial of extubation on three occasions, tracheotomy should be considered.

There are no absolutes, and for some children single-stage surgery should be approached with caution. This includes children who are difficult to intubate, those who have a history of failed single-stage surgery, those who have severe or multilevel airway stenosis, and those who have a history of problems with sedation.

Congenital Anomalies of the Airway

Retrognathia/Glossoptosis

Retrognathia is seen with a variety of conditions, including the Pierre-Robin sequence, Treacher-Collins syndrome, and Stickler syndrome. An associated cleft palate is common in severe cases. The degree of retrognathia is not always a reliable indicator of the degree of obstruction or of the potential problems with tracheal intubation. Although obstructing retrognathia is usually a problem encountered in the neonatal nursery, problems may be encountered years later. Such problems are often triggered by seemingly trivial surgical procedures or with the insidious onset of severe sleep apnea.

For neonates, initial management includes prone positioning, the use of high-flow nasal cannula, and occasionally the use of a nasal trumpet. Continuous positive air pressure is often not successful, as the mask tends to exacerbate the relative retrognathia. Because infants struggle with feeding, nasogastric tube placement is often required. If the airway remains compromised, tracheal intubation is desirable, but, as discussed previously, it may be challenging.

For infants with significant obstructive symptoms or feeding problems, surgical intervention is desirable. Performing a tracheotomy is standard, and, in most children catch-up growth of the mandible will permit decannulation within 1–2 years. If catch-up growth is not apparent by 1 year of age, consideration can be given to mandibular distraction. In some cases, distraction may be an alternative to tracheotomy; however, this remains controversial [1,2]. Even after tracheotomy, some children continue to have symptoms of obstruction, as there is an association with retrognathia and tracheobronchomalacia. Performing flexible bronchoscopy through the tracheotomy tube is diagnostic, and management with CPAP, BiPAP, or positive pressure ventilation may be required. In cases of isolated tracheomalacia, replacing the tracheotomy tube with a longer tube that lies close to carina may be sufficient.

Laryngomalacia

Laryngomalacia is the most frequent cause of stridor in the neonate, and most children are symptomatic at birth or within the first few days of life. Stridor is generally mild, but it is exacerbated by feeding, crying, and lying in a supine position. In 50% of cases, symptoms worsen during the first 6 months of life, and, in virtually all children with laryngomalacia, symptoms resolve by 1 year of age. In less than 5% of cases, severity mandates surgical intervention. In severe cases, symptoms may include apnea, cyanosis, severe retractions, and failure to thrive. Cor pulmonale is seen in very severe cases. There also are some children in whom apnea and cyanosis are not marked but who are clearly obstructed, thus causing family stress and concern. In a subset of these children, intervention also is warranted.

Diagnosis is confirmed by flexible transnasal fiberoptic laryngoscopy. Characteristic findings include short aryepiglottic folds, with prolapse of the cuneiform cartilages. In some cases, a tightly curled (Ω-shaped) epiglottis is also observed. Because of the Bernoulli effect, characteristic collapse of the supraglottic structures is seen on inspiration. Inflammation suggestive of reflux laryngitis is frequently seen. The need for intervention is determined not by the endoscopic appearance of the larynx but rather by the symptoms of the infant.

Children with laryngomalacia rarely present with acute airway compromise. In the 5% of children who require operative management, this may be arranged in a semielective fashion within 1 to 2 weeks of presentation. Preoperative management of gastroesophageal reflux is prudent. Supraglottoplasty (also termed epiglottoplasty) has replaced tracheotomy as the preferred intervention. This is a rapid and effective endoscopic procedure, directed at the infant's specific laryngeal pathology. Both aryepiglottic folds usually are divided. In addition, one or both cuneiform cartilages may be removed. If the aryepiglottic folds alone are divided, postoperative intubation is generally not required; however, overnight tracheal intubation should be considered if more extensive surgery has been performed.

Following supraglottoplasty, overnight observation in the PICU is desirable, as laryngeal edema may compromise the airway, necessitating reintubation. Extubation is usually possible within 24 hr of the surgery. In some children, obstruction persists postoperatively. Repeated fiberoptic laryngoscopy at the bedside can help establish whether this is due to laryngeal edema or persistent laryngomalacia that necessitates further surgery. Reflux management helps manage laryngeal edema. Occasionally, the postoperative appearance of the larynx is adequate, but the infant is still struggling. In such cases, there is sometimes an underlying neurologic component to the laryngomalacia. Although the neurologic problems may be extremely subtle initially, they may become much more evident with time. This group of children is far more likely to require tracheotomy placement [3].

Vocal Cord Paralysis

Vocal cord paralysis is the second most common cause of neonatal stridor. As with laryngomalacia, the diagnosis is established with awake flexible transnasal fiberoptic laryngoscopy. This condition is subdivided into congenital and acquired paralysis and unilateral and bilateral paralysis. In most cases, bilateral vocal cord paralysis is congenital, while unilateral paralysis is an acquired problem caused by damage to the recurrent laryngeal nerve. Because of the length and course of the left recurrent nerve, this is far more likely to be damaged than the right recurrent laryngeal nerve. As such, most children with acquired vocal cord paralysis have unilateral left-sided paralysis.

Congenital cord paralysis is usually idiopathic in nature, but may also be seen with central nervous system pathology, including hydrocephalus and Chiari malformation of the brain stem. It may be reversible if the underlying cause is corrected. Most children with bilateral vocal cord paralysis present with significant airway compromise but excellent voice quality. They usually do not aspirate. Up to 90% of infants with bilateral vocal cord paralysis ultimately require tracheotomy. By contrast, children with unilateral vocal cord paralysis usually have an acceptable airway, but a breathy voice, and are at a slightly higher risk of aspiration.

Diagnosis is made with awake transnasal flexible laryngoscopy. The risk factors for acquired paralysis are patent ductus arteriosus repair, the Norwood cardiac repair, and esophageal surgery, especially tracheoesophageal fistula repair. For older children, thyroid surgery is an additional risk factor.

For an infant with stridor and retractions due to bilateral vocal cord paralysis, tracheotomy is indicated. Stabilization may be achieved with tracheal intubation, CPAP, or high-flow nasal cannula as an alternative temporizing measure. Up to 50% of children with congenital idiopathic bilateral vocal cord paralysis have spontaneous resolution of their paralysis by 1 year of age. Surgical intervention to achieve decannulation is thus usually delayed until after 1 year. Similarly, children with acquired bilateral vocal cord paralysis may have spontaneous recovery several months after recurrent laryngeal nerve injury if the nerve is only stretched or crushed but is otherwise intact.

Most children with unilateral vocal cord paralysis do not require surgical intervention. For those with bilateral paralysis, there are several surgical options because no single surgical approach offers a perfect result. The aim of surgery is to achieve an adequate decannulated airway while maintaining voice and not exacerbating aspiration. Surgical options include laser cordotomy, partial or complete arytenoidectomy (endoscopic or open), vocal process lateralization (open or endoscopically guided), and posterior cricoid cartilage grafting [4,5]. In a child with a tracheotomy, it is often desirable to maintain the tracheotomy to ensure an adequate airway before decannulation. In a child without a tracheotomy, a single-stage procedure can be performed.

Acquired bilateral vocal cord paralysis is usually more recalcitrant to treatment than idiopathic cord paralysis, and more than one procedure may be required to achieve decannulation. For patients who have undergone any such procedures, postextubation stridor may respond to CPAP or high-flow nasal cannula. A child's postoperative risk of aspiration should be assessed by a video swallow study before resuming a normal diet. During the initial weeks following surgery, there is sometimes an increased aspiration risk with certain textures, especially thin fluids.

Subglottic Stenosis

Subglottic stenosis (SGS) can be either congenital or acquired. Congenital SGS is comparatively rare. In the neonate, it is defined as a lumen 4.0 mm in diameter or less at the level of the cricoid. Acquired SGS is much more frequently seen and is normally a sequela of prolonged intubation of the neonate. The cause of congenital SGS is thought to be a failure of the laryngeal lumen to recanalize. This condition is one of a continuum of embryologic failures that include laryngeal atresia, stenosis, and webs. In its mildest form, congenital SGS appears as a normal cricoid with a smaller than average diameter, usually elliptical in shape. Mild SGS may manifest in recurrent upper respiratory infections (often diagnosed as croup) in which minimal subglottic swelling precipitates airway obstruction. In a young child, the greatest obstruction is usually 2–3 mm below the true vocal cords. More severe cases may present with acute airway compromise at delivery. If tracheal intubation is successful, the patient may require intervention before extubation. When intubation cannot be achieved, tracheotomy placement at the time of delivery may be life saving. Important to note, infants typically have surprisingly few symptoms. Even those with grade III SGS may not be symptomatic for weeks or months.

Congenital SGS is often associated with other congenital head and neck lesions and syndromes (e.g., a small larynx in a patient with Down syndrome). After initial management of SGS, the larynx will grow with the patient and may not require further surgical intervention. However, if initial management requires tracheal intubation, the risk of developing an acquired SGS in addition to the underlying congenital SGS is considerable.

Radiologic evaluation of an airway that is not intubated may give the clinician clues about the site and length of the stenosis. Useful imaging modalities include (1) inspiratory and expiratory lateral soft tissue neck films, (2) fluoroscopy to demonstrate the dynamics of the trachea and larynx, and (3) a chest x-ray. The single most important investigation, however, is high-kilovoltage airway films. These films are taken not only to identify the classic *steepling* observed in patients with SGS but also to identify possible tracheal stenosis. The latter condition is generally caused by complete tracheal rings, which may predispose the patient to a life-threatening situation during rigid endoscopy.

Evaluation of SGS, whether congenital, acquired, or a combination of both, requires endoscopic assessment. Endoscopy is necessary for the diagnosis of laryngeal stenosis. Flexible fiberoptic endoscopy provides information on dynamic vocal cord function. Rigid endoscopy with a Hopkins telescope provides the best possible examination. Precise evaluation of the endolarynx should be

carried out, including grading of the subglottic stenosis. Stenosis caused by scarring, granulation tissue, submucosal thickening, or a congenitally abnormal cricoid can be differentiated from SGS with a normal cricoid, but endoscopic measurement with tracheal tubes or bronchoscopes is required for an accurate evaluation.

The greatest risk factor for developing acquired SGS is presently prolonged intubation with an inappropriately large tracheal tube. The appropriate tracheal tube size is not the largest that will fit but rather the smallest that allows for adequate ventilation. Ideally, the tracheal tube should leak air around it, with subglottic pressures below 25–30 cm H_2O. Other cofactors for the development of acquired SGS include gastroesophageal reflux (GER) and eosinophilic esophagitis (EE).

Children with mild acquired SGS may be asymptomatic or minimally symptomatic. Observation rather than intervention may thus be appropriate. This is often the case for children with grades I or II SGS. Those with more severe SGS (grades III and IV), however, are symptomatic, with either tracheal dependency or stridor and exercise intolerance. Unlike congenital SGS, acquired SGS is unlikely to resolve spontaneously and thus requires intervention.

For children with mild symptoms and a minor degree of SGS, endoscopic intervention may be effective. Endoscopic options include radial laser incisions through the stenosis and laryngeal dilatation. More severe forms of SGS are better managed with open airway reconstruction. Laryngotracheal reconstruction using costal cartilage grafts placed through the split lamina of the cricoid cartilage is reliable and has withstood the test of time [6,7]. Costal cartilage grafts may be placed through the anterior lamina of the cricoid cartilage, the posterior lamina of the cricoid cartilage, or both. These procedures may be performed as a two-stage procedure, maintaining the tracheal tube and temporarily placing a suprastomal laryngeal stent above the tracheal tube. Alternatively, in selective cases, a single-stage procedure may be performed, with removal of the tracheal tube on the day of surgery and with the child requiring intubation for a 1–14-day period [8]. More recently, better results have been obtained with cricotracheal resection than with laryngotracheal reconstruction for the management of severe SGS [9]. However, this is a technically demanding procedure that carries a significant risk of complications. Reconstruction of the subglottic airway is a challenging procedure, and the patient should be optimized before undergoing surgery. Preoperative evaluation includes assessment and management of GER, EE, and low-grade tracheal infection, particularly oxacillin-resistant *Staphylococcus aureus* (ORSA) and *Pseudomonas*.

Posterior Laryngeal Clefts

Posterior laryngeal clefts result from a fusion failure of the laryngotracheal groove (failure of the laryngotracheal groove to fuse during embryogenesis). Although these clefts are generally not obstructive in nature, infants with laryngeal clefts sometimes present with significant obstruction. Aspiration is the hallmark clinical feature of this disorder. While gross aspiration may occur with associated apnea, cyanosis, and even pneumonia, often the symptoms are those of microaspiration, with choking episodes, transient cyanosis, and recurrent chest infections. As such, diagnosis may initially be elusive.

Other associated anomalies are common and may be divided into those that affect the airway and those that do not. Associated airway anomalies include tracheomalacia (>80%) and tracheoesophageal fistula (TEF) (20%) formation. Non-airway associations include anogenital anomalies and GER. The most common syndrome associated with posterior laryngeal clefting is Opitz-Frias syndrome, which is characterized by hypertelorism, anogenital anomalies, and posterior laryngeal clefting. Diagnosis is challenging. Although contrast swallow studies may suggest risk of aspiration, definitive diagnosis requires rigid laryngoscopy and bronchoscopy, with the interarytenoid area being specifically probed to determine if a posterior laryngeal cleft is present. Figure 14.1 shows a modification of the Benjamin and Inglis classification system, with cleft types I to V illustrated.

Initial management decisions should consider whether the infant requires tracheotomy placement, gastrostomy tube placement, or Nissen fundoplication. Although none of these is essential, each increases the likelihood of successful cleft repair. Protection against aspiration is also crucial, and nasojejunal feeding may be a useful way of stabilizing an infant. Surgical repair may be performed endoscopically for most type I and some type II clefts; however, longer clefts that extend into the cervical or thoracic trachea require open repair. The transtracheal approach is advocated in that it provides unparalleled exposure of the cleft while protecting the recurrent laryngeal nerves. A two-layer closure is recommended, with the option of performing an interposition graft if warranted;

a useful interposition graft is a free transfer of clavicular or tibial periosteum. The most challenging cleft to repair is the type V cleft, which extends to the carina or beyond. Performing such surgery is anesthetically daunting. Type V clefts are prone to anastomotic breakdown, and the infant often has multiple congenital anomalies [10].

Vascular Compression

Vascular compression of the airway, particularly innominate artery compression, is not uncommon; however, it is usually asymptomatic or minimally symptomatic. Symptomatic vascular compression of the trachea or bronchi is rare but associated with marked symptoms, including biphasic stridor, retractions, a honking cough, and *dying spells*. Symptoms tend to substantially worsen when the child is upset. Forms of vascular compression affecting the trachea include innominate artery compression, double aortic arch, and pulmonary artery sling. Vascular rings resulting from a retroesophageal subclavian artery and a ligamentum arteriosum are less likely to be associated with airway obstruction. Bronchial compression by the pulmonary arteries or aorta may be significant but are more commonly a unilateral problem unless there are associated major cardiac anomalies. The diagnosis of airway compression is best established with rigid bronchoscopy. Thoracic imaging then assists in establishing the relevant vascular anatomy. Imaging modalities include high-resolution computed tomography (CT) imaging with contrast enhancement and three-dimensional reconstruction, magnetic resonance imaging (MRI) and magnetic resonance angiography (MRA), and echocardiography. Less commonly, formal angiography is required. Although the primarily role of imaging is to evaluate the intrathoracic vasculature, excellent images of the airway and the thymus gland may also be obtained.

In a child with an airway compromised by vascular compression, CPAP may provide a limited degree of temporary improvement, as there is often segmental tracheomalacia in the region of the vascular compression. Otherwise, tracheal intubation may be required. Because of the proximity of a vascular structure, prolonged intubation is avoided when possible due to the risk of forming an arterial fistula. Similarly, although tracheotomy will establish an unobstructed airway, there is also an increased risk of a vascular fistula into the airway.

The surgical management of symptomatic vascular compression addresses the specific pathology involved. Innominate artery compression responds well to thymectomy and aortopexy, but, if little thymus is present, an alternative is reimplantation of the innominate artery more proximately on the aortic arch. A double aortic arch requires ligation of the smaller of the two arches, which is usually the left. A pulmonary artery sling is transected at its origin, dissected free, and reimplanted into the pulmonary trunk anterior to the trachea. There is a high incidence of complete tracheal rings in children with a pulmonary artery sling, and these should also be repaired at the time of vascular repair [11].

Alleviating vascular compression will improve the airway; nevertheless, it takes time for the airway to completely normalize. This is a consequence of long-standing vascular compression having adversely affected the normal cartilaginous development of the compressed segment of trachea, with resultant cartilaginous malacia or stenosis. Until the airway normalizes, which may take months, children who are persistently symptomatic may require airway stabilization with a tracheotomy. Although tracheal stabilization with intratracheal stents is alluring under these

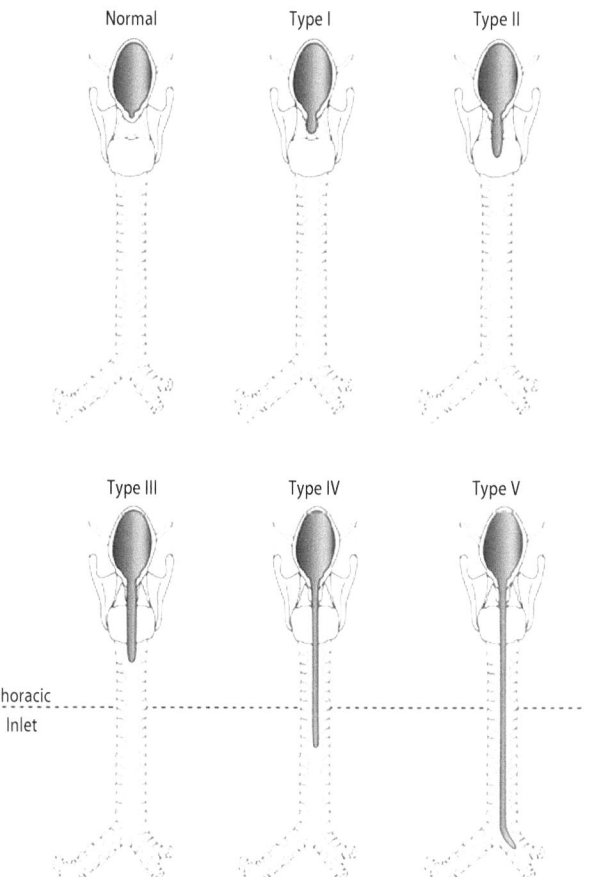

FIGURE 14.1. Classification of posterior laryngeal clefts (a modification of the Benjamin and Inglis classification). The larynx and trachea are viewed from the posterior aspect. Type I: Cleft to but not below the true vocal cords. Type II: Cleft into the cricoid cartilage but not into the cervical trachea. Type III: Cleft through the cricoid into the cervical trachea. Type IV: Cleft into the thoracic trachea. Type V: Cleft to or beyond the carina.

circumstances, the incidence of complications is high. Temporary tracheotomy is generally a more desirable alternative.

Complete Tracheal Rings

Although complete tracheal rings are rare, they are life threatening. They present with insidious worsening of respiratory function over the first few months of life, with stridor, retractions, and marked exacerbation of symptoms during intercurrent upper respiratory tract infections. Children with distal tracheal stenosis usually have a characteristic biphasic wet-sounding breathing pattern that transiently clears with coughing; this pattern is referred to as *washing machine breathing*. The risk of respiratory failure increases with age. Although diagnosis is made with rigid bronchoscopy, an initial high-kilovolt airway film may warn of tracheal narrowing. Bronchoscopy should be performed with great caution, using the smallest possible telescopes, as any airway edema in the region of the stenosis may turn a narrow airway into an extremely critical airway. The location, extent, and degree of stenosis are all relevant; however, if the airway is exceptionally narrow, it may be more prudent just to establish the diagnosis rather than to risk causing post-traumatic edema by forcing a telescope through a stenosis.

Because 50% of children have a tracheal inner diameter of approximately 2 mm at the time of diagnosis, the standard interventions for managing a compromised airway are not applicable. More specifically, the smallest tracheal tube has an outer diameter of 2.9 mm, and the smallest tracheotomy tube has an outer diameter of 3.9 mm; hence, the stenotic segment cannot be intubated. This may leave extracorporeal membrane oxygenation (ECMO) as the only viable alternative for stabilizing the child. This situation is best avoided by performing bronchoscopy with the highest level of care. Over 80% of children with complete tracheal rings have other congenital anomalies, which are generally cardiovascular in origin. As such, investigation should include a high-resolution contrast-enhanced CT scan of the chest and a cardiac echocardiogram. Specifically, a pulmonary artery sling should be excluded, as this is a common association and, if present, should be repaired concurrent with the tracheal repair. Most children with complete tracheal rings require tracheal reconstruction [12]. The recommended surgical technique is the slide tracheoplasty [13]. This approach yields

significantly better results than any other form of tracheal reconstruction and is applicable to all anatomic variants of complete tracheal rings.

References

1. Mandell DL, Yellon, RF, Bradley, JP, et al. Mandibular distraction for micrognathia and severe upper airway obstruction. Arch Otolaryngol Head Neck Surg 2004;130:344–348.
2. Rhee ST, Buchman SR. Pediatric mandibular distraction osteogenesis: the present and the future. J Craniofac Surg 2003;14:803–808.
3. Denoyelle FM, Mondain M, Gresillon N, et al. Failures and complications of supraglottoplasty in children. Arch Otolaryngol Head Neck Surg 2003;129:1077–1080.
4. Miyamoto RC, Parikh SR, Gellad W, et al. Bilateral congenital vocal cord paralysis: a 16-year institutional review. Otolaryngol Head Neck Surg 2005;133:241–245.
5. Hartnick CJ, Brigger MT, Willging JP, et al. Surgery for pediatric vocal cord paralysis: a retrospective review. Ann Otol Rhinol Laryngol 2003;112:1–6.
6. Cotton RT, Gray SD, Miller RP. Update of the Cincinnati experience in pediatric laryngotracheal reconstruction. Laryngoscope 1989; 99: 1111–1116.
7. Cotton RT. The problem of pediatric laryngotracheal stenosis: a clinical and experimental study on the efficacy of autogenous cartilaginous grafts placed between the vertically divided lamina of the cricoid cartilage. Laryngoscope 1991;101:1–34.
8. Gustafson LM, Hartley BE, Liu JH, et al. Single-stage laryngotracheal reconstruction in children: a review of 200 cases. Otolaryngol Head Heck Surg 2000;123:430–434.
9. White DR, Cotton RT, Bean JA, et al. Pediatric cricotracheal resection: surgical outcomes and risk factor analysis. Arch Otolaryngol Head Neck Surg 2005;131:896–899.
10. Rutter MJ, Azizkhan RG, Cotton RT. Posterior laryngeal cleft. In: Ziegler MM, Azizkhan RG, Weber TR, eds. Operative Pediatric Surgery. New York: McGraw-Hill; 2003:313–320.
11. Wright CD. Pediatric tracheal surgery. Chest Surg Clin North Am 2003;13:305–314.
12. Rutter MJ, Cotton RT. Tracheal stenosis and reconstruction. In: Mattei P, ed. Surgical Directives: Pediatric Surgery. Philadelphia: Lippincott, Williams & Wilkins; 2003:151–156.
13. Rutter MJ, Cotton R, Azizkhan R, et al. Slide tracheoplasty for the management of complete tracheal rings. J Pediatr Surg 2003;38:928–934.

15
Status Asthmaticus

Derek S. Wheeler, Kristen Page, and Thomas P. Shanley

Introduction

Asthma is the most common pediatric respiratory disease and remains one of the most common reasons children in the United States require hospitalization. Current statistics suggest that approximately 15 million Americans suffer from this disease, including nearly 5 million children [1]. Asthma poses a significant economic burden to the health care system, accounting for 2 million emergency department visits, 500,000 hospitalizations, and nearly $6 billion in total health care expenditures each year [2–9]. Status asthmaticus, defined as a condition of progressively worsening bronchospasm unresponsive to standard therapy, accounts for a significant number of admissions to the pediatric intensive care unit (PICU) each year. For example, during the 5-year period between 1998 and 2002, status asthmaticus accounted for 6% of all admissions to the PICU at a major tertiary children's medical center (Wheeler, D.S., unpublished data), although only 0.5%–2% of children admitted to the hospital with asthma require intensive care treatment [10–14]. Although recent trends suggest that the incidence of childhood asthma may have reached a plateau, asthma morbidity and mortality continue to rise, especially in certain subsets of the population [4–9,15–19]. As a result, there continues to be great interest in the identification and development of treatment strategies that can effectively manage and improve the outcome of critically ill children diagnosed with status asthmaticus.

Epidemiology

In striking contrast to cancer and heart disease, asthma lacks a standardized, consensus definition and therefore does not lend itself to straightforward epidemiologic study. However, despite this inherent difficulty, the overwhelming preponderance of evidence suggests that the worldwide incidence of asthma is increasing

[18–20]. Since 1980, in fact, the frequency of asthma has approximately doubled [21]. Certainly some of the increases in disease prevalence may be attributed to increased awareness and better reporting, although studies utilizing similar case definitions continue to show an epidemic increase in the incidence of asthma, especially in westernized countries such as the United Kingdom, Australia, and New Zealand; far lower prevalence rates have been observed in India, China, Africa, and other countries in Asia and Eastern Europe [20]. However, several studies demonstrate increasing prevalence rates of asthma in countries as they become more westernized [22,23]. Similar trends have been observed in the United States. For example, the National Center for Health Statistics (NCHS) reported results from the National Health Interview Survey (NHIS) showing that the self-reported prevalence of asthma increased by nearly 75% across all age groups between 1980 and 1994. The greatest increases occurred among preschool children (<5 years), in which the prevalence rate rose by nearly 150% [7]. The prevalence rates are highest among African Americans and children from lower socioeconomic backgrounds [4,7,24,25].

Germane to the present discussion, the morbidity and mortality from asthma appear to be steadily rising in certain high-risk groups of the population [4–9,15–17]. Some investigators have suggested that this apparent increase can be attributed to complications associated with the increased usage of β-agonist therapy, although this probably reflects a greater severity of illness and subsequent need for therapy than an actual cause-and-effect association [26–32]. Rather, the wealth of evidence suggests that undermedication, particularly with regard to the inadequate use of corticosteroids, and lack of recognition of the severity of an asthma attack by both patients and parents (causing a delay in seeking medical care), as well as the health care provider are more important factors [33–39].

There appear to be two clinical subsets of children who die from status asthmaticus [40]. For example, some children with fatal asthma usually have a long history of poorly controlled, severe asthma, often with a previous history of respiratory failure (type I, or *slow onset-late arrival*). This pattern of fatal asthma, which is responsible for the majority of asthma-related deaths, is generally considered preventable, with death occurring secondary to acute respiratory failure and asphyxia or from complications associated with mechanical ventilation [41–46]. Pathologic examination in these cases demonstrates extensive bronchial mucous plugging, edema, and eosinophilic infiltration of the airways. Alternatively,

D.S. Wheeler et al. (eds.), The *Respiratory Tract in Pediatric Critical Illness and Injury*,
DOI 10.1007/978-1-84800-925-7_15, © Springer-Verlag London Limited 2009

TABLE 15.1. Risk factors for potentially fatal asthma.

History of previous attack with
   Severe, rapid progression of symptoms
   Respiratory failure requiring endotracheal
      Intubation or ventilatory support*
   Seizures or loss of consciousness
   Pediatric intensive care unit admission
Attacks precipitated by food allergy
Denial or failure to perceive the severity of illness
Noncompliance
Lack of social support network (dysfunctional family)
Associated psychiatric disorder (e.g., depression)
Nonwhite children (especially african-american and hispanic children)

*May include noninvasive positive pressure ventilation.

some children present with only a mild history of asthma, and often even without a prior history of asthma, experience the sudden onset of bronchospasm, and rapidly progress to cardiac arrest and death (type II, or *fast-onset*) [47–50]. If recognized and managed early, these children respond faster to β-agonists and mechanical ventilatory support compared with children with type I fatal asthma [51]. Pathologic examination in these cases shows *empty* airways devoid of mucous plugging with a greater proportion of neutrophils than eosinophils [52].

Robertson et al. [53] reviewed 51 pediatric deaths from asthma between 1986 and 1989 and found that nearly one-third of these children were judged to have mild asthma with no prior hospitalizations for asthma. Sixty-three percent of these children experienced a sudden collapse within minutes of the onset of symptoms, and 75% died before reaching the hospital. Only 25% of these children had an acute progression of chronic, poorly controlled asthma that resulted in eventual death. The authors of this study concluded that only 39% of these deaths were preventable by earlier recognition and intervention. Over a 6-year period at the Hospital for Sick Children in Toronto, 89 children were admitted to the PICU for status asthmaticus. Three children died in the PICU from hypoxic–ischemic encephalopathy following out-of-hospital cardiac arrest [13]. Kravis and Kolski [54] reported a case series of 13 deaths secondary to asthma. Only one child died following admission to the hospital. Similarly, nearly 50% of asthmatic children in another study died before reaching the hospital, with the time from the onset of symptoms to death less than 1 hr in 21% and less than 2 hr in 50% of these cases, respectively [55,56]. These series further underscore the need for early recognition for children at risk for type II fast-onset, sudden asphyxial asthma. Accordingly, several authors have attempted to define characteristics or *risk factors* of children who die of asthma (Table 15.1) [26,33–35,37,47,48,53,55,57–65].

Pathogenesis

Asthma was widely viewed as a neurologic disorder in the 19th and early 20th century caused largely by emotional disturbances and anxiety [66]. Asthma is now considered a disease of inflammation, and, over the past decade, tremendous gains have been made with regard to our understanding about the pathogenesis of asthma. This mechanistic insight has been driven by attempts to identify the etiology of the two principal hallmarks of asthma, airway (or bronchial) hyperresponsiveness (AHR) and inflammation. By

employing both animal models and well-designed clinical studies, investigators have continued to identify not only the cellular and mediator participants in asthma but also the genetic influences regulating this common disease entity.

Immunopathogenesis

Asthma frequently begins during early childhood and is often associated with atopy, the genetic susceptibility to produce IgE specific to common airborne allergens (e.g., house dust, animal dander). Children with asthma respond to these airborne allergens with an increase in activated, $CD4^+$ T helper (Th) cells. The immunologic response to a particular allergen depends to a significant extent on the type of Th cells that accumulate in the airways. Atopic children tend to respond with a T helper type 2 (Th2) immune response, whereas nonatopic children demonstrate a T helper type 1 (Th1)-skewed response. The Th1 and Th2 cells are effector T cells that develop from naïve T cells upon activation by antigens presented by antigen-presenting cells (APCs) and are characterized by different cytokine production.

Dendritic cells (DCs) are potent APCs and have a central role in initiating the primary immune response [67,68]. Respiratory DCs form a tightly meshed network throughout the airway epithelium and are situated to monitor the external environment [69,70]. Respiratory DCs prime Th2 immune responses to inhaled antigens and initiate allergic airway inflammation [71,72]. Th2 cells produce interleukin (IL)-4, IL-5, IL-6, IL-9, and IL-13 and are involved in activating B cells for the production of immunoglobulins, particularly IgE. Conversely, Th1 cells produce interferon (IFN)-γ, IL-2, and lymphotoxin. T helper type 1 responses stimulate macrophage activation and delayed-type hypersensitivity reactions, whereas Th2 responses stimulate antibody-mediated responses and activation of mast cells and eosinophils (see later). Of interest, Th1 cytokines suppress the development of Th2 cells, and vice versa. The marked increase in the incidence of asthma has been attributed by some investigators to a cleaner environment and reduced bacterial burden during early childhood, leading to a shift in the normal development of the immune response and a shift toward a Th2-dominant immune response to allergens, the so-called hygiene hypothesis. Although such a theory is attractive, it does not explain the parallel rise in the incidence of classic Th1 diseases such as type I diabetes mellitus. A detailed account of the hygiene hypothesis is clearly beyond the scope of the present discussion, although several excellent reviews are available to the interested reader [21,73–75].

As discussed earlier, induction of a Th2 response increases the level of IgE, IL-4, IL-5, IL-9, and IL-13 in the serum of patients with asthma, and increased levels of these cytokines are found in patients with acute asthma [21,74]. Increased IgE levels correlate with asthma severity and may be a risk factor for nonallergic asthma [76,77]. Immunoglobulin E antibodies bind to a high-affinity Fc receptor (FcεRI) that is expressed on mast cells, basophils, and eosinophils. IgE–FcεRI crosslinking results in (1) release of preformed vasoactive mediators (histamine, mast cell tryptase, leukotrienes B4 and C4); (2) upregulation of cytokine expression (tumor necrosis factor (TNF)-α, IL-4, IL-5, and IL-13); and (3) synthesis of prostaglandins. Interleukin-4 induces IgE-type–specific B cells and proliferation and activation of mast cells. Interleukin-5 plays an essential role in enhancing eosinophilic accumulation and activation. Recent evidence suggests that IL-13 is especially critical to the immunopathogenesis of asthma [21,74]. All of the features result in the main pathophysiologic components of the asthmatic response—airway inflammation, bronchial AHR, airway remodeling, and reversible airway obstruction.

Airway Inflammation

Historically, the first evidence that implicated a role for inflammation in asthma was obtained from postmortem lung examinations from patients who died with status asthmaticus [78]. Hyperinflated lungs, plugging of bronchi, excessive mucus, edematous or denuded epithelium, and cellular infiltration with neutrophils, eosinophils, and desquamated epithelial cells all were observed in these studies. More recently, samples obtained by bronchoalveolar lavage (BAL) have confirmed the consistent presence of inflammatory cells that have been more specifically identified to include neutrophils, eosinophils, mast cells, and B and T lymphocytes [79]. Because many of these cell types are not present in the lung normally, it was hypothesized and determined that activation of the residential APCs, principally the DCs (see earlier), results in further stimulation of Th2 cells [80]. The mechanism by which these cell types are recruited to the lung in asthma has been a major focus of ongoing investigations.

The respiratory epithelium plays a key role in the asthmatic response, as it is the first point of contact between the lung and viruses, aeroallergens, and irritants. The respiratory epithelium is not merely a physical barrier; instead, it plays an active role as a regulator of airway inflammation. Epithelial cells can synthesize and release a wide range of chemoattractants to recruit inflammatory cells into the airways. In addition, airway epithelial cells can synthesize and release factors that are important for the maturation and survival of neutrophils, macrophages, and eosinophils [81–83].

The chemotactic cytokines (*chemokines*) are a group of cytokines that are instrumental in the recruitment of leukocyte populations [84,85]. Chemokines are chemoattractant cytokines that have been divided into four groups, with the vast majority falling into either the CXC or CC groups. The minor groups are represented by single molecules: fractalkaline in the CX3X and lymphotactin in the C group. Members of both the CXC and CC groups have diverse functions during asthmatic responses, including recruitment, cellular activation and degranulation, and differentiation and modulation of the Th1 versus Th2 immune response. Identification of multiple chemokines in the BAL fluid of asthmatic patients has supported the concept that these molecules play a key role in asthma pathogenesis [86,87].

Eosinophils are the most prevalent of the immune cells found in the airway of patients with asthma and release a variety of highly charged cationic proteins, such as eosinophil cationic protein (ECP), eosinophil protein X (EPX), eosinophil-derived neurotoxin (EDN), and major basic protein (MBP), all of which are highly toxic to the respiratory epithelium. Mast cell activation and subsequent release of mediators, such as histamine, chemotactic factors, and arachidonic acid metabolites (notably prostaglandins, thromboxane, leukotrienes, and hydroxyeicosatetraenoic acid) further exacerbates the inflammatory response. It is not entirely clear whether neutrophils contribute to asthma pathophysiology; however, it has been shown that neutrophils seem to be significantly increased in the airways of patients with severe asthma but not in mild asthmatics [88].

Airway smooth muscle (ASM) has previously been thought of as playing a passive role in mediating the inflammatory process to inhaled allergens. However, ASM has recently been shown to synthesize and release a multitude of cytokines, chemokines, growth factors, receptors/surface molecules, and lipid mediators/enzymes [89]. That ASM synthesizes chemokines for T cells, eosinophils, neutrophils, and monocytes suggests accumulation of these inflammatory cells around the ASM. In fact, the ASM of atopic asthmatics expresses the IgE receptor FcεRII [90] as well as receptor ligands to allow for T-cell binding [91].

One particularly interesting facet of asthma research is the relatively recent correlation between exhaled nitric oxide (NO) and the degree of airway inflammation. Nitric oxide is produced by the enzyme inducible nitric oxide synthase (iNOS), and the inflammatory stimuli present in the airways of patients with asthma result in an increase in both the gene expression and activation of iNOS [92]. Exhaled NO levels appear to correlate with the severity of asthma [93], and measurement of exhaled NO offers tremendous promise in monitoring the response to treatment of children with chronic asthma in the outpatient setting, as well as during acute exacerbations in the hospital setting [93–97].

Airway Hyperresponsiveness

Airway hyperresponsiveness is an exaggerated bronchoconstrictor response following exposure to allergens, irritants, viral infections, cold air, or exercise. Airway hyperresponsiveness can be measured by inhalation challenge with methacholine or histamine. The degree of AHR generally correlates with the clinical severity of asthma [98]. A genetic linkage between histamine airway responsiveness and a predisposition for the development of asthma has been suggested [reviewed in 99]. Changes in the airway morphology (i.e., epithelial cell damage, thickening of the basement membrane, release of mediators mainly from the increased number of eosinophils) may result in thickening of the airway wall. Using high-resolution computed tomography (CT), bronchial wall thickening has been shown to be more extensive in patients with asthma than in healthy controls, regardless of the severity of the disease [100].

Interleukin-4, IL-5, and IL-13 all seem to play an important role in AHR most likely through their role in IgE synthesis and eosinophil differentiation and activation [80]. Immunoglobulin binds to the FcεR receptors on mast cells, resulting in the release of a variety of chemokines and cytokines from mast cells. In addition, mast cells contain a number of preformed mediators, such as histamine, prostaglandin D2, leukotriene C4, and platelet-activating factor, as well as the proteases mast cell tryptase, carboxypeptidase A, and chymase. These mediators have been shown to enhance the activation of inflammatory cells, cause microvascular leakage, increase mucus production, and induce bronchoconstriction [101]. Airway hyperresponsiveness, as measured by the forced expiratory volume in 1 second (FEV_1), was reduced in a clinical trial in patients treated with an antibody against IgE [102]. However, another study showed that IgE-deficient mice develop AHR following exposure to *Aspergillus fumigatus* [103]. These data suggest that, although IgE levels may play a role in AHR, other mechanisms are likely to be involved.

Airway Remodeling

The airways are continuously exposed to triggers that mediate the remodeling phenotype, including tobacco smoke, viruses, bacteria, and allergens [104–106]. The extent of remodeling and the clinical consequences are still under debate, although relatively few asthmatics are found without any detectable remodeling of the airways. One study documented significant airway remodeling in children with severe asthma as young as 6 years of age [107]. Pathologically, airway remodeling appears to have a variety of features that include alterations of the airway epithelium, increased ASM mass, mucous gland hyperplasia, increased collagen deposition and persistence of chronic inflammatory cellular infiltrates [108–110].

As early as 1922, it was documented that asthmatic patients had significantly more ASM cell mass [111]. Airway smooth muscle cell hyperplasia and hypertrophy have both been shown to play a role in increased ASM cell mass. T helper type 2 CD4+ cells have also been shown to play a role in both ASM and epithelial remodeling after allergen challenge [reviewed in 112]. The role of subepithelial fibrosis, characterized by the enhanced accumulation of fibronectin and types I, III, and V collagens, in asthma severity is still unknown. Although fibrosis was shown to correlate with a decline in FEV_1 [113], another study showed that collagen deposition in the airways of patients with severe asthma was not significantly different from that in either patients with mild asthma or controls [114]. Thickening and hyalinization of the basement membrane along with infiltration of the submucosa with lymphocytes has been detected in bronchial biopsy specimens from children with moderate asthma [115]. There is increasing evidence that the epithelium in asthmatics is abnormal and has enhanced susceptibility to injury. Many investigators have found that the bronchial epithelium in asthma is structurally disturbed with epithelial disruption from the basement membrane and epithelial shedding [116]. In addition, the expression of CD44 and epidermal growth factor receptor (EGFR) is significantly increased in the asthmatic epithelium consistent with the hypothesis that epithelial damage and airway remodeling are consistent features of bronchial asthma [117,118].

Airflow Obstruction

Airflow obstruction can be caused by a variety of changes, including acute bronchoconstriction, airway edema, chronic mucous plug formation, and airway remodeling. Acute bronchoconstriction is the consequence of IgE-dependent mediator release upon exposure to aeroallergens and is the primary component of the early asthmatic response. Airway edema occurs 6–24 hr following an allergen challenge and is referred to as the *late asthmatic response*. Mucus production, which is an important component of host defense, represents an important cause of airway obstruction when secreted in excess. During asthma exacerbations, most patients have a significant increase in mucin [119], and chronic mucous plug formation consists of an exudate of serum proteins and cell debris that may take weeks to resolve. Fatal asthma is commonly associated with goblet cell hyperplasia and airway occlusion from mucous plugs [120,121]. Adoptive transfer of Th2 cells, but not Th1 cells, into the lungs of naïve mice caused goblet cell hyperplasia and mucin production, although the mechanism by which Th2 cytokines induce goblet cell hyperplasia is uncertain [122]. Airway remodeling is associated with structural changes due to long-standing inflammation and may profoundly affect the extent of reversibility of airway obstruction.

Pathophysiology

Severe airway obstruction resulting from inflammation, bronchoconstriction, and excessive mucus production is at the heart of the gas exchange abnormalities and symptomatology in children with status asthmaticus. The marked increase in airway resistance leads to a dramatic increase in the work of breathing and may be characterized by marked reductions in FEV_1, FEV_1/FVC, and FVC_{25-75} [123–125]. As the degree of airway obstruction worsens, expiration becomes active rather than passive. Inspiration often occurs before termination of the previous expiration, resulting in air-trapping and lung hyperinflation [126,127]. Residual volume and functional residual capacity are increased, with the increase in residual volume exceeding that of the increase in functional residual capacity [126,128–130]. Total lung capacity is also increased to a variable extent [126,129]. The increase in lung volumes during an acute asthma exacerbation may increase the caliber of the airways and temporarily improve the resistive work of breathing [131,132], although at a significant mechanical disadvantage [133,134].

Air-trapping and lung hyperinflation lead to an intrinsic positive end-expiratory pressure ($PEEP_i$) or *auto PEEP* [135], a phenomenon also termed *dynamic hyperinflation*. Dynamic hyperinflation has several adverse effects on the cardiovascular and respiratory systems. For example, the increased lung volumes shift tidal breathing to a less compliant portion of the pressure–volume curve. In addition, flattening of the diaphragm produces an additional mechanical disadvantage. Dynamic hyperinflation also results in premature closure of the airways, which produces a further increase in airways resistance, thereby worsening gas exchange. These factors collectively increase the work of breathing and increase the physiologic dead space. The gas exchange abnormalities produced by dynamic hyperinflation result in ventilation–perfusion mismatch.

The effects of dynamic hyperinflation on cardiorespiratory interactions are quite complex suffice it to say that right ventricular afterload is increased by a combination of factors, including lung hyperinflation (increased pulmonary vascular resistance), hypoxic pulmonary vasoconstriction (ventilation–perfusion mismatch), and acidosis. During expiration, the increase in intrathoracic pressure secondary to dynamic hyperinflation impedes systemic venous return, thereby worsening left ventricular preload. During inspiration, the large negative intrathoracic pressures required to overcome airways resistance markedly increase left ventricular afterload [40,136]. These changes are detected clinically as an increase in the pulsus paradoxus (see later).

Clinical Manifestations

The initial clinical assessment of the child presenting with status asthmaticus should focus on the major organ systems and will provide important clues to the potential for progression to respiratory failure. A quick assessment of the child's neurologic status may demonstrate early signs of hypoxia, which can include restlessness, irritability, confusion, anxiety, and an inability to recognize parents. Conversely, the child who is awake, alert, and cooperative is less likely to deteriorate acutely. Furthermore, the child with impending respiratory failure often prefers a sitting or tripod position in an unconscious effort to maximize diaphragmatic excursion [137]. Although tachypnea is the usual compensatory response to hypoxia, bradypnea in the context of status asthmaticus is an ominous finding. Grunting, nasal flaring, retractions, and use of the accessory muscles of breathing are often present. The presence of dyscoordinate, *seesaw* breathing, which if severe will manifest as paradoxical movement of the thoracic cage during breathing (i.e., the chest moves inward during inspiration), is often a harbinger of impending respiratory failure. The older child may be able to communicate the complaints of dyspnea and *air hunger*, although if airway obstruction is severe the child will often speak only in short phrases or even single words.

Tachycardia is the usual physiologic response in status asthmaticus, which may result from a combination of factors, including anxiety, acidosis, fever (if present), and hypoxia. Pulsus paradoxus (over a 10 mm Hg change in systolic blood pressure between inspiration and expiration) is often present in severe airway obstruction and represents a useful prognostic measure of respiratory compromise [138]. Recent advances in the technology of monitoring devices have resulted in dramatic improvements in the precision and accuracy of determining the pulsus paradoxus and may further strengthen its utility as an objective, effort-independent sign in children with status asthmaticus [139–142].

Pulse oximetry provides for a rapid determination of the arterial oxygen saturation, often called the *fifth vital sign*. The newer generation of pulse oximeters allow for a reasonable estimation of arterial oxygen saturation (SaO_2) even under poor monitoring conditions (motion artifact, poor peripheral perfusion, etc.). The SaO_2 may be useful to differentiate between patients who are likely to improve with therapy and those who are likely to progress to respiratory failure. For example, an increase in oxygen saturation following albuterol nebulization predicts patients who are likely to improve [143], and respiratory failure rarely occurs in patients with an oxygen saturation >92% on initial presentation [144]. The degree of hypoxemia significantly correlates with the degree of airway obstruction, as determined by the FEV_1 [145–147]. Furthermore, hypoxemia appears, at least in some studies, to be an independent risk factor for both hospitalization and increased length of stay [148–154].

Hypoxemia is multifactorial in origin, resulting from a combination of factors including ventilation–perfusion mismatch, alveolar hypoventilation, and hypercarbia (although, by the alveolar gas equation, clinically significant hypoxemia, i.e., PaO_2 <60 mm Hg, does not occur under normal conditions, breathing ambient air at sea level until a $PaCO_2$ >72 mm Hg is attained) [155]. Significant hypoxemia, however, is relatively uncommon in children with status asthmaticus [136,156–158]. For example, one study documented a significant correlation between SaO_2 and FEV_1 ($r^2 = 0.59$), although the range of SaO_2 for any given FEV_1 was quite variable, and some children had significant airways obstruction despite normal SaO_2 [146]. The mean SaO_2 of 150 children presenting to the emergency department with status asthmaticus who subsequently required hospitalization was approximately 93% [149]. A large, multicenter trial involving over 1,000 children presenting to the emergency department with status asthmaticus documented a mean SaO_2 of 95 ± 4%. In this particular study, the mean SaO_2 for the 241 children who subsequently required hospitalization was 93 ± 5% ($p < 0.001$ compared with children not requiring hospitalization) [154,159]. Therefore, the presence of significant hypoxemia should alert the physician to search for some additional underlying cause, such as diffuse atelectasis secondary to mucous plugging, pneumonia, or pneumothorax [160].

The degree of airway obstruction is rapidly determined by assessment of pulmonary function using the FEV_1 and the peak expiratory flow rate (PEFR). The PEFR is defined as the greatest flow that can be attained during a forced expiration starting from total lung capacity (i.e., complete lung inflation) and is often utilized as a measure for monitoring the severity of illness upon initial presentation and in response to therapy. The PEFR is easily obtained using a hand-held spirometer, and this is endorsed by the National Asthma Education Program [161,162]. The test is effort dependent, so the accuracy and reliability of the results rely heavily on close supervision. Interpretation of test results should be made only after correction for age and sex. Generally, however, PEFR is 70% to 90% of baseline or predicted normal in mild exacerbations, 50% to 70% of baseline or predicted normal in moderate exacerbations, and <50% of baseline or predicted normal in severe exacerbations. It should be noted that adequate PEFR measurements are often difficult to obtain in children during an acute asthma episode, especially those with an exacerbation severe enough to warrant admission to the PICU [163]. For this reason, PEFR assessment should not delay therapy for a critically ill child, and attempts at PEFR assessment should be discontinued if the child's clinical condition deteriorates during testing.

Based on a rapid assessment, the physician caring for the child with status asthmaticus should be able to have a reasonable impression of the severity of airway obstruction (Table 15.2). The modified Becker Clinical Asthma Score (Table 15.3) is a clinical asthma score that was originally developed by Becker et al. [164] and later modified by DiGiulio et al. [165]. This widely used score assesses the severity of an acute asthma exacerbation based on the acuity of physical signs for four clinical characteristics (respiratory rate, wheezing, inspiratory/expiratory ratio, and accessory muscle use) and assigns a score for each variable ranging from 0 to 12 (0 indicating minimal disease severity).

Although arterial blood gas (ABG) analysis is not predictive of outcome, it may be useful in the initial evaluation and triage of children with status asthmaticus to the PICU. Typical ABG results during an acute asthma exacerbation show normal PaO_2 and respiratory alkalosis, although hypoxemia with PaO_2 approaching 60 mm Hg may be observed in moderate to severe exacerbations [166]. However, serial ABG analyses are more useful in following response to treatment compared with a single measurement. Although the initial $PaCO_2$ may be slightly below normal, a progressive increase in $PaCO_2$ is considered an early warning sign of severe airway obstruction and impending respiratory failure.

Metabolic acidosis is well described in both adults and children with status asthmaticus [167–174]. The majority of studies suggest that the metabolic acidosis reported in these patients is secondary to accumulation of lactic acid, presumably from the prolonged and markedly increased work of breathing (with coincident respiratory muscle fatigue) associated with status asthmaticus. Additional factors include tissue hypoxia secondary to (1) oxygen supply/demand imbalance in respiratory muscles (i.e., insufficient oxygen delivery to meet excessive oxygen demands), (2) dehydration accompanying status asthmaticus from both poor oral intake and increased insensible losses through the respiratory tract, (3) ventilation–perfusion mismatching (rarely sufficient to produce tissue hypoxia, however), and (4) decreased cardiac output associated with hyperinflation. Alternatively, stimulation of β-adrenergic receptors by endogenous catecholamines and β-agonists results in increased glycolysis and lipolysis, potentially leading to excess lactic acidemia through excess substrate utilization [170,174]. Okrent et al. [175] noted the presence of metabolic acidosis in 10/22 adults with status asthmaticus,

TABLE 15.2. Assessment of the severity of acute asthma.

Mild	Moderate	Severe
History		
Intermittent wheezing	Frequent hospitalizations (no intensive care unit admissions)	Previous pediatric intensive care unit admission
Few hospitalizations	Chronic medications ≤2 treatments	Chronic medications ≥2 treatments
No chronic medications		
Physical examination		
CNS		
Absence of CNS signs	Anxious, restless, irritable	Coma, seizures
		Inability to recognize parents
Respiratory system		
No cyanosis in room air	Cyanosis on <1.0 FiO_2	Cyanosis on 1.0 FiO_2
Good air entry with wheezes	Decreased air entry with wheezes	Silent chest
Speaks in full sentences	Speaks in phrases or partial sentences	Speaks only in single words or short phrases
	Tachycardia	Heart rate greatly increased or slightly decreased
Cardiovascular system	Pulsus paradoxus 10–20 mm Hg	Pulsus paradoxus >20 mm Hg
Tachycardia		
No pulsus paradoxus		
Pulmonary function tests		
PEFR		
70%–90% predicted or baseline	50%–70% predicted or baseline	<50% predicted or baseline
FEV_1/FVC		
85%	75%	45%
Laboratory data		
Pulse oximetry		
>95%	90%–95%	<90%
Blood gases		
PaO_2 >80	PaO_2 60–80	PaO_2 >60
$PaCO_2$ <35	$PaCO_2$ <50	$PaCO_2$ >50

Note: CNS, central nervous system; PERF, peak expiratory flow rate.

all of whom had a nonanion gap acidosis with normal whole blood lactate levels. They suggested that the nonanion gap metabolic acidosis in these patients was caused by the excessive renal bicarbonate excretion that occurred as a renal compensatory response to a preceding period of hyperventilation and subsequent respiratory alkalosis.

Hypokalemia is the most common electrolyte abnormality in children with status asthmaticus and is a well-recognized complication of β-agonist administration [170,176–186]. In addition, the glucocorticosteroids used in the management of asthma can possess unwanted mineralocorticoid effects, leading to hypokalemia [182,186]. Children with status asthmaticus are often dehydrated because of increased insensible fluid losses from the respiratory tract, coupled with poor oral intake of fluids. Dehydration may produce thicker, more tenacious bronchial secretions, leading to worsening bronchial mucous plugging. Although the majority of children require intravenous fluid rehydration, overzealous fluid

administration may lead to fluid retention and pulmonary edema. Children with status asthmaticus have elevated plasma antidiuretic hormone levels and are at risk for hyponatremia and fluid overload if given large volumes of hypotonic fluid [187,188]. In addition, the high negative transpulmonary pressures associated with status asthmaticus promote fluid accumulation around the respiratory bronchioles [189], leading to pulmonary edema and worsening respiratory status.

Chest radiographs are generally not helpful in the diagnosis and management of children with mild and uncomplicated asthma [160,190–200]. The majority of chest radiographs of children with asthma show atelectasis or hyperinflation/hyperaeration. For example, in a study by Brooks et al. [190], only 7 of 128 children with acute asthma had a clinically significant x-ray finding, three of which were suspected on clinical assessment alone. Further, Tsai et al. [160] prospectively reviewed 445 children presenting to the emergency department with acute asthma and found no significant correlations among radiographic findings on chest x-ray and duration of hypoxemia, hospital length of stay, or admission to the PICU, even for those children who were hypoxemic. Most of the aforementioned studies, however, excluded children who were admitted to the PICU. Although objective data are lacking, we believe that chest radiographs should be obtained for every child with status asthmaticus requiring admission to the PICU to examine for evidence of infection or air-leak syndromes secondary to hyperinflation. In addition, chest radiographs should be obtained for children with suspected foreign body aspiration or for those not responding appropriately to treatment. Hypoinflation on chest radiograph is highly correlated with disease severity [201] and may warrant more intensive monitoring and treatment.

TABLE 15.3. The modified Becker score for assessing asthma severity.

Score	Respiratory rate	Wheezing	Inspiratory: expiratory ratio	Accessory muscle use
0	<30	None	1:1.5	None
1	30–40	Terminal expiration	1:2.0	One site*
2	41–50	Entire expiration	1:3.0	Two sites
3	>50	Inspiration and entire expiration	>1:3	Three sites or neck strap use

*Site refers to chest wall musculature, such as intercostal and subcostal muscles.

Management

Several studies have shown that a protocolized, systematic approach to the treatment of children who are admitted to the hospital with status asthmaticus will result in improved outcomes and lower hospital costs. For example, in a recent study the use of an asthma clinical pathway significantly shortened the hospital stay (36 hr vs. 71 hrs, $p < 0.001$) and decreased total hospital costs ($1,685 vs. $2,829, $p < 0.001$) compared with traditional inpatient management [202]. McDowell et al. [203] demonstrated a significantly shorter length of stay for children managed on a clinical pathway compared with traditional management, although the study was poorly randomized. Children randomized to the asthma pathway were significantly older and more likely to be white, both factors that impact asthma severity. In addition, the trial excluded children who required admission to the PICU. Wazeka et al. [204], however, demonstrated significant cost-savings and decreased length of stay without an increased rate of readmission following the implementation of an asthma clinical pathway. Notably, children remained on the pathway even if they required admission to the PICU. Further studies that specifically include patients in the PICU are required before the results of these studies can be translated into everyday PICU practice. In addition, experience has shown that implementation of a clinical pathway requires a real commitment of resources, training, and education by all health care providers involved, and the benefits may not be realized initially [205].

Oxygen

The administration of supplemental oxygen is considered standard therapy for children with status asthmaticus [161]. As discussed above, hypoxemia, when present, is multifactorial in origin, resulting from a combination of factors including ventilation–perfusion mismatch, alveolar hypoventilation, and hypercarbia [155], although again, significant hypoxemia is relatively uncommon in children with status asthmaticus [136,156–158]. When present, hypoxemia may produce pulmonary hypertension (via hypoxic pulmonary vasoconstriction, the pulmonary vasculature's normal response to alveolar hypoxia), worsen bronchoconstriction, and decrease oxygen delivery to the muscles of respiration in the face of tremendous metabolic demand.

A recent study of adult asthmatics suggested that administration of 100% oxygen adversely influenced CO_2 elimination [206]. Upon initial presentation, the 37 subjects had moderate-to-severe airway obstruction (FEV_1 49.1 ± 3.6% predicted), hypocarbia ($PaCO_2$ 36.8 ± 1.1 mm Hg), hypoxemia (PaO_2 70.2 ± 2.5 mm Hg), and respiratory alkalosis (pH, 7.43 ± 0.01). During administration of 100% oxygen, gas exchange worsened as manifested by a mean increase in $PaCO_2$ of 4.1 ± 0.6 mm Hg ($p = 0.0003$) in 25 subjects (67.6%). The tendency to develop worsening gas exchange was the greatest for those subjects with the most severe airway obstruction. The potential significance and underlying mechanism of this phenomenon remains to be elucidated, although as yet there are no pediatric studies demonstrating similar occurrences. For now, it seems prudent to administer supplemental oxygen to maintain SaO_2 >92%. It should be mentioned, however, that some bronchodilators, particularly the β-agonists, reduce hypoxic pulmonary vasoconstriction and thus worsen hypoxemia, at least initially [207–209]. Therefore, these medications should be administered concurrently with supplemental oxygen rather than air [159,208,210].

Systemic Corticosteroids

With the recognition that airway inflammation plays a prominent role in the pathophysiology of status asthmaticus, corticosteroids are now standard treatment for children with status asthmaticus. The use of corticosteroids in the treatment of acute asthma is well-established, and numerous clinical trials with both children and adults demonstrate the benefits of corticosteroids in improving PEFR, decreasing the need for β-agonists, and reducing the rate of hospital admission [211–219]. A meta-analysis by Rowe et al. [217] reviewed 30 randomized, controlled trials that evaluated the administration of corticosteroids in children and adults with status asthmaticus. Early administration of corticosteroids reduced hospital admission and improved pulmonary function in both children and adults. A Cochrane Collaboration review of seven randomized, controlled clinical trials involving a total of 426 children (274 with oral prednisone vs. placebo, 106 with intravenous steroids vs. placebo, and 46 with nebulized budesonide vs. prednisolone) concluded that administration of systemic corticosteroids produce some improvements for children admitted to hospital with acute asthma. In this review, a significant number of children treated with corticosteroids were discharged early after admission (<4hr). The length of stay was shorter for the steroid groups, although there were no significant differences between groups in pulmonary function or oxygen saturation measurements. In addition, children treated with steroids in the hospital were less likely to relapse within 1 to 3 months following discharge. Based on the wealth of available evidence, expert opinion and published guidelines [161,162,220] recommend the administration of corticosteroids in the routine management of status asthmaticus within the initial 48 hours of treatment.

The standard recommended dosage of corticosteroid (methylprednisolone 2–4 mg/kg/day divided every 6 hr intravenously) will maintain a minimal plasma steroid concentration of 100–150 μg cortisol/100 mL [221]. However, the optimal dosing of systemic corticosteroids for children with status asthmaticus remains an unresolved issue. Several studies with both children [212,222] and adults [223–226] suggest that *high-dose* corticosteroid therapy offers few advantages over *low-dose* corticosteroids in the treatment of status asthmaticus. In addition, although the currently available evidence does not support the use of inhaled corticosteroids in lieu of systemic corticosteroids (administered intravenously, by mouth, or intramuscularly) for the treatment of status asthmaticus [220,227–230], oral administration appears to be equally efficacious to intravenous or intramuscular administration [231–233]. However, oral corticosteroids are generally not recommended for children with severe status asthmaticus and impending respiratory failure.

The peak antiinflammatory effects of corticosteroids usually become evident between 6 and 12 hours after administration of the first dose [234]. Early administration of corticosteroids in the emergency department should therefore be associated with more rapid improvement in pulmonary function and reduce the need for hospitalization. For example, Scarfone et al. [218] reported that administration of oral prednisone within 4 hr of initial presentation to the emergency department reduced the need for hospitalization of children with status asthmaticus. Tal et al. [215] showed a significantly lower rate of hospitalization for children treated with intramuscular methylprednisolone in the emergency department compared with placebo. Although additional studies contradict these findings [235,236], a Cochrane Collaboration review of 12 randomized, controlled studies involving 863 patients, including both children and adults, suggested that administration of corticosteroids within 1 hr of presentation to the emergency department significantly reduced admission rates. These benefits appeared greatest for patients with more severe exacerbations [237]. Despite the lack of studies specifically addressing the administration of corticosteroids in children with status asthmaticus and impending respiratory failure, the available evidence would suggest that timely administration of corticosteroids in this population would provide early benefits.

Although corticosteroids are widely used in the treatment of asthma, the molecular mechanisms responsible for their antiinflammatory effects remain under active investigation. Corticosteroids are believed to inhibit proinflammatory gene expression, at least partially through a mechanism involving the transcription factor nuclear factor (NF)-κB [238–241]. This would appear to account for at least some of the delayed onset of action for corticosteroids in acute asthma discussed earlier, as the antiinflammatory effects require inhibition of gene expression (so-called genomic effects of corticosteroids). Additional studies have suggested that corticosteroids upregulate β-adrenergic receptor gene expression and enhance β-adrenergic signaling pathways in ASM cells [242,243]. Consistent with these mechanisms that depend on new gene expression, the available clinical evidence suggests that systemic corticosteroids require between 6 and 24 hr in order to produce a maximal antiinflammatory therapeutic effect [234,237,244]. However, so-called nongenomic effects (i.e., effects that do not require new gene expression) have also been reported, possibly through membrane-stabilizing effects or effects on ion channels [245–248]. These nongenomic effects are more or less immediate and may account for at least some of the beneficial effects associated with early administration of corticosteroids in the emergency department.

Inhaled Corticosteroids

As discussed earlier, the currently available evidence does not support the use of inhaled corticosteroids in lieu of systemic corticosteroids (administered intravenously, by mouth, or intramuscularly) for the treatment of status asthmaticus [220,227–230]. Perhaps obstruction of the lower airways (i.e., mucous plugging and bronchospasm) limits the distal delivery of even the most potent inhaled corticosteroids, minimizing their effectiveness. However, several recent studies suggest an adjunctive role for inhaled corticosteroids in the management of children with status asthmaticus. Matthews et al. [227] compared nebulized budesonide (2 mg every 8 hr) with oral prednisolone (2 mg/kg at entry and again at 24 hr) in 46 children admitted to hospital with severe asthma exacerbation. After 24 hr of treatment, FEV_1 improved significantly compared with baseline in children who received nebulized budesonide compared with the prednisolone group (no significant difference). Subjective measurements such as dyspnea, cough severity, and wheezing also decreased significantly in the nebulized budesonide group [227]. Similarly, Devidayal et al. [228] compared nebulized budesonide (800 μg every 30 min for 3 hr) to oral prednisolone (2 mg/kg) in 80 children with acute asthma exacerbations in the emergency department. Oxygen saturation, respiratory rate, pulmonary index, and respiratory distress score improved significantly in the budesonide group compared with the prednisolone group. Significantly more children in the budesonide group than in the prednisolone group were ready for discharge from the emergency department at 2 hr. Five children in the prednisolone group

required admission to the hospital compared with only one child in the budesonide group, though the difference was not statistically significant. Scarfone et al. [229] compared a single dose of nebulized dexamethasone (1.5 mg/kg) with oral prednisone (2 mg/kg) in 111 children with acute asthma. Although there were no significant differences in hospital admission rates between the two groups, significantly more children in the nebulized dexamethasone group were ready for discharge from the emergency department at 2 hr [229]. Similar findings have been noted in studies of adults with acute asthma [249,250]. In contrast to these studies, Schuh et al. [230] compared a single dose of inhaled fluticasone propionate (FP; 2 mg) with oral prednisone (2 mg/kg) in 100 children with severe acute asthma and found that FEV_1 improved significantly in the oral prednisone group compared with the FP group. More importantly, 16 (31%) children in the FP group required hospital admission compared with 5 (10%) children in the oral prednisone group ($p = 0.01$).

Unfortunately, there are no prospective, randomized, controlled studies on which to base recommendations for the use of inhaled corticosteroids in critically ill children with status asthmaticus admitted to the PICU. The evidence presented would suggest that children admitted to the PICU with status asthmaticus may benefit from the use of inhaled corticosteroids. Regardless, the currently available evidence does not support the use of inhaled corticosteroids in lieu of systemic corticosteroids (administered intravenously, by mouth, or intramuscularly), and the possible synergistic effects versus adverse effects with combined administration of inhaled corticosteroids and systemic corticosteroids in this population are not known.

β-Adrenergic Agonists

Table 15.4 provides details on the bronchodilators currently used in the management of status asthmaticus.

Epinephrine

Subcutaneous epinephrine has been used for decades for the treatment of status asthmaticus and was once considered the treatment of choice [251–253]. However, subcutaneous epinephrine has fallen out of favor in recent years, largely because of the widespread availability, ease of administration (painless aerosol vs. painful injection), and efficacy of relatively newer β-adrenergic agonists such as albuterol [254–258]. However, many experts still believe that subcutaneous epinephrine continues to have a role in the treatment of critically ill children with impending respiratory failure secondary to status asthmaticus [203,259–263]. Subcutaneous administration of epinephrine (0.01 mL/kg of 1:1,000 concentration or 1 mg/mL, maximum dose 0.3–0.5 mL) or terbutaline (0.01 mL/kg of 1:1,000 concentration or 1 mg/mL, maximum dose 0.3–0.5 mL) should be considered in children who are rapidly decompensating despite inhaled β-adrenergic agonists (see later) and in children who are unable to cooperate with inhalational therapy secondary to anxiety, altered mental status, or apnea. Subcutaneous epinephrine may be administered every 20 min for three doses. Terbutaline loses its β-selectivity when administered subcutaneously and offers no advantages over epinephrine [264]. Severe air flow obstruction may be relieved by subcutaneous epinephrine to a degree sufficient to allow adequate delivery of aerosolized β-adrenergic agonists to the distal airways, thereby allowing these agents to take effect. Subcutaneous terbutaline and subcutaneous epinephrine appear to be

TABLE 15.4. Bronchodilators currently used in the management of status asthmaticus.

Agent	Parenteral	Aerosol
Epinephrine hydrochloride	Subcutaneous 1 : 1,000, 1 mg/mL 0.01 mL/kg/dose every 15–20 min; may be repeated three times if clinically indicated	No current indications*

Albuterol (salbutamol)	Intravenous
	5–15 μg/kg/dose intermittent dose
	-or-
	1 μg/kg loading dose followed by continuous infusion at
	    0.2 μg/kg/min; dose may be increased by 0.1 μg/kg/min
	    increments to clinical improvement or greater than 20%
	    increase in heart rate
		Intermittent
		0.5% solution, 5 mg/mL
		2.5 mg in 2.5 mL 0.9% saline
		0.5% solution, 5 mg/mL
		0.1–0.3 mg/kg in 2.5 mL 0.9% saline
		Continuous, 10–20 mg/hr

Terbutaline sulfate	Subcutaneous
	1 : 1,000 or 1 mg/mL
	0.01 mL/kg (0.01 mg/kg), maximum dose 0.3– 0.5 mL every
	    15–20 min; may be repeated three times if clinically indicated
	Intravenous
	1 mg/mL
	2–10 μg/kg loading dose followed by continuous infusion at
	    0.5 μg/kg/min; dose may be increased by 0.1–0.2 μg/kg/min
	    increments as clinically indicated every 15–30 min; doses as
	    high as 10 μg/kg/min have been reported
		Intermittent
		1 mg/mL
		0.01–0.03 mL/kg every 4–6 hr (minimum dose 0.1 mL, maximum dose
		    2.5 mL)

Ipratropium bromide	Not available in parenteral form	Intermittent Infants and children: 250 μg every 20 min for three doses, then every 2–4 hr Adolescents: 500 μg every 20 min for three doses, then every 2–4 hr

Magnesium sulfate	Intravenous
	50–75 mg/kg (maximum dose 2 g) every 4–6 hr
	-or-
	50–75 mg/kg loading dose followed by continuous infusion at
	    10–20 mg/kg/hr
	Titrated to keep serum magnesium 4–5.5 mg/dL
		Intermittent
		Magnesium used as a vehicle for albuterol in lieu of 0.9% saline (dose
		    varies among several studies)

Ketamine	Intravenous 2 mg/kg loading dose followed by continuous infusion at 1–2 mg/kg/hr	Not available

*Racemic epinephrine has not been studied in this population.

equal in terms of efficacy and safety profile. Concerns regarding the safety of these agents are largely unfounded, as subcutaneous administration of epinephrine or terbutaline is well tolerated even by adult patients older than 40–50 years with no history of cardiovascular disease (angina or recent myocardial infarction).

Albuterol (Salbutamol)

Several studies have demonstrated the superior efficacy of inhaled β₂-agonists compared with subcutaneous epinephrine in the treatment of status asthmaticus [256,257,265–267]. Littner et al. [268] prospectively compared the bronchodilatory effects of albuterol with inhaled isoproterenol in 11 children presenting with acute asthma, noting that albuterol produced more significant bronchodilation with fewer side effects. However, although a fixed dose of nebulized albuterol (2.5 mg in 2.5 mL saline) appears to be just as efficacious as a dose calculated for bodyweight (0.1 mg/kg body weight) in children with moderate asthma exacerbations [269], higher doses of albuterol (0.30 mg/kg) appear to be more efficacious than lower doses (0.15 mg/kg, 0.05 mg/kg) in children with severe airway obstruction [270,271]. Furthermore, although the duration of action appears to be dose dependent [272], sequential inhalation of these agents produces a more rapid, greater improvement in airway obstruction than nebulizing higher doses less frequently [273,274]. Frequent nebulization is presumed to lead to better drug

delivery to the distal airways, although significant systemic absorption of albuterol has been demonstrated as well, which may account for some of the observed bronchodilatory effects [275–277]. Based on the available evidence, the consensus is that frequent albuterol nebulization should be considered standard therapy for children presenting with status asthmaticus [161].

Several studies have compared the efficacy of small-volume nebulizers versus metered dose inhalers (MDI) with spacers for the treatment of acute asthma exacerbations in children [278]. Although nebulizers allow the concurrent administration of supplemental oxygen, some studies have suggested that close to 90% of the drug is lost to the atmosphere [279]. Drug delivery is maximized with the use of a mouthpiece versus a facemask, flow rates of 6–8 L/min, and total solution volumes of 3–4 mL [280,281]. The available evidence suggests that there are no differences between MDIs with spacers compared with nebulizers, regardless of the severity of the acute asthma exacerbation [278,282], and either option appears reasonable in at least the emergency department setting. We remain convinced, however, that continuous albuterol nebulization is the most appropriate choice for the management of critically ill children with status asthmaticus (see next).

Continuous albuterol nebulization has been shown to be more effective in children with status asthmaticus and impending respiratory failure [283–289]. Continuous nebulization provides sustained stimulation of the β-adrenergic receptors in the airways, thereby preventing the rebound bronchospasm that can occur with intermittent nebulization. In addition, continuous nebulization of albuterol may promote progressive bronchodilation, thereby improving drug delivery in the distal airways. Finally, systemic absorption of albuterol resulting from continuous nebulization may account for a portion of its bronchodilatory effects [275–277].

Although continuous nebulization of albuterol appears to be safe, side effects such as muscle cramps, hypokalemia, and hyperglycemia commonly occur. Katz et al. [285] documented elevated serum creatine phosphokinase (CPK)-MB concentrations in 2 of 19 patients receiving continuous nebulized albuterol. Seven patients developed nonspecific T-wave changes on ECG, although no patients developed sings of myocardial ischemia or cardiac arrhythmias other than sinus tachycardia. Craig et al. [288] documented elevated serum CPK concentrations in 3 of 17 patients receiving continuous nebulized albuterol. Only one of these three patients had elevated serum CPK-MB concentrations, and none of these patients developed signs of myocardial ischemia or cardiac arrhythmias. The significance of these findings is unclear at present. Several investigators have documented elevated serum CPK-MB concentrations in healthy volunteers following vigorous exercise [290–292], and Choi [293] suggested that the excess work of breathing associated with severe airway obstruction is similar to vigorous exercise. Therefore, the elevated CPK concentrations in these patients may not be indicative of myocardial injury. For these reasons, prudence recommends that continuous nebulized albuterol should be administered only in a closely monitored setting.

It should be mentioned that in experimental studies, higher doses of albuterol decreased the DNA binding affinity of the steroid receptor to the glucocorticoid response element, thereby perpetuating airway inflammation through the inhibition of the antiinflammatory response to both endogenously and exogenously administered corticosteroids [294–296]. These data, if duplicated, may partially explain the resistance of some children with status asthmaticus to β-agonists, resulting in the need for other, additional agents working via different mechanisms.

Terbutaline

The first National Asthma Education Program (NAEP) Expert Panel Report recommended the use of systemic β-agonists, such as terbutaline, for the treatment of severe, life-threatening asthma exacerbations [162]. Since the publication of these guidelines, there have been relatively few studies assessing the efficacy of terbutaline in either children or adults with status asthmaticus, and this recommendation was removed in the subsequent revision of the NAEP guidelines in 1997 [161]. Terbutaline is a selective β_2-receptor adrenergic agonist that has been administered to children with status asthmaticus via the subcutaneous [255,297], nebulized [298–300), and parenteral routes [299,301–305]. There are currently no prospective, randomized, placebo-controlled trials on the use of terbutaline in either children or adults with status asthmaticus. In certain cases, children with status asthmaticus may fail to respond to continuous, nebulized albuterol, in part because of the inability of the albuterol to reach its site of action within the lung secondary to severe bronchospasm and mucous plugging [306]. However, several adult trials have failed to show any difference between continuous, nebulized terbutaline and intravenously administered terbutaline [307–309]. Regardless, terbutaline appears to be relatively safe [303,310] and may offer some benefit, although additional studies

will be required before it can be routinely recommended in the treatment of children with status asthmaticus.

Levalbuterol

Albuterol in reality exists as a 50:50 mixture of two mirror-image enantiomers—the active R-albuterol and S-albuterol. In contrast, levalbuterol (Xopenex®) is pure R-albuterol and is currently available as a solution for nebulization. Emerging data suggest that S-albuterol may have deleterious effects—in fact, S-albuterol is thought to promote bronchoconstriction [282]—so that administration of only the R-enantiomer appears to be an appropriate treatment rationale. However, the majority of studies in children with acute exacerbations of asthma suggest that there is no clinical benefit to the use of levalbuterol versus racemic albuterol [311–313]. Carl et al. [314] noted that children treated with levalbuterol had a lower hospitalization rate than children treated with albuterol in a randomized trial involving over 500 children. However, this study has several methodologic flaws that could have potentially biased the results, especially when considered in the context of more recent trials, suggesting no clinical benefits to using levalbuterol versus racemic albuterol. Given the overwhelming difference in cost, until more conclusive evidence is available, racemic albuterol should be preferentially used in the treatment of children with status asthmaticus.

Isoproterenol

Isoproterenol is a nonselective β-agonist that is no longer clinically used for the treatment of status asthmaticus, and it is mentioned here for historical interest. Isoproterenol is a potent bronchodilator when administered either by aerosol (0.5% solution, 5 mg/mL; 0.01–0.03 mL/kg diluted with 1.5 mL saline every 2–6 hr) or continuous intravenous infusion (0.02% solution, 0.2 mg/mL; 0.05–0.1 μg/kg/min, increased by 0.05–0.1 μg/kg/min every 15–20 min until clinical response or greater than 20% increase in heart rate) [268,315–322]. However, isoproterenol was associated with tachyarrhythmias and myocardial ischemia and was removed from clinical use when albuterol became widely available [54,323–326].

Intravenous Albuterol

Intravenous albuterol is not currently available for clinical use in the United States. However, following a similar rationale for the use of either subcutaneous epinephrine or intravenous terbutaline (see earlier), intravenous administration of albuterol via either bolus (5–15 μg/kg) or continuous infusion (1 μg/kg loading dose followed by 0.2 μg/kg/min increased by 0.1 μg/kg/min to clinical improvement or greater than 20% increase in heart rate) is widely used outside of the United States and has been studied in both children and adults with status asthmaticus [327–332]. However, one study suggested that there was no clinical differences between intravenous albuterol and intravenous aminophylline in 44 children presenting to the emergency department with status asthmaticus [331]. Intravenous albuterol may also be associated with an increased incidence of side effects, including tremors, nausea/vomiting, and tachyarrhythmias [333].

Ipratropium Bromide

The autonomic nervous system is intimately involved in the regulation of ASM tone and mucous secretion. The parasympathetic nerve fibers, which are generally confined to the larger, central airways, stimulate bronchoconstriction and increased mucous secretion (mediated through the neurotransmitter acetylcholine). In contrast, the sympathetic nerve fibers are distributed more peripherally in the smaller airways and stimulate bronchodilation [334]. This dual-innervation suggests that a therapeutic strategy aimed at both the cholinergic and adrenergic pathways would be beneficial in the treatment of status asthmaticus. There are at least three subtypes of muscarinic receptors in the human airways: M_1, M_2, and M_3 [335,336]. The M_1 subtype is localized to the parasympathetic ganglion and mediates cholinergic transmission. The prejunctional M_2 receptors inhibit the release of acetylcholine and serve as a negative feedback mechanism, thereby limiting bronchoconstriction. Conversely, stimulation of the M_3 receptors, which are localized to ASM and submucosal glands, results in bronchoconstriction and increased mucous production. The M_2 receptors are thought to be dysfunctional in patients with asthma, especially following viral infection, resulting in unopposed M_1 and M_3 activity, producing excessive bronchoconstriction [337].

The nonselective, muscarinic antagonist ipratropium bromide is a quaternary ammonium atropine derivative that has been used successfully in the treatment of chronic obstructive pulmonary disease (COPD) and chronic asthma (see Table 15.4). Increasing evidence suggests a synergistic reduction in airflow obstruction in both children and adults when treated with both ipratropium bromide and albuterol [334,338,339]. For example, three recent studies showed that the addition of ipratropium bromide to albuterol aerosols in children presenting to the emergency department with status asthmaticus significantly reduced the rate of hospital admission [340—342]. However, two studies in children hospitalized with acute asthma suggested that the addition of ipratropium to standard therapy offered no additional benefit [343,344]. However, there are no studies of ipratropium bromide combined with standard therapy for critically ill children who are admitted to the PICU with status asthmaticus. Given the low risk of adverse effects and until more definitive evidence is available, the addition of ipratropium bromide to standard therapy appears reasonable for this population.

Magnesium

Roselló and Plá [345] first reported the use of magnesium for the treatment of acute asthma in 1936. Since that time, magnesium has been shown to be a direct bronchodilator [346–349], and numerous case reports [350–352] have noted clinical efficacy in patients with respiratory failure complicating status asthmaticus. The mechanism of action by which magnesium produces bronchodilation in asthma is not entirely clear. Magnesium administration may serve to replace an underlying magnesium deficiency. Several studies have shown that patients with status asthmaticus have an underlying hypomagnesemia [353–357], and frequent β-agonist therapy has been demonstrated to result in decreased magnesium levels [358]. Alternatively, magnesium may act as a pharmacologic agent via one of several potential mechanisms (Table 15.5). Regardless of the exact mechanism, it is clear that magnesium acts principally as a calcium antagonist, directly inhibiting calcium uptake in smooth muscle cells, thereby resulting in smooth muscle relaxation [359–365].

Several randomized, controlled trials comparing the effects of placebo versus either nebulized [366,367] or intravenous magnesium sulfate [368,369] in adults with status asthmaticus have been

TABLE 15.5. Potential mechanisms of magnesium bronchodilation in status asthmaticus.

Magnesium acts as a calcium antagonist
Decreases amount of calcium available for myosin light chain phosphorylation
Competes with calcium at its binding sites
Increases activity of the magnesium-calcium atpase (extruding calcium from cell)
Promotes calcium uptake by the sarcoplasmic reticulum
Magnesium acts at the level of the neuromuscular junction
Decreases acetylcholine release
Diminishes the depolarizing action of acetylcholine
Depresses excitability of smooth muscle membrane
Magnesium is necessary cofactor in β-adrenergic signal transduction
Magnesium decreases superoxide production by neutrophils
Magnesium inhibits histamine release (via inhibition of mast cell degranulation)
Magnesium directly inhibits smooth muscle contraction (mechanism?)

conducted, although the results have been conflicting. The experience in children, however, has been somewhat more favorable. Pabon et al. [370] presented their experience with the use of intravenous magnesium sulfate in four children with status asthmaticus admitted to the PICU. All four patients responded favorably to magnesium without any adverse effects. Five small, prospective, randomized, controlled trials comparing intravenous magnesium and placebo in children presenting to the emergency department with status asthmaticus have been conducted since that time [371–375]. Four of these trials [371–373,375] demonstrated significant improvements in respiratory function (as measured variably by PEFR, FEV_1, FVC, and/or CAS [clinical asthma score]), as well as a decreased number of hospital admissions in children who were randomized to the magnesium groups. Scarfone et al. [374], on the other hand, failed to demonstrate any significant differences in these parameters between the magnesium and placebo groups. Two subsequent meta-analyses of these five studies concluded that magnesium sulfate provides additional benefit to children with status asthmaticus when added to a regimen of frequent, nebulized β-adrenergic agonists and corticosteroids [376,377].

The correct dose and frequency of administration have not been adequately defined (see Table 15.4). However, there is evidence to suggest that increasing the serum magnesium level >4 mg/dL is necessary to produce effective bronchodilation [346,348]. Onset of action is quite rapid (within minutes), and the effects last for approximately 2 hr [346,348,378]. Side effects appear to depend on the serum magnesium concentration. Mild effects include nausea, vomiting, facial flushing, and dry mouth. At serum magnesium levels >12 mg/dL, loss of deep tendon reflexes, muscle weakness, and respiratory depression, as well as cardiac conduction defects, may be seen [346,348,379].

Theophylline

Theophylline has been used as a bronchodilator for the treatment of reversible obstructive airway disease for many years and was once considered the bronchodilator of choice for the management of acute asthma. A study conducted in 1971 demonstrated a significant improvement in the FEV_1 in hospitalized children managed with aminophylline, hydrocortisone, and phenylephrine and isoproterenol aerosols compared with children managed with hydrocortisone and aerosols alone [380]. Although theophylline has been

TABLE 15.6. Dosing guidelines for intravenous theophylline.

Loading dose (in patients not currently receiving aminophylline or
    theophylline)
    6 mg/kg (based on aminophylline) administered over 20–30 min

Continuous infusion
    6 Weeks to 6 months: 0.5 mg/kg/hr
    6 Months to 1 year: 0.6–0.7 mg/kg/hr
    1–9 Years: 1–1.2 mg/kg/hr
    9–12 Years and young adult smokers: 0.9 mg/kg/hr
    12–16 Years: 0.7 mg/kg/hr
    Adults (healthy, nonsmoking): 0.7 mg/kg/hr
    Older patients and patients with cor pulmonale, congestive heart failure,
      or liver failure: 0.25 mg/kg/hr

Note: Serum theophylline levels should be obtained 3 hours after the initial loading dose and every 12–24 hours thereafter. The dose should be adjusted to maintain serum theophylline concentrations between 12 and 20 μg/mL:

- If the serum theophylline concentration <12 μg/mL, a repeat bolus of theophylline (based on the assumption that 1 mg/kg will increase the serum theophylline concentration approximately 2 μg/mL) should be administered and the continuous infusion should be increased by 10%.
- If the serum theophylline concentration is between 12 and 16 μg/mL, no changes are made.
- If the serum theophylline concentration is >16 μg/mL, the continuous infusion is decreased by 10%.
- If the serum theophylline concentration is >22 μg/mL, the continuous infusion should be discontinued until the concentration falls below 20 μg/mL.

effective in the management of chronic asthma, its role in the treatment of hospitalized children diagnosed with status asthmaticus has become less clear, particularly for the critically ill (Table 15.6). In addition, as specific inhaled β₂-adrenergic agonists, such as albuterol, have become readily available, the use of theophylline in this population has declined further. Several studies in hospitalized children diagnosed with mild to moderate status asthmaticus have failed to demonstrate any added benefit when theophylline or aminophylline was added to a standard regimen of frequently nebulized β-agonists and intravenously administered corticosteroids [165,381–386]. A recently published meta-analysis of these trials concluded that any benefits associated with the use of theophylline in treating children with mild to moderate status asthmaticus were slight and that the available evidence suggested a detrimental effect with theophylline treatment as measured by an increased number of albuterol treatments and hospital length of stay [387]. As a result of these studies, the NAEP Expert Panel 2 revised its original guidelines and concluded that methylxanthines are not recommended for the treatment of hospitalized children with status asthmaticus [161]. The aforementioned studies, however, excluded children from participation if they were diagnosed with impending respiratory failure or if they required admission to the PICU. In sum, current recommendations, proscribing the use of theophylline are not based on analysis of treatment data in critically ill children with status asthmaticus, and the efficacy of theophylline for critically ill children with status asthmaticus remains to be established.

Theophylline may offer several potential advantages for the treatment of status asthmaticus in the PICU population. For example, theophylline produces bronchodilation and improves air flow without adversely affecting ventilation–perfusion matching [388]. The use of intravenous β-agonists, such as terbutaline, can worsen pulmonary gas exchange, despite improved air flow because

TABLE 15.7. Theophylline toxicity.

Theophylline serum concentration (mg/ml)*	Adverse reactions
15–25	Gastrointestinal upset, gastroesophageal reflux, diarrhea, nausea, vomiting, abdominal pain, nervousness, headache, insomnia, agitation, dizziness, muscle cramp, tremor
25–35	Tachycardia, occasional premature ventricular contractions
>35	Ventricular tachycardia, frequent premature ventricular contractions, seizure

*Adverse effects do not necessarily occur according to serum levels. Arrhythmia and seizure can occur without seeing the other adverse effects.

of the effect of hypoxic pulmonary vasoconstriction [389,390]. Theophylline's diuretic effects may also reduce excess alveolar fluid and microvascular permeability [388,391]. Finally, theophylline increases respiratory drive, improves mucociliary clearance, reduces pulmonary vascular resistance, and improves contractility of the diaphragm, all of which may benefit the tenuous child with impending respiratory failure secondary to status asthmaticus [388].

Three recent trials have examined the effects of theophylline when added to the standard treatment regimen of β-agonists, corticosteroids, and oxygen in critically ill children who were admitted to the PICU with status asthmaticus [392–394]. Notably, two of these trials included children who developed respiratory failure and required mechanical ventilation [392,393]. These studies suggest that theophylline continues to have a role in the management of severe acute exacerbations of asthma in children; however, other therapies with a lower risk of adverse effects (Table 15.7) should be utilized first. In addition, serum theophylline concentrations should be followed closely, as several conditions (Table 15.8) and medications (Table 15.9) affect theophylline clearance.

Helium–Oxygen

According to Hagen-Poiseuille's law, the change in air flow resulting from a reduction in airway diameter is directly proportional to the airway radius elevated to the fourth power. While airway resistance is inversely proportional to the radius of the airway to the *fourth power* when there is laminar flow, resistance is inversely proportional to the *fifth power* when there is turbulent flow. The therapeutic use of helium–oxygen mixtures in children with asthma therefore appears reasonable based on the physical properties of helium. Helium reduces the Reynolds number and renders turbulent flow less likely to occur in the small airways [395,396].

TABLE 15.8. Clinical factors reported to affect theophylline clearance.

Decreased level	Increased level
Smoking (cigarettes, marijuana)	Acute pulmonary edema
High protein/low carbohydrate diet	Cor pulmonale
Charcoal-broiled beef	Congestive heart failure
	Hypothyroidism
	Cessation of smoking (after chronic use)
	Fever
	Liver dysfunction
	Acute renal failure
	Shock
	Acute viral illness

TABLE 15.9. Medications affecting theophylline clearance resulting in either increased or decreased serum levels.

Decreased level	Increased level
Aminoglutethimide	Alcohol
Carbamazepine	Allopurinol (>600 mg/day)
Isoproterenol (IV)	Beta-blockers
Isoniazid*	Calcium channel blockers
Ketoconazole	Cimetidine
Loop diuretics*	Ciprofloxacin
Nevirapine	Clarithromycin
Phenobarbital	Corticosteroids
Phenytoin	Disulfiram
Rifampin	Ephedrine
Ritonavir	Erythromycin
Sulfinpyrazone	Esmolol
Sympathomimetics	Influenza virus vaccine
	Interferon, human recombinant alpha 2-a and 2-b
	Isoniazid*
	Loop diuretics*
	Methotrexate
	Mexiletine
	Oral contraceptives
	Propafenone
	Propranolol
	Tacrine
	Thiabendazole
	Thyroid hormones
	Troleandomycin (TAO®)
	Verapamil
	Zileuton

*Both increased and decreased theophylline levels have been reported.

Several small series and anecdotal reports suggest that helium–oxygen decreases the work of breathing and improves respiratory mechanics in both tracheally intubated and nonintubated children with status asthmaticus [397–403]. A Cochrane Database review, however, recently concluded that the available evidence does not currently support a role for the administration of helium–oxygen mixtures to emergency department patients with moderate to severe acute asthma [404]. A recently published trial (not included in the above Cochrane Database review) suggests that continuous albuterol nebulized with helium–oxygen mixtures results in a greater clinical improvement compared with continuous albuterol nebulized with 100% oxygen [405]. Thirty children were randomly assigned to receive continuously nebulized albuterol (15 mg/hr) delivered by either heliox or oxygen using a nonrebreathing face mask. There was a statistically significant improvement in pulmonary index score at 240 min in the heliox group compared with the oxygen group. In addition, the heliox group was discharged from the emergency department sooner [405]. The utility of helium–oxygen for children for the treatment of status asthmaticus and acute respiratory failure remains unproven, although, until more definitive evidence is available, helium–oxygen remains a reasonable therapeutic alternative in this critically ill population.

Ketamine

Ketamine is a dissociative anesthetic agent that causes bronchodilation secondary to a combination of factors, including the drug-induced release of endogenous catecholamines, inhibition of vagal tone, and direct muscle relaxation [406,407]. For these reasons, it is the induction agent of choice for the tracheal intubation of children with asthma. Although ketamine has been used successfully for the treatment of refractory bronchospasm in intubated patients [408–414], there is controversy surrounding its use in nonintubated patients because of its propensity to increase pulmonary secretions, cause occasional laryngospasm, and induce hallucinations. Numerous case reports and anecdotes [408,415–417], as well as a recently completed prospective study in children [418], however, suggest that ketamine may be a safe and efficacious adjunct to standard therapy in the treatment of children with status asthmaticus and impending respiratory failure. Ketamine should only be used in a monitored setting, however, and additional prospective, randomized, controlled trials demonstrating its efficacy and safety in this setting are justified [419].

Leukotriene Modifying Agents

Leukotriene modifying agents (LMAs) are a relatively new class of asthma medications that are approved for use in the chronic treatment of moderate-to-severe asthma. The LMAs are biologically active fatty acids generated from arachidonic acid (AA) by the enzyme 5-lipoxygenase. 5-Lipoxygenase generates leukotriene (LT) A4 (LTA4) from AA. LTA4 is metabolized to LTC4, LTD4, and LTE4 (the so-called slow-reacting substances of anaphylaxis). The LTs produce bronchoconstriction, stimulate mucous secretion, decrease mucociliary clearance, increase vascular permeability, and recruit eosinophils and basophils into the airway, thereby perpetuating the airway inflammation that is the hallmark of asthma [420]. The LTs are 1,000 times more potent than either histamine or methacholine in airway challenge tests [421]. Activation of LT pathways during acute asthma exacerbations, as determined by urinary LTE4 levels, appears to strongly correlate with the degree of airway obstruction [422].

Several LMAs are currently available, each working via different mechanisms. Zileuton blocks LTA4 synthesis by directly inhibiting 5-lipoxygenase, while montelukast and zafirlukast are LT receptor antagonists. Currently, only montelukast and zafirlukast are approved for use in children. Although slightly less effective than inhaled corticosteroids, the LMAs have demonstrated efficacy in reducing the symptoms of chronic asthma. In addition, there is evidence suggesting that the LMAs produce a rapid improvement in FEV_1, an effect that seems to be additive to the effects of β-agonists [423–426] and inhaled corticosteroids [427]. For this reason, there has been growing interest in using these agents for the treatment of status asthmaticus, although only a few studies exist for adults [428–430] and no current studies exist for children. The preliminary data appear promising, but further work needs to be done before these agents can achieve widespread use in this setting.

Mechanical Ventilation

Status asthmaticus leading to respiratory failure is an important cause of morbidity and mortality because of the potential risks of barotrauma and cardiovascular instability associated with the use of mechanical ventilation in these children [11,63,431–435]. Given these risks, many experts feel that mechanical ventilation should be avoided at all costs [63,431], frequently viewing this modality as *a last ditch effort* or the *therapy of last resort*. Although the decision to tracheally intubate a child with status asthmaticus should not be taken lightly, the potential benefits of ventilatory support, especially when used carefully and judiciously with appropriate goals in mind, appear to outweigh the potential adverse effects. Noninvasive positive pressure ventilation is an attractive modality that may obviate the need for tracheal intubation [436].

There are few absolute indications for tracheal intubation in children with status asthmaticus (e.g., coma, cardiac arrest), although failure to maintain adequate oxygen saturations, a worsening metabolic acidosis, and decreasing mental status are all signs that respiratory arrest is imminent. The decision to tracheally intubate should be based on the clinical examination and not the results of an arterial blood gas. These children are quite ill, and a rapid-sequence intubation technique should be performed by the most experienced physician available. Ketamine (2 mg/kg intravenous [IV]) is an excellent choice for an induction agent because of its bronchodilatory properties, although propofol (2 mg/kg IV) may be an effective alternative as well. Neuromuscular blockade with either succinylcholine (if there are no contraindications to its use) or high-dose vecuronium (0.3 mg/kg IV) produces acceptable conditions for laryngoscopy and tracheal intubation within 1–3 min. These children will require high inspiratory pressures, and the use of a cuffed tracheal tube is justifiably preferable in this scenario [48,63,434]. More than half of the complications in patients requiring mechanical ventilation for status asthmaticus occur at or around the time of tracheal intubation [63] and include hypoxemia, hypotension, and cardiac arrest. Hyperventilation should be avoided, and hypotension should improve with volume resuscitation and slowing the respiratory rate to avoid further air-trapping and dynamic hyperinflation. A tension pneumothorax should be considered if these measures fail to relieve hypotension and hypoxemia—in these cases, needle thoracentesis is life saving.

The goal of mechanical ventilation is to maintain acceptable oxygenation, avoid complications, and *buy time* to allow the corticosteroids and bronchodilators to break the cycle of bronchospasm and airways inflammation. Mechanical ventilation should *not* be targeted toward the results of an arterial blood gas! A landmark article by Darioli and Perett in 1984 introduced the concept of *permissive hypercapnia*, in which low tidal volumes and respiratory rates were used in adult asthmatics, dramatically reducing the frequency of barotraumas and death compared with historical controls [437]. Similarly, strategies that emphasize the use of *low* tidal volumes (8–10 mL/kg), short inspiratory times (0.75–1.5 sec) and correspondingly longer expiratory times to allow adequate time for emptying, and lower-than-normal respiratory rates in children with status asthmaticus result in improved survival [433–435]. The degree of hypercapnia that can be safely tolerated is not known. Several case reports of severe acute hypercapnia in children with reported $PaCO_2$ as high as 269 mm Hg, usually associated with near-fatal status asthmaticus, have been reported in the literature [438]. Sodium bicarbonate can be administered to maintain a relatively physiologic pH [431,439] and in some cases may even reduce $PaCO_2$ [440].

The most appropriate mode of mechanical ventilatory support may differ among patients and their stages of illness. Pressure control [441], volume control [433,434,442], and pressure support [443] ventilation have all been used in children with status asthmaticus. Each mode of ventilation has its advantages and disadvantages. We generally prefer a pressure-regulated volume-control mode (PRVC) because of the advantage of delivering a constant tidal volume, even in the face of changing lung compliance and airways resistance, using a decelerating flow pattern that minimizes peak inspiratory pressures. A PRVC can be delivered in a

synchronized, intermittent mandatory ventilation (SIMV) mode with the Servo *i* ventilator (Siemens, Inc.). The use of PEEP in this population remains controversial, and many experts continue to recommend against using PEEP because of the concerns for more air trapping and auto PEEP [444]. However, low-level PEEP may minimize dynamic airway collapse and decrease trigger work in spontaneously breathing patients [63,136,445–447]. We generally set external PEEP just below auto PEEP, as determined by an end-expiratory hold maneuver.

Additional, potentially life-saving techniques of invasive support have been reported in the literature but have not been adequately studied. For example, tracheal gas insufflation is a method that may reduce the physiologic dead space and improve ventilation [448,449]. The use of high-frequency oscillatory ventilation in children with acute respiratory failure secondary to status asthmaticus has also been described [450]. Finally, extracorporeal life support may be potentially life-saving for children with refractory status asthmaticus [398,451–456].

Volatile Anesthetics

Inhalational anesthetics were used for the treatment of status asthmaticus and acute respiratory failure as early as 1939 [457]. The bronchodilatory properties of these agents are well known, and proposed mechanisms include direct stimulation of the β-adrenergic receptor, direct relaxation of bronchial smooth muscle, inhibition of the release and action of bronchoactive mediators (e.g., histamine, acetylcholine), and depression of vagally mediated airway reflexes [458]. In addition, preliminary studies in certain animal models suggest that inhalational anesthetics may mediate bronchodilation via an epithelial-dependent mechanism involving either nitric oxide or a prostanoid [459,460]. Halothane appears to be particularly effective [461–463], although concerns regarding its potential toxicity, including direct myocardial depression, hypotension, and arrhythmias, have limited its use in this setting. These adverse effects may be further potentiated in children with status asthmaticus who will have some degree of hypoxia, hypercapnia, and acidosis and who are frequently managed with the concomitant administration of β-adrenergic agents and/or theophylline [464]. Inhalational anesthetics may also precipitate malignant hyperthermia and require special, expensive equipment to administer, monitor, and scavenge gases.

The use of isoflurane in status asthmaticus and acute respiratory failure offers several advantages over halothane. Isoflurane has a low blood-gas solubility coefficient such that the depth of anesthesia can be rapidly titrated and recovery from anesthesia is relatively short. Isoflurane produces less myocardial depression and is less arrhythmogenic compared with other inhalational anesthetics such as halothane. Given its role as a general anesthetic, concomitant administration of sedation/analgesia and neuromuscular blockade is not necessary. Finally, although isoflurane produces dose-dependent hypotension via direct vasodilation, there is a compensatory increase in heart rate so that cardiac output is relatively preserved [442,465,466]. In addition, the hypotension is usually responsive to volume resuscitation.

Isoflurane has been used with some success in both children and adults with status asthmaticus refractory to conventional therapy [442,467–472]. Based on these data and on the theoretical advantages discussed earlier, we currently favor isoflurane over other inhalational anesthetics such as halothane. Isoflurane should only be administered in consultation with an anesthesiologist using either an anesthesia machine or vaporizer custom-fitted to a standard PICU ventilator—we have used the Servo 900D ventilator (Siemens, Inc.) [442]. An inline volatile gas analyzer is necessary for monitoring the inspiratory and expiratory concentrations of isoflurane. Finally, a system to scavenge exhaled gases is necessary. We generally start therapy with 1%–2% isoflurane and increase the dose by 0.1% every 15 min until a therapeutic effect is achieved (decrease in positive inspiratory pressure ≤35 cm H_2O with tidal volumes 8–10 mL/kg with improving air entry on clinical examination). Sedation, analgesia, and neuromuscular blockade are discontinued, as this dose of isoflurane provides adequate anesthesia. Other therapeutic agents, such as albuterol, corticosteroids, magnesium, and terbutaline, are continued. Isoflurane undergoes minimal metabolism, although prolonged isoflurane has been associated with an increase in plasma fluoride concentration because of the release of fluoride ions [465]. Fluoride concentrations >50 μmol/L are nephrotoxic [473], although subclinical nephrotoxicity may occur at lower levels with prolonged exposure [474,475]. Renal function should therefore be monitored closely.

References

1. Redd SC. Asthma in the United States: burden and current theories. Environ Health Perspect 2002;110(Suppl 4):557–560.
2. Smith DH, Malone DC, Lawson KA, Okamoto LJ, Battista C, Saunders WB. A national estimate of the economic costs of asthma. Am J Respir Crit Care Med 1997;156:787–793.
3. Lozano P, Sullivan SD, Smith DH, Weiss KB. The economic burden of asthma in US children: estimates from the National Medical Expenditure Survey. J Allergy Clin Immunol 1999;104:957–963.
4. Weitzman M, Gortmaker SL, Sobol AM, Perrin JM. Recent trends in the prevalence and severity of childhood asthma. JAMA 1992;268:2673–2677.
5. Control CfD. Asthma mortality and hospitalization among children and young adults: United States, 1980–1993. JAMA 1996;275:1535–1537.
6. Goodman DC, Stukel TA, Chang C. Trends in pediatric asthma hospitalization rates: regional and socioeconomic differences. Pediatrics 1998;101:208–213.
7. Mannino DM, Homa DM, Akinbami LJ, Moorman JE, Gwynn C, Redd SC. Surveillance for asthma: United States, 1980–1999. Morbid Mortal Wkly Rep CDC Surveill Summ 2002;51:1–13.
8. Mannino DM, Homa DM, Pertowski CA, Ashizawa A, Nixon LL, Johnson CA, et al. Surveillance for asthma: United States, 1960–1995. Morbid Mortal Wkly Rep CDC Surveill Summ 1998;47:1–27.
9. Akinbami LJ, Schoendorf KC. Trends in childhood asthma: prevalence, health care utilization, and mortality. Pediatrics 2002;110:315–322.
10. Pirie J, Cox P, Johnson D, Schuh S. Changes in treatment and outcomes of children receiving care in the intensive care unit for severe acute asthma. Pediatr Emerg Care 1998;14:104–108.
11. Paret G, Kornecki A, Szeinberg A, Vardi A, Barzilai A, Augarten A, et al. Severe acute asthma in a community hospital pediatric intensive care unit: a ten years' experience. Ann Allergy Asthma Immunol 1998;80:339–344.
12. Osundwa VM, Dawod S. Four-year experience with bronchial asthma in a pediatric intensive care unit. Ann Allergy 1992;69:518–520.
13. Stein R, Canny GJ, Bohn DJ, Reisman JJ, Levison H. Severe acute asthma in the pediatric intensive care unit: six years' experience. Pediatrics 1989;83:1023–1028.
14. Shugg AW, Kerr S, Butt WW. Mechanical ventilation of paediatric patients with asthma: short and long term prognosis. J Paediatr Child Health 1990;26:343–346.
15. Russo MJ, McConnochie KM, McBride JT, Szilagyi PG, Brooks AM, Roghmann KJ. Increase in admission threshold explains stable asthma hospitalization rates. Pediatrics 1999;104(3 Pt 1):454–462.
16. Sly RM. Decrease in asthma mortality in the United States. Ann Allergy Asthma Immunol 2000;85:121–127.
17. Wennergren G, Strannegard IL. Asthma hospitalizations continue to decrease in schoolchildren but hospitalization rates for wheezing remain high in young children. Acta Paediatr 2002;91:1239–1245.
18. Committee TIS. International Survey of Asthma and Allergy in Childhood: worldwide variation in prevalence of symptoms of asthma, allergic conjunctivitis, and atopic eczema. Lancet 1998;351:1225–1232.
19. Burney P, Chinn S, Jarvis D. Variations in the prevalence of respiratory symptoms, self-reported asthma attacks, and use of asthma medication in the European Community Respiratory Health Survey (ECRHS). Eur Respir J 1996;9:687–695.
20. Keller MB, Lowenstein SR. Epidemiology of asthma. Semin Respir Crit Care Med 2002;23:317–329.
21. Elias JA, Lee CG, Ma B, Homer RJ, Zhu Z. New insights into the pathogenesis of asthma. J Clin Invest 2003;111:291–297.
22. Van Niekerk CH, Weinberg EG, Shore SC, Heese HV, Van Schalkwyk J. Prevalence of asthma: a comparative study of urban and rural Xhosa children. Clin Allergy 1979;9:319–324.
23. Von Mutius E, Weiland SK, Fritzsch C, Duhme H, Keil U. Increasing prevalence of hay fever and atopy in Leipzig, East Germany. Lancet 1998;351:862–866.
24. Schwartz J, Gold D, Dockery DW, Weiss ST, Speizer FE. Predictors of asthma and persistent wheeze in a national sample of children in the United States: association with social class, perinatal events, and race. Am Rev Respir Dis 1990;142:555–562.
25. Lwebuga-Mukasa JS, Dunn-Georgious E. The prevalence of asthma in children of elementary school age in western New York. J Urban Health 2000;77:745–761.
26. Ernst P, Habbick B, Suissa S, Hemmelgarn B, Cockroft D, Buist AS, et al. Is the association between inhaled beta-agonist use and life-threatening asthma because of confounding by severity? Am Rev Respir Dis 1993;148:75–79.
27. Suissa S, Blais L, Ernst P. Patterns of increasing beta-agonist use and the risk of fatal or near-fatal asthma. Eur Respir J 1994;7:1602–1609.
28. Suissa S, Ernst P, Boivin JF, Horwitz RI, Habbick B, Cockroft D, et al. A cohort analysis of excess mortality in asthma and the use of inhaled beta-agonists. Am J Respir Crit Care Med 1994;149:604–610.
29. McFadden ER, Jr. The beta2-agonist controversy revisited. Ann Allergy Asthma Immunol 1995;75:173–176.
30. Rea HH, Garrett JE, Lanes SF, Birmann BM, Kolbe J. The association between asthma drugs and severe life-threatening attacks. Chest 1996;110:1446–1451.
31. Lanes SF, Birmann B, Raiford D, Walker AM. International trends in sales of inhaled fenoterol, all inhaled beta-agonists, and asthma mortality, 1970–1992. J Clin Epidemiol 1997;50:321–328.
32. Williams C, Crossland L, Finnerty J, Crane J, Holgate S, Pearce N, et al. Case–control study of salmeterol and near-fatal attacks of asthma. Thorax 1998;53:7–13.
33. Sears MR, Rea HH, Beaglehole R, Gillies AJ, Holst PE, O'Donnell TV, et al. Deaths from asthma in New Zealand. N Z Med J 1985;98:271–275.
34. Sears MR, Rea HH, Fenwick J, Beaglehole R, Gillies AJ, Holst PE, et al. Deaths from asthma in New Zealand. Arch Dis Child 1986;61:6–10.
35. Sears MR, Rea HH, Rothwell RP, O'Donnell TV, Holst PE, Gillies AJ, et al. Asthma mortality comparison between New Zealand and England. BMJ 1986;293:1342–1345.
36. Ernst P, Spitzer WO, Suissa S, Cockroft D, Habbick B, Horwitz RI, et al. Risk of fatal and near-fatal asthma in relation to inhaled corticosteroids use. JAMA 1992;268:3462–3464.
37. Suissa S, Ernst P. Optical illusions from visual data analysis: example of the New Zealand asthma mortality epidemic. J Clin Epidemiol 1997;50:1079–1088.

38. Suissa S, Ernst P. Inhaled corticosteroids: impact on asthma morbidity and mortality. J Allergy Clin Immunol 2001;107:937–944.
39. Suissa S, Ernst P, Benvanoun S, Baltzan M, Cai B. Low-dose inhaled corticosteroids and the prevention of death from asthma. N Engl J Med 2000;343:332–336.
40. Papiris S, Kotanidou A, Malagari K, Roussols C. Clinical review: severe asthma. Critical Care 2002;6:30–44.
41. McFadden ER, Jr., Warren EL. Observations on asthma mortality. Ann Intern Med 1997;127:142–147.
42. Benatar SR. Fatal asthma. N Engl J Med 1986;314:423–429.
43. McFadden ER, Jr. Fatal and near-fatal asthma. N Engl J Med 1991;324:409–411.
44. Association BT. Death due to asthma. BMJ 1982;285:1251–1255.
45. Molfino NA, Nannini LJ, Martelli AN, Slutsky AS. Respiratory arrest in near-fatal asthma. N Engl J Med 1991;324:285–288.
46. Strunk RC. Sudden death in asthma. Am J Respir Crit Care Med 1993;148:550–552.
47. Strunk RC. Identification of the fatality-prone subject with asthma. J Allergy Clin Immunol 1989;83:477–485.
48. DeNicola LK, Monem GF, Gayle MO, Kissoon N. Treatment of critical status asthmaticus in children. Pediatr Clin North Am 1994;41(6):1293–324.
49. Wasserfallen J-B, Schaller M-D, Feihl F, Perret CH. Sudden asphyxic asthma: a distinct entity? Am Rev Respir Dis 1990;142:108–111.
50. Sur S, Crotty TB, Kephart GM, Hyma BA, Colby TV, Reed CE, et al. Sudden-onset fatal asthma. A distinct entity with few eosinophils and relatively more neutrophils in the airway submucosa? Am J Respir Crit Care Med 1993;148:713–719.
51. Maffei FA, van der Jagt EW, Powers KS, Standage SW, Connolly HV, Harmon WG, et al. Duration of mechanical ventilation in life-threatening pediatric asthma: description of an acute asphyxial subgroup. Pediatrics 2004;114(3):762–767.
52. Reid LM. The presence or absence of bronchial mucus in fatal asthma. J Allergy Clin Immunol 1987;80(Suppl):415–419.
53. Robertson CF, Rubinfeld AR, Bowes G. Pediatric asthma deaths in Victoria: the mild are at risk. Pediatr Pulmonol 1992;13:95–100.
54. Kravis LP, Kolski GB. Unexpected death in childhood asthma. A review of 13 deaths in ambulatory patients. Am J Dis Child 1985;139(6):558–563.
55. Fletcher HJ, Ibrahim SA, Speight N. Survey of asthma deaths in the northern region, 1970–1985. Arch Dis Child 1990;65:163–167.
56. Matsui T, Baba M. Death from asthma in children. Acta Paediatr Jpn 1990;32:205–208.
57. Mountain RD, Sahn SA. Clinical features and outcome in patients with acute asthma presenting with hypercapnia. Am Rev Respir Dis 1988;138:535–539.
58. Strunk RC, Mrazek DA, Fuhrman GS, LaBrecque JF. Physiologic and psychological characteristics associated with deaths due to asthma in childhood: a case-controlled study. JAMA 1985;254:1193–1198.
59. Strunk RC, Mrazek DA. Deaths from asthma in childhood: can they be predicted? N Engl Reg Allergy Proc 1986;7:454–461.
60. Birkhead G, Attaway NJ, Strunk RC, Townsend MC, Teutsch S. Investigation of a cluster of deaths of adolescents from asthma: evidence implicating inadequate treatment and poor patient adherence with medications. J Allergy Clin Immunol 1989;84(4 pt 1):484–491.
61. Martin AJ, Campbell DA, Gluyas PA, Coates JR, Ruffin RE, Roder DM, et al. Characteristics of near-fatal asthma in childhood. Pediatr Pulmonol 1995;20:1–8.
62. Patterson R, Greenberger PA, Patterson DR. Potentially fatal asthma: the problem of noncompliance. Ann Allergy 1991;67(2 pt 1):138–142.
63. Werner HA. Status asthmaticus in children: a review. Chest 2001;119:1913–1929.
64. Male I, Richter H, Seddon P. Children's perception of breathlessness in acute asthma. Arch Dis Child 2000;83:325–329.
65. Belessis Y, Dixon S, Thomsen A, Duffy B, Rawlinson W, Henry R, et al. Risk factors for an intensive care unit admission in children with asthma. Pediatr Pulmonol 2004;37:201–209.
66. Thomas M, Griffths C. Asthma and panic: scope for intervention? Am J Respir Crit Care Med 2005;171:1197–1198.
67. Steinman RM. The dendritic cell system and its role in immunogenicity. Ann Rev Immunol 1991;9:271–296.
68. Banchereau J, Steinman RM. Dendritic cells and the control of immunity. Nature 1998;392:245–252.
69. Sertl K, Takemura T, Tschachler E, Ferrans VJ, Kaliner MA, Shevach EM. Dendritic cells with antigen-presenting capability reside in airway epithelium, lung parenchyma, and visceral pleura. J Exp Med 1986;163:436–451.
70. Holt PG, Schon-Hegrad MA. Localization of T cells, macrophages, and dendritic cells in rat respiratory tract tissue: implications for immune function studies. Immunology 1987;62:349–356.
71. Havenith CE, Van MPP, Breedijk AJ, Beelen RH, Hoefsmit EC. Migration of dendritic cells into the draining lymph nodes of the lung after intratracheal instillation. Am J Respir Cell Mol Biol 1993;9:484–488.
72. Lambrecht BN, Salomon B, Klatzmann D, Pauwels RA. Dendritic cells are required for the development of chronic eosinophilic airway inflammation in response to inhaled antigen in sensitized mice. J Immunol 1998;160:4090–4097.
73. Kay AB. Allergy and allergic diseases. N Engl J Med 2001;344:30–37.
74. Prescott SL. New concepts of cytokines in asthma: is the Th2/Th1 paradigm out the window? J Paediatr Child Health 2003;39:575–579.
75. Busse WW, Lemanske J, R.F. Asthma. N Engl J Med 2001;344:350–362.
76. Sears MR, Burrows B, Flannery EM, Herbison GP, Hewitt CJ, Holdaway MD. Relation between airway responsiveness and serum IgG in children with asthma and apparently normal children. N Engl J Med 1991;325:1067–1071.
77. Beeh KM, Ksoll M, Buhl R. Elevation of total serum immunoglobulin E is associated with asthma in nonallergic individuals. Eur Respir J 2000;16:609–614.
78. Kaliner MA, Blennerhassett J, Austen FK, eds. Bronchial Asthma. New York: Grune and Stratton; 1976.
79. Gerblich AA, Salik H, Schuyler MR. Dynamic T-cell changes in peripheral blood and bronchoalveolar lavage after antigen provocation in asthmatics. Am Rev Respir Dis 1991;143:533–539.
80. Wills-Karp M. Immunologic basic of antigen-induced airway hyperresponsiveness. Annu Rev Immunol 1999;17:255–281.
81. Cox G, Ohtoshi T, Vancheri C, Denburg JA, Dolovich J, Gauldie J, et al. Promotion of eosinophil survival by human bronchial epithelial cells and its modulation by steroids. Am J Respir Cell Mol Biol 1991;4:525–531.
82. Cox G, Gauldie J, Jordana M. Bronchial epithelial cell–derived cytokines (G-CSF and GM-CSF) promote the survival of peripheral blood neutrophils in vitro. Am J Respir Cell Mol Biol 1992;7:507–513.
83. Xing Z, Ohtoshi T, Ralph P, Gauldie J, Jordana M. Human upper airway structural cell-derived cytokines support human peripheral blood monocyte survival: a potential mechanism for monocyte/macrophage accumulation in the tissue. Am J Respir Cell Mol Biol 1992;6:212–218.
84. Bisset LR, Schmid-Grendelmeier P. Chemokines and their receptors in the pathogenesis of allergic asthma: progress and perspective. Curr Opin Pulmonol Med 2005;11:35–42.
85. Miller AL, Lukacs NW. Chemokine receptors: understanding their role in asthmatic disease. Immunol Allergy Clin North Am 2004;24:667–683.
86. Mathew A, MacLean JA, DeHaan E, Tager AM, Green FH, Luster AD. Signal transducer and activator of transcription 6 controls chemokine production and T helper cell type 2 cell trafficking in allergic pulmonary inflammation. J Exp Med 2001;193(9):1087–1096.
87. Mathew A, Medoff BD, Carafone AD, Luster AD. Cutting edge: Th2 cell trafficking into the allergic lung is dependent on chemoattractant receptor signaling. J Immunol 2002;169(2):651–655.
88. Ennis M. Neutrophils in asthma pathophysiology. Curr Allergy Asthma Rep 2003;3:159–165.

89. Chung KF. Airway smooth muscle cells: contributing to and regulating airway mucosal inflammation? Eur Respir J 2000;15:961–968.

90. Hakonarson H, Carter C, Kim C, Grunstein MM. Altered expression and action of the low-affinity IgE receptor FcepsilonRII (CD23) in asthmatic airway smooth muscle. J Allergy Clin Immunol 1999;104:575–584.

91. Hakonarson H, Kim C, Whelan R, Campbell D, Grunstein MM. Bidirectional activation between human airway smooth muscle cells and T lymphocytes: role in induction of altered airway responsiveness. J Immunol 2001;166:293–303.

92. Hamid Q, Springall DR, Riveros-Moreno V, Chanez P, Howart P, Redington A, et al. Induction of nitric oxide synthase in asthma. Lancet 1993;342:1510–1513.

93. DeNicola LK, Kissoon N, Duckworth LJ, Blake KV, Murphy SP, Silkoff PE. Exhaled nitric oxide as an indicator of severity of asthmatic inflammation. Pediatr Emerg Care 2000;16:290–295.

94. Lanz MJ, Leung DY, White CW. Comparison of exhaled nitric oxide to spirometry during emergency treatment of asthma exacerbations with glucocorticoids in children. Ann Allergy Asthma Immunol 1999;82:161–164.

95. Baraldi E, Dario C, Ongaro R, Scollo M, Azzolin NM, Panza N, et al. Exhaled nitric oxide concentrations during treatment of wheezing exacerbation in infants and young children. Am J Respir Crit Care Med 1999;159:1284–1288.

96. Massaro AF, Gaston B, Kita D, Fanta C, Stamler JS, Drazen JM. Expired nitric oxide levels during treatment of acute asthma. Am J Respir Crit Care Med 1995;152:800–803.

97. Nelson BV, Sears S, Woods J, Ling CY, Hunt J, Clapper LM, et al. Expired nitric oxide as a marker for childhood asthma. J Pediatr 1997;130:423–427.

98. Murray AB, Ferguison AC, Morrison B. Airway responsiveness to histamine as a test for overall severity of asthma in children. J Allergy Clin Immunol 1981;68:119–124.

99. O'Byrne PM, Inman MD. Airway hyperresponsiveness. Chest 2003;123:411S–416S.

100. Lee YM, Park JS, Hwang JH, Park SW, Uh ST, Kim YH, et al. High-resolution CT findings in patients with near-fatal asthma: comparison of patients with mild-to-severe asthma and normal control subjects and changes in airway abnormalities following steroid treatment. Chest 2004;126:1840–1848.

101. Metcalfe DD, Baram D, Mekori YA. Mast cells. Physiol Rev 1997;77:1033–1079.

102. Fahy JV, Fleming HE, Wong HH, Liu JT, Su JQ, Reimann F, et al. The effect of an anti-IgE monoclonal antibody on the early- and late-phase responses to allergen inhalation in asthmatic subjects. Am J Respir Crit Care Med 1997;155:1828–1824.

103. Mehlhop PD, van de Rijn M, Goldberg AB, Brewer JB, Kurup VP, Martin TR, et al. Allergen-induced bronchial hyperreactivity and eosinophilic inflammation occur in the absence of IgE in a mouse model of asthma. Proc Natl Acad Sci USA 1997;94:1344–1349.

104. Holtzmann MJ, Morton JD, Shornick LP, Tyner JW, O'Sullivan MP, Antao A, et al. Immunity, inflammation, and remodeling in the airway epithelial barrier: epithelial–viral–allergic paradigm. Physiol Rev 2002;82:19–46.

105. Reed CE. The natural history of asthma in adults: the problem of irreversibility. J Allergy Clin Immunol 1999;103:539–547.

106. Holgate ST, Lackie P, Wilson S, Roche W, Davis D. Bronchial epithelium as a key regulator of airway allergens sensitization and remodeling in asthma. Am J Respir Crit Care Med 2000;162:S113–S117.

107. Jenkins HA, Cool C, Szefler SJ, Covar R, Brugman S, Gelfand EW, et al. Histopathology of severe childhood asthma: a case series. Chest 2003;124:32–41.

108. Cutz E, Levison H, Cooper DM. Ultrastructure of airways in children with asthma. Histopathology 1978;2(6):407–421.

109. Park JW, Hong YK, Kim CW, Kim DK, Choe KO, Hong CS. High-resolution computed tomography in patients with bronchial asthma: correlation with clinical features, pulmonary functions, and bronchial hyperresponsiveness. J Invest Allergy Clin Immunol 1997;7:186–192.

110. Aikawa T, Shimura S, Sasaki H, Ebina M, Takishima T. Marked goblet cell hyperplasia with mucus accumulation in the airways of patients who died of severe acute asthma attack. Chest 1992;101:916–921.

111. Huber HL, Koessler KK. The pathology of bronchial asthma. Arch Intern Med 1922;30:689–760.

112. Hirst SJ, Martin JG, Bonacci JV, Chan V, Fixman ED, Hamid QA, et al. Proliferative aspects of airway smooth muscle. J Allergy Clin Immunol 2004;114:S2–S17.

113. Chetta A, Foresi A, Del Donno M, Bertorelli G, Pesci A, Olivieri D. Airways remodeling is a distinctive feature of asthma and is related to severity of disease. Chest 1997;111:852–857.

114. Chu HW, Halliday JL, Martin RJ, Leung DY, Szefler SJ, Wenzel SE. Collagen deposition in large airways may not differentiate severe asthma from milder forms of the disease. Am J Respir Crit Care Med 1998;158:1936–1944.

115. Cokugras H, Akcakaya N, Seckin I, Camcioglu Y, Sarimurat N, Aksoy F. Ultrastructural examination of bronchial biopsy specimens from children with moderate asthma. Thorax 2001;56:25–29.

116. Montefort S, Roche WR, Holgate ST. Bronchial epithelial shedding in asthmatics and non-asthmatics. Respir Med 1993;87:9–11.

117. Lackie PM, Baker JE, Gunthert U, Holgate ST. Expression of CD44 isoforms is increased in the airway epithelium of asthmatic subjects. Am J Respir Cell Mol Biol 1997;16:14–22.

118. Puddicombe SM, Polosa R, Richter A, Krishna MT, Howart PH, Holgate ST, et al. Involvement of the epidermal growth factor receptor in epithelial repair in asthma. FASEB J 2000;14:1362–1374.

119. Openshaw PJ, Turner-Warwick M. Observations on sputum production in patients with variable airflow obstruction: implications for the diagnosis of asthma and chronic bronchitis. Respir Med 1989;83:25–31.

120. Houston JC, De Navasquez S, Trounce JR. A clinical and pathologic study of fatal cases of status asthmaticus. Thorax 1953;8:207–213.

121. Dunnil MS. The pathology of asthma with special reference to changes in the bronchial mucosa. J Clin Pathol 1960;13:27–33.

122. Cohn L, Homer RJ, Marinov A, Rankin J, Bottomly K. Induction of airway mucus production by T helper 2 (Th2) cells: a critical role for interleukin-4 in cell recruitment but not mucus production. J Exp Med 1997;186:1737–1747.

123. Society ATSER. Respiratory mechanics in infants: physiologic evaluation in health and disease. Am Rev Respir Dis 1993;147:474–496.

124. Ducharme FM, Davis GM. Measurement of respiratory resistance in the emergency department: feasibility in young children with acute asthma. Chest 1997;111:1519–1525.

125. Enright PL, Lebowitz MD, Cockroft D. Physiologic measures: pulmonary function tests. Asthma outcome. Am J Respir Crit Care Med 1994;149:S9–S18.

126. Peress L, Sybrecht G, Macklem PT. The mechanism of increase in total lung capacity during acute asthma. Am J Med 1976;61:165–169.

127. Cormier Y, Lecours R, Legris C. Mechanisms of hyperinflation in asthma. Eur Respir J 1990;3:619–624.

128. Woolcock AJ, Read J. Lung volumes in exacerbations of asthma. Am J Med 1966;41:259–273.

129. Holmes PW, Campbell AH, Barter CE. Acute changes of lung volumes and lung mechanics in asthma and in normal subjects. Thorax 1978;33:394–400.

130. Pellegrino R, Brusasco V. On the causes of lung hyperinflation during bronchoconstriction. Eur Respir J 1997;10:468–475.

131. Martin J, Powell E, Shore S, Emrich J, Engel LA. The role of respiratory muscles in the hyperinflation of bronchial asthma. Am Rev Respir Dis 1980;121:441–447.

132. Wheatley JR, West S, Cala SJ, Engel LA. The effect of hyperinflation on respiratory muscle work in acute induced asthma. Eur Respir J 1990;3:625–632.

133. Collett PW, Engel LA. Influence of lung volume on oxygen cost of resistive breathing. J Appl Physiol 1986;61:16–24.

134. Weiner P, Suo J, Fernandez E, Cherniack RM. The effect of hyperinflation on respiratory muscle strength and efficiency in healthy subjects and patients with asthma. Am Rev Respir Dis 1990;141: 1501–1505.

135. Aldrich TK, Hendler JM, Vizioli LD, Park M, Multz AS, Shapiro SM. Intrinsic positive end-expiratory pressure in ambulatory patients with airways obstruction. Am Rev Respir Dis 1993;147:845–849.

136. Bohn D, Kissoon N. Acute asthma. Pediatr Crit Care Med 2001; 2:151–163.

137. Wade OL, Gilson JC. Effect of posture on diaphragmatic movement and vital capacity in normal subjects. Thorax 1951;6:103–126.

138. Frey B, Freezer N. Diagnostic value and pathophysiologic basis of pulsus paradoxus in infants and children with respiratory disease. Pediatr Pulmonol 2001;31:138–143.

139. Frey B, Butt W. Pulse oximetry for assessment of pulsus paradoxus: a clinical study in children. Intensive Care Med 1999;24:242–246.

140. Hartert TV, Wheeler AP, Sheller JR. Use of pulse oximetry to recognize severity of airflow obstruction in obstructive airway disease: Correlation with pulsus paradoxus. Chest 1999;115:475–481.

141. Jay GD, Onuma K, Davis R, Chen M-H, Mansell A, Steele D. Analysis of physician ability in the measurement of pulsus paradoxus by sphygmomanometry. Chest 2000;118:348–352.

142. Rayner JR, Steele DW, Ziad A, Shaikhouni A, Jay GD. Continuous and non-invasive pulsus paradoxus monitoring. Acad Emerg Med 2003; 10:566–567.

143. Cook T, Stone G. Pediatric asthma: A correlation of clinical treatment and oxygen saturation. Hawaii Med J 1995;54:665–668.

144. Carruthers DM, Harrison BD. Arterial blood gas analysis or oxygen saturation in the assessment of acute asthma? Thorax 1995;50:186–188.

145. McFadden ER, Lyons HA. Arterial blood gas tensions in asthma. N Engl J Med 1968;278:1027–1032.

146. Kerem E, Canny G, Tibshirani R, Reisman J, Bentur L, Schuh S, et al. Clinical–physiologic correlations in acute asthma of childhood. Pediatrics 1991;87:481–486.

147. Sole D, Komatsu MK, Carvalho KV, Naspitz CK. Pulse oximetry in the evaluation of the severity of acute asthma and/or wheezing in children. J Asthma 1999;36:327–333.

148. Yamamoto LG, Wiebe RA, Rosen LM, Ringwood JW, Uechi CM, Miller NC, et al. Oxygen saturation changes during the pediatric emergency department treatment of wheezing. Am J Emerg Med 1992;10:274–284.

149. Geelhoed GC, Landau LI, LeSouëf PN. Evaluation of SaO₂ as a predictor of outcome in 280 children presenting with acute asthma. Ann Emerg Med 1994;23:1236–1241.

150. Cook T, Stone G. Pediatric asthma—a correlation of clinical treatment and oxygen saturation. Hawaii Med J 1995;54:665–668.

151. Morray B, Redding G. Factors associated with prolonged hospitalization of children with asthma. Arch Pediatr Adolesc Med 1995;149: 276–279.

152. Hilliard TN, Witten H, Male IA, Hewer SL, Seddon PC. Management of acute childhood asthma: a prospective multicentre study. Eur Respir J 2000;15:1102–1105.

153. Keogh KA, Macarthur C, Parkin PC, Stephens D, Arseneault R, Tennis O, et al. Predictors of hospitalization in children with acute asthma. J Pediatr 2001;139:273–277.

154. Keahey L, Bulloch B, Becker AB, Pollack CV Jr, Clark S, Camargo CA Jr. Initial oxygen saturation as a predictor of admission in children presenting to the emergency department with acute asthma. Ann Emerg Med 2002;40:300–307.

155. Hori T. Pathophysiological analysis of hypoxaemia during severe acute asthma. Arch Dis Child 1985;60:640–643.

156. Simpson H, Forfar JO, Grubb DJ. Arterial blood gas tensions and pH in acute asthma in childhood. BMJ 1968;3:460–464.

157. Downes JJ, Wood DW, Striker TW, Pittman JC. Arterial blood gas and acid–base disorders in infants and children with status asthmaticus. Pediatrics 1968;42(2):238–249.

158. Weng TR, Langer HM, Featherby EA, Levison H. Arterial blood gas tensions and acid–base balance in symptomatic and asymptomatic asthma in childhood. Am Rev Respir Dis 1970;101:274–282.

159. Rodriguez-Roisin R. Gas exchange abnormalities in asthma. Lung 1990;168(Suppl):599–605.

160. Tsai S-L, Crain EF, Silver EJ, Goldman HS. What can we learn from chest radiographs in hypoxemic asthmatics? Pediatr Radiol 2002;32: 498–504.

161. National Heart Lung and Blood Institute: National Asthma Education Program. National Asthma Education and Prevention Program Expert Panel Report 2: Guidelines for the Diagnosis and Management of Asthma. Bethesda, MD: U.S. Department of Health and Human Services; 1997.

162. National Heart Lung and Blood Institute: National Asthma Education Program. National Asthma Education Program Expert Panel Report. Executive Summary: Guidelines for the Diagnosis and Management of Asthma. Bethesda, MD: U.S. Department of Health and Human Services; 1991.

163. Gorelick MH, Stevens MW, Schultz T, Scribano PV. Difficulty in obtaining peak expiratory flow measurements in children with acute asthma. Pediatr Emerg Care 2004;20:22–26.

164. Becker AB, Nelson NA, Simons FER. The pulmonary index: assessment of a clinical score for asthma. Am J Dis Child 1984;138:574–576.

165. DiGuilio GA, Kercsmar CM, Krug SE, Alpert SE, Marx CM. Hospital treatment of asthma: lack of benefit from theophylline given in addition to nebulized albuterol and intravenously administered corticosteroid. J Pediatr 1993;122:464–469.

166. Obata T, Kimura Y, Iikura Y. Relationship between arterial blood gas tensions and a clinical score in asthmatic children. Ann Allergy 1992;68:530–532.

167. Roncoroni AJ, Adrogue HJ, De Obrutsky CW, Marchisio ML, Herrera MR. Metabolic acidosis in status asthmaticus. Respiration 1976; 33(2):85–94.

168. Appel D, Rubenstein R, Schrager K, Williams MH, Jr. Lactic acidosis in severe asthma. Am J Med 1983;75:580–584.

169. Mountain RD, Heffner JE, Brackett NC, Jr, Sahn SA. Acid–base disturbances in acute asthma. Chest 1990;98:651–655.

170. Assadi FK. Therapy of acute bronchospasm. Complicated by lactic acidosis and hypokalemia. Clin Pediatr (Phila) 1989;28(6):258–260.

171. Braden GL, Johnston SS, Germain MJ, Fitzgibbons JP, Dawson JA. Lactic acidosis associated with the therapy of acute bronchospasm. N Engl J Med 1985;313:890–891.

172. Rabbat A, Laaban JP, Boussairi A, Rochemaure J. Hyperlactatemia during acute severe asthma. Intensive Care Med 1998;24:85–94.

173. Yousef E, McGeady SJ. Lactic acidosis and status asthmaticus: how common in pediatrics? Ann Allergy Asthma Immunol 2002;89(6):585–588.

174. Manthous CA. Lactic acidosis in status asthmaticus: three cases and review of the literature. Chest 2001;119:1599–1602.

175. Okrent DG, Tessler S, Twersky RA, Tashkin DP. Metabolic acidosis not due to lactic acidosis in patients with severe acute asthma. Crit Care Med 1987;15:1098–1101.

176. DaCruz D, Holburn C. Serum potassium responses to nebulized salbutamol administered during an acute asthmatic attack. Arch Emerg Med 1989;6(1):22–26.

177. Du Plooy WJ, Hay L, Kahler CP, Schutte PJ, Brandt HD. The dose-related hyper- and hypokalaemic effects of salbutamol and its arrhythmogenic potential. Br J Pharmacol 1994;111(1):73–76.

178. Haalboom JR, Deenstra M, Struyvenberg A. Hypokalaemia induced by inhalation of fenoterol. Lancet 1985;1(8438):1125–1127.

179. Haddad S, Arabi Y, Shimemeri AA. Hypokalemic paralysis mimicking Guillain-Barré syndrome and causing acute respiratory failure. Middle East J Anesthesiol 2004;17(5):891–897.

180. Haffner CA, Kendall MJ. Metabolic effects of beta 2-agonists. J Clin Pharm Ther 1992;17(3):155–164.

181. Hung CH, Hua YM, Lee MY, Tsai YG, Yang KD. Evaluation of different nebulized bronchodilators on clinical efficacy and hypokalemia in asthmatic children. Acta Paediatr Taiwan 2001;42(5):287–290.

182. Kolski GB, Cunningham AS, Niemec PW Jr, Davignon GF Jr, Freehafer JG. Hypokalemia and respiratory arrest in an infant with status asthmaticus. J Pediatr 1988;112:304–307.

183. Singhi S, Marudkar A. Hypokalemia in a pediatric intensive care unit. Indian Pediatr 1996;33(1):9–14.

184. Singhi SC, Jayashree K, Sarkar B. Hypokalaemia following nebulized salbutamol in children with acute attack of bronchial asthma. J Paediatr Child Health 1996;32(6):495–497.

185. Smith SR, Kendall MJ. Potentiation of the adverse effects of intravenous terbutaline by oral theophylline. Br J Clin Pharmacol 1986; 21(4):451–453.

186. Tsai WS, Wu CP, Hsu YJ, Lin SH. Life-threatening hypokalemia in an asthmatic patient treated with high-dose hydrocortisone. Am J Med Sci 2004;327:152–155.

187. Singleton R, Moel DI, Cohn RA. Preliminary observation of impaired water excretion in treated status asthmaticus. Am J Dis Child 1986; 140(1):59–61.

188. Iikura Y, Odajima Y, Akazawa A, Nagakura T, Kishida M, Akimoto K. Antidiuretic hormone in acute asthma in children: effects of medication on serum levels and clinical course. Allergy Proc 1989;10(3):197–201.

189. Stalcup SA, Mellins RB. Mechanical forces producing pulmonary edema in acute asthma. N Engl J Med 1977;297:592–596.

190. Brooks LJ, Cloutier MM, Afshani E. Significance of roentgenographic abnormalities in children hospitalized for asthma. Chest 1982;82:315–318.

191. Alario AJ, McCarthy PL, Markovitz R, Kornguth P, Rosenfield N, Leventhal JM. Usefulness of chest radiographs in children with acute lower respiratory tract disease. J Pediatr 1987;111(2):187–193.

192. Gay BB Jr. Radiologic evaluation of the nontraumatized child with respiratory distress. Radiol Clin North Am 1978;16(1):91–112.

193. Gershel JC, Goldman HS, Stein RE, Shelov SP, Ziprkowski M. The usefulness of chest radiographs in first asthma attacks. N Engl J Med 1983;309:336–339.

194. Ismail Y, Loo CS, Zahary MK. The value of routine chest radiographs in acute asthma admissions. Singapore Med J 1994;35(2):171–172.

195. Kita Y, Sahara H, Yoshita Y, Shibata K, Ishise J, Kobayashi T. Status asthmaticus complicated by atelectasis in a child. Am J Emerg Med 1995;13(2):164–167.

196. Mahabee-Gittens EM, Bachman DT, Shapiro ED, Dowd MD. Chest radiographs in the pediatric emergency department for children < or =18 months of age with wheezing. Clin Pediatr (Phila) 1999;38(7):395–399.

197. Press S, Lipkind RS. A treatment protocol of the acute asthma patient in a pediatric emergency department. Clin Pediatr (Phila) 1991;30(10):573–577.

198. Roback MG, Dreitlein DA. Chest radiograph in the evaluation of first time wheezing episodes: review of current clinical practice and efficacy. Pediatr Emerg Care 1998;14(3):181–184.

199. Rushton AR. The role of the chest radiograph in the management of childhood asthma. Clin Pediatr (Phila) 1982;21(6):325–328.

200. Zieverink SE, Harper AP, Holden RW, Klatte EC, Brittain H. Emergency room radiography of asthma: an efficacy study. Radiology 1982;145(1):27–29.

201. Spottswood SE, Allison KZ, Lopatina OA, Sethi NN, Narla LD, Lowry PA, et al. The clinical significance of lung hypoexpansion in acute childhood asthma. Pediatr Radiol 2004;34(4):322–325.

202. Kelly CS, Andersen CL, Pestian JP, Wenger AD, Finch AB, Strope GL, et al. Improved outcomes for hospitalized asthmatic children using a clinical pathway. Ann Allergy Asthma Immunol 2000;84(5):509–516.

203. McDowell KM, Chatburn RL, Myers TR, O'Riordan MA, Kercsmar CM. A cost-saving algorithm for children hospitalized for status asthmaticus. Arch Pediatr Adolesc Med 1998;152(10):977–984.

204. Wazeka A, Valacer DJ, Cooper M, Caplan DW, DiMaio M. Impact of a pediatric asthma clinical pathway on hospital cost and length of stay. Pediatr Pulmonol 2001;32:211–216.

205. Kwan-Gett TS, Lozano P, Mullin K, Marcuse EK. One-year experience with an inpatient asthma clinical pathway. Arch Pediatr Adolesc Med 1997;151:684–689.

206. Chien JW, Ciufo R, Novak R, Skowronski M, Nelson J, Coreno A, et al. Uncontrolled oxygen administration and respiratory failure in acute asthma. Chest 2000;117:728–733.

207. Tal A, Pasterkamp H, Leahy F. Arterial oxygen desaturation following salbutamol inhalation in acute asthma. Chest 1984;86:868–869.

208. Douglas JG, Rafferty P, Fergusson RJ. Nebulised salbutamol without oxygen in severe acute asthma: How effective and how safe? Thorax 1985;40:180–183.

209. Connett G, Lenney W. Prolonged hypoxaemia after nebulised salbutamol. Thorax 1993;48:574–575.

210. Gleeson JG, Green S, Price JF. Air or oxygen as driving gas for nebulized salbutamol. Arch Dis Child 1988;63:900–904.

211. Collins JV, Jones D. Corticosteroids in the treatment of severe acute asthma (status asthmaticus). Acta Tuberc Pneumol Belg 1977;68(1):63–73.

212. Harfi H, Hanissian AS, Crawford LV. Treatment of status asthmaticus in children with high doses and conventional doses of methylprednisolone. Pediatrics 1978;61(6):829–831.

213. Pierson WE, Bierman CW, Kelley VC. A double-blind trial of corticosteroid therapy in status asthmaticus. Pediatrics 1974;54(3):282–288.

214. Younger RE, Gerber PS, Herrod HG, Cohen RM, Crawford LV. Intravenous methylprednisolone efficacy in status asthmaticus of childhood. Pediatrics 1987;80(2):225–230.

215. Tal A, Levy N, Bierman JE. Methylprednisolone therapy for acute asthma in infants and toddlers: a controlled clinical trial. Pediatrics 1990;86:350–356.

216. Shapiro GG, Furukawa CT, Pierson WE, Gardinier R, Bierman CW. Double-blind evaluation of methylprednisolone versus placebo for acute asthma episodes. Pediatrics 1983;71:510–514.

217. Rowe BH, Keller JL, Oxman AD. Effectiveness of steroid therapy in acute exacerbations of asthma: a meta-analysis. Am J Emerg Med 1992;10:301–310.

218. Scarfone RJ, Fuchs SM, Nager AL, Shane SA. Controlled trial of oral prednisone in the emergency department treatment of children with acute asthma. Pediatrics 1993;92:513–518.

219. Kattan M, Gurwitz D, Levison H. Corticosteroids in status asthmaticus. J Pediatr 1980;96(3 Pt 2):596–599.

220. Smith M, Iqbal S, Elliot TM, Everard M, Rowe BH. Corticosteroids for hospitalised children with acute asthma. Cochrane Database Syst Rev 2003;CD002886.

221. Collins JV, Clark TJ, Harris PW, Townsend J. Intravenous corticosteroids in treatment of acute bronchial asthma. Lancet 1970;21:1047–1049.

222. Langton Hewer S, Hobbs J, Reid F, Lenney W. Prednisolone in acute childhood asthma: clinical response to three dosages. Respir Med 1998;92:541–546.

223. Raimondi AC, Figueroa-Casa JC, Roncoroni AJ. Comparison between high and moderate doses of hydrocortisone in the treatment of status asthmaticus. Chest 1986;89:832–835.

224. Britton MG, Collins JV, Brown D, Fairhurst NP, Lambert RG. High-dose corticosteroids in severe acute asthma. BMJ 1976;2:73–74.

225. Emerman CL, Cydulka RK. A randomized comparison of 100-mg vs 500-mg dose of methylprednisolone in the treatment of acute asthma. Chest 1995;107:1559–1563.

226. Marquette CH, Stach B, Cardot E, Bervar JF, Saulnier F, Lafitte JJ, et al. High-dose and low-dose systemic corticosteroids are equally efficient in acute severe asthma. Eur Respir J 1995;8:22–27.

227. Matthews EE, Curtis PD, McLain BI, Morris LS, Turbitt ML. Nebulized budesonide versus oral steroid in severe exacerbations of childhood asthma. Acta Paediatr 1999;88:841–843.

228. Devidayal, Singhi S, Kumar L, Jayshree M. Efficacy of nebulized budesonide compared to oral prednisolone in acute bronchial asthma. Acta Paediatr 1999;88:835–840.

229. Scarfone RJ, Loiselle JM, Wiley JF, II, Decker JM, Henretig FM, Joffe MD. Nebulized dexamethasone versus oral prednisone in the emergency treatment of asthmatic children. Ann Emerg Med 1995;26: 480–486.

230. Schuh S, Reisman J, Alshehri M, Dupuis A, Corey M, Arseneault R, et al. A comparison of inhaled fluticasone and oral prednisone for children with severe acute asthma. N Engl J Med 2000;343:689–694.

231. Becker JM, Arora A, Scarfone RJ, Spector ND, Fontana-Penn ME, Gracely E, et al. Oral versus intravenous corticosteroids in children hospitalized with asthma. J Allergy Clin Immunol 1999;103:586–590.

232. Barnett PJ, Caputo GL, Baskin M, Kupperman N. Intravenous versus oral corticosteroids in the management of acute asthma in children. Ann Emerg Med 1997;29:212–217.

233. Klig JE, Hodge D, III, Rutherford MW. Symptomatic improvement following emergency department management of asthma: a pilot study of intramuscular dexamethasone versus oral prednisone. J Asthma 1997;34:419–425.

234. Klaustermeyer WB, Hale FC. The physiologic effect of an intravenous glucocorticoid in bronchial asthma. Ann Allergy 1976;37:80–86.

235. Wolfson DH, Nypaver MM, Blaser M, Hogan A, Evans RI, Davis AT. A controlled trial of methylprednisolone in the early emergency department treatment of acute asthma in children. Pediatr Emerg Care 1994;10:335–338.

236. Rodrigo C, Rodrigo G. Early administration of hydrocortisone in the emergency room treatment of acute asthma: a controlled clinical trial. Respir Med 1994;88:755–761.

237. Rowe BH, Spooner C, Ducharme FM, Bretzlaff JA, Bota GW. Early emergency department treatment of acute asthma with systemic corticosteroids. Cochrane Database Syst Rev 2001;1: CD002178.

238. Blackwell TS, Christman JW. The role of nuclear factor-kappa B in cytokine gene regulation. Am J Respir Crit Care Med 1997;17:3–9.

239. Barnes PJ, Karin M. Nuclear factor-kappa B—a pivotal transcription factor in chronic inflammatory diseases. N Engl J Med 1997;336:1066–1071.

240. Hayashi R, Wada H, Ito K, Adcock IM. Effects of glucocorticoids on gene transcription. Eur J Pharmacol 2004;500:51–62.

241. Barnes PJ, Adcock IM. How do corticosteroids work in asthma? Ann Intern Med 2003;139:359–370.

242. Schramm CM. Beta-adrenergic relaxation of rabbit tracheal smooth muscle: a receptor deficit that improves with corticosteroid administration. J Pharmacol Exp Ther 2000;292:280–287.

243. Kalavantavanich K, Schramm CM. Dexamethasone potentiates high-affinity beta-agonist binding and g(s) alpha protein expression in airway smooth muscle. Am J Physiol Lung Cell Mol Physiol 2000;278: L1101–L1106.

244. Rodrigo C, Rodrigo G. Corticosteroids in the emergency department therapy of acute adult asthma: an evidence-based evaluation. Chest 1999;116:285–295.

245. Liu L, Wang YX, Zhou J, Long F, Sun HW, Liu Y, et al. Rapid non-genomic inhibitory effects of glucocorticoids on human neutrophil degranulation. Inflamm Res 2005;54:37–41.

246. Pitzalis C, Pipitone N, Perretti M. Regulation of leukocyte–endothelial interactions by glucocorticoids. Ann NY Acad Sci 2002;966: 108–118.

247. Croxtall JD, van Hal PT, Choudhury Q, Gilroy DW, Flower RJ. Different glucocorticoids vary in their genomic and non-genomic mechanism of action in A549 cells. Br J Pharmacol 2002;135:511–519.

248. Townley RG, Suliaman F. The mechanism of corticosteroids in treating asthma. Ann Allergy 1987;58:1–6.

249. Rodrigo G, Rodrigo C. Inhaled flunisolide for acute severe asthma. Am J Respir Crit Care Med 1998;157:698–703.

250. Rodrigo GJ. Comparison of inhaled fluticasone with intravenous hydrocortisone in the treatment of adult acute asthma. Am J Respir Crit Care Med 2005;171:1231–1236.

251. Siegel SC, Richards W. Status asthmaticus in children. Int Anesthesiol Clin 1971;9(1):99–115.

252. Bocles JS. Status asthmaticus. Med Clin North Am 1970;54(2):493–509.

253. Kampschulte S, Marcy J, Safar P. Simplified physiologic management of status asthmaticus in children. Crit Care Med 1973;1(2):69–74.

254. Becker AB, Nelson NA, Simons FE. Inhaled salbutamol (albuterol) vs injected epinephrine in the treatment of acute asthma in children. J Pediatr 1983;102:465–469.

255. Simons FE, Gillies JD. Dose response of subcutaneous terbutaline and epinephrine in children with acute asthma. Am J Dis Child 1981; 135:214–217.

256. Tinkelman DG, Vanderpool GE, Carroll MS, Lotner GZ, Spangler DL. Comparison of nebulized terbutaline and subcutaneous epinephrine in the treatment of acute asthma. Ann Allergy 1983;50:398–401.

257. Uden DL, Goetz DR, Kohen DP, Fifield GC. Comparison of nebulized terbutaline and subcutaneous epinephrine in the treatment of acute asthma. Ann Emerg Med 1985;14:229–232.

258. Victoria MS, Battista CJ, Nangia BS. Comparison between epinephrine and terbutaline injections in the acute management of asthma. J Asthma 1989;26:287–290.

259. Appel D, Karpel JP, Sherman M. Epinephrine improves expiratory flow rates in patients with asthma who do not respond to inhaled metaproterenol sulfate. J Allergy Clin Immunol 1989;84:90–98.

260. Kornberg AE, Zuckerman S, Welliver JR, Mezzadri F, Aquino N. Effect of injected long-acting epinephrine in addition to aerosolized albuterol in the treatment of acute asthma in children. Pediatr Emerg Care 1991;7:1–3.

261. Lin YZ, Hsieh KH, Chang LF, Chu CY. Terbutaline nebulization and epinephrine injection in treating acute asthmatic children. Pediatr Allergy Immunol 1996;7:95–99.

262. Safdar B, Cone DC, Pham KT. Subcutaneous epinephrine in the pre-hospital setting. Prehosp Emerg Care 2001;5:200–207.

263. Sharma A, Madan A. Subcutaneous epinephrine vs nebulized salbutamol in asthma. Indian J Pediatr 2001;68:1127–1130.

264. Amory DW, Burnham SC, Cheney FW. Comparison of the cardiopulmonary effects of subcutaneously administered epinephrine and terbutaline in patients with reversible airway obstruction. Chest 1975;67:279–286.

265. Schwartz AL, Lipton JM, Warburton D, Johnson LB, Twarog FJ. Management of acute asthma in childhood. A randomized evaluation of beta-adrenergic agents. Am J Dis Child 1980;134:474–478.

266. Ben-Zvi Z, Lam C, Hoffman J, Teets-Grimm K, Kattan M. An evaluation of the initial treatment of acute asthma. Pediatrics 1982;70: 348–353.

267. Becker AB, Nelson NA, Simons FER. Inhaled salbutamol vs injected epinephrine in the treatment of acute asthma in children. J Pediatr 1983;102:465–469.

268. Littner MR, Tashkin DP, Siegel SC, Katz R. Double-blind comparison of acute effects of inhaled albuterol, isoproterenol, and placebo on cardiopulmonary function and gas exchange in asthmatic children. Ann Allergy 1983;50:309–316.

269. Oberklaid F, Mellis CM, Souef PN, Geelhoed GC, Maccarrone AL. A comparison of a bodyweight dose versus a fixed dose of nebulised salbutamol in acute asthma in children. Med J Aust 1993;158:751–753.

270. Schuh S, Parkin P, Rajan A, Canny G, Healy R, Rieder M, et al. High-versus low-dose frequently administered nebulised albuterol in children with severe acute asthma. Pediatrics 1989;83:513–518.

271. Schuh S, Reider MJ, Canny G, Pender E, Forbes T, Tan YK, et al. Nebulised albuterol in acute childhood asthma: comparison of two doses. Pediatrics 1990;86:509–513.

272. Reilly PA, Yahav J, Mindorff C, Kazim F, Levison H. Dose response characteristics of nebulized fenoterol in asthmatic children. J Pediatr 1983;103:121–126.

273. Heimer D, Shim C, Williams MH Jr. The effect of sequential inhalations of metaproterenol aerosol in asthma. J Allergy Clin Immunol 1980;66:75–77.

274. Robertson CF, Smith F, Beck R, Levison H. Response to frequent low doses of nebulized salbutamol in acute asthma. J Pediatr 1985;106:672–674.

275. Penna AC, Dawson KP. Nebulised salbutamol; systemic absorption could be important in achieving bronchodilation. J Asthma 1993;30:105–107.

276. Penna AC, Dawson KP, Manglick P. Extremely high plasma salbutamol concentrations in three children treated for acute asthma. Aust J Hosp Pharm 1993;23:165–167.

277. Penna AC, Dawson KP, Manglick P, Tam J. Systemic absorption following nebuliser delivery in acute asthma. Acta Paediatr 1993;82:963–966.

278. Amirav I, Newhouse MT. Metered-dose inhaler accessory devices in acute asthma. Arch Pediatr Adolesc Med 1997;151:876–882.

279. Rubilar L, Castro-Rodriguez JA, Girardi G. Randomized trial of salbutamol via metered-dose inhaler with spacer versus nebulizer for acute wheezing in children less than 2 years of age. Pediatr Pulmonol 2000;29:264–269.

280. Clay MM, Pavia D, Newman SP, Lennard-Jones T, Clarke SW. Assessment of jet nebulisers for lung aerosol therapy. Lancet 1983;2:592–594.

281. Hess D, Horney D, Snyder T. Medication-delivery performance of eight small-volume, hand-held nebulizers: Effects of diluent volume, gas, flow rate, and nebulizer model. Respir Care 1989;34:717–723.

282. Scarfone RJ, Friedlaender EY. Beta-2-agonists in acute asthma: the evolving state of the art. Pediatr Emerg Care 2002;18:442–447.

283. Ba M, Thivierge RL, Lapierre JG, Gaudreault P, Spier S, Lamarre A. Effects of continuous inhalation of salbutamol in acute asthma [abstr]. Am Rev Respir Dis 1987;135:A326.

284. Salazar RO, Joos TH, Nickles PA, Pierantoni WN. Treatment of status asthmaticus with continuous nebulized albuterol therapy in children [abstr]. J Allergy Clin Immunol 1990;85:A210.

285. Katz RW, Kelly HW, Crowley MR, Grad R, McWilliams BC, Murphy SJ. Safety of continuous nebulized albuterol for bronchospasm in infants and children. Pediatrics 1993;92:666–669.

286. Papo MC, Frank J, Thompson AE. A prospective, randomized study of continuous versus intermittent nebulized albuterol for severe status asthmaticus in children. Crit Care Med 1993;21(10):1479–1486.

287. Singh M, Kumar L. Continuous nebulised salbutamol and oral once a day prednisolone in status asthmaticus. Arch Dis Child 1993;69(4):416–419.

288. Craig VL, Bigos D, Brilli RJ. Efficacy and safety of continuous albuterol nebulization in children with severe status asthmaticus. Pediatr Emerg Care 1996;12(1):1–5.

289. Montgomery VL, Eid NS. Low-dose beta-agonist continuous nebulization therapy for status asthmaticus in children. J Asthma 1994;31(3):201–207.

290. Siegel AJ, Silverman LM, Holman BL. Elevated creatine kinase isoenzyme level in marathon runners. Normal myocardial scintigrams suggest noncardiac source. JAMA 1981;246:2049–2051.

291. Siegel AJ, Silverman LM, Lopez RE. Creatine kinase elevations in marathon runners: relationship to training and competition. Yale J Biol Med 1980;53:275–279.

292. Jaffe AS, Garfinkel BT, Ritter CS, Sobel BE. Plasma MB creatine kinase after vigorous exercise in professional athletes. Am J Cardiol 1984;53:856–858.

293. Choi YS. Serum enzyme monitoring in asthma patients [letter]. Pediatrics 1992;90:279–280.

294. Adcock IM, Peters MJ, Brown CR, Stevens DA, Barnes PJ. High concentrations of beta-adrenergic agonists inhibit DNA binding of glucocorticoids in human lungs in vitro. Biochem Soc Trans 1995;23:217S.

295. Peters MJ, Adcock IM, Brown CR, Barnes PJ. ß-Agonist inhibition of steroid receptor DNA binding activity in human lung [abstr]. Am Rev Respir Dis 1993;147:A772.

296. Peters MJ, Adcock IM, Brown CR, Barnes PJ. Beta-adrenoreceptor agonists interfere with glucocorticoid receptor DNA binding in rat lung. Eur J Pharmacol 1995;289:275–281.

297. Pang LM, Rodriguez-Martinez F, Davis WJ, Mellins RB. Terbutaline in the treatment of status asthmaticus. Chest 1977;72(4):469–473.

298. Moler FW, Hurwitz ME, Custer JR. Improvement in clinical asthma score and PaCO2 in children with severe asthma treated with continuously nebulized terbutaline. J Allergy Clin Immunol 1988;81:1101–1109.

299. Moler FW, Johnson CE, Van Laanen C, Palmisano JM, Nasr SZ, Akingbola O. Continuous versus nebulized terbutaline: plasma levels and effects. Am J Respir Crit Care Med 1995;151:602–606.

300. Portnoy J, Aggarwal J. Continuous terbutaline nebulization for the treatment of severe exacerbations of asthma in children. Ann Allergy 1988;60:368–371.

301. Hultquist C, Lindberg C, Nyberg B, Kjellman B, Wettrell G. Kinetics of terbutaline in asthmatic children. Eur J Respir Dis Suppl 1984;134:195–203.

302. Tipton WR, Nelson HS. Frequent parenteral terbutaline in the treatment of status asthmaticus in children. Ann Allergy 1987;58(4):252–256.

303. Stephanopoulos DE, Monge R, Schell KH, Wyckoff P, Peterson BM. Continuous intravenous terbutaline for pediatric status asthmaticus. Crit Care Med 1998;26(10):1744–1748.

304. Fuglsang G, Pedersen S, Borgstrom L. Dose–response relationships of intravenously administered terbutaline in children with asthma. J Pediatr 1989;114:315–320.

305. Hultquist C, Lindberg C, Nyberg L, Kjellman B, Wettrell G. Pharmacokinetics of intravenous terbutaline in asthmatic children. Dev Pharmacol Ther 1989;13:11–20.

306. O'Connell MB, Iber C. Continuous intravenous terbutaline infusions for adult patients with status asthmaticus. Ann Allergy 1990;64:213–219.

307. Pierce RJ, Payne CR, Williams SJ, Denison DM, Clark TJ. Comparison of intravenous and inhaled terbutaline in the treatment of asthma. Chest 1981;79:506–511.

308. Williams SJ, Winner SJ, Clark TJ. Comparison of inhaled and intravenous terbutaline in acute severe asthma. Thorax 1981;36:629–632.

309. Van Renterghem D, Lamont H, Elinck W, Pauwels R, Van Der Straeten M. Intravenous versus nebulized terbutaline in patients with acute severe asthma; a double-blind randomized study. Ann Allergy 1987;59:313–316.

310. Chiang VW, Burns JP, Rifai N, Lipshultz SE, Adams MJ, Weiner DL. Cardiac toxicity of intravenous terbutaline for the treatment of severe asthma in children: a prospective assessment. J Pediatr 2000;137:73–77.

311. Hardasmalani MD, DeBari V, Bithoney WG, Gold N. Levalbuterol versus racemic albuterol in the treatment of acute exacerbation of asthma in children. Pediatr Emerg Care 2005;21:415–419.

312. Ralston ME, Euwema MS, Knecht KR, Ziolkowski TJ, Coakley TA, Cline SM. Comparison of levalbuterol and racemic albuterol combined with ipratropium bromide in acute pediatric asthma: a randomized, controlled trial. J Emerg Med 2005;29:29–35.

313. Qureshi F, Zaritsky A, Welch C, Meadows T, Burke BL. Clinical efficacy of racemic albuterol versus levalbuterol for the treatment of acute pediatric asthma. Ann Emerg Med 2005;46:29–36.

314. Carl JC, Myers TR, Kirchner HL, Kercsmar CM. Comparison of racemic albuterol and levalbuterol for treatment of acute asthma. J Pediatr 2003;143:731–736.

315. Steiner P, Rao M, Ehrlich R, Padre R. The use of intravenous isoproterenol in the treatment of status asthmaticus. J Asthma Res 1975;12(4):215–219.

316. Herman JJ, Noah ZL, Moody RR. Use of intravenous isoproterenol for status asthmaticus in children. Crit Care Med 1983;11(9):716–720.

317. Parry WH, Martorano F, Cotton EK. Management of life-threatening asthma with intravenous isoproterenol infusions. Am J Dis Child 1976;130(1):39–42.

318. Victoria MS, Tayaba RG, Nangia BS. Isoproterenol infusion in the management of respiratory failure in children with status asthmaticus: experience in a small community hospital and review of the literature. J Asthma 1991;28(2):103–108.

319. Newman LJ, Richards W, Church JA. Isoetharine-isoproterenol: a comparison of effects in childhood status asthmaticus. Ann Allergy 1982;48(4):230232.

320. Downes JJ, Wood DW, Harwood I, Sheinkopf HN, Raphaely RC. Intravenous isoproterenol infusion in children with severe hypercapnia due to status asthmaticus. Effects on ventilation, circulation, and clinical score. Crit Care Med 1973;1(2):63–68.

321. Phanichyakarn P, Pongpanich B, Ayudthya PS, Vongpraomas C, Krisarin C, Vongvivat K, et al. Intravenous isoproterenol infusion in asthmatic attacks and life threatening status asthmaticus in Thai children. J Med Assoc Thai 1978;61(9):529–535.

322. Wood DW, Downes JJ. Intravenous isoproterenol in the treatment of respiratory failure in childhood status asthmaticus. Ann Allergy 1973;31(12):607–610.

323. Maguire JF, Geha RS, Umetsu DT. Myocardial specific creatine phosphokinase isoenzyme elevation in children with asthma treated with intravenous isoproterenol. J Allergy Clin Immunol 1986;78(4 Pt 1): 631–636.

324. Mikhail MS, Hunsinger SY, Goodwin SR, Loughlin GM. Myocardial ischemia complicating therapy of status asthmaticus. Clin Pediatr (Phila) 1987;26(8):419–421.

325. Maguire JF, O'Rourke PP, Colan SD, Geha RS, Crone R. Cardiotoxicity during treatment of severe childhood asthma. Pediatrics 1991; 88(6):1180–1186.

326. Matson JR, Loughlin GM, Strunk RC. Myocardial ischemia complicating the use of isoproterenol in asthmatic children. J Pediatr 1978; 92:776–778.

327. Bohn D, Kalloghlian A, Jenkins J, Edmonds J, Barker G. Intravenous salbutamol in the treatment of status asthmaticus in children. Crit Care Med 1984;12(10):892–896.

328. Browne GJ, Penna AC, Phung X, Soo M. Randomised trial of intravenous salbutamol in early management of acute severe asthma in children. Lancet 1997;349:301–305.

329. Browne GJ, Lam LT. Single-dose intravenous salbutamol bolus for managing children with acute severe asthma in the emergency department: reanalysis of data. Pediatr Crit Care Med 2002;3:117–123.

330. Sellers WF, Messahel B. Rapidly repeated intravenous boluses of salbutamol for acute severe asthma. Anaesthesia 2003;58:680–683.

331. Roberts G, Newsom D, Gomez K, Raffles A, Saglani S, Begent J, et al. Intravenous salbutamol bolus compared with an aminophylline infusion in children with severe asthma: a randomised controlled trial. Thorax 2003;58:306–310.

332. Browne GJ, Trieu L, Van Asperen P. Randomized, double-blind, placebo-controlled trial of intravenous salbutamol and nebulized ipratropium bromide in early management of severe acute asthma in children presenting to an emergency department. Crit Care Med 2002;30:448–453.

333. Habashy D, Lam LT, Browne GJ. The administration of beta2-agonists for paediatric asthma and its adverse reaction in Australian and New Zealand emergency departments: a cross-sectional survey. Eur J Emerg Med 2003;10(3):219–224.

334. Rodrigo GJ, Rodrigo C. The role of anticholinergics in acute asthma treatment: an evidence-based evaluation. Chest 2002;121:1977–1987.

335. Barnes PJ, Minette P, Maclagan J. Muscarinic receptor subtypes in the airways. Trends Pharmacol Sci 1988;9:412–416.

336. Barnes PJ. Muscarinic receptor subtypes in airways. Life Sci 1993; 52:529–536.

337. Fryer AD, Jacoby DB. Effect of inflammatory cell mediators on M2 muscarinic receptors in the lungs. Life Sci 1993;52:529–536.

338. Rowe BH, Travers AH, Holroyd BR, Kelly KD, Bota GW. Nebulized ipratropium bromide in acute pediatric asthma: does it reduce hospital admissions among children presenting to the emergency department? Ann Emerg Med 1999;34:75–85.

339. Aaron SD. The use of ipratropium bromide for the management of acute asthma exacerbation in adults and children: a systematic review. J Asthma 2001;38:521–530.

340. Schuh S, Johnson DW, Callahan S, Canny G, Levison H. Efficacy of frequent nebulized ipratropium bromide added to frequent high-dose albuterol therapy in severe childhood asthma. J Pediatr 1995;126:639–645.

341. Qureshi F, Pestian J, Davis P, Zaritsky A. Effect of nebulized ipratropium on the hospitalization rates of children with asthma. N Engl J Med 1998;339:1030–1035.

342. Zorc JJ, Pusic MV, Ogborn CJ, Lebet R, Duggan AK. Ipratropium bromide added to asthma treatment in the pediatric emergency department. Pediatrics 1999;103:748–752.

343. Goggin N, Macarthur C, Parkin PC. Randomized trial of the addition of ipratropium bromide to albuterol and corticosteroid therapy in children hospitalized because of an acute asthma exacerbation. Arch Pediatr Adolesc Med 2001;155:1329–1334.

344. Craven D, Kercsmar CM, Myers TR, O'Riordan MA, Golonka G, Moore S. Ipratropium bromide plus nebulized albuterol for the treatment of hospitalized children with acute asthma. J Pediatr 2001;138(1):51–58.

345. Roselló HJ, Plá JC. Sulfato de magnesio en la crisis de asthma. Prensa Med Argent 1936;23:1677–1680.

346. Okayama H, Aikawa T, Okayama M, Sasaki H, Mue S, Takishima T. Bronchodilating effects of intravenous magnesium sulfate in bronchial asthma. JAMA 1987;257:1076–1078.

347. Rolla G, Bucca C, Caria E, Arossa W, Bugiani M, Cesano L, et al. Acute effect of intravenous magnesium sulfate on airway obstruction of asthmatic patients. Ann Allergy 1988;61:388–391.

348. Noppen M, Vanmaele L, Impens N, Schandevyl W. Bronchodilating effect of intravenous magnesium sulfate in acute severe bronchial asthma. Chest 1990;97:373–376.

349. Dominguez LJ, Barbagallo M, Di Lorenzo G, Drago A, Scola S, Morici G, et al. Bronchial reactivity and intracellular magnesium: a possible mechanism for the bronchodilating effects of magnesium in asthma. Clin Sci (Lond) 1998;95:137–142.

350. McNamara RM, Spivey WH, Skobeloff E, Jacubowitz S. Intravenous magnesium sulfate in the management of acute respiratory failure complicating asthma. Ann Emerg Med 1989;18:197–199.

351. Kuitert LM, Kletchko SL. Intravenous magnesium sulfate in acute, life-threatening asthma. Ann Emerg Med 1991;20:1243–1245.

352. Sydow M, Crozier TA, Zielmann S, Radke J, Burchardi H. High-dose intravenous magnesium sulfate in the management of life-threatening status asthmaticus. Intensive Care Med 1993;19:467–471.

353. Kakish KS. Serum magnesium levels in asthmatic children during and between exacerbations. Arch Pediatr Adolesc Med 2001;155(2):181–183.

354. Zervas E, Papatheodorou G, Psathakis K, Panagou P, Georgatou N, Loukides S. Reduced intracellular Mg concentrations in patients with acute asthma. Chest 2003;123:113–118.

355. Falkner D, Glauser J, Allen M. Serum magnesium levels in asthmatic patients during exacerbations of asthma. Am J Emerg Med 1992; 10:1–3.

356. Emelyanov A, Fedoseev G, Barnes PJ. Reduced intracellular magnesium concentrations in asthmatic patients. Eur Respir J 1999;13: 38–40.

357. Hashimoto Y, Nishimura Y, Maeda H, Yokoyama M. Assessment of magnesium status in patients with bronchial asthma. J Asthma 2000;37:489–496.

358. Bodenhamer J, Bergstrom R, Brown D, Gabow P, Marx JA, Lowenstein SR. Frequently nebulized beta-agonists for asthma: effects on serum electrolytes. Ann Emerg Med 1992;21:1337–1342.

359. de Castillo J, Engbaek L. The nature of the neuromuscular block produced by magnesium. J Physiol 1954;124:370–384.

360. Altura BM, Altura BT, Waldemar Y. Prostaglandin-induced relaxations and contractions of arterial smooth muscle: effects of magnesium ions. Artery 1976;2:326–336.

361. Iseri LT, French JH. Magnesium: Nature's physiologic calcium blocker. Am Heart J 1984;108:188–193.

362. Brandt DR, Ross EM. Catecholamine-stimulated GTPase cycle: multiple sites of regulation by beta-adrenergic receptor and Mg^{2+} studied in reconstituted receptor-Gs vesicles. J Biol Chem 1986;261:1656–1664.

363. Spivey WH, Skobeloff EM, Levin RM. Effect of magnesium chloride on rabbit bronchial smooth muscle. Ann Emerg Med 1990;19:1107–1112.

364. Ransnas LA, Jasper JR, Leiber D, Insel PA. Beta-adrenergic-receptor-mediated dissociation and membrane release of the Gs protein in S49 lymphoma-cell membranes. Dependence on Mg^{2+} and GTP. Biochem J 1992;283:519–524.

365. Cairns CB, Kraft M. Magnesium attenuates the neutrophil respiratory burst in adult asthmatic patients. Acad Emerg Med 1996;3:1093–1097.

366. Mangat HS, D'Souza GA, Jacob MS. Nebulized magnesium sulfate versus nebulized salbutamol in acute bronchial asthma: a clinical trial. Eur Respir J 1998;12:341–344.

367. Nannini LJ Jr, Pendino JC, Corna RA, Mannarino S, Quispe R. Magnesium sulfate as a vehicle for nebulized salbutamol in acute asthma. Am J Med 1998;108:193–197.

368. Rowe BH, Bretzlaff JA, Bourdon C, Bota GW, Camargo CA Jr. Intravenous magnesium sulfate treatment for acute asthma in the emergency department: a systematic review of the literature. Ann Emerg Med 2000;36:181–190.

369. Rodrigo G, Rodrigo C, Burschtin O. Efficacy of magnesium sulfate in acute adult asthma: a meta-analysis of randomized trials. Am J Emerg Med 2000;18:216–221.

370. Pabon H, Monem G, Kissoon N. Safety and efficacy of magnesium sulfate infusions in children with status asthmaticus. Pediatr Emerg Care 1994;10(4):200–203.

371. Ciarallo L, Sauer AH, Shannon MW. Intravenous magnesium therapy for moderate to severe pediatric asthma: results of a randomized, placebo-controlled trial. J Pediatr 1996;129:809–814.

372. Devi PR, Kumar L, Singhi SC, Prasad R, Singh M. Intravenous magnesium sulfate in acute severe asthma not responding to conventional therapy. Indian Pediatr 1997;34:389–397.

373. Gurkan F, Haspolat K, Bosnak M, Dikici B, Derman O, Ece A. Intravenous magnesium sulfate in the management of moderate to severe acute asthmatic children nonresponding to conventional therapy. Eur J Emerg Med 1999;6:201–205.

374. Scarfone RJ, Loiselle JM, Joffe MD, Mull CC, Stiller S, Thompson K, et al. A randomized trial of magnesium in the emergency department treatment of children with asthma. Ann Emerg Med 2000;36:572–578.

375. Ciarallo L, Broussea D, Reinert S. Higher-dose intravenous magnesium therapy for children with moderate to severe acute asthma. Arch Pediatr Adolesc Med 2000;154:979–983.

376. Markovitz B. Does magnesium sulphate have a role in the management of paediatric status asthmaticus? Arch Dis Child 2002;86(5):381–382.

377. Cheuk DK, Chau TC, Lee SL. A meta-analysis on intravenous magnesium sulphate for treating acute asthma. Arch Dis Child 2005;90:74–77.

378. Skobeloff EM, Spivey WH, McNamara RM, Greenspon L. Intravenous magnesium sulfate for the treatment of acute asthma in the emergency department. JAMA 1989;262:1210–1213.

379. Skorodin MS, Freebeck PC, Yetter B, Nelson JE, Van de Graff WB, Walsh JM. Magnesium sulfate potentiates several cardiovascular and metabolic actions of terbutaline. Chest 1994;105:701–705.

380. Pierson WE, Bierman CW, Stamm SJ, Van Arsdel PP Jr. Double-blind trial of aminophylline in status asthmaticus. Pediatrics 1971;48(4):642–646.

381. Hambleton G, Stone MJ. Comparison of IV salbutamol with IV aminophylline in the treatment of severe, acute asthma in childhood. Arch Dis Child 1979;54:391–402.

382. Carter E, Cruz M, Chesrown S, Shieh G, Reilly K, Hendeles L. Efficacy of intravenously administered theophylline in children hospitalized with severe asthma. J Pediatr 1993;122:470–476.

383. Strauss RE, Wertheim DL, Bonagura VR, Valacer DJ. Aminophylline therapy does not improve outcome and increases adverse effects in children hospitalized with acute asthmatic exacerbations. Pediatrics 1994;93:205–210.

384. Bien JP, Bloom MD, Evans RL, Specker B, O'Brien KP. Intravenous theophylline in pediatric status asthmaticus. A prospective, randomized, double-blind, placebo-controlled trial. Clin Pediatr (Phila) 1995;34(9):475–481.

385. Needleman JP, Kaifer MC, Nold JT, Shuster PE, Redding MM, Gladstein J. Theophylline does not shorten hospital stay for children admitted for asthma. Arch Pediatr Adolesc Med 1995;149:206–209.

386. Nuhoglu Y, Dai A, Barlan IB, Basaran MM. Efficacy of aminophylline in the treatment of acute asthma exacerbations in children. Ann Allergy Asthma Immunol 1998;80:395–398.

387. Goodman DC, Littenberg B, O'Connor GT, Brooks JG. Theophylline in acute childhood asthma: a meta-analysis of its efficacy. Pediatr Pulmonol 1996;21:211–218.

388. Montserrat JM, Barbera JA, Viegas C, Roca J, Rodriguez-Roisin R. Gas exchange response to intravenous aminophylline in patients with a severe exacerbation of asthma. Eur Respir J 1995;8:28–33.

389. Wagner PD, Dantzker DR, Iacovoni VE, Tomlin WC, West JB. Ventilation–perfusion inequality in asymptomatic asthma. Am Rev Respir Dis 1978;118:511–524.

390. Ballester E, Reyes A, Roca J, Guitart R, Wagner PD, Rodriguez-Roisin R. Ventilation–perfusion mismatching in acute severe asthma: effects of salbutamol and 100% oxygen. Thorax 1989;44:258–267.

391. Bell M, Jackson E, Mi Z, McCombs J, Carcillo J. Low-dose theophylline increases urine output in diuretic-dependent critically ill children. Intensive Care Med 1998;24:1099–1105.

392. Yung M, South M. Randomized controlled trial of aminophylline for severe acute asthma. Arch Dis Child 1998;79:405–410.

393. Ream RS, Loftis LL, Albers GM, Becker BA, Lynch RE, Mink RB. Efficacy of IV theophylline in children with severe status asthmaticus. Chest 2001;119(5):1480–1488.

394. Wheeler DS, Jacobs BR, Kenreigh CA, Bean JA, Hutson TK, Brilli RJ. Theophylline versus terbutaline in treating critically ill children with status asthmaticus: a prospective, randomized, controlled trial. Pediatr Crit Care Med 2005;6:142–147.

395. Ho AM-H, Lee A, Karmakar MK, Dion PW, Chung DC, Contardi LH. Heliox vs air–oxygen mixtures for the treatment of patients with acute asthma: a systematic overview. Chest 2003;123:882–890.

396. Gupta VK, Cheifetz IM. Heliox administration in the pediatric intensive care unit: an evidence-based review. Pediatr Crit Care Med 2005;6:204–211.

397. Kudukis TM, Manthous CA, Schmidt GA, Hall JB, Wylam ME. Inhaled helium–oxygen revisited: effect of inhaled helium–oxygen during the treatment of status asthmaticus in children. J Pediatr 1997;130(2):217–224.

398. Tobias JD, Garrett JS. Therapeutic options for severe, refractory status asthmaticus: inhalational anaesthetic agents, extracorporeal membrane oxygenation and helium/oxygen ventilation. Paediatr Anaesth 1997;7(1):47–57.

399. Gluck EH, Onorato DJ, Castriotta R. Helium–oxygen mixtures in intubated patients with status asthmaticus and respiratory acidosis. Chest 1990;98:693–698.

400. Haynes JM, Sargent RJ, Sweeney EL. Use of heliox to avoid intubation in a child with acute severe asthma and hypercapnia. Am J Crit Care 2003;12:28–30.

401. Abd-Allah SA, Rogers MS, Terry M, Gross M, Perkin RM. Helium-oxygen therapy for pediatric acute severe asthma requiring mechanical ventilation. Pediatr Crit Care Med 2003;4:353–357.

402. Schaeffer EM, Pohlman A, Morgan S, Hall JB. Oxygenation in status asthmaticus improves during ventilation with helium–oxygen. Crit Care Med 1999;27(12):2666–2670.

403. Carter ER, Webb CR, Moffitt DR. Evaluation of heliox in children hospitalized with acute severe asthma. A randomized crossover trial. Chest 1996;109:1256–1261.

404. Rodrigo GJ, Rodrigo C, Pollack CV, Rowe B. Use of helium–oxygen mixtures in the treatment of acute asthma: a systematic review. Chest 2003;123(3):891–896.

405. Kim IK, Phrampus E, Venkataraman S, Pitteti R, Saville A, Corcoran T, et al. Helium/oxygen-driven albuterol nebulization in the treatment of children with moderate to severe asthma exacerbations: a randomized, controlled trial. Pediatrics 2005;116:1127–1133.

406. Huber FC Jr., Gutierrez J, Corssen G. Ketamine: its effect on airway resistance in man. South Med J 1972;65(10):1176–1180.

407. Hirshman CA, Downes H, Farbood A, Bergman NA. Ketamine block of bronchospasm in experimental canine asthma. Br J Anaesth 1979;51(8):713–718.

408. Betts EK, Parkin CE. Use of ketamine in an asthmatic child: a case report. Anesth Analg 1971;50(3):420–421.

409. Fischer MM. Ketamine hydrochloride in severe bronchospasm. Anaesthesia 1977;32(8):771–772.

410. Rock MJ, Reyes de la Rocha S, L'Hommedieu CS, Truemper E. Use of ketamine in asthmatic children to treat respiratory failure refractory to conventional therapy. Crit Care Med 1986;14(5):514–516.

411. L'Hommedieu CS, Arens JJ. The use of ketamine for the emergency intubation of patients with status asthmaticus. Ann Emerg Med 1987;16(5):568–571.

412. Hemming A, MacKenzie I, Finfer S. Response to ketamine in status asthmaticus resistant to maximal medical treatment. Thorax 1994; 49(1):90–91.

413. Nehama J, Pass R, Bechtler-Karsch A, Steinberg C, Notterman DA. Continuous ketamine infusion for the treatment of refractory asthma in a mechanically ventilated infant: case report and review of the pediatric literature. Pediatr Emerg Care 1996;12(4):294–297.

414. Youssef-Ahmed MZ, Silver P, Nimkoff L, Sagy M. Continuous infusion of ketamine in mechanically ventilated children with refractory bronchospasm. Intensive Care Med 1996;22(9):972–976.

415. Strube PJ, Hallam PL. Ketamine by continuous infusion in status asthmaticus. Anaesthesia 1986;41(10):1017–1019.

416. Jahangir SM, Islam F, Aziz L. Ketamine infusion for postoperative analgesia in asthmatics: a comparison with intermittent meperidine. Anesth Analg 1993;76(1):45–49.

417. Sarma VJ. Use of ketamine in acute severe asthma. Acta Anaesthesiol Scand 1992;36(1):106–107.

418. Petrillo TM, Fortenberry JD, Linzer JF, Simon HK. Emergency department use of ketamine in pediatric status asthmaticus. J Asthma 2001;38(8):657–664.

419. Howton JC, Rose J, Duffy S, Zoltanski T, Levitt MA. Randomized, double-blind, placebo-controlled trial of intravenous ketamine in acute asthma. Ann Emerg Med 1996;27(2):170–175.

420. Drazen JM, Israel E, O'Byrne PM. Treatment of asthma with drugs modifying the leukotriene pathway. N Engl J Med 1999;340:197–206.

421. Adelroth E, Morris MM, Hargreave FE, O'Byrne PM. Airway responsiveness to leukotrienes C4 and D4 and to methacholine in patients with asthma and normal controls. N Engl J Med 1986;315:480–484.

422. Green SA, Malice MP, Tanaka W, Tozzi CA, Reiss TF. Increase in urinary leukotriene LTE4 levels in acute asthma: correlation with airflow limitation. Thorax 2004;59:100–104.

423. Gaddy JN, Margolskee DJ, Bush RK, Williams VC, Busse WW. Bronchodilation with a potent and selective leukotriene-D4 antagonist in asthma patients. Am Rev Respir Dis 1992;146:358–363.

424. Reiss TF, Chervinsky P, Dockhorn RJ, Shingo S, Seidenberg B, Edwards TB. Montelukast, a once daily leukotriene receptor antagonist, in the treatment of chronic asthma. A multi-center, randomized, double-blind trial. Arch Intern Med 1998;158:1213–1220.

425. Dempsey OJ, Wilson AM, Sims EJ, Mistry C, Lipworth BJ. Additive bronchoprotective and bronchodilator effects with single doses of salmeterol and montelukast in asthmatic patients receiving inhaled corticosteroids. Chest 2000;117:950–953.

426. Dockhorn RJ, Baumgartner RA, Leff JA, Noonan M, Vandormael K, Stricker W, et al. Comparison of the effects of intravenous and oral montelukast on airway function: a double-blind, placebo-controlled, three period, crossover study in asthmatic patients. Thorax 2000;55:260–265.

427. Reiss TF, Sorkness CA, Stricker W, Botto A, Busse WW, Kundu S, et al. Effects of montelukast, a potent cysteinyl leukotriene receptor antagonist, on bronchodilation in asthmatic patients treated with and without inhaled corticosteroids. Thorax 1997;52:45–48.

428. Silverman RA, Chen Y, Bonuccelli C. Zafirlukast improves emergency department outcomes after an acute asthma episode [abstr]. Ann Emerg Med 1999;34:S1.

429. Camargo CA Jr, Smithline HA, Malice MP, Green SA, Reiss TF. A randomized controlled trial of intravenous montelukast in acute asthma. Am J Respir Crit Care Med 2003;167:528–533.

430. Silverman RA, Nowak RM, Korenblat PE, Skobeloff E, Chen Y, Bonuccelli C, et al. Zafirlukast treatment for acute asthma: evaluation in a randomized, double-blind, multicenter trial. Chest 2004;126:1480–1489.

431. Mansmann HC Jr, Abboud EM, McGeady SJ. Treatment of severe respiratory failure during status asthmaticus in children and adolescents using high flow oxygen and sodium bicarbonate. Ann Allergy Asthma Immunol 1997;78(1):69–73.

432. Newcomb RW, Akhter J. Respiratory failure from asthma. A marker for children with high morbidity and mortality. Am J Dis Child 1988;142:1041–1044.

433. Dworkin G, Kattan M. Mechanical ventilation for status asthmaticus in children. J Pediatr 1989;114(4 Pt 1):545–549.

434. Cox RG, Barker GA, Bohn DJ. Efficacy, results, and complications of mechanical ventilation in children with status asthmaticus. Pediatr Pulmonol 1991;11(2):120–126.

435. Malmstrom K, Kaila M, Korhonen K, Dunder T, Nermes N, Klaukka T, et al. Mechanical ventilation in children with severe asthma. Pediatr Pulmonol 2001;31:405–411.

436. Akingbola OA, Simakajornboon N, Hadley EF Jr, Hopkins RL. Noninvasive positive-pressure ventilation in pediatric status asthmaticus. Pediatr Crit Care Med 2002;3(2):181–184.

437. Darioli R, Perret C. Mechanical controlled hypoventilation in status asthmaticus. Am Rev Respir Dis 1984;129:385–387.

438. Mazzeo AT, Spada A, Pratico C, Lucanto T, Santamaria LB. Hypercapnia: what is the limit in paediatric patients? A case of near-fatal asthma successfully treated by multipharmacological approach. Paediatr Anaesth 2004;14:596–603.

439. Menitove SM, Goldring RM. Combined ventilator and bicarbonate strategy in the management of status asthmaticus. Am J Med 1983; 74:898–901.

440. Buysee CMP, de Jongste JC, de Hoog M. Life-threatening asthma in children: treatment with sodium bicarbonate reduces PCO$_2$. Chest 2005;127:866–870.

441. Sarnaik AP, Daphtary KM, Meert KL, Lieh-Lai MW, Heidemann SM. Pressure-controlled ventilation in children with severe status asthmaticus. Pediatr Crit Care Med 2004;5(2):133–138.

442. Wheeler DS, Clapp CR, Ponaman ML, Bsn HM, Poss WB. Isoflurane therapy for status asthmaticus in children: a case series and protocol. Pediatr Crit Care Med 2000;1(1):55–59.

443. Wetzel RC. Pressure-support ventilation in children with severe asthma. Crit Care Med 1996;24(9):1603–1605.

444. Leatherman JW, Ravenscraft SA. Low measured auto-positive end-expiratory pressure during mechanical ventilation of patients with severe asthma: hidden auto-positive end-expiratory pressure. Crit Care Med 1996;24:541–546.

445. Qvist J, Andersen JB, Pemberton M, Bennike KA. High-level PEEP in severe asthma. N Engl J Med 1982;307:1347–1348.

446. Gay PC, Rodarte JR, Hubmayr RD. The effects of positive expiratory pressure on isovolume flow and dynamic hyperinflation in patients receiving mechanical ventilation. Am Rev Respir Dis 1989;139:621–626.

447. Smith TC, Marini JJ. Impact of PEEP on lung mechanics and work of breathing in severe airflow obstruction. J Appl Physiol 1988;65:1488–1499.

448. Eckmann DM. Ventilatory support by tracheal gas insufflation and chest vibration during bronchoconstriction. Crit Care Med 2000;28: 2533–2539.

449. Nahum A. Tracheal gas insufflation as an adjunct to mechanical ventilation. Respir Clin North Am 2002;8:171–185.

450. Duval EL, van Vught AJ. Status asthmaticus treated by high-frequency oscillatory ventilation. Pediatr Pulmonol 2000;30(4):350–353.

451. Cooper DJ, Tuxen DV, Fisher MM. Extracorporeal life support for status asthmaticus. Chest 1994;106:978–979.

452. Kukita I, Okamoto K, Sato T, Shibata Y, Taki K, Kurose M, et al. Emergency extracorporeal life support for patients with near-fatal status asthmaticus. Am J Emerg Med 1997;15:566–569.

453. Mabuchi N, Takasu H, Ito S, Yamada T, Arakawa M, Hatta M, et al. Successful extracorporeal lung assist (ELCA) for a patient with severe asthma and cardiac arrest. Clin Intensive Care 1991;2:292–294.

454. MacDonnell KF, Moon HS, Sekar TS, Ahlwalia MP. Extracorporeal membrane oxygenator support in a case of severe status asthmaticus. Ann Thorac Surg 1981;31:171–175.

455. Sakai M, Ohteki H, Doi K, Narita Y. Clinical use of extracorporeal lung assist for a patient in status asthmaticus. Ann Thorac Surg 1996;62: 885–887.

456. Tajimi K, Kasai T, Nakatani T, Kobayashi T. Extracorporeal lung assist for patient with hypercapnia due to status asthmaticus. Intensive Care Med 1988;14:588–589.

457. Meyer NE, Schotz S. Relief of intractable bronchial asthma with cyclopropane anesthesia: report of case. J Allergy 1939;10:239–240.

458. Hirshman CA, Edelstein G, Peetz S, Wayne R, Downes H. Mechanism of action of inhalational anesthetics on airways. Anesthesiology 1982;56:107–111.

459. Park KW, Dai HB, Lowenstein E, Kocher ON, Sellke FW. Isoflurane- and halothane-mediated dilation of distal bronchi in the rat depends on the epithelium. Anesthesiology 1997;86:1078–1087.

460. Park KW, Dai HB, Lowenstein E, Sellke FW. Epithelial dependence of the bronchodilatory effect of sevoflurane and desflurane in rat distal bronchi. Anesth Analg 1998;86:646–651.

461. Gold MI, Helrich M. Pulmonary mechanics during general anesthesia: V. Status asthmaticus. Anesthesiology 1970;32:422–428.

462. Echeverria M, Gelb AW, Wexler HR, Ahmad D, Kenefick P. Enflurane and halothane in status asthmaticus. Chest 1986;89:152–154.

463. O'Rourke PP, Crone PK. Halothane in status asthmaticus. Crit Care Med 1982;10:341–343.

464. Saulnier FF, Durocher AV, Deturck RA, Lefebvre MC, Wattel FE. Respiratory and hemodynamic effects of halothane in status asthmaticus. Intensive Care Med 1990;16:104–107.

465. Eger EI. Isoflurane: A review. Anesthesiology 1981;55:559–576.

466. Pearson J. Prolonged anesthesia with isoflurane. Anesth Analg 1985;64:92–93.

467. Parnass SM, Feld JM, Chamberlin WH, Segil LJ. Status asthmaticus treated with isoflurane and enflurane. Anesth Analg 1987;66:193–195.

468. Rice M, Hatherill M, Murdoch IA. Rapid response to isoflurane in refractory status asthmaticus. Arch Dis Child 1998;78(4):395–396.

469. Best A, Wenstone R, Murphy P. Prolonged use of isoflurane in asthma. Can J Anaesth 1994;41:452–453.

470. Johnston RG, Noseworthy TW, Friesen EG, Yule HA, Shustack A. Isoflurane therapy for status asthmaticus in children and adults. Chest 1990;97(3):698–701.

471. Bierman MI, Brown M, Muren O, Keenan RL, Glauser FL. Prolonged isoflurane anesthesia in status asthmaticus. Crit Care Med 1986;14: 832–833.

472. Otte RW, Fireman P. Isoflurane anesthesia for the treatment of refractory status asthmaticus. Ann Allergy 1991;66(4):305–309.

473. Mazze RI, Calverly RK, Smith NT. Inorganic fluoride nephrotoxicity: prolonged enflurane and halothane anesthesia in volunteers. Anesthesiology 1977;46:265–271.

474. Truog RD, Rice SA. Inorganic fluoride and prolonged isoflurane anesthesia in the intensive care unit. Anesth Analg 1989;69:843–845.

475. Spencer EM, Willats SM, Prys-Roberts C. Plasma inorganic fluoride concentrations during and after prolonged (>24 h) isoflurane sedation: effect on renal function. Anesthesiology 1991;73:731–737.

16
Bronchiolitis

Ann Marie LeVine

Introduction

Disorders of the lower respiratory tract account for significant morbidity and mortality in children. Viral bronchiolitis is the most common lower respiratory tract infection (LRTI) in children less than 12 months of age and is the most frequent cause of hospitalization of infants under 6 months of age. Respiratory syncytial virus (RSV) is the most common pathogen, with parainfluenza virus, adenovirus, influenza virus, rhinoviruses, and, most recently, human metapneumovirus accounting for the majority of the remainder of acute viral LRTI. Nearly 100% of children in the United States are infected with RSV by 2 or 3 years of age, and, although RSV infection usually results in a mild, self-limited respiratory illness, approximately 1% of infants require hospitalization. There is evidence to suggest that bronchiolitis hospitalizations have increased during the past two decades. For example, from 1980 through 1996, more than 1.6 million children under the age of 5 years were hospitalized for bronchiolitis in the United States alone [1,2] The majority of these children (nearly 81%) were under 1 year of age. During this time period, the rate of hospitalizations increased, especially for young infants less than 6 months of age [1,2]. Perhaps just as important, RSV infection early in life has been associated with long-term respiratory problems and wheezing later in life.

Respiratory syncytial virus is a pleomorphic, enveloped, cytoplasmic virus containing single-stranded, negative-sense RNA and is classified in the genus *Pneumovirus*, which belongs to the family Paramyxoviridae. The Paramyxoviridae family also includes two other genera, Paramyxovirus (containing parainfluenza virus types 1, 2, and 3 and mumps virus) and Morbillivirus. The surface proteins of RSV that induce protective antibodies are the major antigenic determinants, including the disulfide-bonded glycoprotein (F, fusion protein), which mediates viral penetration and syncytium formation, and the large glycoprotein (G, attachment protein), which mediates viral attachment [3].

The clinical picture of RSV infection varies according to age. Respiratory syncytial virus has the potential to cause disease in all age groups, although infection in older infants and children is usually less severe. The primary infection at 6 weeks to 2 years of age is usually symptomatic and involves the lower respiratory tract. Asymptomatic primary RSV infection in children is rare. Repeated infecting in older children is usually less severe. Respiratory tract infections are frequently associated with expiratory wheezing, pneumonia, and acute otitis media. Respiratory syncytial virus infections in neonates differ from those in older children, as neonates do not often exhibit wheezing, and apnea may be the only symptom of infection. Pneumonia is the most common manifestation in elderly subjects. Isolated upper respiratory tract infections associated with RSV have been noted in older children and adults with rhinorrhea, nasal congestion, pharyngitis, and cough [4].

The diagnostic criteria for bronchiolitis vary among centers. In general, bronchiolitis presents clinically in infants less than 12 months old who, after a brief prodrome of upper respiratory symptoms, display wheezing, dyspnea, respiratory distress, poor feeding, tachypnea (>50/min), and radiologic evidence of hyperaeration of the lung. Auscultation of the chest often reveals fine crepitation. The symptoms and signs resolve within a few days to a week after the onset of illness. Infants under 6 weeks old and those with underlying illnesses often need longer hospitalization [3].

Epidemiology

In the northern hemisphere, annual outbreaks of RSV infection typically occur between October and May, with the peak in January and February. Infections with RSV occur in 50%–67% of infants in the first year of life, causing wheezing in about 30% of those infected. Approximately 2% of all infants will be hospitalized. The proportion of hospitalizations associated with bronchiolitis among children younger than 1 year of age has increased from 22.2% in 1980 to 47.4% in 1996 [1], and RSV bronchiolitis had been documented as the leading cause of hospital admissions for infants younger than 1 year of age [5]. Fatalities are uncommon in the United States among otherwise healthy children. However,

D.S. Wheeler et al. (eds.), The *Respiratory Tract in Pediatric Critical Illness and Injury,*
DOI 10.1007/978-1-84800-925-7_16, © Springer-Verlag London Limited 2009

mortality is more frequent in those with underlying heart or lung diseases, in immunocompromised children, and in the developing world [6]. Of RSV hospitalized infants, only 10% require mechanical ventilation [7]; however, more than half of RSV-hospitalized infants and a large percentage of infants who require mechanical ventilation and even die from RSV infection were previously healthy [8]. Overall, the mortality associated with primary RSV infection in otherwise healthy children is estimated to be 0.005% to 0.020%. In hospitalized children, mortality rates are estimated to range from 1% to 3%. However, considerably higher mortality rates have been observed for children with cardiopulmonary abnormalities and in immunosuppressed patients [6].

Pathology

Respiratory syncytial virus infection results in loss of epithelial cilia and sloughing of epithelial cells in the airway. The pathologic features include collections of desquamated airway epithelial cells, polymorphonuclear cells, and lymphocytes within the airway and cellular infiltration and edema around the airway, with very little alveolar infiltration of inflammatory cells. Desquamation of airway epithelial cells and inflammation are more extensive in bronchiolitis than in asthma. In acute bronchiolitis, sloughed epithelial cells, neutrophils, and lymphocytes appear to be the major contributors to airway obstruction. The complete plugging of some airways and partial plugging of others may lead to localized atelectasis of some units of lung parenchyma and overdistention of other units. This patchwork of overdistention and underdistention is a common finding on chest radiographs in infants with bronchiolitis (Figure 16.1). The imbalance of ventilation and perfusion results in hypoxemia that can be in part aided by the administration of oxygen [9,10].

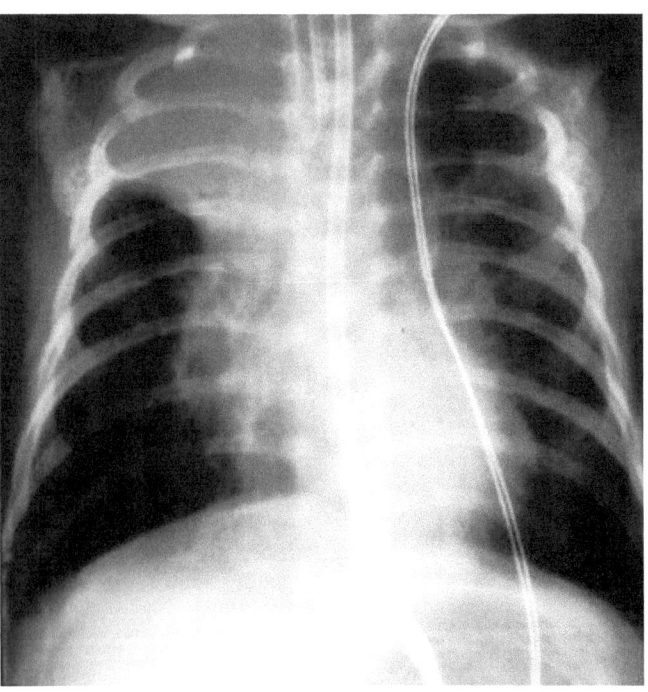

FIGURE 16.1. Chest radiograph of an infant with the clinical syndrome of acute bronchiolitis.

In fatal cases of bronchiolitis, pathologic changes in the lung include detachment and necrosis of the epithelium, airway wall edema, infiltration of the airway wall and of the interstitium with leukocytes (predominantly macrophages and lymphocytes), and plugging of the airway with mucus and cellular debris. The plugs may completely obstruct terminal bronchioles and extend into the alveoli. There is no evidence of smooth muscle hypertrophy in bronchiolitis.

Immunology

Antibody-Mediated Immunity

Passively acquired maternal immunoglobulins protect newborns against RSV infection during the first 2 months of life. However, the presence of maternal antibodies decreases gradually during the first 6 months of life, leaving most infants unprotected against RSV between 2 and 4 months of age [11]. Humoral responses are stronger if primary infection occurs after 6 months of age. These responses are also enhanced after each subsequent episode of reinfection throughout life.

Cell-Mediated Immunity

Epithelial cells and alveolar macrophages are key players in the activation of cellular immunity after RSV infection. These cells release multiple chemical substances, including chemokines, proinflammatory cytokines, and mediators. These include interleukin (IL)-1, tumor necrosis factor-α, IL-6, IL-8 (CXCL8), macrophage inflammatory protein (MIP)-1α (CCL3), and RANTES (regulated upon activation, normal T cell expressed and secreted) (CCL5) [12]. Release of these cytokines and chemokines appears to be at least partially responsible for airway inflammation and bronchial hyperresponsiveness, as well as upper respiratory symptoms. When these chemical mediators are released into the airway, recruited cells prolong the inflammatory response with further cytokine/chemokine release that attracts and upregulates other inflammatory cells. The release of these chemical substances may persist for months after clinical evidence of infection has disappeared.

The response of helper T (Th) cells plays an important role in RSV infection. T cells produce proinflammatory mediators categorized as type 1 cytokines (Th1) or type 2 (Th2) cytokines. Type 1 cells secrete IL-2, interferon (IFN)-γ, and lymphotoxin, whereas Th2 cells produce IL-4, IL-5, IL-6, and IL-13. Interleukin-4 and IL-5 promote both IgE production and eosinophilia. When there is an imbalance in Th1 and Th2 responses, disease severity appears to be enhanced [13].

Infants who recover from RSV lower respiratory tract infection have an increased risk of recurrent wheezing during early childhood. Recurrent wheezing is accompanied by functional abnormalities of the airways, such as airway hyperresponsiveness. Infection with RSV may be one factor, although other host and environmental factors may also contribute to the development, suggesting that it may only indirectly predispose children to postbronchiolitic wheezing and asthma [14]. Overall, children are more likely to wheeze or develop asthma if they have been passively exposed to cigarette smoke, if they develop atopic disease, and if RSV infection induces peripheral blood eosinophilia. Only indirectly does RSV appear to cause childhood wheezing and asthma [14].

Management

Efforts aimed at developing successful therapeutics to combat RSV infection have been in progress for decades. Despite attempts at vaccine, drug development, and antiviral regimens, there are still no effective treatments for RSV infections. Typically, infants hospitalized for RSV are given supplemental oxygen and provided a suitable thermal environment in which oxygen consumption will be minimized. Attention is paid to hydration status, and mucus is periodically suctioned to remove excess nasopharyngeal secretions.

Fluid Replacement

Adequate fluid replacement should be ensured, and the route of administration varies among units. The increased fluid demand of patients with bronchiolitis because of fever, tachypnea, and inadequate intake because of respiratory difficulty makes the parenteral administration of fluids often necessary. Interestingly, infants with bronchiolitis have a transient increased risk of swallowing dysfunction and aspiration that may alter the natural history of the disease and generate further morbidity. Moreover, aspiration might play a role when rapid deterioration occurs in infants with bronchiolitis [15].

Antibiotics

Because viruses are the primary agents in bronchiolitis, antibiotics should not influence the course of the disease, and no evidence supports the use of antibiotics for bronchiolitis or RSV pneumonia. The risk of concurrent serious bacterial infections in infants with bronchiolitis is low (<2%) [16]. The bacterial infection work-up should be restricted to those severely ill-appearing infants with underlying high-risk factors (chronic cardiac or pulmonary disease, immunodeficiency) and/or those with atypical signs and symptoms (e.g., recrudescence or persistence of fever, development of radiologic infiltrates, prolonged respiratory distress) [17].

Antiviral Agents: Ribavirin

Ribavirin is a synthetic guanosine analogue with a broad spectrum of antiviral activity against RSV, influenza types A and B, parainfluenza virus, adenovirus, measles virus, hepatitis virus, and a number of other viruses. It is a virustatic agent that inhibits viral replication during the active replication phase [18]. Aerosolized ribavirin is the only antiviral agent currently approved for treatment of RSV bronchiolitis in hospitalized infants. Early trials with ribavirin suggested that ribavirin was effective in improving the clinical condition in infants with RSV bronchiolitis [19]; however, the uncertainty about the drug arose because of possible teratogenicity, high costs, problems with its administration, and less than persuasive clinical effects. In 1996, the American Academy of Pediatrics published recommendations for the use of ribavirin that advised it be used at the discretion of the physicians caring for infants at high risk of severe disease, including those with complicated congenital heart disease, bronchopulmonary dysplasia and other chronic lung disease or immunosuppressive conditions, previously healthy premature infants, those younger than 6 weeks, and those who are severely ill [20].

A randomized, controlled trial showed that ribavirin does not significantly reduce mortality rate or risk of deterioration in previously healthy infants undergoing mechanical ventilation for RSV bronchiolitis [21]. These results were in agreement with other published studies [22]. A study evaluating the long-term morbidity of RSV bronchiolitis showed that early (<5 days of the course of illness) ribavirin treatment in combination with bronchodilators and systemic steroids resulted in a reduction of incidence and severity of reactive airway disease as well as respiratory illness-related hospitalization during a 1-year follow-up period. However, previous studies with longer follow-up periods after discharge (5 years) did not find these positive results [23,24].

Given the concerns about cost, safety, and limited positive effects, decisions about ribavirin aerosol therapy should be based on the clinical circumstances and the experiences of the health care team. If the decision is made to administer ribavirin, treatment should probably be initiated early in order to achieve its maximal potential benefits and administered according to the "high dose," short-duration regimen (60 mg/mL over three 2-hr periods for a total of 6 g/100mL every 24 hr) in a nebulized form [25].

Immunotherapy

Standard and Enriched Immunoglobulins

Aerosolized or intravenous administration of standard immunoglobulins has shown no benefit in patients with bronchiolitis. Respiratory syncytial virus immunoglobulin (RSV-IGIV; RespiGam, MedImune, Inc.), an immunoglobulin preparation enriched with high titers of anti-RSV antibodies, did not affect clinical outcome in previously healthy RSV-infected infants, although there was a trend toward fewer days of mechanical ventilation and shorter intensive care stay in infants with more severe disease [6]. Respiratory syncytial virus immunoglobulin has not been shown to have a role in the treatment of RSV bronchiolitis.

Monoclonal Antibodies: Palivizumab

Palivizumab is a genetically engineered, humanized monoclonal antibody directed at the F glycoprotein of RSV. Currently, palivizumab is approved for RSV prophylaxis for high-risk infants as defined by American Academy of Pediatrics criteria. Palivizumab has been demonstrated to be approximately 50% effective in reducing the need for hospitalization for RSV related illness when given to high-risk infants (those born prematurely with or without chronic lung disease of prematurity) throughout the RSV epidemic season [27]. A randomized, controlled trail with mechanically ventilated RSV-infected infants showed that a single dose of palivizumab resulted in reduced viral load in tracheal aspirates, but the clinical outcome was not changed [28]. Thus, current evidence does not support the use of palivizumab for acute RSV bronchiolitis.

Antiinflammatory Agents: Corticosteroids

The antiinflammatory actions of steroids have been examined to potentially reduce airway edema and the duration of bronchiolitis symptoms; however, no study has demonstrated a conclusive benefit in this setting. Inhaled or systemic corticosteroids do not provide significant short- or long-term benefits for healthy infants with the first episode of acute viral bronchiolitis [29–31]. However, a study examining high-dose dexamethasone 1 mg/kg by mouth initiated within 4 hr of therapy and continued for 5 days revealed benefit for infants with moderate-to-severe disease by reducing the rate of hospitalization and improving the respiratory status measured by a respiratory assessment score [32]. Further studies with larger populations will be needed to determine the effects of corticosteroids on severely affected and/or high-risk patients and to define optimal dosing strategies before incorporating corticosteroids into standard practice.

Antileukotrienes: Montelukast

Cysteinyl-leukotrienes (cys-LTs) are potent proinflammatory mediators that cause increased mucosal blood flow and mucosal edema through increased vascular permeability and interstitial transport of macromolecules. Cysteinyl-LTs are released during RSV airway infection and represent a potential target for treating RSV bronchiolitis [33].

Montelukast reduced lung symptoms, primarily cough, in patients with RSV bronchiolitis [34]. Studies are currently investigating the use of montelukast in young infants with severe bronchiolitis.

Bronchodilators

The use of bronchodilators for bronchiolitis is likely explained by the similarity of symptoms and signs between bronchiolitis and asthma; however, the primary pathology in bronchiolitis is not airway smooth muscle constriction. Despite the widespread use for acute viral bronchiolitis, bronchodilators have not been universally accepted in this setting.

β_2-Agonists

A meta-analysis examined the effectiveness of bronchodilators in patients with bronchiolitis and found only a modest short-term improvement in clinical scores, without changes in oxygen saturation, rate of hospitalization, or length of hospital stay [35]. There is no evidence to support the indiscriminate use of inhaled β_2-agonists for acute viral bronchiolitis. It is possible that a subset of patients with recurrent wheezing and/or asthmatics may respond to a therapeutic trial. Lack of significant improvement within 60 min of a trial with inhalation therapy should lead to its discontinuation [36].

Adrenergics: Epinephrine

Epinephrine has bronchodilatory effects and in addition may be efficacious in bronchiolitis because of its α-adrenergic effects resulting in pulmonary arteriolar vasoconstriction, decreasing mucosal edema, and increasing airway caliber. Studies comparing epinephrine to β$_2$-agonists or placebo revealed a greater short-term benefit for infants receiving epinephrine. Epinephrine enhanced clinical score and oxygenation, improved respiratory function, and reduced hospitalization rate [37,38]. Some studies failed to find advantages from the use of epinephrine [39,40]. A randomized, double-blind, controlled trial comparing nebulized single-isomer epinephrine with placebo in 194 infants with clinical diagnosis of bronchiolitis found no significant difference in length of hospital stay. This trial did not demonstrate benefit in either short-term or long-term clinical outcomes from nebulized epinephrine for infants hospitalized with acute bronchiolitis [41]. If inhaled epinephrine is considered, this therapy should be discontinued if there is no

significant improvement in clinical assessment within 30 min after the first treatment.

Anticholinergics: Ipratropium Bromide

Parasympathetic stimulation does not appear to contribute substantially to airway obstruction in bronchiolitis. Ipratropium bromide alone or added to albuterol therapy has not been demonstrated to be efficacious in the management of acute viral bronchiolitis [42,43].

Helium–oxygen Gas Mixture

Helium–oxygen (heliox) mixture has a substantially lower density than air–oxygen mixture, enabling helium–oxygen to reduce the driving pressure required by turbulent flow conditions and preserve laminar flow at high flow rates by reducing the Reynolds number [44]. This effect makes it particularly beneficial for patients with airway obstruction and turbulent gas flow. Short-term heliox therapy for infants with acute bronchiolitis resulted in a significant improvement in the clinical asthma score, with the most severe disease at baseline demonstrating the greatest decrease in severity score [45]. A prospective study examining humidified 70% helium and 30% oxygen mixture delivered by a nonrebreather reservoir facemask demonstrated improved clinical status as reflected by clinical scoring and reduced tachycardia and tachypnea. The onset of the beneficial response to heliox compared with conventional therapy occurred within the first hour of its administration and was maintained as long as heliox therapy was continued. In addition, the length of stay in the pediatric intensive care unit was shorter in infants treated with heliox [46]. The results of these studies suggest that heliox is effective in improving the respiratory condition of infants with acute bronchiolitis in a safe, noninvasive, and simple manner; however, long-term prospective studies are needed to establish its therapeutic role in bronchiolitis.

Nitric Oxide

Inhaled nitric oxide has pulmonary vasodilatory and bronchodilatory properties that may be useful in bronchiolitis especially in patients with severe bronchoconstriction and/or pulmonary hypertension. However, the bronchodilatory effect of nitric oxide is weak, and the incidence of pulmonary hypertension is low. Case reports describe a positive response in oxygenation when inhaled nitric oxide was added to conventional and high-frequency ventilation [47,48]. However, outside of these reports, studies assessing inhaled nitric oxide with bronchiolitis have not shown benefit [49]. Therefore, there is no specific role for nitric oxide in the routine treatment of acute bronchiolitis.

Exogenous Surfactant

Infants with bronchiolitis have a deficiency and/or a functional abnormality in endogenous surfactant [50]. Surfactant plays a role in the prevention of small airway collapse; therefore, its replacement may be useful in mechanically ventilated infants with bronchiolitis. Studies of administering surfactant to previously healthy infants mechanically ventilated for acute respiratory failure caused by RSV infection, complicated with atelectasis or pneumonia, demonstrated improved gas exchange and respiratory mechanics, shortened time on mechanical ventilation, and decreased length of stay in the intensive care unit [51]. Additional studies are necessary to further explore the potential of exogenous surfactant in high-risk groups and to determine optimal timing and dosage.

Mechanical Ventilation

The majority of children requiring intensive care are high-risk infants with chronic lung disease, congenital heart disease, and/or ex-premature infants. Indications for intensive care include recurrent apnea, slow irregular breathing, reduced conscious level, shock, exhaustion, hypoxia despite high-inspired oxygen, and respiratory acidosis (pH < 7.2). A trial of continuous positive airway pressure (CPAP) is sometimes effective and may avoid the need for intermittent positive pressure ventilation (IPPV) [52]. However, the majority of deteriorating infants required IPPV. Ventilatory strategies vary from child to child, but it is essential for infants with significant air trapping on chest x-ray to allow adequate expiratory times and thus avoid hyperinflation. Permissive hypercapnia will reduce barotrauma. The majority of patients are successfully ventilated by IPPV, but if gas exchange remains problematic, high-frequency oscillatory ventilation may be effective [53]. For children whose clinical condition is deteriorating despite maximal respiratory support, extracorporeal membrane oxygenation (ECMO) should be considered [54].

Infection Control

Infection-control measures should accompany medical care to protect patients and providers from RSV nosocomial infections. Isolating suspected cases, segregating case cohorts, and using dedicated stethoscopes and other instruments or supplies for each patient can be effective in reducing transmission. Washing hands before entering and leaving the room and using gloves and masks that cover the nose and eyes are effective means of infection control [55].

Genetic Predisposition

Investigators have begun to identify particular genetic polymorphisms that are overrepresented in infants with severe RSV disease. Linked variants of three Th2 cytokine genes, IL-4, IL-13, and IL-5, are associated with more severe RSV disease [56]. Interleukin-8, a member of the CXC chemokine family, contributes to the activation and migration of neutrophils, and polymorphisms near the IL-8 gene were significantly increased in infants with bronchiolitis, especially those without known risk factors [57]. Respiratory syncytial virus attachment protein G binds to CX3CR, the specific receptor for the CX3C chemokines fractalkine, which has been shown to facilitate RSV infection. Polymorphisms in this gene have been identified; however, it is not clear at this time whether there is an association with severe RSV disease [58]. The toll-like family of proteins are a link between immune stimulants produced by microorganisms and the initiation of host defense. Toll-like receptor 4 (TLR4) and CD14 are the major receptors for lipopolysaccharide (LPS) and have been shown to interact with RSV [9]. Common TLR4 mutations have been associated with severe RSV bronchiolitis [60].

Surfactant proteins (SP) A and D are members of the "collectin" (collagen-like) family involved in host defense, and they bind and enhance clearance of RSV [61]. Polymorphism in these genes might confer a higher susceptibility to viral disease in the airways. Genotype analyses for SP-A and SP-D polymorphism have revealed alleles that are overrepresented in RSV-infected infants compared with control subjects [62,63].

Conclusion

Respiratory syncytial virus infection occurs in predictable, annual outbreaks, and most infants with bronchiolitis who do not have underlying conditions can be managed successfully as outpatients. Nonetheless, hospitalization rates for lower respiratory tract disease in many young children appear to be increasing. As more children and adults become immunocompromised as a result of the increasing use of organ transplantation and chemotherapeutic agents, greater attention is likely to be focused on the importance of RSV as an opportunistic pathogen. At present, the only option for prevention of RSV infection in high-risk patients is passive immunoprophylaxis. To substantially decrease the overall burden of RSV disease in children, a vaccine will be required.

References

1. Shay DK, Holman RC, Newman RD, Liu LL, Stout JW, Anderson LJ. Bronchiolitis-associated hospitalizations among US children, 1980–1996. JAMA 1999;282(15):1440–1446.
2. Shay DK, Holman RC, Roosevelt GE, Clarke MJ, Anderson LJ. Bronchiolitis-associated mortality and estimates of respiratory syncytial virus-associated deaths among US children, 1979–1997. J Infect Dis 2001;183(1):16–22.
3. Welliver RC. Respiratory syncytial virus and other respiratory viruses. Pediatr Infect Dis J 2003;22(2 Suppl):S6–S12.
4. Ogra PL. Respiratory syncytial virus: the virus, the disease and the immune response. Paediatr Respir Rev 2004;5(Suppl A):S119–S126.
5. Leader S, Kohlhase K. Respiratory syncytial virus-coded pediatric hospitalizations, 1997 to 1999. Pediatr Infect Dis J 2002;21(7):629–632.
6. Meissner HC. Selected populations at increased risk from respiratory syncytial virus infection. Pediatr Infect Dis J 2003;22(2 Suppl): S40–S45.
7. Wang EE, Law BJ, Stephens D. Pediatric Investigators Collaborative Network on Infections in Canada (PICNIC) prospective study of risk factors and outcomes in patients hospitalized with respiratory syncytial viral lower respiratory tract infection. J Pediatr 1995;126(2):212–219.
8. Buckingham SC, Quasney MW, Bush AJ, DeVincenzo JP. Respiratory syncytial virus infections in the pediatric intensive care unit: clinical characteristics and risk factors for adverse outcomes. Pediatr Crit Care Med 2001;2(4):318–323.
9. Aherne W, Bird T, Court SD, Gardner PS, McQuillin J. Pathological changes in virus infections of the lower respiratory tract in children. J Clin Pathol 1970;23(1):7–18.
10. Gardner PS, Turk DC, Aherne WA, Bird T, Holdaway MD, Court SD. Deaths associated with respiratory tract infection in childhood. BMJ 1967;4(575):316–320.
11. Englund J, Glezen WP, Piedra PA. Maternal immunization against viral disease. Vaccine 1998;16(14–15):1456–1463.
12. McNamara PS, Flanagan BF, Selby AM, Hart CA, Smyth RL. Pro- and anti-inflammatory responses in respiratory syncytial virus bronchiolitis. Eur Respir J 2004;23(1):106–112.
13. Legg JP, Hussain IR, Warner JA, Johnston SL, Warner JO. Type 1 and type 2 cytokine imbalance in acute respiratory syncytial virus bronchiolitis. Am J Respir Crit Care Med 2003;168(6):633–639.

14. Bont L, Aalderen WM, Kimpen JL. Long-term consequences of respiratory syncytial virus (RSV) bronchiolitis. Paediatr Respir Rev 2000;1(3):221–227.
15. Hernandez E, Khoshoo V, Thoppil D, Edell D, Ross G. Aspiration: a factor in rapidly deteriorating bronchiolitis in previously healthy infants? Pediatr Pulmonol 2002;33(1):30–31.
16. Hall CB, Powell KR, Schnabel KC, Gala CL, Pincus PH. Risk of secondary bacterial infection in infants hospitalized with respiratory syncytial viral infection. J Pediatr 1988;113(2):266–271.
17. Antonow JA, Hansen K, McKinstry CA, Byington CL. Sepsis evaluations in hospitalized infants with bronchiolitis. Pediatr Infect Dis J 1998;17(3):231–236.
18. Lugo RA, Nahata MC. Pathogenesis and treatment of bronchiolitis. Clin Pharmacol 1993;12(2):95–116.
19. Barry W, Cockburn F, Cornall R, Price JF, Sutherland G, Vardag A. Ribavirin aerosol for acute bronchiolitis. Arch Dis Child 1986;61(6):593–597.
20. Reassessment of the indications for ribavirin therapy in respiratory syncytial virus infections. American Academy of Pediatrics Committee on Infectious Diseases. Pediatrics 1996;97(1):137–140.
21. Moler FW, Steinhart CM, Ohmit SE, Stidham GL. Effectiveness of ribavirin in otherwise well infants with respiratory syncytial virus-associated respiratory failure. Pediatric Critical Study Group. J Pediatr 1996;128(3):422–428.
22. Guerguerian AM, Gauthier M, Lebel MH, Farrell CA, Lacroix J. Ribavirin in ventilated respiratory syncytial virus bronchiolitis. A randomized, placebo-controlled trial. Am J Respir Crit Care Med 1999;160(3):829–834.
23. Krilov LR, Mandel FS, Barone SR, Fagin JC. Follow-up of children with respiratory syncytial virus bronchiolitis in 1986 and 1987: potential effect of ribavirin on long term pulmonary function. The Bronchiolitis Study Group. Pediatr Infect Dis J 1997;16(3):273–276.
24. Long CE, Voter KZ, Barker WH, Hall CB. Long term follow-up of children hospitalized with respiratory syncytial virus lower respiratory tract infection and randomly treated with ribavirin or placebo. Pediatr Infect Dis J 1997;16(11):1023–1028.
25. Englund JA, Piedra PA, Ahn YM, Gilbert BE, Hiatt P. High-dose, short-duration ribavirin aerosol therapy compared with standard ribavirin therapy in children with suspected respiratory syncytial virus infection. J Pediatr 1994;125(4):635–641.
26. Rodriguez WJ, Gruber WC, Welliver RC, Groothuis JR, Simoes EA, Meissner HC, et al. Respiratory syncytial virus (RSV) immune globulin intravenous therapy for RSV lower respiratory tract infection in infants and young children at high risk for severe RSV infections: Respiratory Syncytial Virus Immune Globulin Study Group. Pediatrics 1997;99(3):454–461.
27. The IMpact-RSV Study Group. Palivizumab, a humanized respiratory syncytial virus monoclonal antibody, reduces hospitalization from respiratory syncytial virus infection in high-risk infants. Pediatrics 1998;102(3):531–537.
28. Malley R, DeVincenzo J, Ramilo O, Dennehy PH, Meissner HC, Gruber WC, et al. Reduction of respiratory syncytial virus (RSV) in tracheal aspirates in intubated infants by use of humanized monoclonal antibody to RSV F protein. J Infect Dis 1998;178(6):1555–1561.
29. De Boeck K, Van der Aa N, Van Lierde S, Corbeel L, Eeckels R. Respiratory syncytial virus bronchiolitis: a double-blind dexamethasone efficacy study. J Pediatr 1997;131(6):919–921.
30. Richter H, Seddon P. Early nebulized budesonide in the treatment of bronchiolitis and the prevention of postbronchiolitic wheezing. J Pediatr 1998;132(5):849–853.
31. Bulow SM, Nir M, Levin E, Friis B, Thomsen LL, Nielsen JE, et al. Prednisolone treatment of respiratory syncytial virus infection: a randomized controlled trial of 147 infants. Pediatrics 1999;104(6):e77.
32. Schuh S, Coates AL, Binnie R, Allin T, Goia C, Corey M, et al. Efficacy of oral dexamethasone in outpatients with acute bronchiolitis. J Pediatr 2002;140(1):27–32.
33. Volovitz B, Welliver RC, De Castro G, Krystofik DA, Ogra PL. The release of leukotrienes in the respiratory tract during infection with respiratory syncytial virus: role in obstructive airway disease. Pediatr Res 1988;24(4):504–507.
34. Bisgaard H. A randomized trial of montelukast in respiratory syncytial virus postbronchiolitis. Am J Respir Crit Care Med 2003;167(3):379–383.
35. Flores G, Horwitz RI. Efficacy of beta2-agonists in bronchiolitis: a reappraisal and meta-analysis. Pediatrics 1997;100(2 Pt 1):233–239.
36. Wright RB, Pomerantz WJ, Luria JW. New approaches to respiratory infections in children. Bronchiolitis and croup. Emerg Med Clin North Am 2002;20(1):93–114.
37. Sanchez I, De Koster J, Powell RE, Wolstein R, Chernick V. Effect of racemic epinephrine and salbutamol on clinical score and pulmonary mechanics in infants with bronchiolitis. J Pediatr 1993;122(1):145–151.
38. Numa AH, Williams GD, Dakin CJ. The effect of nebulized epinephrine on respiratory mechanics and gas exchange in bronchiolitis. Am J Respir Crit Care Med 2001;164(1):86–91.
39. Patel H, Platt RW, Pekeles GS, Ducharme FM. A randomized, controlled trial of the effectiveness of nebulized therapy with epinephrine compared with albuterol and saline in infants hospitalized for acute viral bronchiolitis. J Pediatr 2002;141(6):818–824.
40. Abul-Ainine A, Luyt D. Short term effects of adrenaline in bronchiolitis: a randomised controlled trial. Arch Dis Child 2002;86(4):276–279.
41. Wainwright C, Altamirano L, Cheney M, Cheney J, Barber S, Price D, et al. A multicenter, randomized, double-blind, controlled trial of nebulized epinephrine in infants with acute bronchiolitis. N Engl J Med 2003;349(1):27–35.
42. Schuh S, Johnson D, Canny G, Reisman J, Shields M, Kovesi T, et al. Efficacy of adding nebulized ipratropium bromide to nebulized albuterol therapy in acute bronchiolitis. Pediatrics 1992;90(6):920–923.
43. Rubin BK, Albers GM. Use of anticholinergic bronchodilation in children. Am J Med 1996;100(1A):49S–53S.
44. Papamoschou D. Theoretical validation of the respiratory benefits of helium-oxygen mixtures. Respir Physiol 1995;99(1):183–190.
45. Hollman G, Shen G, Zeng L, Yngsdal-Krenz R, Perloff W, Zimmerman J, et al. Helium–oxygen improves Clinical Asthma Scores in children with acute bronchiolitis. Crit Care Med 1998;26(10):1731–1736.
46. Martinon-Torres F, Rodriguez-Nunez A, Martinon-Sanchez JM. Heliox therapy in infants with acute bronchiolitis. Pediatrics 2002;109(1):68–73.
47. Leclerc F, Riou Y, Martinot A, Storme L, Hue V, Flurin V, et al. Inhaled nitric oxide for a severe respiratory syncytial virus infection in an infant with bronchopulmonary dysplasia. Intensive Care Med 1994;20(7):511–512.
48. Hoehn T, Krause M, Krueger M, Hentschel R. Treatment of respiratory failure with inhaled nitric oxide and high-frequency ventilation in an infant with respiratory syncytial virus pneumonia and bronchopulmonary dysplasia. Respiration 1998;65(6):477–480.
49. Patel NR, Hammer J, Nichani S, Numa A, Newth CJ. Effect of inhaled nitric oxide on respiratory mechanics in ventilated infants with RSV bronchiolitis. Intensive Care Med 1999;25(1):81–87.
50. LeVine AM, Lotze A, Stanley S, Stroud C, O'Donnell R, Whitsett J, et al. Surfactant content in children with inflammatory lung disease. Crit Care Med 1996;24(6):1062–1067.
51. Luchetti M, Ferrero F, Gallini C, Natale A, Pigna A, Tortorolo L, et al. Multicenter, randomized, controlled study of porcine surfactant in severe respiratory syncytial virus-induced respiratory failure. Pediatr Crit Care Med 2002;3(3):261–268.
52. Soong WJ, Hwang B, Tang RB. Continuous positive airway pressure by nasal prongs in bronchiolitis. Pediatr Pulmonol 1993;16(3):163–166.
53. Duval EL, Leroy PL, Gemke RJ, van Vught AJ. High-frequency oscillatory ventilation in RSV bronchiolitis patients. Respir Med 1999;93(6):435–440.
54. Khan JY, Kerr SJ, Tometzki A, Tyszczuk L, West J, Sosnowski A, et al. Role of ECMO in the treatment of respiratory syncytial virus bronchi-

olitis: a collaborative report. Arch Dis Child Fetal Neonatal Ed 1995;73(2):F91–F94.

55. Madge P, Paton JY, McColl JH, Mackie PL. Prospective controlled study of four infection-control procedures to prevent nosocomial infection with respiratory syncytial virus. Lancet 1992;340(8827):1079–1083.

56. Choi EH, Lee HJ, Yoo T, Chanock SJ. A common haplotype of interleukin-4 gene IL4 is associated with severe respiratory syncytial virus disease in Korean children. J Infect Dis 2002;186(9):1207–1211.

57. Hacking D, Knight JC, Rockett K, Brown H, Frampton J, Kwiatkowski DP, et al. Increased in vivo transcription of an IL-8 haplotype associated with respiratory syncytial virus disease-susceptibility. Genes Immun 2004;5(4):274–282.

58. Tripp RA, Jones LP, Haynes LM, Zheng H, Murphy PM, Anderson LJ. CX3C chemokine mimicry by respiratory syncytial virus G glycoprotein. Nat Immunol 2001;2(8):732–738.

59. Kurt-Jones EA, Popova L, Kwinn L, Haynes LM, Jones LP, Tripp RA, et al. Pattern recognition receptors TLR4 and CD14 mediate response to respiratory syncytial virus. Nat Immunol 2000;1(5):398–401.

60. Tal G, Mandelberg A, Dalal I, Cesar K, Somekh E, Tal A, et al. Association between common toll-like receptor 4 mutations and severe respiratory syncytial virus disease. J Infect Dis 2004;189(11):2057–2063.

61. LeVine AM, Whitsett JA. Pulmonary collectins and innate host defense of the lung. Microbes Infect 2001;3(2):161–166.

62. Lofgren J, Ramet M, Renko M, Marttila R, Hallman M. Association between surfactant protein A gene locus and severe respiratory syncytial virus infection in infants. J Infect Dis 2002;185(3):283–289.

63. Lahti M, Lofgren J, Marttila R, Renko M, Klaavuniemi T, Haataja R, et al. Surfactant protein D gene polymorphism associated with severe respiratory syncytial virus infection. Pediatr Res 2002;51(6):696–699.

17
Pneumonia and Empyema

Imad Y. Haddad and David N. Cornfield

Introduction

Pneumonia is defined as infection and inflammation of the lower respiratory tract in association with parenchymal radiographic opacity. This definition excludes bronchiolitis, tracheitis, neonatal pneumonia, and noninfectious causes of pneumonia and pneumonitis, and these are not discussed in this chapter.

In the pediatric intensive care unit (PICU), several pneumonia types may be encountered. First, a previously healthy child may be admitted to the PICU because of severe community-acquired pneumonia (CAP). The pneumonia is usually caused by organisms that are prevalent in the out-of-hospital environment. Second, patients with genetic or acquired immune deficiency commonly develop severe pneumonia with opportunistic infections that usually do not infect healthy children. These immunocompromised patients commonly have been given chemo-radiotherapy for cancer or are receiving immune-suppressive agents to prevent rejection episodes following solid organ and hematopoietic stem cell transplantation. Third, both previously healthy and immunocompromised patients may acquire nosocomial pneumonia during their hospital stay. Mechanically ventilated patients are at especially high risk to develop nosocomial ventilator-associated pneumonia (VAP). Finally, aspiration pneumonia caused by chronic inoculation of the lower respiratory tract with large amounts of less virulent bacteria in a susceptible host prone to aspiration is also observed in the PICU.

This classification of pneumonia types in the PICU is important because it has major implications on the causative microbial agent and, thus, the choice of initial empiric treatment that may be life saving. This chapter reviews respiratory host defenses that maintain sterility of the lower respiratory tract. In addition, the pathogenesis, classification, and treatment options for pneumonia and empyema in the PICU patient are briefly discussed.

Pulmonary Host Defense

In humans, the lung represents the largest epithelial surface of the body exposed to the external environment. This area is 40-fold larger than the skin. As a consequence, the upper airways and lower lung are continuously exposed to a variety of airborne particles and microbial agents. Despite this constant attack, sterility of the conducting airways, bronchioles, and alveoli is maintained by a complex pulmonary host defense system. Throughout the upper (nasopharynx) and lower (conducting airways and alveolar spaces) respiratory tracts, the innate and adaptive immune systems work synchronously to identify and eliminate foreign non-self particles, including microbes. In invertebrates, the innate system is the sole mechanism of host defense against pathogens, but in higher vertebrates it constitutes the first line of defense. The innate defenses are constitutive, rapid, and nonspecific. The innate system is based on pattern recognition of repetitive molecular patterns shared by microorganisms.

Major advances in innate immunity have focused on the discovery of a series of cell-surface receptors called *toll-like receptors* (TLRs), first described in *Drosophila*, but now at least 11 homologues have been discovered in humans [1] and 13 homologues in mice. Individual TLRs differ in their ligand specificities (Figure 17.1). The interaction between a TLR and a microbial component triggers adaptor proteins and signal molecules, leading to transcription factors activation, production of proinflammatory cytokines, and expression of host defense peptides [2]. Importantly, the innate system and TLR activation also induce co-stimulatory molecules that stimulate and drive the inducible and slower specific adaptive immune system such that antigen-presenting cells present antigen to T helper (Th) cells that differentiate along two pathways: the Th1 pathway, important in cell-mediated immunity, and Th2 pathway involved in humoral responses [3].

Mechanical defenses also play a major role in respiratory host defense. Aerodynamic filtration in the nose and nasopharynx prevents particles that are >10 μm from passing to the lower respiratory tract. Particles from 5 to 10 μm are filtered by impaction in the conducting airways. Material deposited along the airways is removed by the mucociliary system, which starts in the nasopharynx and ends in the terminal bronchioles. Ciliary beating occurs in a precise and well-orchestrated fashion, propelling mucus and deposited organisms toward the oropharynx. A final constituent of the mechanical defense of the respiratory tract is cough. This

D.S. Wheeler et al. (eds.), The *Respiratory Tract in Pediatric Critical Illness and Injury*,
DOI 10.1007/978-1-84800-925-7_17, © Springer-Verlag London Limited 2009

FIGURE 17.1. Toll-like receptors (TLR) and their ligands. LPS, lipopolysaccharide; HSPs, heat shock proteins.

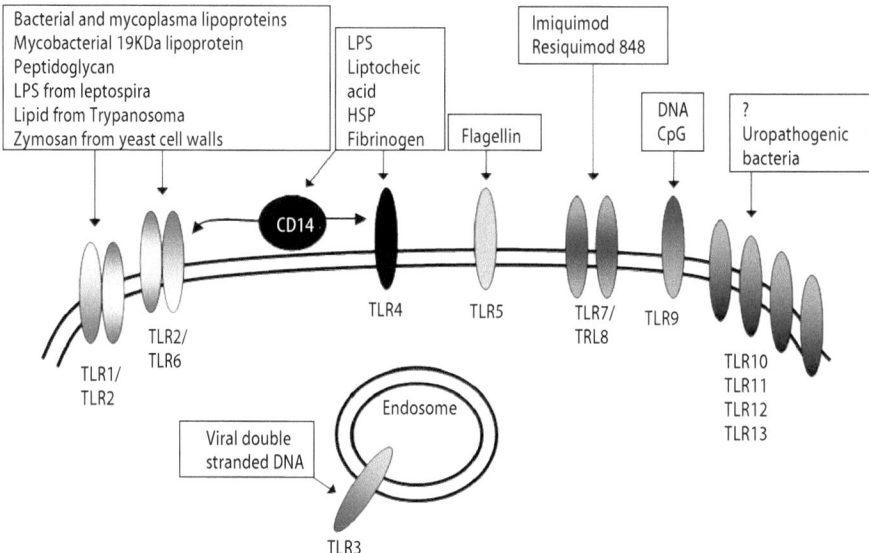

potent expiratory maneuver is of fundamental importance in preventing material from being aspirated into the lungs.

The conducting airways also contain several antimicrobial substances, including immunoglobulins (IgG and secretory IgA), and complement that bind and enhance the elimination of microbial agents. In addition, airway epithelial and alveolar type (AT) II cells secrete several antimicrobial peptides. One of the best characterized families of antimicrobial peptides are the defensins, which are cysteine-rich peptides possessing broad antimicrobial activity [4]. An important recent discovery is the expanding role of respiratory airway epithelium in innate immune defenses by mechanisms that mimic those noted in phagocytic cells. Respiratory epithelial cells, including ATII cells, express TLR and are capable of expressing a variety of cytokines that amplify inflammation. The importance of innate immunity in epithelial cells was confirmed in mice with specific inhibition of nuclear factor (NF) κB activation that was restricted to distal airway epithelial cells. Mice lacking the ability to activate NFκB in epithelial cells exhibited impaired inflammatory response to inhaled LPS [5]. These data provide evidence that distal airway epithelial cells and the signals they transduce play a key physiologic role in lung inflammation in vivo. Alveolar type II cells also secrete surfactant proteins (SP)-A and D. Both SP-A and SP-D are collagen-like lectins (collectins) that agglutinate and/or opsonize pathogens and enhance their phagocytosis by innate immune cells such as alveolar macrophages and neutrophils [6]. Surfactant proteins A and D may have additional immunoregulatory functions [7] and also may exhibit direct bactericidal effects by inducing damage to the bacterial cell membrane [8]. The functions of SP-A and SP-D in host defense are listed in Table 17.1.

In the distal airspaces, alveolar macrophages are the first phagocytic cell type encountered by pathogens entering the lung. Macrophages have the capacity to induce the generation of large amounts

of cytokines, chemokines, matrix metalloproteinases (MMP), nitric oxide, and potent oxidants that participate in antimicrobial defenses. In contrast, interstitial macrophages are located in the lung connective tissue and serve as both phagocytic cells and antigen-processing cells. Tumor necrosis factor (TNF)-α, a macrophage-derived multifunctional cytokine, is expressed early in both patients with and animal models of pneumonia [9]. Microbes also induce macrophages to generate potent chemokines that attract circulating neutrophils and monocytes into the lungs. Cytokines/chemokines amplify inflammatory responses and orchestrate the polarization and transition of innate to adaptive immunity that function to eliminate invading microorganisms [10]. Figure 17.2 summarizes the cellular and secretory peptides that are components of host defense against microbes in the lower respiratory tract. Disorders associated with impaired mechanical, innate, and adaptive host responses that may lead to the development of pneumonia in a susceptible host are listed in Table 17.2.

Pathogenesis

The upper respiratory tract is normally colonized with nonpathogenic bacterial flora, but physical and immunologic host defenses generally ensure that bacteria that gain access to the lower respiratory tract are cleared. Pneumonia occurs because of an impairment of host defenses (as discussed earlier), invasion by a virulent organism, or invasion by an overwhelming inoculum of less virulent organisms. There are five main modes of pathogen entry into the lower respiratory tract.

Inhalation and Droplets

Inhalation of infectious particles is probably the most important pathogenic mechanism in the development of CAP, with particular importance in pneumonia of those caused by *Legionella* species and *Mycobacterium tuberculosis*. Contact with contaminated fomites also may be important in the acquisition of viral agents, especially respiratory syncytial virus. The viral agents that cause pneumonia proliferate and spread by contiguity to involve lower and more distal portions of the respiratory tract. Inhalation is also a common cause of pneumonia caused by contaminated ventilator tubes.

TABLE 17.1. Functions of lung collectins SP-A and SP-D in host defense.

	SP-A	SP-D
Agglutination	+	++
Opsonization	++	+
Reduced viral infectivity	+	++
Modulation of inflammation	+	+

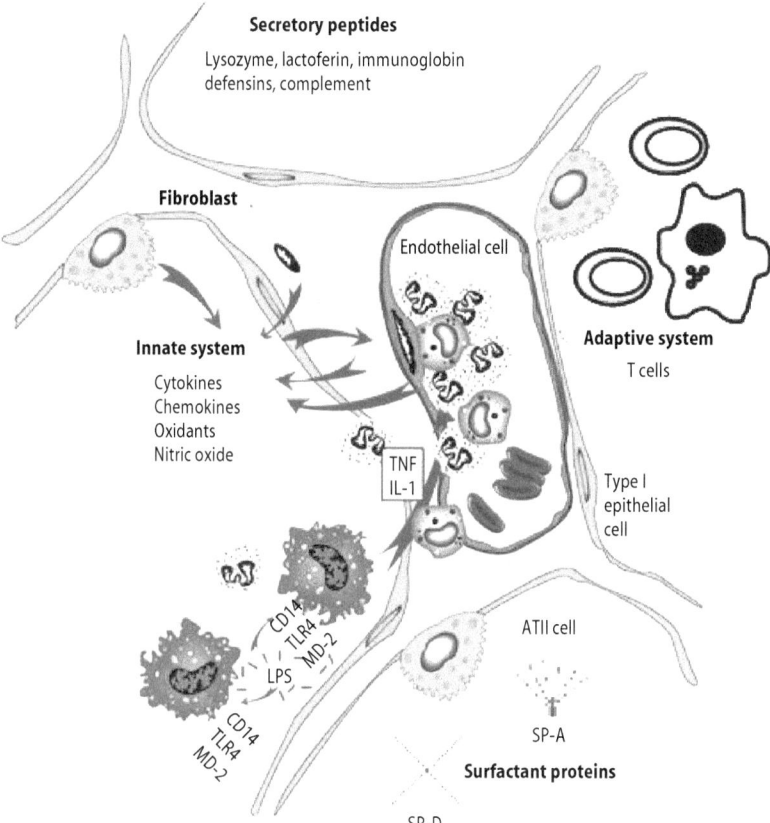

Secretory peptides

Lysozyme, lactoferin, immunoglobin
defensins, complement

Fibroblast

Endothelial cell

Innate system

Cytokines
Chemokines
Oxidants
Nitric oxide

Adaptive system

T cells

TNF
IL-1

Type I
epithelial
cell

CD14
TLR4
MD-2

LPS

ATII cell

CD14
TLR4
MD-2

SP-A

Surfactant proteins

SP-D

FIGURE 17.2. Cellular and secretory peptides involved in antimicrobial innate and adaptive host defense systems.

Aspiration

In addition to inhalation, pneumonia arises following the aspiration of microorganisms from the oral cavity or nasopharynx. Invasive disease most commonly occurs upon acquisition of a new serotype of the organism with which the patient has not had previous experience. Most episodes of VAP are thought to develop from the aspiration of oropharyngeal secretions containing potentially pathogenic organisms. Aspiration of gastric secretions may also contribute, although likely to a lesser degree. Tracheal intubation interrupts the body's anatomic and physiologic defenses against aspiration, making mechanical ventilation a major risk factor for VAP. The term *aspiration pneumonia* should be reserved for pneumonia or pneumonitis resulting from the aspiration of large amounts of gastric or oropharyngeal contents that may contain a large inoculum of relatively nonvirulent bacteria. The pathogens that commonly produce CAP or VAP, such as *Streptococcus pneumoniae*, Gram-negative bacilli, and *Staphylococcus aureus*, are relatively virulent bacteria so that only a small inoculum is required and the aspiration is usually subtle.

Hematogenous Spread

In immunocompromised individuals, an additional mode of pneumonia acquisition is bacteremia and sepsis. Hematogenous deposition of bacteria is responsible for some cases of pneumonia caused by *Staph. aureus*, *Pseudomonas aeruginosa*, and *Escherichia coli*.

Reactivation

Reactivation of pathogens can take place in the setting of deficits of cell-mediated immunity. Pathogens such as *Pneumocystis carinii/jiroveci*, *M. tuberculosis*, and cytomegalovirus (CMV) may remain latent for many years after exposure, with flares of active disease in the face of immune compromise. Reactivation tuberculosis occasionally occurs in immunocompetent hosts.

TABLE 17.2. Conditions associated with impaired pulmonary host defense.

Mechanical defenses	Phagocytic function	Cellular immunity (T cells)	Humoral immunity (B cells)
Impaired cough	Inherited	Inherited	Inherited
	Chronic granulomatous disease	Severe combined immunodeficiency syndrome	X-linked agammaglobulinemia
	Chediak-Higashi syndrome	DiGeorge syndrome	Common variable immunodeficiency
	Leukocyte adhesion deficiency	Wiskott-Aldrich syndrome	IgA deficiency
		Ataxia telangiectasia	IgG subclass deficiency
Impaired mucociliary function	Acquired	Acquired	Acquired
Primary ciliary dyskinesia	Neutropenia	Immunosuppressive medications	Steroids
Cystic fibrosis		Acquired immunodeficiency syndrome	Excessive pleural or peritoneal fluids losses
		Graft-versus-host disease	Nephrotic syndrome

Direct Injury and Inflammation

Direct inoculation rarely occurs as a result of surgery or bronchoscopy but may play a role in the development of pneumonia in patients supported with mechanical ventilation. The direct extension of infection to the lung from contiguous areas such as the pleural or subdiaphragmatic spaces is rare.

Pneumonia Types in the Pediatric Intensive Care Unit

Community-Acquired Pneumonia

Definitions and Main Features

Community-acquired pneumonia refers to pneumonia in a previously healthy person who acquired the infection outside a hospital. It is one of the most common serious infections in children, with an incidence of 34 to 40 cases per 1,000 children in the industrialized world [11]. A subset of these patients will require PICU admission. Admission to the intensive care unit should be considered for patients with persistent hypoxemia despite oxygen therapy, recurrent apnea, signs of respiratory fatigue with or without mental status changes, or evidence of compensated or decompensated shock. Infants less than 6 months of age and children with comorbid conditions such as bronchopulmonary dysplasia, cystic fibrosis, neuromuscular disorders, congenital heart disease, and immunodeficiency disorders have limited respiratory reserves and, therefore, are at increased risk for respiratory failure during a pneumonia episode.

For the adult population, the American and British Thoracic Societies have developed guidelines for hospital and ICU admissions for patients with severe CAP [12]. According to the American Thoracic Society Guidelines, admission to the ICU is needed for patients with severe CAP, defined as the presence of either one of two major criteria, or the presence of two of three minor criteria. The major criteria include need for mechanical ventilation and septic shock; the minor criteria include systolic blood pressure ≤90 mm Hg, multilobar disease, and a PaO_2/FiO_2 ratio <250. In addition, a Pneumonia Severity Index (PSI) score identifies adults at increased risk of medical complications and death [13]. However, similar guidelines or scores to grade the severity of pneumonia in children have not been developed.

Specific Pathogens

Children admitted to the PICU because of CAP are more commonly infected with bacterial than viral pathogens. *Streptococcus pneumoniae* is the most commonly identified bacterial cause of CAP in infants and children older than 1 month. Pneumonias caused by group A *Streptococcus* and *Staph. aureus* are less frequent. *Haemophilus influenzae* pneumonia has become uncommon following the widespread use of *Haemophilus* influenza type B immunization. Viruses are identified most often in children <5 years of age. Respiratory syncytial virus is the most common viral etiology during infancy, with adenovirus, influenza virus, parainfluenza virus, and the recently described human metapneumonovirus (14) also not infrequently detected. *Mycoplasma pneumoniae* and *Chlamydia pneumoniae* are more common in older children and adolescents [11].

In May 1993 an outbreak of an acute febrile illness associated with respiratory failure, shock, and high mortality was identified by investigators from the Centers for Disease Control and Prevention (CDC) as being caused by a hantavirus. In the United States, 95% of the cases occurred west of the Mississippi after environmental exposure to infected deer mouse saliva, urine, or feces. In addition, a novel coronavirus was identified as the causative agent of severe acute respiratory syndrome (SARS), a new respiratory illness that affects adults and children, although the severity of the disease is less in children than in adults [15]. Another cause of severe pneumonia that should be considered is tuberculosis. A history of contact with a person with pulmonary tuberculosis is usually elicited. Finally, uncommon causes of CAP in otherwise healthy children are fungal infections including *Coccidiodes immitis*, *Histoplasma capsulatum*, and *Blastomyces dermatitidis*. These organisms should be included in the differential diagnosis as a cause of pneumonia only if there is a history of residence or travel to an area of endemic infection.

Occasionally, infection with *Strep. pneumoniae* [16] and *Mycoplasma pneumoniae* [17] can cause necrotic pneumonia secondary to an invasive organism or exaggerated host immune response. Compared to patients with pneumonia and parapneumonic effusions, children who developed necrotizing pneumonia exhibited a more protracted hospital course associated with higher rates of complications, including bronchopleural fistulas and need for thoracotomy for fistula repair or lobectomy. None of the necrotizing pneumonia patients were immune deficient [18].

Approach

The diagnosis of CAP is usually made based on the presence of respiratory symptoms (cough, retractions) in a febrile and tachypneic child. The presence of infiltrates on chest radiographs confirms the diagnosis of pneumonia. Infiltrates are generally either interstitial or alveolar. Although alveolar infiltrates are more commonly observed during bacterial pneumonia [19], in most studies, the pattern of infiltrates has not been shown to correctly differentiate viral from bacterial pneumonia [20]. Chest radiographs will also detect the presence of pleural effusions, pneumatoceles which are observed during staphylococcal pneumonia, or presence of air–fluid levels indicative of abscess formation.

After initial stabilization, diagnostic testing should be performed rapidly, avoiding delays in the administration of initial empiric therapy. In addition to a chest radiograph, an admitted patient should have a complete blood count and differential and routine blood chemistry testing (including glucose, serum sodium, liver and renal function tests, and electrolytes). All admitted patients should have oxygen saturation assessed by pulse oximetry and supplemental oxygen administered as needed. Arterial blood gas should be measured in any patient with severe illness to assess both the level oxygenation and the degree of carbon dioxide retention.

For critically ill patients with pneumonia, an aggressive approach to determine the causative microbial agent is warranted. Microbiologic confirmation is ultimately obtained for approximately 30%–50% of children with CAP [21]. If a pleural effusion is present, aspiration of pleural fluid for Gram stain and culture prior to starting antibiotics is valuable. Blood culture may reveal organisms in up to 30% of patients with bacterial pneumonia [22]. Sputum collection is usually not practical for infants and children, and bacterial organisms recovered from the nasopharynx do not accurately predict the etiology of pneumonia. However, recovery of viruses and other atypical pathogens from the nasopharynx is more predictive. Bacterial organisms recovered from tracheal secretions obtained through an endotracheal tube may or may not reflect the causative agent(s) responsible for lower respiratory tract infection. Specimens are considered appropriate for examination if they contain ≤10 epithelial cells and ≥25 polymorphonuclear leukocytes under low power [23]. The primary purpose of tracheal aspirate samples is to visualize a bacterial morphology of an organism that was not anticipated so that appropriate drugs can be added to the initial antibiotic regimen (e.g., *Staph. aureus* or an enteric Gram-negative antibiotic). Bronchoalveolar lavage (BAL) has been shown to be a rapid, relatively safe, and relatively noninvasive diagnostic procedure to obtain lower respiratory tract samples for microbial identification and analysis.

Other techniques that can be used to identify pathogens include antigen detection of bacteria and viruses using immunofluorescence, polymerase chain reaction, and serology such as cold agglutination test for *M. pneumonia*. The specificity of the cold agglutination test for *M. pneumonia* is almost absolute, although the sensitivity is only about 50%. Detection of *Mycoplasma* IgM by enzyme-linked immunoabsorbant assay (ELISA) is a sensitive technique and should be considered for children [24].

Pneumonia in the Immunocompromised Host

Definitions and Main Features

Immunocompromised patients are those whose immune mechanisms are deficient because of congenital immune deficiency syndromes, acquired immunologic disorders, or exposure to cytotoxic chemotherapy and steroids. In addition, recipients of solid organ and hematopoietic stem cell transplantation (HSCT) are frequently given life-long treatment with immunosuppressive agents designed to prevent graft rejection or graft-versus-host disease. Patients who develop severe neutropenia (i.e., an absolute neutrophil count ≤500 cells/mL) or lymphopenia for prolonged periods of time are at greatest risk to develop a variety of infectious complications, including life-threatening pneumonia. The lung is the predominant site of opportunistic infection in the immunocompromised patient [25].

Pathogens

Immunosuppressed patients are predisposed to develop infections by ubiquitous microorganisms that do not normally cause disease in healthy people. They are also more susceptible to the usual causes of pneumonia, which can affect anyone. The sequence in which different organisms appear in the immunosuppressed and post-transplant recipients is fairly characteristic. Nosocomial bacterial infections remain the most common cause of pneumonia during the early post-transplant, neutropenic phase. *Staphylococcus aureus* and Gram-negative pathogens predominate. In addition, fungal infections with *Candida* and *Aspergillus* species are not uncommonly seen during a severe neutropenic phase. The second period, from 1 to 6 months after solid organ transplant, is the time when opportunistic infections more commonly associated with transplantation, including *Nocardia*, *P. carinii/jiroveci*, and CMV are observed [26]. During the third period, after 6 months, patients are categorized into different risk groups depending on the level of function of their allograft and the degree of immunosuppression they have received. Those who are on minimal immunosuppression therapy are subject mainly to the same pathogens as the rest of the community. Those with allograft dysfunction and ongoing heavy immunosuppressive therapy remain subject to all of the opportunistic infections seen during the second period. Lung transplant recipients who develop bronchiolitis obliterans and HSCT recipients who develop graft-versus-host disease remain especially at risk for infections [26].

Approach

Pulmonary infiltrates in the immunocompromised host may be caused by a variety of organisms, and may have noninfectious causes. Because progression to respiratory failure may be rapid, an aggressive approach to diagnosis and treatment is necessary to limit morbidity and mortality. Initial broad-spectrum therapy is important, with alterations of the empiric regimen once the clinical situation has stabilized and more diagnostic information has been obtained. In the immunocompromised host, BAL procedure should be performed promptly to rule out infectious etiologies. Table 17.3

TABLE 17.3. Evaluation of bronchoalveolar lavage in immunocompromised hosts.

Stains	Culture	Antigen determinations	Cytology
KOH	Bacterial	*Legionella*	Cell count and differential
	Routine aerobic	Respiratory syncytial virus	
	Legionella	Cytomegalovirus	
	Nocardia		
	Mycobacterium		
Gram's	Viral		
	Cytomegalovirus shell vial		
	Respiratory syncytial virus		
	Influenza		
	Parainfluenza		
	Adenovirus		
	Enteroviruses		
Silver methenamine	Fugal		
Pneumocystis carinii	*Aspergillus*		
Fungi	*Candida*		
Wright	*Chlamydia*		
Chlamydia inclusions			
Hematoxylin and eosin			
Oil-Red-O			
Lipid-laden macrophage index			

lists suggested BAL fluids analysis studies and cultures. Bronchoalveolar lavage is very helpful in the diagnosis of *P. carinii/jiroveci*, CMV, tuberculosis, and some fungal infections. However, the ability of BAL fluids analysis and culture to detect invasive aspergillosis, one of the most lethal infectious complication after transplantation, is limited [27]. The diagnostic yield for *Aspergillus* species infection has been enhanced by the recently developed ELISA that detects galactomannan, a fungal cell wall component released during invasive disease [28]. Histopathologic analysis and culture of open lung biopsy specimens may provide accurate determination for the cause of pulmonary infiltrates in pediatric patients [29]. However, open lung biopsy is associated with a significant surgical risk in critically ill patients. Open lung biopsy is most effective and least risky when performed early in the course of patients who develop nodular infiltrates that require rapid differentiation between fungal infections and more benign lesions [30].

Chemoprophylaxis against opportunistic infections is an important component of management of the post-transplant immunosuppressed patients. Before the widespread introduction of chemoprophylaxis, *P. carinii* pneumonia (PCP) was observed to be a common opportunistic infection among transplant recipients. With the administration of low-dose trimethoprim–sulfamethoxazole or an alternative prophylactic agent such as pentamidine, PCP can be effectively prevented [31]. Prophylaxis is also recommended for CMV in high-risk CMV seronegative recipients. Such prophylaxis includes intravenous ganciclovir for 14 days, followed by oral ganciclovir capsules for three months [32].

Aspiration Pneumonia

Definitions and Main Features

Aspiration pneumonia refers to the pulmonary consequences resulting from the abnormal entry of fluid, formula, or endogenous secretions into the lower airways. There is usually compromise in host defenses that protect the lower airways, including glottic closure, cough reflex, and other clearing mechanisms. Histories of seizure, anesthesia, or other episode of reduced level of consciousness, neurologic disease, dysphagia, or gastroesophageal reflux are all risk factors for aspiration. The risk of aspiration is especially high after removal of an endotracheal tube because of the residual effects of sedative drugs, the presence of a nasogastric tube, and swallowing dysfunction related to alterations of upper-airway sensitivity, glottic injury, and laryngeal muscular dysfunction [33]. Aspiration pneumonia may be classified into three clinical syndromes: chemical pneumonitis, bacterial infection, and airway obstruction. In animal models, development of chemical pneumonitis requires a 1 to 4 mL/kg inoculum of fluid with a pH of 2.5 to initiate an inflammatory reaction that may lead to pulmonary fibrosis [34]. Bacteria, present in the aspirated oropharyngeal and gastric secretions, may also lead to pneumonia. Aspiration pneumonia may involve particulate matter or foreign body, which, in addition to causing airway obstruction or reflux airway closure, may synergistically contribute to acid-induced lung injury [34].

Pathogens

True aspiration pneumonia, by convention, usually refers to an infection caused by less virulent bacteria, primarily anaerobes, which are common constituents of the normal flora in a susceptible host prone to aspiration. Pneumonia is commonly caused by oropharyngeal flora, including anaerobic Gram-negative bacilli (*Bacteroides fragilis*, *Fusobacterium nucleatum*, *Peptostreptococcus*, and *Prevotella*) and anaerobic Gram-positive bacilli (*Clostridium*, *Eubacterium*, *Actinomyces*, *Lactobacillus*, and *Propionibacterium*).

Approach

Aspiration usually occurs when the patient is supine during or immediately after feeding. In the supine position the right upper lobe is the most dependent part of the lung and is most frequently affected. Commonly, impaired airway protective responses are observed. The presence of tracheoesophageal malformations should be investigated if recurrent aspiration is noted in an otherwise healthy infant.

The clinical presentation and course of chemical pneumonitis after inhalation of gastric contents ranges from mild and self-limited to severe and life threatening, depending on the nature of the aspirate and the underlying condition of the host. In the absence of witnessed inhalation of vomit, diagnosis is difficult and requires a high index of suspicion in a patient who has risk factors for aspiration. In the absence of an obvious predisposition, the abrupt onset of a self-limited illness characterized by dyspnea, cyanosis, and low-grade fever associated with diffuse rales, hypoxemia, and alveolar infiltrates in dependent lobes should suggest aspiration [35]. If BAL is performed, assessment of lipid-laden macrophage index using Oil-Red-O stain is helpful in confirming the diagnosis [36]. The presence of foul-smelling putrid discharge in sputum or pleural fluid is regarded as diagnostic of anaerobic infection. Patients often have prolonged fever and productive cough, frequently showing blood in the sputum, which indicates necrosis (tissue death) in the lung. If aspiration is persistent, fibrosis and bronchiectasis may result.

A number of interventions (e.g., positioning, dietary changes, drugs, oral hygiene, tube feeding) have been proposed to prevent aspiration Patients with an observed aspiration should have immediate tracheal suction or bronchoscopy to clear fluids and particulate matter that may cause obstruction. The use of corticosteroids in the treatment of chemical pneumonitis is controversial [37], and antibiotics should not be used early in the course unless a superimposed bacterial infection is suspected.

Nosocomial and Ventilator-Associated Pneumonia

Definitions and Main Features

The National Nosocomial Infection Surveillance (NNIS) program sponsored by the CDC defines VAP as pneumonia in patients who have been on mechanical ventilation for >48 hr and have developed new and persistent radiographic evidence of focal infiltrates. In addition, patients had to have two of the following: temperature >38′C, leukocytosis (white blood cell >12,000/mm^3), and purulent sputum (>25 white blood cells/high-powered field on tracheal aspirate Gram stain). After blood stream infections, VAP is the second most common cause of nosocomial infections in PICUs. The mean VAP rate in children ranges from 6 to 12/1,000 ventilator days, accounting for 20%–50% of hospital-acquired infections [38,39]. Infections acquired in the PICU are associated with a significantly increased risk of death [40].

Pathogens

Nosocomial pneumonia and VAP are typically categorized as either early onset (occurring in the first 3–4 days of mechanical ventilation) or late onset. This distinction is important microbiologically. Early-onset nosocomial pneumonia and VAP are commonly caused by antibiotic-sensitive, community-acquired organisms (e.g., *Strep. pneumoniae*, and *Staph. aureus*). Late-onset nosocomial pneumonia and VAP are commonly caused by anti-biotic-resistant nosocomial organisms (e.g., *P. aeruginosa*, methicillin-resistant *Staph. aureus*, *Acinetobacter* species, and *Enterobacter* species). During the winter respiratory viral season, all patients in a medical care environment are at risk for disease due to respiratory syncytial virus, parainfluenza, and influenza viruses. Legionnaire's disease is a multisystem illness with pneumonia caused by *Legionella* species usually present in contaminated water. Legionnaire's disease is less common in children than adults.

Approach

Compared with postmortem lung biopsies and culture results, the use of clinical criteria to diagnose VAP (lung infiltrates, leukocytosis, purulent secretions, fever) had a sensitivity of 69% and a specificity of 75% [41]. Clearly, a number of noninfectious causes of fever and pulmonary infiltrates can also occur in these patients, making the above clinical criteria nonspecific for the diagnosis of VAP. Lung infiltrates may be caused by pulmonary hemorrhage, chemical aspiration, or atelectasis. Fever may be caused by a drug reaction, extrapulmonary infection, or blood transfusion. Autopsy results in a series of patients with acute lung injury demonstrated that clinical criteria alone led to an incorrect diagnosis of VAP in 29% of clinically suspected cases [42]. These limitations have encouraged the use of invasive approaches to sample and culture material from the lower respiratory tract for accurate diagnosis of VAP.

Ventilator-associated pneumonia is most accurately diagnosed by quantitative culture and microscopic examination of lower respiratory tract secretions, which are best obtained by bronchoscopy and BAL [43]. Cultures of tracheal aspirates are not very useful in establishing the cause of VAP [44]. Although such cultures are highly sensitive, their specificity is low even when they are cultured quantitatively [45]. Combining clinical and bacteriologic evaluation is probably the best way to achieve the objectives of correctly diagnosing VAP and appropriately using antimicrobial agents. The main aims of this diagnostic approach are to rapidly identify patients with true lung bacterial infection, to select appropriate initial antimicrobial therapy, to adjust therapy based on antibiotic sensitivities, and to withhold antibiotics from patients without VAP. Guidelines for the prevention of VAP in children are lacking, but data extrapolated from adult studies support routine elevation of head of bed 30°, appropriate use of sedatives and muscle relaxants, and adequate oral and circuit hygiene [46].

Empyema

Definitions and Main Features

Empyema is the presence of purulent material containing polymorphonuclear leukocytes and fibrin in the pleural cavity. Empyema is usually a complication of inadequately treated bacterial CAP, although it may occur after trauma, thoracic surgery, or intrathoracic esophageal perforation. Although parapneumonic pleural effusions are noted in up to 34&–40% of children with pneumonia, empyema is rare, present in 1%–2% of cases [47]. The formation of an empyema can be divided into three stages: exudative, fibrinopurulent, and organizing. During the exudative stage, pus accumu-

lates. This is followed by fibrin deposition and loculation of pleural fluid known as the fibrinopurulent stage. The organizing stage is characterized by fibroblast proliferation; at this time there is the potential for lung entrapment by scarring [48].

Typically, the pleural fluid in empyema is exudative, caused by protein leakage from the capillaries because of increased permeability and increased hydrostatic pressure during the inflammatory process. Although the distinction between transudates and exudates is sometimes difficult to make, several features favor an exudative process. If at least one of the following three criteria is present, the fluid is virtually always an exudate: (1) pleural fluid protein >2.9g/dL or protein/serum protein ratio greater than 0.5; (2) pleural fluid lactate dehydrogenase (LDH)/serum LDH ratio greater than 0.6; and/or (3) pleural fluid LDH greater than two thirds the serum LDH [49,50].

Pathogens

The most common organisms that cause empyema in children are Strep. pneumoniae, *Staph. aureus*, and group A streptococci. *Haemophilus influenzae* is rarely encountered since the advent of the *H. influenzae* B vaccine. *Mycoplasma pneumoniae* and viruses can rarely result in exudative pleural effusions. In a series of 72 pediatric patients with empyema, 24% were secondary to anaerobic infection [51]. These data highlight the importance of anaerobic bacteria in selected cases of empyema in children and adolescents. In addition, tuberculosis should always be considered in the differential diagnosis, and a purified protein derivative test should be performed.

Approach

The differential diagnosis of patients with pleural effusions is shown in Table 17.4. The presence of fever associated with clinical signs of bacterial pneumonia is a clue to an underlying pneumonia as the cause of the effusion. A lateral decubitus radiograph, ultrasonography, or computed tomography may differentiate whether the fluid is loculated. A sample of the fluid should be obtained by thoracentesis in order to determine if the effusion is a transudate versus exudate. Pleural cultures are positive in approximately one half of pediatric patients with empyema. Blood culture and urine latex agglutination may help to identify a bacterial pathogen. A pneumatocele or pneumothorax seen on chest film suggests *Staph. aureus* as the cause of the empyema.

Until a specific organism is identified, empiric antibiotic therapy should be instituted. This might include a third-generation cephalosporin and antistaphylococcal β-lactamase–resistant penicillin. Antibiotics can be adjusted once an organism is identified. Antibiotic therapy should be intravenous until the patient becomes afebrile and then should be continued orally for an additional 2–3 weeks.

TABLE 17.4. Causes of pleural effusion.

Transudate	Exudate
Parapneumonic effusions	Empyema
Congestive heart failure	Neoplasms
Nephrotic syndrome	Connective tissue disorder
Cirrhosis	Pancreatitis
Ascites	Esophageal perforation
Hypothyroidism	Chylothorax

There is major debate as to the proper adjuvant treatment of children with empyema. Prospective, randomized and controlled studies of children with empyema are lacking. With the exception of starting appropriate or empiric antibiotics, there is no consensus on when and in whom to place a chest tube, instill fibrinolytic agents, or take to the operating room [52]. In 1992, Light suggested that chest tubes should be inserted if the pleural fluid is gross pus, if the Gram stain of the pleural fluid is positive, if the pleural fluid glucose level is below 40 mg/dL, or if the pleural fluid pH level is less than 7.00 [53]. If drainage with a chest tube is unsatisfactory, either urokinase or tissue plasminogen activator (tPA) should be injected intrapleurally [54,55]. If drainage is still unsatisfactory, a decortication should be considered [56]. A stage-related approach to the management of empyema is perhaps most efficacious and cost-effective [57]. In the exudative stage, conservative treatment using tube drainage may suffice. Fibrinolytic treatment may be useful during the fibrinopurulent stage. In contrast, aggressive treatment using surgical decortication may be necessary during the organizing stage.

With the advent of video-assisted thoracoscopy (VATS), these traditional approaches to management of empyema in children are being challenged. Video-assisted techniques offer distinct advantages in the accurate staging of the disease process, effectiveness of management of organizing pleural disease, and post-operative patient comfort [58]. In a retrospective study, the performance of early VATS (<48hr after admission) in children with empyema was associated with significantly decreased length of hospital stay compared with performance of late VATS (>48hr after admission) [59].

Children treated for empyema generally recover and have no residual sequelae. Radiographs at the time of discharge usually show pleural thickening that later resolves. Follow-up pulmonary function tests and physical examination are also usually normal or consistent with mild restrictive disease [60].

General Treatment Principles

Antimicrobial Therapy

Most epidemiologic investigations have clearly demonstrated that the indiscriminate administration of antibiotic agents to patients in the PICU has contributed to the emergence of multiresistant pathogens with potentially increased morbidity and mortality. The prevalence of penicillin-resistant strains of *Strep. pneumoniae*, methicillin-resistant *Staph. aureus*, vancomycin-resistant *Enterococcus*, and Gram-negative bacteria producing extended-spectrum β-lactamase is increasing. Despite these concerns, it is clear that patient survival may improve if pneumonia is correctly and rapidly treated. In adults, inappropriate initial antibiotic therapy is strongly associated with fatality [61]. Therefore, it may be concluded that empiric antibiotics for the treatment of severe pneumonia are indicated.

The choice of antibiotics is based on several factors, including the age of the patient, the type of pneumonia, and the local resistant patterns of predominant bacterial pathogens. Suggested choices for initial empiric antibiotic coverage for pneumonia in the PICU are listed in Table 17.5. Aspiration pneumonia occurring in the community can be treated with ampicillin-sulbactam. Empiric treatment for pneumonia in immunocompromised hosts requires broad-spectrum Gram-positive and Gram-negative coverage.

TABLE 17.5. Common bacterial causes and empiric antibiotic therapy for pneumonia in the pediatric intensive care unit.

	Community-acquired pneumonia	Ventilator-associated pneumonia
Usual pathogens	Infant *Streptococcus pneumoniae* *Staphylococcus aureus* Child and adolescent *Streptococcus pneumoniae* *Mycoplasma, Chlamydia*	Gram positive *Staphylococcus aureus* Methicillin-resistant *Staphylococcus aureus* (MRSA) Gram negative *Klebsiella pneumoniae* *Pseudomonas aeruginosa* *Escherichia coli* *Serratia marcescens* *Acinotobacter* sp. *Stenotrophomonas maltophilia*
Recommended initial treatment	Infant: Cefuroxime+ cloxacillin Child and adolescent Cefuroxime + erythromycin	Ticarcillin-clavulanate or Piperacillin-tazobactam + aminoglycoside Alternatives Vancomycin (if MRSA present) Ceftazidime+ aminoglycoside (if suspect *Pseudomonas*)

Immunocompromised patients are especially susceptible to a variety of life-threatening opportunistic viral and fungal pneumonias that require prompt diagnosis and aggressive treatment. For example, trimethoprim-sulfamethoxazole or pentamidine should be given for *P. carinii/jiroveci*, amphotericin B or caspofungin for *Candida* and *Aspergillus species*, acyclovir for herpes, amantadine for influenza, ganciclovir or foscarnet for CMV, and ribavirin for severe respiratory syncytial virus. Empiric regimens may need to be modified once results of cultures and antibiotic susceptibility testing are available.

Antiinflammatory Approach

The inflammatory response to infection is necessary for host defense but can contribute to the systemic toxicity and lung injury that may result from pneumonia. In some settings, adjunctive treatment of lower respiratory infections with antiinflammatory agents can reduce morbidity. Corticosteroids have a well-documented role in the management of *P. carinii/jiroveci* pneumonia. In a multicenter trial, infusion of hydrocortisone significantly decreased length of hospital stay and prevented mortality in adult patients with CAP [62]. Corticosteroids also may be effective under some circumstances in the treatment of inflammatory sequelae of respiratory tract infection, such as tuberculous pleurisy and bronchiolitis obliterans organizing pneumonia (BOOP). Strategies targeting specific cytokines have not been effective to date but remain active areas of investigation. Enhanced understanding of the interactions of pathogen components with TLRs may be helpful one day in controlling and containing infectious diseases.

Vaccines

Immunization has reduced the incidence of several serious childhood diseases. Immunization against influenza and increasingly resistant pneumococci can play a critical role in the prevention of pneumonia, particularly in immunocompromised patients.

References

1. Kaisho T, Akira S. Pleiotropic function of toll-like receptors. Microbes Infect 2004;6:1388–1394.

2. Skerrett SJ, Liggitt HD, Hajjar AM, Wilson CB. Myeloid differentiation factor 88 is essential for pulmonary host defense against *Pseudomonas aeruginosa* but not *Staphylococcus aureus*. J Immunol 2004;172: 3377–3381.

3. Pasare C, Medzhitov R. Toll-like receptors: linking innate and adaptive immunity. Adv Exp Med Biol 2005;560:11–18.

4. Schonwetter BS, Stolzenberg ED, Zasloff MA. Epithelial antibiotics induced at sites of inflammation. Science 1995;267:1645–1648.

5. Skerrett SJ, Liggitt HD, Hajjar AM, Ernst RK, Miller SI, Wilson CB. Respiratory epithelial cells regulate lung inflammation in response to inhaled endotoxin. Am J Physiol Lung Cell Mol Physiol 2004;287: L143–L152.

6. Wright JR. Host defense functions of pulmonary surfactant. Biol Neonate 2004;85:326–332.

7. Yang S, Milla C, Panoskaltsis-Mortari A, Ingbar DH, Blazar BR, Haddad IY. Human surfactant protein a suppresses T cell–dependent inflammation and attenuates the manifestations of idiopathic pneumonia syndrome in mice. Am J Respir Cell Mol Biol 2001;24:527–536.

8. Schaeffer LM, McCormack FX, Wu H, Weiss AA. Interactions of pulmonary collectins with Bordetella bronchiseptica and Bordetella pertussis lipopolysaccharide elucidate the structural basis of their antimicrobial activities. Infect Immun 2004;72:7124–7130.

9. Mehrad B, Strieter RM, Standiford TJ. Role of TNF-alpha in pulmonary host defense in murine invasive aspergillosis. J Immunol 1999;162: 1633–1640.

10. Strieter RM, Belperio JA, Keane MP. Host innate defenses in the lung: the role of cytokines. Curr Opin Infect Dis 2003;16:193–198.

11. McIntosh K. Community-acquired pneumonia in children. N Engl J Med 2002;346:429–437.

12. Niederman MS, Bass JB Jr, Campbell GD, Fein AM, Grossman RF, Mandell LA, Marrie TJ, Sarosi GA, Torres A, Yu VL. Guidelines for the initial management of adults with community-acquired pneumonia: diagnosis, assessment of severity, and initial antimicrobial therapy. American Thoracic Society. Medical Section of the American Lung Association. Am Rev Respir Dis 1993;148:1418–1426.

13. Fine MJ, Auble TE, Yealy DM, Hanusa BH, Weissfeld LA, Singer DE, Coley CM, Marrie TJ, Kapoor WN. A prediction rule to identify low-risk patients with community-acquired pneumonia. N Engl J Med 1997;336:243–250.

14. Williams JV, Harris PA, Tollefson SJ, Halburnt-Rush LL, Pingsterhaus JM, Edwards KM, Wright PF, Crowe JE, Jr. Human metapneumovirus and lower respiratory tract disease in otherwise healthy infants and children. N Engl J Med 2004;350:443–450.

15. Hon KL, Leung CW, Cheng WT, Chan PK, Chu WC, Kwan YW, Li AM, Fong NC, Ng PC, Chiu MC, et al. Clinical presentations and outcome of severe acute respiratory syndrome in children. Lancet 2003; 361:1701–1703.

16. Hsieh YC, Hsueh PR, Lu CY, Lee PI, Lee CY, Huang LM. Clinical manifestations and molecular epidemiology of necrotizing pneumonia and empyema caused by *Streptococcus pneumoniae* in children in Taiwan. Clin Infect Dis 2004;38:830–835.

17. Wang RS, Wang SY, Hsieh KS, Chiou YH, Huang IF, Cheng MF, Chiou CC. Necrotizing pneumonitis caused by *Mycoplasma pneumoniae* in pediatric patients: report of five cases and review of literature. Pediatr Infect Dis J 2004;23:564–567.

18. Hacimustafaoglu M, Celebi S, Sarimehmet H, Gurpinar A, Ercan I. Necrotizing pneumonia in children. Acta Paediatr 2004;93:1172–1177.

19. Korppi M, Kiekara O, Heiskanen-Kosma T, Soimakallio S. Comparison of radiological findings and microbial aetiology of childhood pneumonia. Acta Paediatr 1993;82:360–363.

20. Bettenay FA, de Campo JF, McCrossin DB. Differentiating bacterial from viral pneumonias in children. Pediatr Radiol 1988;18:453–454.

21. Heiskanen-Kosma T, Korppi M, Jokinen C, Kurki S, Heiskanen L, Juvonen H, Kallinen S, Sten M, Tarkiainen A, Ronnberg PR, et al. Etiology of childhood pneumonia: serologic results of a prospective, population-based study. Pediatr Infect Dis J 1998;17:986–991.

22. Donowitz GR, Mandell GL. Acute pneumonia. In: Mandell GL, Douglas RG, Bennet JF, eds. Principles and Practice of Infectious Diseases. New York: Churchill Livingstone; 1990:540–544.

23. Murray PR, Washington JA. Microscopic and bacteriologic analysis of expectorated sputum. Mayo Clin Proc 1975;50:339–344.

24. Uphoff CC, Brauer S, Grunicke D, Gignac SM, MacLeod RA, Quentmeier H, Steube K, Tummler M, Voges M, Wagner B, et al. Sensitivity and specificity of five different mycoplasma detection assays. Leukemia 1992;6:335–341.

25. Fishman JA, Rubin RH. Infection in organ-transplant recipients. N Engl J Med 1998;338:1741–1751.

26. Kotloff RM, Ahya VN, Crawford SW. Pulmonary complications of solid organ and hematopoietic stem cell transplantation. Am J Respir Crit Care Med 2004;170:22–48.

27. Jantunen E, Piilonen A, Volin L, Parkkali T, Koukila-Kahkola P, Ruutu T, Ruutu P. Diagnostic aspects of invasive *Aspergillus* infections in allogeneic BMT recipients. Bone Marrow Transplant 2000;25:867–871.

28. Maertens J, Glasmacher A, Selleslag D, Ngai A, Ryan D, Layton M, Taylor A, Sable C, Kartsonis N. Evaluation of serum sandwich enzyme-linked immunosorbent assay for circulating galactomannan during caspofungin therapy: results from the caspofungin invasive aspergillosis study. Clin Infect Dis 2005;41:e9–e14.

29. Hayes-Jordan A, Benaim E, Richardson S, Joglar J, Srivastava DK, Bowman L, Shochat SJ. Open lung biopsy in pediatric bone marrow transplant patients. J Pediatr Surg 2002;37:446–452.

30. Gulbahce HE, Pambuccian SE, Jessurun J, Woodard P, Steiner ME, Manivel JC, Hite S, Ramsay NK, Baker KS. Pulmonary nodular lesions in bone marrow transplant recipients: impact of histologic diagnosis on patient management and prognosis. Am J Clin Pathol 2004;121: 205–210.

31. Gordon SM, LaRosa SP, Kalmadi S, Arroliga AC, Avery RK, Truesdell-LaRosa L, Longworth DL. Should prophylaxis for *Pneumocystis carinii* pneumonia in solid organ transplant recipients ever be discontinued? Clin Infect Dis 1999;28:240–246.

32. Pescovitz MD, Brook B, Jindal RM, Leapman SB, Milgrom ML, Filo RS. Oral ganciclovir in pediatric transplant recipients: a pharmacokinetic study. Clin Transplant 1997;11:613–617.

33. Tolep K, Getch CL, Criner GJ. Swallowing dysfunction in patients receiving prolonged mechanical ventilation. Chest 1996;109:167–172.

34. Knight PR, Rutter T, Tait AR, Coleman E, Johnson K. Pathogenesis of gastric particulate lung injury: a comparison and interaction with acidic pneumonitis. Anesth Analg 1993;77:754–760.

35. DePaso WJ. Aspiration pneumonia. Clin Chest Med 1991;12:269–284.

36. Corwin RW, Irwin RS. The lipid-laden alveolar macrophage as a marker of aspiration in parenchymal lung disease. Am Rev Respir Dis 1985; 132:576–581.

37. Wolfe JE, Bone RC, Ruth WE. Effects of corticosteroids in the treatment of patients with gastric aspiration. Am J Med 1977;63:719–722.

38. Tablan OC, Anderson LJ, Besser R, Bridges C, Hajjeh R. Guidelines for preventing health-care–associated pneumonia, 2003: recommendations of CDC and the Healthcare Infection Control Practices Advisory Committee. MMWR Recomm Rep 2004;53:1–36.

39. Richards MJ, Edwards JR, Culver DH, Gaynes RP. Nosocomial infections in pediatric intensive care units in the United States. National Nosocomial Infections Surveillance System. Pediatrics 1999;103:e39.

40. Garrett DO, McKibben P, Levine G, Jarvis WR. Prevalence of nosocomial infections in pediatric intensive care unit patients at US Children's Hospitals [abstr]. Fourth Decennial International Conference on Nosocomial and Healthcare-Associated Infections March 5–9, 2000.

41. Fabregas N, Ewig S, Torres A, El-Ebiary M, Ramirez J, de la Bellacasa JP, Bauer T, Cabello H. Clinical diagnosis of ventilator associated pneumonia revisited: comparative validation using immediate post-mortem lung biopsies. Thorax 1999;54:867–873.

42. Andrews CP, Coalson JJ, Smith JD, Johanson WG Jr. Diagnosis of noso-comial bacterial pneumonia in acute, diffuse lung injury. Chest 1981;80:254–258.

43. Meduri GU, Wunderink RG, Leeper KV, Beals DH. Management of bacterial pneumonia in ventilated patients. Protected bronchoalveolar lavage as a diagnostic tool. Chest 1992;101:500–508.

44. Meduri GU. Diagnosis and differential diagnosis of ventilator-associated pneumonia. Clin Chest Med 1995;16:61–93.

45. Marquette CH, Georges H, Wallet F, Ramon P, Saulnier F, Neviere R, Mathieu D, Rime A, Tonnel AB. Diagnostic efficiency of endotracheal aspirates with quantitative bacterial cultures in intubated patients with suspected pneumonia. Comparison with the protected specimen brush. Am Rev Respir Dis 1993;148:138–144.

46. Kollef MH. The prevention of ventilator-associated pneumonia. N Engl J Med 1999;340:627–634.

47. Bryant RE, Salmon CJ. Pleural empyema. Clin Infect Dis 1996;22:747–762.

48. Antony VB, Mohammed KA. Pathophysiology of pleural space infections. Semin Respir Infect 1999;14:9–17.

49. Light RW, MacGregor MI, Luchsinger PC, Ball WC Jr. Pleural effusions: the diagnostic separation of transudates and exudates. Ann Intern Med 1972;77:507–513.

50. Heffner JE, Brown LK, Barbieri CA. Diagnostic value of tests that dis-criminate between exudative and transudative pleural effusions. Primary Study Investigators. Chest 1997;111:970–980.

51. Brook I. Microbiology of empyema in children and adolescents. Pedi-atrics 1990;85:722–726.

52. Chen CF, Soong WJ, Lee YS, Jeng MJ, Lin MY, Hwang B. Thoracic empyema in children: early surgical intervention hastens recovery. Acta Paediatr Taiwan 2003;44:93–97.

53. Light RW. Pleural diseases. Dis Mon 1992;38:261–331.

54. Barnes NP, Hull J, Thomson AH. Medical management of parapneu-monic pleural disease. Pediatr Pulmonol 2005;39:127–134.

55. Ray TL, Berkenbosch JW, Russo P, Tobias JD. Tissue plasminogen acti-vator as an adjuvant therapy for pleural empyema in pediatric patients. J Intensive Care Med 2004;19:44–50.

56. Ozcelik C, Ulku R, Onat S, Ozcelik Z, Inci I, Satici O. Management of postpneumonic empyemas in children. Eur J Cardiothorac Surg 2004;25:1072–1078.

57. Meier AH, Smith B, Raghavan A, Moss RL, Harrison M, Skarsgard E. Rational treatment of empyema in children. Arch Surg 2000;135:907–912.

58. Chen CY, Chen JS, Huang LM, Lee PI, Lu CY, Lee YC, Lu FL. Favorable outcome of parapneumonic empyema in children managed by primary video-assisted thoracoscopic debridement. J Formos Med Assoc 2003;102:845–850.

59. Schultz KD, Fan LL, Pinsky J, Ochoa L, Smith EO, Kaplan SL, Brandt ML. The changing face of pleural empyemas in children: epidemiology and management. Pediatrics 2004;113:1735–1740.

60. McLaughlin FJ, Goldmann DA, Rosenbaum DM, Harris GB, Schuster SR, Strieder DJ. Empyema in children: clinical course and long-term follow-up. Pediatrics 1984;73:587–593.

61. Iregui M, Ward S, Sherman G, Fraser VJ, Kollef MH. Clinical impor-tance of delays in the initiation of appropriate antibiotic treatment for ventilator-associated pneumonia. Chest 2002;122:262–268.

62. Confalonieri M, Urbino R, Potena A, Piattella M, Parigi P, Puccio G, Della PR, Giorgio C, Blasi F, Umberger R, et al. Hydrocortisone infusion for severe community-acquired pneumonia: a preliminary randomized study. Am J Respir Crit Care Med 2005;171:242–248.

18
Pediatric Lung Transplantation

David N. Cornfield and Imad Y. Haddad

Introduction

Since the initial report of lung transplantation in a human being in 1963 [1], incremental advances in surgical technique, immunology, organ procurement, and preservation have enabled lung transplantation to become increasingly accepted and employed as a viable therapeutic option to address end-stage lung disease in infants and children [2–5]. Throughout the world, more than 17,500 lung and heart–lung transplantations have been performed in adults [6], but only 1,200 lung and heart–lung transplantations have been performed in children [4]. The disparity between children and adults derives from the smaller number of children relative to adults in the general population as well as from the natural history of lung disease in children to improve with growth. Nonetheless, increasing success in the area of pediatric lung transplantation has prompted medical centers throughout the world to create and maintain programs in lung transplantation. At present there are approximately 25 medical centers in the United States that perform lung transplantation in any given year [4,5]. Consequently, many pediatric intensivists with relatively little prior clinical experience managing children after lung transplantation may be responsible for the care and management of children with newly transplanted lungs. The objective of this chapter is to outline and review the immediate postoperative care and acute clinical problems of children who have undergone lung transplantation.

Historical Perspective

The first lung transplantation, reported in 1963, although ethically compromised, was technically successful. The 58-year-old convicted felon recipient had metastatic bronchial carcinoma. The donor had experienced severe and substantial myocardial infarction, and consent for an autopsy, not an organ explantation, was procured. Renal failure was the proximate cause of death 18 days following transplantation [1]. In 1966, the first lobar lung transplantation was performed by Shinoi and colleagues at the Tokyo Medical College. The transplanted lobe remained in place for 18 days, providing essential pulmonary support during a period of time when the patient may have otherwise died from hypoxemia [7].

Throughout the 1970s, the promise of lung transplantation went unrealized, largely as a result of insufficient integrity of the bronchial anastomoses. Two separate but related changes in the approach to lung transplantation fundamentally altered the course of pediatric lung transplantation. First, the advent of a corticosteroid-sparing approach to perioperative immune suppression in lung transplantation dramatically decreased the incidence of dehiscence of the bronchial anastomoses [8,9]. The introduction of cyclosporine obviated the need for high-dose corticosteroid therapy. To further mitigate the potential of breakdown of the bronchial anastomoses, an innovative group of surgeons demonstrated that wrapping the omentum around the bronchial anastomoses led to the development of viable arterial circulation to the bronchus within 4 days after transplantation [9,10]. In recent years, pericardial tissue has been used with similar efficacy [11].

The refinement in surgical techniques and improved understanding of the immunobiology of graft–host interactions allowed for increased application of lung transplantation to the pediatric population. In recent years, approximately 60 children have undergone lung transplantation annually. Given that there are roughly 25 medical centers that perform pediatric lung transplantation, each center is performing an average of two to three procedures each year. Two-thirds of the children undergoing lung transplantation are between 11 and 17 years of age (Figure 18.1) [4–6].

In general, the most frequent indication for lung transplantation is cystic fibrosis (CF) (Table 18.1). One third of all children less than 10 years of age have undergone lung transplantation as a result of CF, but the number increases to almost 70% for children between ages 11 and 17 years [4]. However, improvement in the care of children with CF has decreased the need for lung transplantation in children. For children less than 1 year of age, congenital heart disease remains the leading indication for pediatric lung transplantation, followed by primary pulmonary hypertension and pulmonary vascular disease. Additional indications in the infant

D.S. Wheeler et al. (eds.), The *Respiratory Tract in Pediatric Critical Illness and Injury*,
DOI 10.1007/978-1-84800-925-7_18, © Springer-Verlag London Limited 2009

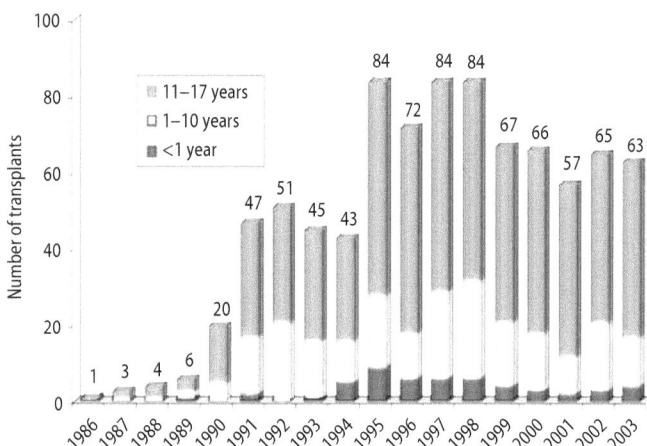

FIGURE 18.1. Age distribution of pediatric lung recipients by year of transplant from January 1986 to June 2003. (From Boucek et al. [4]. Copyright 2005 from International Society for Heart and Lung Transplantation. Reprinted with permission.)

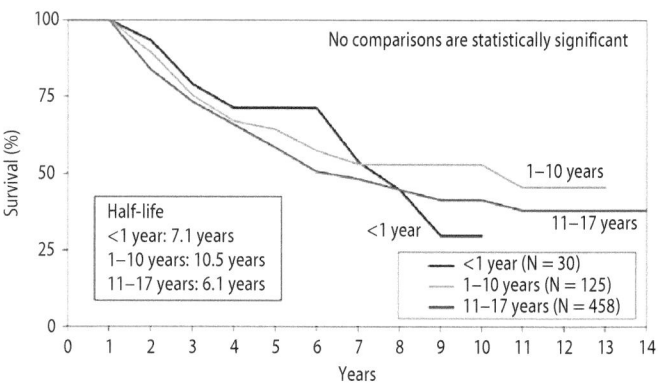

FIGURE 18.2. Kaplan-Meier survival curve of lung transplant recipients by age at time of transplant. (between January 1988 and June 2003). There is no difference in length of survival between eras. (From Boucek et al. [4]. Copyright 2005 from International Society for Heart and Lung Transplantation. Reprinted with permission.)

population include alveolar proteinosis, surfactant protein B deficiency, and interstitial pneumonias [4,5,12].

Despite recent improvements in clinical outcome, morbidity and mortality rates for patients undergoing lung transplantation remain high. Interestingly, when mortality rates from three different eras in pediatric lung transplantation are compared, there is no difference in mortality rate [4]. Fifty percent survival is 3.7 years for pediatric lung transplant recipients. However, when patients who died within the first year after transplant are removed from the analysis, 50% survival increases to 6.7 years (Figure 18.2) [13]. Survival is compromised by the development of bronchiolitis obliterans [14], which is associated with both acute and chronic rejection [13]. Within 5 years of the transplantation, less than 50% of transplant recipients are free from bronchiolitis obliterans (Figure 18.3). Hence, significant emphasis has been given to the identification of clinical tools to minimize both acute and chronic graft dysfunction is particularly important.

Surgical Approach

Currently, bilateral sequential lung transplant is the most frequently performed lung transplant procedure in children. The sequential procedure allows for each lung to be implanted separately and calls for a transthoracic approach via a *clamshell incision*. The main stem bronchi and left and right pulmonary arteries are connected via end-to-end anastomoses. Two pulmonary veins with intact atrial connections are harvested from each donor lung. Each left atrial patch is sewn onto the recipient heart. Among the advantages of the bilateral sequential lung transplantation is the ability to minimize cardiopulmonary bypass (CPB) time, thereby reducing CPB-related complications. The more optimal visualization of the pleural cavities afforded by the clamshell incision is of particular benefit for patients with pleural adhesions as a result of chronic inflammation as occurs in CF. Furthermore, the approach allows for another recipient to receive the heart, thereby benefiting at least two recipients from a single donor [2,3,15,16].

Although combined heart–lung transplantation had been a favored surgical approach, improved surgical techniques as well as the profound scarcity of donor organs have led to a dramatic decrease in the frequency of heart–lung transplantation. Throughout the 1990s, the number of patients undergoing heart–lung transplantation has steadily declined, with only 15 patients undergoing the procedure in 1999 [5]. Moreover, the recognition that right-sided heart failure associated with pulmonary hypertension resolves following lung transplantation has obviated the need for heart transplantation to address pulmonary hypertension [17,18].

TABLE 18.1. Leading indications for pediatric lung transplantations performed between January 1991 and June 2004.

Diagnosis	Age < 1 year	Age 1–10 year
Cystic fibrosis		72 (36.5%)
Primary pulmonary hypertension	7 (13.7%)	26 (13.2%)
Congenital heart disease	24 (47.1%)	21 (10.7%)
Idiopathic pulmonary fibrosis		12 (6.1%)
Pulmonary vascular disease	7 (13.7%)	6 (3.0%)
Re-transplant: non-obliterative bronchiolitis	3 (5.9%)	8 (4.1%)
Re-transplant: obliterative bronchiolitis		11 (5.6%)
Interstitial pneumonitis	3 (5.9%)	7 (3.6%)
Obliterative bronchiolitis (not re-transplant)		9 (4.6%)
Bronchiectasis		2 (1.0%)
Other	7 (13.7%)	23 (11.7%)

Source: Boucek et al. [4].

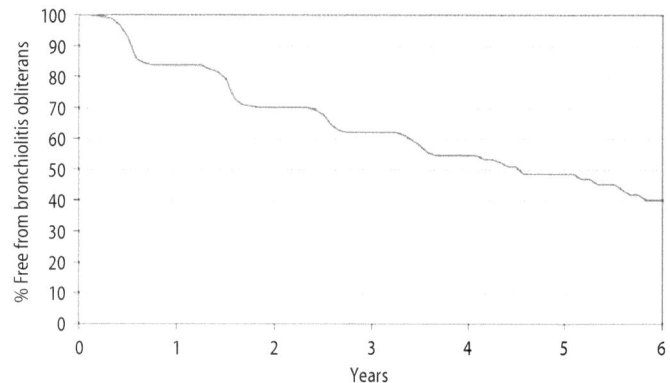

FIGURE 18.3. Freedom from bronchiolitis obliterans for pediatric lung recipients (follow-up: April 1994 to June 2004). (From Boucek et al. [4]. Copyright 2005 from International Society from Heart and Lung Transplantations Reprinted with permission.)

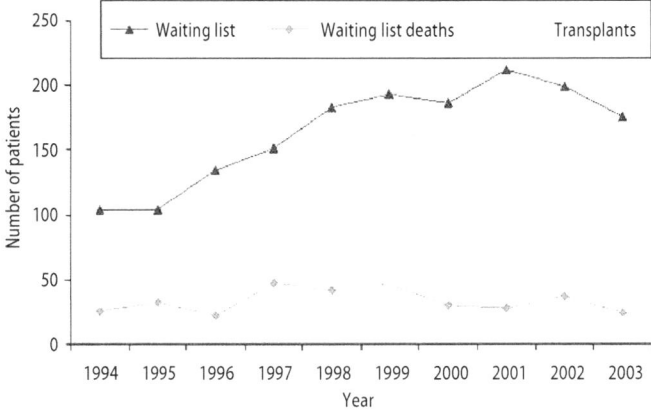

Figure 18.4. Number of pediatric patients waiting on list, transplanted, or dying on wait list from January 1994 to June 2003. (From Reproduce with permission from http://www. ustransplant.org/annual_reports/2004/figure_v_16.gif.)

In addition, the emergence of several medical therapies for pulmonary hypertension has led to a decrease in the number of patients undergoing lung transplantation to address pulmonary hypertension [19].

Single-lung transplantation is infrequently applied to the pediatric population [5]. Recent data indicate that the survival of patients undergoing single-lung transplantation is decreased compared with patients who undergo bilateral single-lung transplantation [4]. Moreover, given that the plurality of pediatric lung transplants are undertaken to address CF, single-lung transplantation would leave an immunosuppressed host with a significant bacterial burden in the native lung. Thus, both the transplanted lung and the patient would be at significant risk of infectious disease. Because the potential for growth of transplanted lung tissue remains unknown, providing a child with the greatest possible surface area for gas exchange might mitigate against the potential that no growth of the transplanted lungs occurs following transplantation.

Owing largely to the scarcity of donor organs, as reflected in the number of children dying while waiting for transplantation (Figure 18.4), living related donor transplantation has developed as a viable strategy for transplantation [20,21]. Since the advent of the technique, 240 people have received living related lobar lung transplantation (Transplantation Registry). Nationally, 38% of the recipients are children. Although the majority of the experience is in California (58%), there are only seven centers in the United States performing the procedure at present. In living related lobar lung transplantation, two separate donors undergo lower lobectomy. The lobes are implanted, becoming the right and left lungs of the recipient. It is essential that the size of the recipient be well matched to the donor lobes. An optimal size of the recipient is critical as lobes from an adult are generally too large for children younger than 7 years. Conversely, it is difficult to procure sufficient lung tissue from only two single lobes to satisfy the metabolic and ventilatory requirements of adolescents significantly taller than 65 inches [20,21]. Although the outcomes have been highly favorable, generally comparable with the outcomes in cadaveric transplantation, the very real risk that donors experience superimposed on the technical challenges associated with the procedure have prevented the procedure from being more widely adopted [22].

Pediatric Intensive Care Management

Immediate postoperative care is focused on careful respiratory and hemodynamic management. Pulmonary care in the perioperative period emphasizes reestablishment of functional residual capacity in the transplanted lung. Aggressive tracheobronchial toilet, chest physiotherapy, and even flexible bronchoscopy may play important roles in mobilizing secretions and ensuring patency of the airways and the integrity of the surgical anastomoses. Mechanical ventilation is generally necessary for less than 48 hr but may be prolonged in the event of graft dysfunction. To minimize oxygen-radical–related injury to the lungs, the fraction of inspired oxygen is rapidly decreased to <0.60 while maintaining systemic arterial saturation at 94% or greater. In determining a ventilator strategy, tidal volumes should be limited to <8 mL/kg and the plateau inspiratory pressure <30 cm H_2O [23]. The use of sufficient positive end-expiratory pressure to fully recruit and maintain the functional residual capacity of the newly transplanted lungs is of critical importance. Inhalational nitric oxide has been shown to improve oxygenation in the presence of acute graft dysfunction, likely as a result of enhanced ventilation and perfusion matching. Recent data suggest that perioperative use of inhaled nitric oxide may decrease the incidence of acute rejection in the initial 28 days after transplantation, implying that inhalational nitric oxide may have an immune modulatory role [24].

Hemodynamic status must be closely monitored. Vascular permeability and myocardial function may be adversely affected by cardiopulmonary bypass, necessitating inotropic support in the perioperative period. Hemodynamic instability may be exacerbated by diminished intravascular volume, even in the presence of an increase in total body water as low serum oncotic pressure may be present owing to the compromised nutritional status of the recipients before transplantation. Central venous pressure monitoring is beneficial in order to optimize cardiac output. In managing patients postoperatively, early recognition of compromised renal function is essential, as the prescription of all medications excreted and metabolized by the kidneys will need to be promptly altered.

Recipients may experience early and severe graft dysfunction. Early graft dysfunction may result from injury to the donor organ because of prolonged ischemic time, exaggerated reperfusion injury, or lung injury that occurred before organ harvest. The incidence of early graft dysfunction is estimated to be between 10% and 35%. The clinical presentation of early graft dysfunction is entirely consistent with noncardiogenic pulmonary edema or acute respiratory distress syndrome as manifested by elevated alveolar-arteriolar gradient, compromised pulmonary parenchymal compliance, ventilation and perfusion inequality, and subsequent hypoxemia caused by intrapulmonary shunting and/or impaired diffusion. Biopsy of the transplanted organ is likely to reveal diffuse alveolar damage. Experience at several transplant centers suggests that most grafts will recover if the recipient can be supported for a sufficient period of time. Treatment entails optimal ventilator management as well as diuretic support in an effort to minimize total body water. Hence, in the face of severe graft dysfunction, extracorporeal membrane oxygenation has been employed as a therapeutic modality [25]. Recent data indicate that inclusion of nitric oxide donors in the preservation solution or exposure to inhaled nitric oxide before organ harvest may decrease the incidence of acute graft dysfunction [26,27]. In addition, recent data demonstrate that low-potassium–

containing dextran preservative solutions mitigate against the development of severe reperfusion injury [28].

The postoperative course is not infrequently complicated by technical problems associated with the surgery. At many centers the patency of the airway anastomoses is routinely assessed within 24 hr of return to the pediatric intensive care unit with flexible bronchoscopy. Whereas the vascular anastomoses are more difficult to assess, arterial anastomoses are generally amenable to inspection with nuclear medicine studies. To assess the venous anastomoses, transesophageal echocardiography may be necessary. Despite the need to attend to these issues, postoperative bleeding remains the most frequent cause for reoperation [16].

Vocal cord paresis and diaphragmatic paresis can be potential complications of virtually any major thoracic surgery. However, the clinical symptoms entailed by these issues are generally not apparent until after extubation. Although it is unusual for these injuries to occur concomitantly, both derive from injuries to the nerve at the time of surgery. Vocal cord paralysis or paresis results from recurrent injury to the laryngeal nerve, and phrenic nerve injury leads to diaphragmatic paralysis or paresis [29]. The likelihood of phrenic nerve injury seems to be increased in patients who have had prior thoracic surgery, although most of these injuries resolve within several weeks of surgery [30]. In the event that hemidiaphragmatic function is severely compromised, as evidenced by paradoxical movement with inspiration and atelectasis shortly after extubation, serious consideration should be given to early diaphragmatic plication as the risk of infection in the affected lung is quite high [31]. Vocal cord paresis or paralysis is difficult to assess in the periextubation period as it may take several days for vocal cord function to be fully replete following removal of a tracheal tube even in the absence of true injury to the vocal cords or recurrent laryngeal nerve injury. Thus, definitive treatment decisions should be deferred until vocal function evaluation can be performed at least 72 hr after extubation [29].

Immunobiology

Acute cellular rejection of the transplanted lungs occurs in almost two thirds of children who undergo lung transplantation. The clinical manifestations of rejection include fever, dyspnea, and hypoxia. Chest radiograph findings are relatively nonspecific but include perihilar infiltrates and effusions. Pulmonary function testing indicates increasing air flow obstruction. The distinction between infection and rejection generally requires bronchoscopic evaluation wherein bronchoalveolar lavage and transbronchial biopsies are performed. Transbronchial biopsies are obtained from only a single lung as the risk of pneumothorax is not insubstantial. Adequate evaluation for the potential of rejection mandates the procurement of approximately 12 specimens from at least two lobes of an ipsilateral lung [32]. Histologic evaluation of the specimens leads to the assignment of a grade, with A0 indicating an absence of rejection. Grade A4 indicates severe rejection [33]. Perivascular lymphocytic infiltration is the histologic hallmark of rejection, but, with more severe rejection, the airways demonstrate significant inflammatory infiltration. The clear relationship between acute rejection episodes and the development of bronchiolitis obliterans mandates treatment for such occurrences even in the absence of overt signs and symptoms of rejection [34].

Induction in the perioperative period with either a cytolytic agent or an interleuken-2 receptor antagonist has been shown to diminish the likelihood of rejection episodes [35]. Acute rejection generally mandates treatment with high-dose intravenous corticosteroid treatment. The response to therapy is rapid, with evidence of clinical improvement within days. Standard dosing is intravenous methylprednisolone at a dose of 10–15 mg/kg for 3–5 days. The dose is rapidly tapered over a 3-week time period. Subjective improvement occurs with diminished dyspnea. Objective evidence of improvement includes improved oxygenation, increases in pulmonary function, and resolution of infiltrates on chest radiograph. Should rejection persist despite steroid therapy, treatment is undertaken with monoclonal antibodies. The incidence of acute rejection is greatest in the first 6 months following transplantation and diminishes progressively over time.

Infectious Diseases

The lungs are in continuous contact with the environment and are therefore readily accessible as a portal of entry for infectious pathogens. Normally, mobilization of secretions, the mucociliary clearance, cough, and both cellular and molecular defense mechanisms prevent invasive infection. However, the compromised immune function superimposed on the difficulties in mobilizing secretions in the perioperative lung transplant recipient predisposes to infection. The pharmacologically induced compromise in immune function renders any infection life threatening. Thus, the index of suspicion for infection must be high and the threshold for initiating broad-spectrum antibiotic therapy low. The similarities in the signs and symptoms for both rejection and infection mandate liberal use of bronchoscopy to distinguish between these two alternatives [36]. Even in the absence of transbronchial biopsies, bronchoalveolar lavage can be helpful to preclude infection [37].

As opportunistic infections in the lung transplant population are particularly problematic, prophylactic treatment with antiviral and anti-*Pneumocystis carinii* therapeutic agents has become a standard component of infection. Prophylactic treatment with ganciclovir has been adopted by some transplant centers [38]. However, whether such strategies diminish the incidence of bronchiolitis obliterans or result in antiviral resistant infections is not known. With the advent of gene-based diagnostic modalities, and the corresponding enhancement in diagnostic sensitivity, treatment has become more focused. Despite effective antiviral therapy, cytomegalovirus infection remains a source of both morbidity and mortality. Cytomegalovirus infection is associated with an increased incidence of both acute and chronic rejection.

Aspergillosis is a particularly problematic infectious pathogen in the pediatric lung transplant population [39]. A significant number of children with cystic fibrosis, the majority of all children undergoing lung transplantation, are colonized with aspergillosis. Many of the children with cystic fibrosis and aspergillosis have allergic bronchopulmonary aspergillosis (ABPA). In the patients with CF, ABPA is treated with steroids because, if left unchecked, it leads to central saccular bronchiectasis and air flow obstruction. However, in the presence of immune compromise, aspergillosis can become invasive, resulting in disseminated infection that can manifest in the lungs, brain, or other solid organs [40]. Thus, consideration should be given to treating children colonized with *Aspergillus* with antifungal therapy before transplantation [41] in order to diminish the infectious burden and thereby mitigate the likelihood of disseminated infection in the perioperative period when immune suppression is most vigorous [42].

Neurologic Compromise

Following lung transplantation, patients generally return to the pediatric intensive care unit intubated and mechanically ventilated. While mechanical ventilation is ongoing, high-dose opiates are used for analgesia and benzodiazepines for amnestic properties in the perioperative period. As drug metabolism is often altered in the perioperative period because of compromised renal function and low total body protein levels, the effects of these agents on the central nervous system may be exaggerated. The assessment of neurologic status may therefore be more complicated. In addition, the agents most responsible for modulating immune function, the calcineurin phosphatase inhibitors FK 506 and cyclosporine, cause cerebral vasoconstriction and may possess idiosyncratic effects on the central nervous system that include tremors, seizures, an altered level of consciousness, and even obtundation [43]. Magnetic resonance imaging studies demonstrate characteristic findings. Interestingly, although the neurologic toxicity is attributed to the calcineurin phosphatase inhibitors, no linear relationship between the serum levels of the agents and neurologic toxicity has been demonstrated [44]. Nonetheless, the presence of neurologic toxicity mandates a change from one agent to the other. There is no consensus on the need to treat with anticonvulsant therapy. The determination to do so is contingent on the overall clinical presentation.

Post-Transplant Lymphoproliferative Disease

Post-transplant lymphoproliferative disease (PTLD) is a serious, sometimes fatal complication that occurs following lung transplantation. Primary Epstein-Barr virus (EBV) infection represents a major risk factor for the development of PTLD following lung transplantation, as seroconversion significantly increases the risk for PTLD [45]. Recent data support the use of prophylactic antiviral therapy in seronegative patients. Given that children are likely to be seronegative at the time of transplantation, timely initiation of prophylactic antiviral therapy may be of great benefit [46]. Clinically, PTLD may present as lymphadenopathy, fever, malaise, or as mass lesions. Diagnosis can be directed with quantitative polymerase chain reactions, EBV titers, and biopsy of lymph nodes or affected tissues. Treatment includes a reduction in immune suppression and the initiation of monoclonal antibodies designed to specifically target CD20 surface markers on B cells [47]. Patients treated with diminished immune suppression in concert with anti-CD20 antibodies have achieved remission in a relatively short time frame, thereby mitigating the risk to the graft and minimizing the infectious risks necessarily entailed by chemotherapy.

Drug Interactions

In the perioperative period, most pediatric lung transplant recipients are being treated with multiple medications. In initiating or discontinuing therapy, careful consideration must be undertaken to ensure that unintended consequences do not accrue. This is especially true in the context of medications that are metabolized via the cytochrome P450 pathway in the liver. Macrolide antibiotics, oral antifungal agents, and antiepileptic agents will have

significant effects on the metabolism of both tacrolimus and cyclosporine [48]. Moreover, standard measures of renal function may provide unjustified reassurance as glomerular filtration rate may be significantly diminished despite relatively normal serum levels of blood urea nitrogen and creatinine [49]. Given that children undergoing lung transplantation have been chronically ill for many years before the transplantation, the presence of compromised renal function is not surprising. Accordingly, treatment with nephrotoxic agents must be undertaken with careful consideration.

Conclusion

Lung transplantation is an increasingly well-accepted treatment for children with end-stage lung disease resulting from many causes. Improved surgical technique has brought transplantation to a broader set of patients. The advent of living related lung transplant programs holds the promise that lung transplantation will be more readily available in the future than has been the case in the past. Nonetheless, long-term survival rates remain significantly lower than for transplantation of other solid organs. In order for lung transplantation to realize its full promise, better understanding of and treatment for chronic rejection and bronchiolitis obliterans must be realized. Notwithstanding such limitations, lung transplantation has demonstrated progressively improved outcomes. With ongoing and incremental improvements in care, lung transplantation is likely to become more frequent and available at more centers in the future than has been the case in the past. As such, providers of pediatric critical care will need to be even more familiar with the nuances of care surrounding the child undergoing lung transplantation than has been the case in the past.

References

1. Hardy J, Webb W, Dalton M, Walker G. Lung homotransplantations in man. JAMA 1963;186:99–108.
2. Starnes V, Marshall S, Lewiston N, Theodore J, Stinson E, Shumway N. Heart-lung transplantation in infants, children, and adolescents. J Pediatr Surg 1991;26:434–438.
3. Spray T, Mallory G, Canter C, Huddleston C. Pediatric lung transplantation. J Thorac Cardiovasc Surg 1994;107:990–1000.
4. Boucek MM, Edwards LB, Keck BM, Trulock EP, Taylor DO, Hertz MI. Registry of the International Society for Heart and Lung Transplantation: eighth official pediatric report-2005. J Heart Lung Transplant 2005;24(8):968–982.
5. Boucek MM, Edwards LB, Keck BM, Trulock EP, Taylor DO, Hertz MI. Pediatric Registry Report, Registry for the International Society for Heart and Lung Transplantation: seventh official pediatric report—2004. J Heart Lung Transplant 2004;23:933–947.
6. Hertz MI, Taylor DO, Trulock EP, Boucek MM, Mohacsi PJ, Edwards LB, et al. The Registry of the International Society for Heart and Lung Transplantation: nineteenth official report—2002. J Heart Lung Transplantation 2002;21(9):950–970.
7. Mendeloff EN. The history of pediatric heart and lung transplantation. Pediatric Transplantation 2002;4(6):270–279.
8. Goldberg M, Lima O, Morgan E, et al. A comparison between cyclosporine A and methylprednisolone plus azathioprine on bronchial healing following canine lung transplantation. J Thorac Cardiovasc Surg 1983; 85:821–826.
9. Cooper J, Pearson F, Patterson G, Todd T, Ginsberg R, Goldberg M. Technique of successful lung transplantation in humans. J Thorac Cardiovasc Surg 1987;93(2):173–181.

10. Lima O, Goldberg M, Peters WJ, et al. Bronchial omentopexy in canine lung allotransplantation. J Thorac Cardiovasc Surg 1982;83(3):418–421.

11. Pasque MK, Cooper JD, Kaiser LR, Haydock DA, Triantofillou A, Trulock EP. Improved technique for bilateral lung transplantation: rationale and clinical experience. Ann Thorac Surg 1990;49(5):785–791.

12. Sweet S, Spray T, Huddleston C, Mendeloff E, Canter C, Balzer D. Pediatric lung transplantation in St. Louis Children's Hospital, 1990–1995. Am J Respir Crit Care Med 1997;155(3):1027–1035.

13. Boucek MM, Edwards LB, Keck BM, Trulock EP, Taylor DO, Hertz MI. Registry for the International Society for Heart and Lung Transplantation: seventh official pediatric report—2004. J Heart Lung Transplant. 2004;23(8):933–947.

14. Kurland G, Michelson P. Bronchiolitis obliterans in children. Pediatr Pulmonol 2005;39(3):193–208.

15. Bolman R, Shumway SJ, Estrin JA, Hertz MI. Lung and heart-lung transplantation. Evolution and new applications. Ann Surg 1991;214(4):456–468.

16. Arcasoy SM, Kotloff RM. Lung transplantation [review]. N Engl J Med 1999;340:1081–1091.

17. Pasque M, Trulock E, Cooper J, Triantifillou A, Huddleston C, Rosenbloom M, et al. Single lung transplantation for pulmonary hypertension. Single institution experience in 54 patients. Circulation 1995;92(8):2252–2258.

18. Ivy D. Diagnosis and treatment of severe pediatric pulmonary hypertension. Cardiol Rev 2001;9(4):227–237.

19. Rosenzweig E, Widlitz A, Barst R. Pulmonary arterial hypertension in children. Pediatr Pulmonol 2004;38(1):2–22.

20. Starnes VA, Barr ML, Cohen RG. Lobar transplantation: indications, technique, and outcome. J Thorac Cardiovasc Surg 1994;108(3):403–410.

21. Starnes VA, Woo MS, MacLaughlin EF, Horn MV, Wong PC, Rowland JM, et al. Comparison of outcomes between living donor and cadaveric lung transplantation in children. Ann Thorac Surg 1999;68(6):2279–2283.

22. Woo MS, MacLaughlin EF, Horn MV, Wong PC, Rowland JM, Barr ML, et al. Living donor lobar lung transplantation: the pediatric experience. Pediatric Transplantation 1998;2(3):185–190.

23. Frank J, Mathay M. Science review: mechanisms of ventilator induced injury. Crit Care 2003;7(3):233–241.

24. Cornfield DN, Milla CE, Barbato JE, Haddad IY, Park S. Inhaled nitric decreases acute graft rejection in the first 28 days after lung transplantation. J Heart Lung Transplant 2003;22(8):903–907.

25. Meyers BF, Sundt III TM, Henry S, Trulock EP, Guthrie T, Cooper JD, et al. Selective use of extracorporeal membrane oxygenation is warranted after lung transplantation. J Cardiovasc Surg 2000;120(1):20–26.

26. Fujino S, Nagahiro AN, Triantafillou AN, Boasquevisque CH, Yano M, et al. Inhaled nitric oxide at the time of harvest improves early graft function. Ann Thorac Surg 1997;63:1383–1389.

27. Fujino S, Nagahiro I, Yamashita M, Yano M, Schmid R, et al. Preharvest nitroprusside flush improves posttransplantation lung function. J Heart Lung Transplant 1997;16:1073–1080.

28. Fischer S, Matte-Martyn A, De Perrot M, Waddell TK, Sekine Y, Hutcheon M, et al. Low-potassium Dextran preservation solution improves lung function after human lung transplantation. J Thorac Cardiovasc Surg 2001;121(3):594–596.

29. Fan LL, Campbell DN, Clarke DR, Washington RL, et al. Paralyzed left vocal cord associated with ligation of patent ductus arteriosus. J Thorac Cardiovasc Surg 1989;98(4):611–613.

30. Grocott HP, Clark JA, Homi HM, Sharma A. "Other" neurologic complications after cardiac surgery. Semin Cardiothorac Vasc Anesth 2004;8(3):213–226.

31. de Leeuw M, Williams JM, Freedom RM, Williams WG, Shemie SD, McCrindle BW. Impact of diaphragmatic paralysis after cardiothoracic surgery in children. J Thorac Cardiovasc Surg 1999;118(3):510–517.

32. Hopkins PM, Aboyoun CL, Chhajed PN, Malouf MA, Plit ML, Rainer SP, et al. Prospective analysis of 1,235 transbronchial lung biopsies in lung transplant recipients. J Heart Lung Transplant 2002;21(10):1062–1067.

33. Yousem S, Berry GJ, Cagle PT, Chamberlain D, Husain AN, Hruban RH, et al. A revision of the 1990 Working Formulation for the classification of pulmonary allograft rejection: Lung Rejection Study Group (LRSG). J Heart Lung Transplant 1996;15:1–15.

34. Sharples LD, McNeil K, Stewart S, Wallwork J. Risk factors for bronchiolitis obliterans: a systematic review of recent publications. J Heart Lung Transplant 2002;21(2):271–281.

35. Brock MV, Borja MC, Ferber L, Orens JB, Anzcek RA, Krishnan J, et al. Induction therapy in lung transplantation: a prospective, controlled clinical trial comparing OKT3, anti-thymocyte globulin, and daclizumab. J Heart Lung Transplant 2001;20(12):1282–1290.

36. Higenbottam T, Stewart S, Penketh A, Wallwork J. The diagnosis of lung rejection and opportunistic infection by transbronchial lung biopsy. Transplant Proc 1987;19(5):3777–3778.

37. Guilinger RA, Paradis IL, Dauber JH, Yousem SA, Williams PA, Keenan RJ, et al. The importance of bronchoscopy with transbronchial biopsy and bronchoalveolar lavage in the management of lung transplant recipients. Am J Respir Crit Care Med 1995;152(6 Pt 1):2037–2043.

38. Perreas KG, McNeil K, Charman S, Sharples LD, Wreghitt T, Wallwork J. Extended ganciclovir prophylaxis in lung transplantation. J Heart Lung Transplant 2005;24(5):583–587.

39. Dummer JS, Lazariashvilli N, Barnes J, Ninan M, Milstone AP. A survey of anti-fungal management in lung transplantation. J Heart Lung Transplant 2004;23(12):1376–1381.

40. Nunley DR, Ohori P, Grgurich WF, Iacono AT, Williams PA, Keenan RJ, et al. Pulmonary aspergillosis in cystic fibrosis lung transplant recipients. Chest 1998;114(5):1321–1329.

41. Avery RK. Prophylactic strategies before solid-organ transplantation. Curr Opin Infect Dis 2004;17:(4):353–356.

42. Minari A, Husni R, Avery RK, Longworth DL, DeCamp M, Bertin M, et al. The incidence of invasive aspergillosis among solid organ transplant recipients and implications for prophylaxis in lung transplants. Transpl Infect Dis 2002;4(4):195–200.

43. Wong M, Mallory GJ, Goldstein J, Goyal M, Yamada K. Neurologic complications of pediatric lung transplantation. Neurology 1999;53(7):1542–1549.

44. Menegaux F, Keefe E, Andrews B. Neurological complications of liver transplantation in adult versus pediatric liver transplant recipients. Transplantation 1994;58(4):447–450.

45. Davis JE, Sherritt MA, Bharadwaj M, Morrison LE, Elliott SL, Kear LM, et al. Determining virological, serological and immunological parameters of EBV infection in the development of PTLD. Int Immunol 2004;16(7):983–989.

46. Malouf MA, Chhajed PN, Hopkins P, Plit M, Turner J, Glanville AR. Anti-viral prophylaxis reduces the incidence of lymphoproliferative disease in lung transplant recipients. J Heart Lung Transplant 2002;21(5):547–554.

47. Pescovitz MD. The use of rituximab, anti-CD20 monoclonal antibody, in pediatric transplantation. Pediatr Transplant 2004;8(1):9–21.

48. Buckhart G, Canafax D, Yee G. Cyclosporine monitoring. Drug Intel Clin Pharmacol 1986;20(9):649–652.

49. Hellerstein S, Alon U, Warady BA. Creatinine for estimation of glomerular filtration rate. Pediatr Nephrol 1992;6(6):507–511.

19
Neuromuscular Respiratory Failure

Margaret F. Guill and Thomas P. Shanley

Introduction

Chronic respiratory failure is the expected outcome of many congenital neuromuscular disorders, including muscular dystrophy and spinal muscular atrophy. Early in the management process for these diseases, shortly after confirmation of the diagnosis, discussion should begin with parents and guardians about long-term expectations and plans for handling end-of-life issues. Ideally, end-of-life circumstances for these patients, as the disease takes its inexorable toll, are handled outside the critical care setting by appropriate preplanning. However, intercurrent illness may affect respiratory function more dramatically in these children than in others and require acute intervention with the expectation of some degree of reversibility and return to the baseline state. Also, appropriate decisions may not have been made previously in these children to prevent the need for urgent respiratory support, necessitating that this support be provided in the setting of the pediatric intensive care unit (PICU). As a result, it is imperative for PICU staff to familiarize themselves with the mechanisms underlying neuromuscular respiratory failure as well as the therapeutic support applicable to this patient population.

Therapeutic Principles

Management of patients with progressive neuromuscular disease has been improved with the institution of greater options for mechanical support, especially noninvasive strategies. As a result, noninvasive support measures such as mask bilevel positive airway pressure or chest cuirass for negative pressure ventilation are the preferred means of support for patients with chronic progressive neuromuscular disease when possible. Additionally, strict atten-

tion to airway clearance will aid in the prevention or delay of respiratory failure in these chronically ill patients who usually have an ineffective cough. Manual percussion and postural drainage with deep suction can be beneficial. The use of a mechanical in–exsufflator (cough assist device) has been found to be helpful in improving airway clearance. In a retrospective study of 62 children with neuromuscular disease who used the mechanical in–exsufflator in the home setting, 90% found it to be effective in promoting airway clearance and preventing atelectasis and pneumonia [1]. This device has been demonstrated to potentially aid physicians and respiratory therapy staff in successfully weaning such patients from mechanical ventilatory support. Bach et al. have reported successful use of a protocol-driven approach to extubation in spinal muscular atrophy type 1 (SMA-1) patients using a combination of the mechanical in–ex-sufflator and nasal positive pressure ventilation [2,3] A similar protocol has been reported for patients with Duchenne muscular dystrophy (DMD) [4]. In either circumstance, strict attention to airway clearance is the most important goal for preventing respiratory failure or aiding the recovery from an episode of respiratory failure in patients with chronic neuromuscular disorders.

The decision to move from noninvasive ventilation to tracheal intubation for treatment of an acute event must be made with the understanding that there is a strong possibility of long-term ventilator dependence and tracheotomy for patients with progressive neuromuscular disease. In a questionnaire study of pediatric intensivists, physiatrists, and neurologists regarding attitudes about intervention for acute respiratory distress in a child with SMA-1, there was a wide variation in practice among specialties. Intensivists and neurologists were more likely than physiatrists to support noninvasive mechanical ventilation (NIMV) for both acute and chronic management, whereas physiatrists were more likely to support tracheal intubation/tracheostomy for these patients and less likely to promote comfort care only [5]. In another retrospective study of 56 SMA-1 children with respiratory failure presenting before 2 years of age, outcomes were compared for three groups: 16 children with tracheostomy, 33 children with nocturnal NIMV and cough assist plus tracheal intubation for acute infections, and 7 children who died of respiratory failure after tracheal intubation or tracheostomy was rejected [3]. Those children with tracheostomies had fewer hospitalizations before the age of 3 years, but this group also had more hospitalizations after the age of 5 years compared with those children using NIMV. Fifteen of the children with

D.S. Wheeler et al. (eds.), The *Respiratory Tract in Pediatric Critical Illness and Injury*,
DOI 10.1007/978-1-84800-925-7_19, © Springer-Verlag London Limited 2009

tracheostomies required full mechanical ventilatory support 24 hr per day. Those using NIMV had fewer hospitalizations after age 5 years and were more likely to be support-free during waking hours, although 3 of the 31 children in this group who survived beyond 13 months required virtually continuous NIMV. The seven children in the third group died at 5–13 months of age when either the family rejected support or it was not offered [3]. Thus, differing approaches to support provide both advantages and disadvantages over time, so that decisions must be made with the family understanding the dynamic consequences of any therapeutic plan.

Anatomy

Chest Wall

The chest wall consists of respiratory muscles, supportive connective tissue, and the rib cage. The bony structures of the thorax are a framework of ribs, sternum, and vertebral column. There are three groups of muscles of respiration: the diaphragm, the intercostal and accessory muscles, and the abdominal muscles. When contracted, the respiratory muscles enlarge the thoracic cavity and push the abdominal structures downward, thus decreasing the intrathoracic pressure and creating a pressure gradient between the mouth and the lower airway for initiation of air flow [6,7].

Diaphragm

The diaphragm, which is a skeletal muscle under both voluntary and autonomic control, has a crucial role in inspiration. This dome-shaped muscle is attached to the lower ribs and acts as a piston. The primary function of the diaphragm is to support inspiration by expanding the rib cage [6–9]. During normal quiet breathing the diaphragm moves approximately 1–2 cm; however, on forced expiration and at times of increased respiratory demand, the diaphragmatic excursion can be as much as 10 cm. There is some activity of the diaphragm during the early part of expiration (braking action). The innervation of the diaphragm is supplied by the phrenic nerve, which originates from C3–C5 spine segments [7–9]. Injury to the innervation of the diaphragm resulting in either paresis or paralysis causes it to move paradoxically with an upward excursion as opposed to its normal downward movement.

Intercostal and Accessory Muscles

The external intercostal muscles and the interchondral portion of the internal intercostal muscles are inspiratory in nature as their contraction works to elevate the rib cage. The internal intercostal muscles are expiratory as they contract the lower ribs and pull down the anterior part of the lower chest. The innervation of the intercostal muscles is supplied from the first through twelfth thoracic segments [6–8]. The accessory muscles of breathing consist of the scalene (anterior, medial, and posterior) and sternomastoid muscles. Both of these muscle groups have inspiratory function, and they are used at times of increased need (e.g., coughing, exercise, and sneezing) or in pathologic states necessitating increased work of breathing (e.g., asthma exacerbation). There are other muscles that contribute to respiration (ala nasi, upper airway muscles), especially at times of increased demand [7–11]. In certain pathologic states, discoordination of the diaphragm and upper airway muscles occurs and results in the occlusion of upper airway muscles during inspiration to cause obstructive apnea.

Abdominal Muscles

The abdominal muscles utilized during respiratory effort include the rectus abdominus, external and internal oblique muscles, transverse abdominus, and internal intercostal muscles. These muscles are stimulated during the active expiration that occurs with coughing, exercise, and speech, as well as during periods of increased mechanical load, as with acute asthma [6–9].

Force–Length Relationship

Active force is developed as a function of the length of the muscle. Maximal force is generated at the muscle's resting length [7–12]. Any excessive shortening or lengthening of the muscle results in the generation of suboptimal force. When the lungs inflate, inspiratory muscles shorten and expiratory muscles lengthen. As lung volume increases, maximal inspiratory pressure decreases whereas maximal expiratory pressure increases. Hyperinflation of the lungs, frequently seen in diseases associated with airway obstruction, flattens the diaphragm and decreases the ability to generate force. Under this circumstance, the diaphragm is less productive and operates at a mechanical disadvantage [8–12]. The force generated by a respiratory muscle is also a function of the stimulation of the muscle fiber and the velocity of fiber shortening. Force generation increases as muscle stimulation increases to a plateau, after which there is no further increase in force regardless of stimulus frequency. Thus, in the setting of abnormal innervations as is the underlying defect in neuromuscular diseases, muscle shortening is significantly attenuated.

Elastic Properties of the Chest Wall

The interactions between the lung and the chest wall are complex. The tendency of the lung to collapse (inward) is counterbalanced by the outward pull of the chest wall. Functional residual capacity (FRC) in healthy individuals denotes the volume in the lungs at the point where the outward recoil of the chest wall is in equilibrium with the inward recoil of the lungs and occurs at the completion of a normal expiration. At this lung volume no respiratory muscles are contracted [10–13]. The slope of each curve at any given volume represents the compliance at that volume (change of volume per unit pressure). The elastic recoil pressure of the lungs at any given volume differs from the elastic recoil pressure of the chest wall. The sum of these two system compliances denotes the total respiratory system compliance (Figure 19.1 and text below). The static compliance slope (change of volume per unit pressure at no flow) for the respiratory system depends also on body position. This is primarily because of a change in chest wall elastic recoil compliance and the effect of gravity on the diaphragm while lung elastic recoil remains essentially the same. When an individual is in the supine position, the abdominal contents are pushing against the diaphragm and the outward recoil of the chest wall is diminished, resulting in diminished FRC. Therefore, FRC in an individual differs whether the individual is in a sitting or a supine position [10,12]. This change in FRC becomes prominent in conditions such as obesity. Furthermore, respiratory muscle input is sleep stage dependent and differs in wakefulness. In non-REM sleep there is a mild decrease in upper

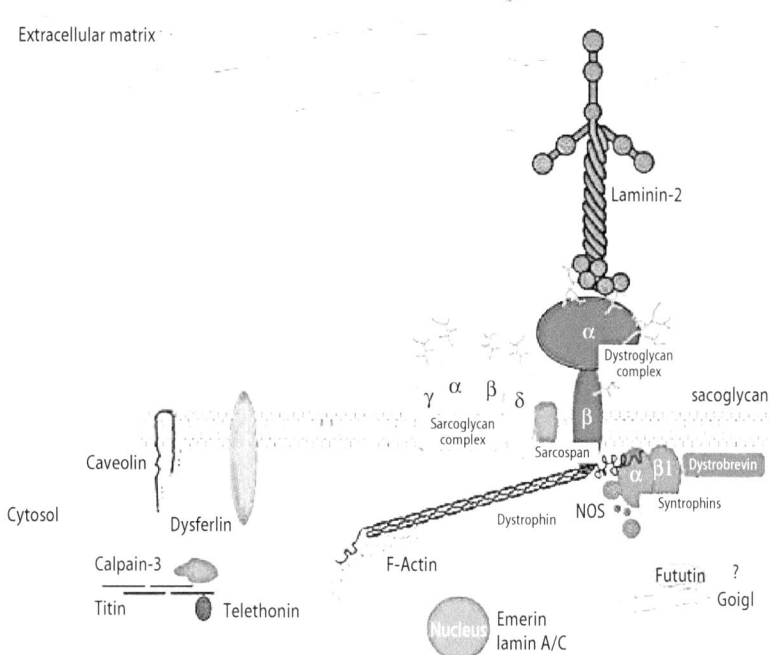

FIGURE 19.1. The dystrophin-associated protein complex in muscle linking the internal cytoskeleton to the extracellular matrix. The DAPC is comprised of sarcoplasmic proteins (α-dystrobrevin, syntrophins and nitric oxide synthase), transmembrane proteins (β-dystroglycan, the sarcoglycan complex, caveolin and dysferin) and extracellular proteins (α-dystroglycan and laminin-2). The amino terminus of dystrophin attaches to F-actin myofilament of skeletal muscle while the carboxy terminus anchors to the sarcolemmal membrane via the dystroglycan complex. Attachment to the extracellular matrix by the dystroglycan complex is mediated by laminin-2. The DAPC is essential in providing a mechanical link between the intracellular cytoskeleton and the extracellular matrix. As a result, the loss of sarcolemmal integrity that results from expression of a mutant, non-functional protein of the DAPC causes muscle fibres to be more susceptible to damage over time and long-term development of weakness associated with muscular dystrophies. (Adapted from Gilchrist [65]).

airway muscle tone and tonic activity of the intercostals, resulting in an increase in upper airway resistance. More changes occur during REM sleep where marked reduction/absence of phasic activity correlates with bursts of rapid eye movements [14]. As is discussed later, changes in the normal chest wall elastic recoil compliance related to underlying neuromuscular diseases can have a profound impact on respiratory function.

Growth and Development

The chest wall, and as a result the whole respiratory system, undergoes complex changes from infancy to adulthood. Specific developmental characteristics of the respiratory system in infants place them at a mechanical disadvantage and at an increased risk for respiratory pump failure [15]. The infant chest wall is highly compliant because of poorly mineralized bone and increased amount of soft cartilage. Chest wall compliance is approximately three to six times that of the lung. In premature infants, chest wall compliance is even higher than in term infants. Chest wall compliance decreases gradually during the first 2 years of life [15–18]. This overall picture is advantageous during birth as it allows the fetus to more easily traverse the birth canal; however, the increased compliance of the infant chest wall may become a functional disadvantage at times of increased mechanical load on the respiratory system. Ossification of the chest wall begins in utero and continues until age 25 [18]. With aging, there is a progressive calcification of the costal cartilages and a change in the elastic properties of the lungs. Total respiratory compliance decreases as the child grows, primarily because of this decrease in the chest wall compliance.

The configuration of the chest wall in infants also differs from that in adults and imposes an additional risk factor for respiratory failure and respiratory pump inefficiency. The hallmark of the infant rib cage is its horizontal orientation and the horizontal position of the diaphragm. By age 10 years the adult pattern of caudal orientation is achieved [14,15,18].

The percentage of muscle fibers differs among adults and full-term and premature infants. With growth, changes occur in the composition, innervation, and mass of muscle fibers. In full-term infants there are approximately 30% of these fibers and only 10% in premature infants. The number of fatigue-resistant fibers increases and reaches adult levels by 1 year of age [19], such that 50%–60% of muscle fibers are composed of fatigue-resistant, slow-twitch, high-oxidative type 1 fibers by adulthood. In addition, higher metabolic rate, immature respiratory control, and greater time spent in rapid eye movement (REM) sleep present additional risks to the infant. In REM sleep the stabilizing intercostal muscles are inhibited, and paradoxical inward motion occurs during inspiration in infants [20]. As a result the respiratory pump in infants is less effective. Compliance of the respiratory system differs between newborns and adults primarily because of differences in chest wall compliance (see Figure 19.1). This has a significant impact on infants' end-expiratory volume (EEV). In healthy children and adults EEV is equivalent to FRC. Because FRC is determined by two opposing forces, the outward recoil of the chest wall and inward recoil of the lungs, infants are predisposed to a low FRC and are at risk for airway closure and atelectasis [10,20–22]. As a defense mechanism against atelectasis, infants actively maintain their FRC above their passively determined EEV by active interruption of expiration. This is achieved by postinspiratory activity of the diaphragm and laryngeal narrowing during expiration [23,24]. Changes in EEV occur during sleep; EEV is particularly diminished in REM sleep [25,26]. At approximately 12 months of age, FRC is no longer actively determined. After 3 years paradoxical motion of the diaphragm in REM is rare or absent, and in adolescents it is completely absent [27].

Assessment of Chest Wall Function

Maximal inspiratory pressure (MIP) and maximal expiratory pressure (MEP) provide objective measurements of respiratory strength in the children who can cooperate and perform spirometry. Maximal inspiratory pressure can be measured with a simple, quick, and noninvasive clinical procedure to determine this index of inspiratory muscle strength both in healthy subjects and in patients with pulmonary or neuromuscular diseases. In the latter group, MIP is indicative of ventilatory capacity and the development of respiratory insufficiency and can also be useful in assessing the degree of abnormality, in monitoring inspiratory muscle weakness over time, and in estimating the success of weaning patients from mechanical ventilators. Recent research supports that MIP increases from 32 weeks to term but thereafter is constant throughout development [28]. In normal individuals, MIP against an occluded airway ranges from 100 to 200 cm H_2O [29–31]. In contrast, MEP continues to increase with age and correlates with cough efficiency. Gender differences are observed, with boys having higher occlusion pressures than girls [29–31].

Transdiaphragmatic pressure is an index of diaphragmatic force and is the difference between pleural and abdominal pressures:

$$Pdi = Pab - Ppl$$

where Pdi is transdiaphragmatic pressure, Pab is abdominal pressure, and Ppl is pleural pressure. The Pdi is decreased in states of diaphragm fatigue as well as in diseases that lead to diaphragmatic paralysis and subsequent pump failure (e.g., central motor neuron diseases, peripheral neuron disease, disease of neuromuscular junction, primary diseases of muscle).

The tension time index (TTI) can be a useful clinical test for assessing respiratory failure. The TTI is obtained by multiplying the ratio of transdiaphragmatic pressure and maximal transdiaphragmatic pressure with the ratio of inspiratory time and respiratory cycle time:

$$TTI = Pdi/Pdi \, max \times Ti/TiTot$$

In normal individuals, TTI is less than 0.1. Increased TTI with values above 0.2 are likely associated with respiratory fatigue [32]. There is a paucity of literature regarding infants, and normative values in this age group have not yet been defined [15]. In neuromuscular disease TTI is increased as Pdi max is decreased, whereas in upper airway obstruction (e.g., croup) Ti is increased. In diseases associated with lower airway obstruction or abnormal lung compliance (asthma, adult respiratory distress syndrome, cystic fibrosis), Pdi is increased to overcome airway resistance [15].

Polysomnography is a valuable tool in the evaluation of early respiratory impairment caused by neuromuscular disease. Sleep represents a vulnerable time for the respiratory pump as breathing undergoes change. The first signs of respiratory insufficiency in respiratory muscle weakness occur in REM sleep in which the accessory muscles of inspiration are inhibited while the diaphragm is relatively spared. Among the first notable abnormalities in children with neuromuscular weaknesses is REM-associated hypoventilation, followed later by hypoventilation in non-REM sleep [14,33].

TABLE 19.1. Neuromuscular conditions with respiratory implications.

Neuropathies
  Acute
    Central nervous system or spinal cord injury
    Phrenic nerve injury
    Infection: poliomyelitis or other enterovirus agent
    Toxin
      Tick paralysis
      Botulism
      Organophosphate poisoning
    Inflammatory
      Guillain-Barré syndrome/acute inflammatory demyelinating polyneuropathy
      Subacute inflammatory demyelinating polyneuropathy
      Acute motor sensory axonal neuropathy (*Campylobacter jejuni* infection)
    Autoimmune: myasthenia gravis
    Other
      Critical illness polyneuropathy
      Acute porphyric neuropathy
  Chronic
    Critical illness polyneuropathy
    Spinal muscular atrophy
      Infantile/Werdnig-Hoffman type 1
      Childhood/Werdnig-Hoffman type II
      Juvenile/Kugelberg-Welander disease
Myopathies
  Acute
    Metabolic: acid maltase deficiency (Pompe disease)
    Inflammatory
      Dermatomyositis
      Polymyositis
    Congenital myotonic dystrophy
    Critical illness myopathy
  Chronic
    Muscular dystrophies
    Myotonic dystrophy
    Congenital and metabolic myopathies

Upper airway obstruction may occur because of weakness of upper airway muscles leading to an increased number of obstructive and central apneas. As the disease progresses, nocturnal desaturation occurs initially in REM sleep and later in non-REM sleep.

Ultimately, respiratory pump failure occurs when the mechanical load exceeds the capacity of the pump, or the pump's intrinsic properties are diminished due to disease. Pulmonary function testing, MIP, MEP, full overnight polysomnography, and serial blood gas measurements along with clinical evaluation likely provide the best assessment of the respiratory pump [14]. Detection of subtle changes using these various modalities in neuromuscular disease states at an earlier time may afford timely institution of preventative interventions.

Disease Classifications

Acute and chronic neuromuscular processes can be characterized as primarily neuropathies or myopathies, as outlined in the Table 19.1. Not all affect respiratory function, and only some are further discussed.

Neuropathies

Central Nervous System or Spinal Cord Injury

Acute respiratory failure caused by neuromotor dysfunction is most often the result of central nervous system (CNS) or spinal cord injury, which may or may not be reversible. Loss of respiratory drive because of CNS injury or of respiratory motor function because of cervical cord injury must be managed with urgent intubation and ventilation to sustain life while determining the cause and potential reversibility of the dysfunction. Unless there is total absence of respiratory function, the signs of failure, even in the acute situation, may be spartan. Tachypnea and tachycardia may be attributed to stimuli other than low vital capacity, and paradoxical motion of the abdomen and chest wall may be missed. A dramatic fall in vital capacity is required before hypoxia ensues. A high index of suspicion for respiratory failure must be maintained, even in the setting of an acute injury [34]. Other causes of respiratory compromise related to motor neuron dysfunction include unilateral phrenic nerve injury related to cardiothoracic surgery in children. This injury can be an important factor in the failure to wean patients from mechanical ventilator support in the postoperative period. Although adults generally tolerate this insult well, diaphragmatic plication may be needed in children to prevent paradoxical diaphragmatic motion and thus permit adequate respiratory function without ventilator support [34]. In the absence of obvious trauma, infectious causes of lower motor neuron dysfunction must be ruled out.

Spinal Muscular Atrophy

The spinal muscular atrophies (SMA) are a group of autosomal recessive disorders that vary in age of onset and severity of manifestations. They are generally grouped into types 1, 2, and 3, based on detection of weakness before 6 months, at 6 to 12 months, and in the second or third year of life, respectively. Diagnosis is based on history, demonstration of proximal weakness with normal muscle enzymes, absence of deep tendon reflexes, and specific patterns on muscle biopsy and electromyography. The site of the neurologic deficit is the motor neurons of the ventral horn of the spinal cord and the motor nuclei of the brain stem [58,59]. Spinal muscular atrophy type 1 is associated with hypotonia from the perinatal period and early feeding and respiratory difficulties. Death from respiratory insufficiency usually occurs within the first decade in SMA-1, even with tracheostomy and respiratory support [59]. Spinal muscular atrophy type 2 patients demonstrate a progressive restrictive pulmonary insufficiency but often survive into the second decade with NIMV. Spinal muscular atrophy type 3 is associated with little impact on respiratory function in childhood. Aggressive pulmonary toilet with chest percussion and airway clearance is the mainstay of therapy as pulmonary function is a critical prognostic factor in all forms of SMA. Use of NIMV is preferable to tracheostomy, when feasible, for its ability to prolong independence from full ventilator support [3,59].

Inflammatory and Immunologically Mediated Neuropathies

Additional illnesses with more insidious onset that often lead to respiratory failure include those related to neurotoxins and the inflammatory and immunologically mediated neuropathies.

Guillain-Barré Syndrome

Guillain-Barré syndrome (GBS) is an inflammatory polyneuropathy of rapid onset that frequently follows an infectious or inflammatory process by days to weeks. It is the most common cause of acute flaccid paralysis in infants and children [48]. There are multiple forms with subtleties of presentation and manifestation. The

season of prevalence is the fall and winter, temporally related to the respiratory virus season in the United States. Most cases in children are classified as acute inflammatory demyelinating polyneuropathy (AIDP), characterized by decreased nerve conduction velocities and amplitudes, delayed distal nerve latency, and nerve conduction blocks. The less common axonal form of GBS, acute motor axonal neuropathy (AMAN), is characterized by lack of electrophysiologic evidence of demyelination and has been associated with preceding *Campylobacter jejuni* infection and antiganglioside antibodies [48].

Cerebrospinal fluid protein is generally elevated in both forms, with little or no pleocytosis. In a 16-year retrospective review of 23 patients, Hung et al. found a biphasic age distribution with no patients under 1 year old. Fourteen of their 23 patients were 1–10 years old, and 9 were 13–17 years old [48]. The evolution of symptoms usually progresses over 1–2 weeks in a central to peripheral pattern. Bulbar muscle weakness may lead to respiratory compromise, and recovery may be prolonged. Respiratory failure may occur in 10% of all patients (children and adults) at presentation and in up to 30% over the course of the disease [49].

Therapy is supportive, including monitoring of pulmonary function and vital signs, good nutrition and skin care, provision of deep vein thrombosis prophylaxis, and pain control. Plasmapheresis or intravenous gammaglobulin (IVIg) given at 0.4 mg/kg/dose for 5 days is the most effective intervention. Intravenous gammaglobulin is thought to shorten the time to first improvement and decrease the hospitalization time [49]. Systemic corticosteroids have not been shown to be helpful in GBS.

In another retrospective study of 23 patients from Turkey, those with the demyelinating form of GBS recovered more quickly after IVIg than those with the axonal form. Mechanical ventilation was required in 7 of the 23 patients, and three of these died of respiratory failure. All who survived were fully recovered at 12 months from the onset of symptoms [50]. On rare occasion, demyelination may extend to the CNS with severe neurologic sequelae [51]. Guillain-Barré syndrome was identified in 1 of 37 children with severe neurologic complications of stem cell transplant [52]. In this child the onset of GBS was fulminant and occurred 8 months posttransplant, with the child dying less than 2 months later of respiratory distress despite plasmapheresis and high-dose IVIg.

Subacute and Chronic Inflammatory Polyneuropathies

Two other inflammatory polyneuropathies share features common with GBS and with each other, but they are distinct entities. Subacute inflammatory demyelinating polyneuropathy (SIDP), first reported—8 weeks. There is electrophysiologic evidence of demyelination, as in GBS, but recurrence is unlikely after initial recovery [54]. In contrast to GBS, SIDP responds to systemic corticosteroids [53,54], and respiratory failure is uncommon. In a review of 16 patients with definite SIDP and 29 with probable SIDP, only four patients (<10%) developed respiratory failure [54]. The most prominent laboratory feature other than electrophysiologic evidence of demyelination was elevated CSF protein (usually >55 mg/dL).

Chronic inflammatory demyelinating polyneuropathy (CIDP) has a delay from onset to nadir of symptoms of greater than 2 months and a tendency to relapse after treatment. Spinal fluid protein may be elevated but less likely so than in GBS or SIDP. Identification of an antecedent infection is less likely, and improvement to full recovery is also less likely [53,54]. The syndrome is thought to be autoimmune in origin, with antibodies against myelin proteins having been reported. Although uncommon in children, it is similar to SIDP in that it is generally steroid responsive; however, plasmapheresis and IVIg have also been used therapeutically.

Diseases of the Neuromuscular Junction

As motor nerves enter the muscle, they divide into multiple terminal axons each of which innervates a single muscle fiber at the neuromuscular junction (NMJ). At the NMJ, neurotransmission is mediated via acetylcholine (Ach) in the following manner. An action potential the traverses the axon to the terminus to open voltage-gated calcium channels on the presynaptic membrane and cause release of the synaptic vesicles containing Ach. Released Ach diffuses across the synaptic cleft to bind to postsynaptic receptors, which mediates opening of sodium-potassium channels and depolarization of the muscle membrane. Once the endplate potential reaches threshold, an action potential is generated and propagates along the muscle membrane, resulting in contraction. A number of disease entities interfere with this neuromuscular transmission and can impair respiratory function.

Myasthenia Gravis

Myasthenia gravis is the most common defect of neuromuscular transmission and is an autoimmune process characterized by the development of antibodies to the postsynaptic Ach receptor. It is most prevalent in women in their second and third decades and in older men, about 10%–15% in association with thymoma [49,55]. Presenting symptoms usually include bulbar dysfunction resulting in dysphagia, dysarthria, and ocular muscle weakness in addition to prominent fatigue, and it commonly progresses to involve trunk and extremity muscles. In a report from Thailand of 27 cases of childhood-onset myasthenia, 92% had ocular symptoms at onset, with 24% of these progressing to generalized symptoms. Two patients (8%) presented with respiratory failure requiring ventilator support [56]. Ninety percent achieved at least partial remission using azathioprine and pyridostigmine, the majority of these having full recovery. None of these children experienced a myasthenic crisis, although 15%–25% of all patients may have this rapid decline in respiratory muscle function triggered by one of a variety of factors [49].

Diagnosis can be confirmed with use of a short-acting anti-Ach (e.g., edrophonium), electromyography, or assaying for anti-Ach receptor antibodies. It is important to note that a majority of patients who are seronegative for anti-Ach receptor antibodies demonstrated antibodies against a related component of the NMK, the muscle-specific receptor tyrosine kinase (MuSK). Treatment is symptomatic with a longer acting anti-Ach, pyridostigmine, although immune-modulating therapies (steroids, azathioprine, cyclophosphamide, high-dose IVIg) can be employed in more severe cases. Plasmapheresis can acutely and temporarily decrease antibody titers in a myasthenic crisis, although these occur infrequently in children. Caution should be used in selection of pharmacologic agents for patients with myasthenia because of the potential for worsening weakness. Paralyzing agents and anesthetics, certain antibiotics, and a long list of other drugs have been associated with either precipitating a myasthenic crisis or worsening underlying disease [57].

Botulism

There are multiple forms of botulism that can occur in both children and adults. Before 1980 the most common type was food-

borne, with ingestion of preformed toxin from food sources, particularly improperly canned foods [41]. Since the late 1970s, the most common form has been infantile or adult intestinal botulism, with toxin generated in the intestines from ingested *Botulinum* spores [42,43]. Botulinum toxin can also be produced in wounds that are infected with spores. Drug addicts may be subject to wound botulism, most recently from spores found in black tar heroin. The toxin is produced after *Clostridium* spores germinate in the intestine or the wound site which is absorbed systemically and binds irreversibly to the presynaptic motor terminals causing irreversible blockade of synaptic vesicle release and therefore inhibits motor activity. The pattern of illness is one of descending paralysis with bulbar weakness. Notably, poor feeding and constipation are frequently presenting symptoms in infants. Older patients may complain of dry mouth and blurred vision, and orthostatic hypotension and urinary retention may be evidenced as a result of autonomic dysfunction [42]. Neither the sensory system nor cognitive function is affected. Diagnosis can often be suspected by history and physical findings and confirmed by identification of the organism in the stool and by characteristic electromyographic findings [44,45].

Treatment of botulism is supportive, identifying the cause and removing the source of spores or toxin. However, mechanical ventilation may be required for several weeks. Failure to recognize the problem and intervene may lead to death from respiratory failure. A human-derived antitoxin (botulism immune globulin intravenous) is available for treatment of infant botulism that reduces morbidity and length of hospitalization [43,45]. It is most effective when administered early in the course, because it works only on circulating toxin, not on that which is already bound to the nerve terminal [42]. There are two equine-derived antitoxins for treatment of food-borne and wound botulism: a trivalent form consisting of antibodies to types A, B, and E and a bivalent form with antibodies to types A and B only. There has been a growing concern for the use of botulinum toxin as a bioterror agent. Aerosolized toxin in a large metropolitan population could potentially cause as many as 50,000 cases of clinical botulism and 30,000 deaths [46]. Children may be more susceptible than adults to the effects of this and other agents of bioterrorism because of their relatively higher metabolic and respiratory rates, their frequent hand to mouth contact, and their proximity to the ground [47].

Tick Paralysis

In the context of ataxia and acute ascending paralysis one most often thinks of GBS (reviewed earlier). However, the possibility of neurologic dysfunction from the toxin of certain female ticks must also be considered. In the United States the common vector is the genus *Dermacentor*, represented by the common dog tick or the wood tick. The neurotoxin is secreted in the saliva of adult female ticks and injected into the host during feeding. The toxin acts on the presynaptic motor terminals, inhibiting the release of acetylcholine [37]. Young children are most often affected and may present with a progressive symptom complex that evolves from vague complaints of restlessness and fatigue to gait instability to an ascending flaccid paralysis over days. The onset of symptoms usually begins 5–7 days after tick attachment [37,38]. Sensory and cognitive functions remain intact. One or more engorged ticks may be easily overlooked, buried in an unexamined skin fold or deep in thick hair [39]. If the tick is discovered and removed, recovery may begin within an hour and be complete within a day or two [38–40].

If not actively sought and discovered, paralysis continues to involve muscles innervated by the cranial nerves, including sternocleidomastoid, facial, lingual, and ocular muscles, and up to 10% of patients may succumb from respiratory failure [37,39,40].

Lambert-Eaton Myasthenic Syndrome

Although rare in childhood, Lambert-Eaton myasthenic syndrome is an autoimmune disorder resulting from antibodies directed against the voltage-gated calcium channel of the presynaptic membrane. This effectively decreases the release of Ach such that the endplate potential is insufficient to trigger an action potential. Most cases are associated with malignancies, particularly small cell carcinoma of the lung. Typical clinical features include fatigue, proximal limb weakness, areflexia, and dysautonomia, and it occasionally progresses to respiratory insufficiency, although sensation remains intact. Diagnosis is confirmed by antibody testing but is often suspected on the basis of electrodiagnostic testing that reveals an increased motor response with maximum exercise, which is a unique feature of this disease. Treatment remains symptomatic (with pyridostigmine, steroids, and/or IVIg) and supportive.

Myopathies

Acute Myopathies

The acute inflammatory myopathies *dermatomyositis and polymyositis* usually affect proximal muscle and rarely respiratory muscle function. Presentation is usually with symmetric proximal muscle weakness and elevated skeletal muscle enzymes. Muscle biopsy demonstrates both inflammation and muscle fiber necrosis. Respiratory compromise in these patients is multifactorial, with chronic aspiration related to dysphagia, interstitial lung disease, and an inflammatory alveolitis causing more respiratory failure than the muscle weakness itself [49,60]. Treatment is with antiinflammatory agents, primarily corticosteroids.

Congenital Myotonic Dystrophy

Congenital myotonic dystrophy represents the early onset of a condition that more commonly affects young adults [61]. Autosomal dominant myotonic dystrophy may have an earlier onset over repeated generations in a kindred, called *genetic anticipation*, during which the causative triplet repeats expand. It can present in the neonatal period with weakness and respiratory distress. Congenital myotonic dystrophy was previously thought to have a high mortality rate, especially if ventilation was required for more than 30 days. A recent retrospective review identified better than expected long-term outcomes, even when ventilation was required for more than 6 months. In a group of 20 children with congenital myotonic dystrophy, eight were ventilated for 35–812 days. Three of these died at 8 months, 10 months, and 11 years of age; however, five of the eight survived for follow ups of 5–13 years. Those children requiring longer ventilation had greater resuscitation needs at birth than the four requiring no ventilation or the eight who were ventilated for <30 days [61].

Critical Illness Myopathy/Steroid Myopathy

An iatrogenic myopathy may result from the treatment of critical illness, particularly severe asthma. Critical illness myopathy occurs most often in the adult population requiring ventilator support for air flow obstruction and managed with both high-dose steroids and neuromuscular blockade [49]. In a prospective study of 830 PICU admissions, 14 (1.7%) developed generalized weakness and four had repeated failures in attempted extubation [62]. All required ventilation for a mean of 260 hr (range 11–552 hr); 12 of 14 required more than 5 days of ventilation. Of note, 3 of 14 were less than 3 years old and the remainders were over 10 years old. Only one patient had asthma, and eight were solid organ or bone marrow transplant recipients. Twelve of the 14 patients had multiorgan system failure. One died during the PICU stay, and two additional patients died within 3 months of the episode but of complications relating to the underlying condition, not of the muscle weakness itself; however, both persisted in having severe proximal muscle weakness after discharge from the intensive care unit. Muscle biopsies show atrophy and vacuolization [49] or thick filament loss [62] but no evidence of inflammation.

The combination of high-dose systemic corticosteroids and neuromuscular blockade in patients with severe respiratory compromise appears to be the primary setting for this complication of life-saving therapy [49]. Post-transplant patients who are also receiving high-dose steroids appear to be disproportionately represented in the pediatric study [62]. There is no treatment other than physical therapy and muscular rehabilitation. It has been suggested that limitation of full neuromuscular blockade or allowing periods of muscle activity may help decrease both the risk and severity of muscle injury [36,49].

Chronic Myopathies

Muscular Dystrophies

The muscular dystrophies are divided into groups based on the onset of symptoms: infant, early childhood, late childhood, and adolescent onset [63,64]. Infantile onset is characterized by symptoms before 1 year of age with generalized muscle weakness and hypotonia. Diaphragm weakness leads to respiratory compromise, and death usually occurs in the early 20s. In early childhood dystrophies, symptoms begin between 1 and 5 years of age. They may be subdivided into two phenotypes: a rapidly progressive type with loss of ambulation by early adolescence and death at 20–30 years of age (including DMD); and a slowly progressive type with independent walking affected late or not at all and death not until >50 years of age (some limb-girdle dystrophies). In the late childhood onset dystrophies, symptoms begin between 6 and 12 years of age, with three subtypes based on ambulation ability, respiratory impact, and life expectancy [63].

The underlying molecular cause of DMD has been elegantly worked out in the past decade and relates to a deletion or duplication of the dystrophin gene on chromosome X(p21) leading to an X-linked inheritance pattern. Dystrophin is a large molecule on the sarcolemmal membrane and an integral part of the so-called dystrophin-associated glycoprotein (DAG) complex which is necessary for maintaining the structural integrity of the sarcolemmal membrane [65].

Prediction of respiratory compromise in DMD is directly related to lung function. In a review of 523 pulmonary function tests in 58 adolescent and young adult patients who had a minimum follow up of 2 years, the age when the forced vital capacity (FVC) fell to less than 1 L was a marker of mortality in that 5-year survival rate was only 8% after this objective decline in FVC [66]. There was no difference in maximal achieved vital capacity between those dying at less than 20 years of age and those living beyond 20 years, nor was there a difference in the rate of decline of absolute FVC per year. However, those who died before age 20 years had a greater decline in the percent predicted FVC per year [66]. Sleep hypoventilation is another marker of impending respiratory failure in DMD. Hukins and Hillman [67] found relationships between spirometry and awake blood gas parameters that suggested the need for sleep evaluation and potential NIMV intervention when forced expiratory volume in one second (FEV_1) was <40% predicted or $PaCO_2$ was >45 mm Hg or base excess was >4 mmol/L, with the base excess being the most sensitive predictor of sleep hypoventilation. Initiation of nocturnal NIMV in these patients was associated with a decrease in daytime $PaCO_2$ despite continuing decline in FEV_1 [67].

Systemic corticosteroids have been used to preserve muscle function and delay respiratory compromise in DMD [68]. Animal studies in the mouse model have suggested that treatment with prednisone decreases collagen deposition in the diaphragm and thus decreases fibrosis and muscle dysfunction [69]. Based on findings with the mouse model of DMD, the benefit of prednisone is thought to be due to suppression of both transforming growth factor-β (TGF-β), which is important in collagen production, and the inflammatory cytokine tumor necrosis factor (TNF)-α [69]. Several studies have looked at doses of prednisone from 0.75 mg/kg/day to 1.5 mg/kg every other day for periods from 3 to 36 months. All suggested improved strength and function [68]. However, side effects of long-term steroids are significant. Recent studies suggest delay of scoliosis and maintenance of ambulation with doses tailored to minimize side effects [70–72]. Genetic therapies and pharmacologic modification of intrinsic genetic dysfunction are also therapies being evaluated for this population, although results have been disappointing to date [73].

Metabolic Myopathies

A number of inborn errors of metabolism affect muscle function; however, they most often present as recurrent rhabdomyolysis or incapacitating, exercise-induced myalgia and do not significantly impair respiratory function. A notable exception is acid maltase deficiency in which deficiency of this lysosomal enzyme that releases glucose from maltase and glycogen results in hypotonia and respiratory muscle weakness in the infantile form. Although treatment is largely supportive, premature death usually by the end of the second decade is most often caused by respiratory failure. Finally, it is important to note that any number of mitochondrial encephalomyopathies can result in progressive skeletal myopathy ultimately affecting the respiratory muscles. However, these diseases (e.g., Kearns-Sayre syndrome; mitochondrial encephalomyopathy, lactic acidosis, and stroke-like episodes [MELALS]; and myoclonus epilepsy with ragged red fibers [MERRF]) are multisystem disorders with a variety of presentations beyond the scope of this chapter.

Conclusion

The presentation and management of neuromuscular disorders is variable, and signs of respiratory failure may be few until severe compromise has occurred. For most there is no definitive treatment, only recognition and support. For some, preparation of the patient and family for a progressive course of respiratory failure is the only option. In both acute and chronic management of respiratory failure in patients with neuromuscular dysfunction, strict attention to airway clearance and support with noninvasive ventilation are the major tools available in the physician's armamentarium.

References

1. Miske LJ, Hickey EM, Kolb SJ, Weiner DJ, Panitch HB. Use of the mechanical in-exsufflator in pediatric patients with neuromuscular disease and impaired cough. Chest 2004;125:1406–1412.
2. Bach JR, Niranjan V, Weaver B. Spinal muscular atrophy type 1—a noninvasive respiratory management approach. Chest 2000;117:1100–1105.
3. Bach JR, Baird JS, Plosky D, Navado J, Weaver B. Spinal muscular atrophy type 1: management and outcomes. Pediatr Pulmonol 2002;34:16–22.
4. Gomez-Merino E. Duchenne muscular dystrophy: prolongation of life by noninvasive ventilation and mechanically assisted coughing. Am J Phys Med Rehabil 2002;81:411–415.
5. Hardart MKM, Burns JP, Truog RD. Respiratory support in spinal muscular atrophy type 1: a survey of physician practices and attitudes. Pediatrics 2002;110:e24.
6. Murray JF. Respiratory muscles. In: The Normal Lung, 2nd ed. Murray JF, ed. Philadelphia: WB Saunders; 1986:121–138.
7. Derenne JP, Macklem PT, Roussos C: The respiratory muscles: mechanics, control and pathophysiology. Parts I, II and III. Am Rev Respir Dis 1978;118–133, 373–390, 581–601.
8. DeTroyer A, Loring SH. Action of respiratory muscles. In: Mecklem PT, Mead J, eds. Handbook of Physiology: The Respiratory System—Mechanics of Breathing, vol III. Bethesda, MD: American Physiological Society; 1986:453.
9. Roussos C, Macklem PT. The respiratory muscles. N Engl J Med 1982;307:786–792.
10. Agostini E, Mead J. Statics of the respiratory system. In: Fenn WO, Rahn H, eds. Handbook of Physiology, vol 1. Washington, DC: American Physiological Society, 1964:401.
11. Altose MD. Pulmonary mechanics. In: Fisherman AP, ed. Pulmonary Disease and Disorders, vol 1, 2nd ed. New York: McGraw-Hill; 1988:171–184.
12. D'Angelo E. Statics of the chest wall. In: Roussos C, Macklem PT, eds. Thorax, part A. New York: Dekker; 1985:259–295.
13. Agostini E. Mechanics of the pleural pressure space. In: Macklem PT, Mead J, eds. Mechanics of Breathing, part 2, Handbook of Physiology, sec 3: The Respiratory System, vol 32. Bethesda, MD: American Physiological Society; 1964:531–559.
14. Rosen CL. Maturation of breathing during sleep. In: Louglin G, Carroll J, Marcus C, eds. Sleep and Breathing in Children, 1st ed. New York: Dekker; 2000:181–205.
15. Allen J, Gripp K. Development of thoracic cage. In: Chernick-Mellins, eds. Basic Mechanisms of Pediatric Respiratory Disease, 2nd ed. London: BC Decker; 2002:124–138.
16. Papastomelos C, Panitch H, England S, Allen J. Developmental changes in chest wall compliance in infancy and early childhood. J Appl Physiol 1995;78:179–184.
17. Gerhardt T, Bancalari E. Chest wall compliance in full term and premature infants. Acta Paediatr Scand 1980;69:359–364.
18. Openshaw P, Edwards S, Helms P. Changes in rib cage geometry during childhood. Thorax 1984;39:624–627.
19. Keens TG, Bryan AC, Levison H, Ianuzzo CD. Developmental pattern of muscle fiber types in human ventilatory muscles. J Appl Physiol Respir Environ Exerc Physiol 1978;44:909–913.

20. Gaultier C, Praud JP, Canet E, Delaperche MF, D'Allest AM. Paradoxical inward rib cage motion during rapid eye movement sleep in infants and young children. J Dev Physiol 1987;9:391–397.

21. Gaultier C. Cardiorespiratory adaptation during sleep in infants and children. Pediatr Pulmonol 1995;19:105–117.

22. England S, Gaultier C, Bryan A. Chest wall mechanics in the newborn. In: Roussos C, ed. The Thorax: Lung Biology in Health and Disease, 2nd ed. New York: Dekker, 1995:1541–1556.

23. Kosch PC, Stark AR. Dynamic maintenance of end-expiratory lung volume in full term infants. J Appl Physiol 1984;57:1126–1133.

24. Kosch PC, Hutchison AA, Wozniak JA, et al. Posterior cricoarytenoid and diaphragm activities during tidal breathing in neonates. J Appl Physiol 1988;64:1968–1978.

25. Collin AA, Wohl ME, Mead J, Ratjen FA, Glass G, Stark AR. Transition from dynamically maintained to relaxed end-expiratory volume in human infants. J Appl Physiol 1989;67:2107–2111.

26. Stark AR, Cohlan BA, Waggener TB, Frantz ID III, Kosch PC. Regulation of end-expiratory lung volume during sleep in premature infants. J Appl Physiol 1987;62:1117–1123.

27. Tabachnik E, Muller NL, Bryan AC, Levsion H. Changes in ventilation and chest wall mechanics during sleep in normal adolescents. J Appl Physiol 1981;51:557–564.

28. Dimitoru G, Greenough A, Dyke H, Rafferty GF. Maximal airway pressures during crying in healthy preterm and term neonates. Early Hum Dev 2000;57:149–156.

29. Gaultier C, Zinman R. Maximal static pressures in healthy children. Respir Physiol 1983;51:45–61.

30. Shardonofsky FR, Perez-Chada D, Carmuega E, Milic-Emili J. Airway pressures during crying in healthy infants. Pediatr Pulmonol 1989;6:14–18.

31. Wagener JS, Hibbert ME, Landau LI. Maximal respiratory pressures in children. Am Rev Respir Dis 1984;129:873–875.

32. Rochester DF, Arora NS. Respiratory muscle failure. Med Clin North Am 1983;67:573–597.

33. Allen J. Respiratory function in children with neuromuscular disease. Monaldi Arch Chest Dis 1996;51:230–235.

34. MacDuff A, Grand IS. Critical care management of neuromuscular disease, including long term ventilation. Curr Opin Crit Care 2003;9:106–112.

35. Padman R. Respiratory management of pediatric patients with spinal cord injuries: retrospective review of the duPont experience. Neurorehabil Neural Repair 2003;17:32–36.

36. Lorin S, Nierman DM. Critical illness neuromuscular abnormalities. Crit Care Clin 2002;18:553–568.

37. Greenstein P. Tick paralysis. Med Clin North Am 2002;86:441–446.

38. Gordon BM, Giza CC. Tick paralysis presenting in an urban environment. Pediatr Neurol 2004;30:122–124.

39. Felz MW, Smith CD, Swift TR. Brief report: a six year old girl with tick paralysis. N Engl J Med 2000;342:90–94.

40. Li Z, Turner RP. Pediatric tick paralysis: discussion of two cases and literature review. Pediatr Neurol 2004;31:304–307.

41. Armada M, Love S, Barrett E, Monroe J, Peery D, Sobel J. Foodborne botulism in a six month old infant caused by home canned baby food. Ann Emerg Med 2003;42:226–229.

42. Marks, JD. Medical aspects of biologic toxins. Anesthesiol Clin North Am 2004;22:509–532.

43. American Academy of Pediatrics. Botulism. In: Pickering LK, ed. Pediatric Red Book: 2003 Report of the Committee on Infectious Diseases, 26th ed. Elk Grove Village, IL: American Academy of Pediatrics; 2003:243–246.

44. Cox N, Hinkle R. Infant botulism. Am Fam Physician 2002;65:1388–1392.

45. Fox CK, Keet CA, Strober JB. Recent advances in infant botulism. Pediatr Neurol 2005;32:149–154.

46. St John R, Finlay B, Blau C. Bioterrorism in Canada: an economic assessment of preventive and postattack exposure. Can J Infect Dis 2001;12:275–284.

47. Leissner KB, Holzman RS, McCann ME. Bioterrorism in children: unique concerns with infection control and vaccination. Anesthesiol Clin North Am 2004;22(3):563–577.

48. Hung PL, Chang WN, Huang LT, et al. A clinical and electrophysiologic survey of childhood Guillian-Barre syndrome. Pediatr Neurol 2004;30:86–91.

49. Marinelli, WA, Leatherman JW. Neuromuscular disorders in the intensive care unit. Crit Care Clin 2002;18:915–929.

50. Tekgul, H, Serdaroglu G, Tutuncuoglu S. Outcome of axonal and demyelinating forms of Guillian-Barre syndrome in children. Pediatr Neurol 2003;28:295–299.

51. Tan MJ, Chattophadyay AK, Griffiths PD, Baxter PS. Acute central and peripheral demyelination associated with *Mycoplasma pneumoniae*. Pediatr Neurol 2003;29:239–241.

52. Facari M, Lanino E, Dini G, et al. Severe neurologic complications after hematopoietic stem cell transplantation in children. Neurology 2002;59:1895–1904.

53. Colan RV, Snead OC, Oh SJ, Benton JW. Steroid-responsive polyneuropathy with subacute onset in childhood. J Pediatr 1980;97:374–377.

54. Oh SJ, Kurokawa K, de Almeida DF, Ryan HF, Claussen GC. Subacute inflammatory demyelinating polyneuropathy. Neurology 2003;61:507–1512.

55. Chitnis T, Khoury SJ. Immunologic neuromuscular disorders. J Allergy Clin Immunol 2003;111:(Suppl 2):S656–668.

56. Raksadawan N. Childhood onset myasthenia gravis. J Med Assoc Thai 2002;85(Suppl 2):S769–777.

57. Bertorini TE. Perisurgical management of patients with neuromuscular disorders. Neurol Clin North Am 2004;22:293–313.

58. Gozal D. Pulmonary manifestations of neuromuscular disease with special reference to Duchenne muscular dystrophy and spinal muscular atrophy. Pediatr Pulmonol 2000;29:141–150.

59. Ioos C, Leclair-Richard D, Mrad S, Barois A, Estournet-Mathiaud B. Respiratory capacity course in patients with infantile spinal muscular atrophy. Chest 2004;126:831–837.

60. Prahalad S, Bohnsack JF, Maloney CG, Leslie KO. Fatal acute fibrinous and organizing pneumonia in a child with juvenile dermatomyositis. J Pediatr 2005;146:289–292.

61. Campbell C, Sherloc R, Jacob P, Blayney M. Congenital myotonic dystrophy: assisted ventilation duration and outcome. Pediatrics 2004;113:811–816.

62. Papazian O, Alfonso I. Adolescents with muscular dystrophies. Adolesc Med 2002;13:511–535.

63. Banwell BJ, Mildner RJ, Hassall AC, Becker LE, Vajsar J, Shemie SD. Muscle weakness in critically ill children. Neurology 2003;61:1779–1782.

64. Wagner KR. Genetic diseases of muscle. Neurol Clin North Am 2002;20:645–678.

65. Gilchrist JM. Overview of neuromuscular disorders affecting respiratory function. Semin Respir Crit Care Med 2002;23:191–200.

66. Phillips MF, Quinlivan RCM, Edwards RHT, Claverley PMA. Changes in spirometry over time as a prognostic marker in patients with Duchenne muscular dystrophy. Am J Respir Crit Care Med 2001;164:2191–2194.

67. Hukins CA, Hillman DR. Daytime predictors of sleep hypoventilation in Duchenne muscular dystrophy. Am J Respir Crit Care Med 2001;161:166–170.

68. Moxley RT, Ashwal S, Pandya S, et al. Practice parameter: corticosteroid treatment of Duchenne dystrophy. Neurology 2005;64:13–20.

69. Gosselin LE, McCormick KM. Targeting the immune system to improve ventilatory function in muscular dystrophy. Med Sci Sports Exerc 2004;36:44–51.

70. Alman BA. Steroid treatment and the development of scoliosis in males with Duchenne muscular dystrophy. J Bone Joint Surg Am 2004;86:519–524.

71. Yilmaz O. Prednisolone therapy in Duchenne muscular dystrophy prolongs ambulation and prevents scoliosis. Eur J Neurol 2004;11:541–544.

72. Beenakker EA. Intermittent prednisone therapy in Duchenne muscular dystrophy: a randomized controlled trial. Arch Neurol 2005;62:128–132.

73. Kapsa R, Kornberg AJ, Byrne E. Novel therapies for Duchenne muscular dystrophy. Lancet Neurol 2003;2:299–310.

20
Diseases of the Pulmonary Vascular System

Peter Oishi and Jeffrey R. Fineman

Introduction

Although historically considered the *lesser circulation*, pathology of the pulmonary circulation is a great source of pediatric morbidity and mortality. This is most commonly displayed in neonates with persistent pulmonary hypertension; neonates, infants, and children with congenital heart disease; and adolescents and young adults with primary pulmonary hypertension. Recent evidence indicates that normal pulmonary vascular tone is regulated by a complex interaction of vasoactive substances that are locally produced by the vascular endothelium [1–6]. These substances, such as nitric oxide (NO) and endothelin-1 (ET-1), are capable of producing vascular relaxation and/or constriction, modulating the propensity of blood to clot, and inducing and/or inhibiting smooth muscle cell migration and replication [6–20]. In fact, mounting data implicate endothelial injury and the subsequent aberration in the endogenous production of these substances in the pathophysiology of pulmonary hypertensive disorders [21–25]. This chapter discusses the normal regulation of the fetal, transitional, and postnatal pulmonary circulations, the pathophysiology of pediatric pulmonary hypertensive disorders, and new therapeutic and preventative strategies for pulmonary hypertension. Particular emphasis is placed on the role of the pulmonary vascular endothelium in these processes and treatment modalities.

Regulation of the Fetal, Transitional, and Postnatal Pulmonary Circulations

The Normal Fetal Circulation

In the fetus, gas exchange occurs in the placenta and pulmonary blood flow is low, measuring approximately 100 mL/100 g wet lung weight in the near-term lamb [26]. The majority of right ventricular output, which represents two thirds of total combined ventricular output, is diverted away from the lungs through the widely patent ductus arteriosus to the descending thoracic aorta [27]. Midway through gestation, pulmonary blood flow is approximately 3%–4% of the total combined ventricular output. This value increases progressively, reaching about 6% at 80% gestation, when the release of surface active material into lung fluid begins and up to a maximum of 8%–10% at or near term [21,28,29]. Fetal pulmonary arterial pressure also increases with advancing gestation. At term, mean pulmonary arterial pressure is about 50 mm Hg, generally exceeding the mean descending aortic pressure by 1–2 mm Hg [28,30]. Pulmonary vascular resistance, which is extremely high in early gestation, falls progressively as pulmonary arterial development advances, which increases the cross-sectional area of the pulmonary circulation; however, the pulmonary vascular resistance of the fetus is still much higher than that of the neonate after birth [27,31]. A number of mechanisms have been implicated in the maintenance of the high pulmonary vascular resistance and pulmonary arterial pressure during fetal life. These include mechanical factors, the low oxygen tension of fetal pulmonary and systemic blood, leukotrienes, thromboxane, ET-1, NO, prostaglandin (PG) I_2, platelet-derived growth factor (PDGF), and K^+ channels (32).

The Transitional Circulation

The transition from the fetal to the neonatal pulmonary circulation is marked by a dramatic fall in pulmonary vascular resistance and rise in pulmonary blood flow, which increases 8–10-fold (up to 300–400 mL/min/kg body weight). These changes are associated with the initiation of ventilation of the lungs and the subsequent increase in pulmonary and systemic arterial blood oxygen tensions. The increase in pulmonary blood flow increases pulmonary venous return and left atrial pressure, allowing the foramen ovale to close. In addition, the ductus arteriosus constricts, functionally closing within several hours after birth, which effectively separates the pulmonary and systemic circulations. Mean pulmonary arterial pressure decreases, and by 24 hr of age is approximately 50% of mean systemic arterial pressure. Under normal conditions, adult values are reached 2–6 weeks after birth [29].

The decrease in pulmonary vascular resistance with ventilation and oxygenation at birth is regulated by a complex and incompletely understood interplay between metabolic and mechanical factors. In experiments, physical expansion of the fetal lamb lung without changing oxygen tension increases fetal pulmonary blood

D.S. Wheeler et al. (eds.), The *Respiratory Tract in Pediatric Critical Illness and Injury*,
DOI 10.1007/978-1-84800-925-7_20, © Springer-Verlag London Limited 2009

flow and decreases pulmonary vascular resistance but not to newborn values [33]. A proportion of this decrease relates to alterations in the physical architecture of the alveoli and small pulmonary vessels that occur with mechanical distention [34]. In addition, physical expansion of the lung results in the release of vasoactive substances, such as PGI_2, which increases pulmonary blood flow and decreases pulmonary vascular resistance in the fetal goat and lamb independent of the changes in oxygen tension [35–40].

When ventilation is accompanied by changes in oxygen tension (i.e., ventilation with ambient air or supplemental oxygen), fetal pulmonary blood flow increases and pulmonary vascular resistance falls to newborn values. The exact mechanisms of this oxygen-induced pulmonary vasodilation remain unclear. Alveolar and/or arterial oxygen may directly dilate pulmonary resistance vessels or may trigger the release of vasoactive substances, such as PGI_2 or NO. In fact, data indicate that NO, in particular, participates in the decrease in pulmonary vascular resistance that accompanies increases in alveolar and arterial oxygen tension [7,12] However, despite its important role, inhibition of NO does not impair the immediate fall in pulmonary vascular resistance seen after birth, further suggesting that multiple mechanisms are involved in this transitional physiology. In fact, recent data implicate fluid shear forces across endothelial cells, which result in the production of both NO and PGI_2, as an additional mechanism by which vasodilation occurs after birth [32]. It is possible that this particular mechanism acts to maintain pulmonary vasodilation once it has been established by the mechanisms described earlier.

In general, the dramatic increase in pulmonary blood flow with the initiation of ventilation and oxygenation at birth reflects a shift from active pulmonary vasoconstriction in the fetus to active pulmonary vasodilatation in the newborn. Failure to undergo this normal transition contributes substantially to the pathophysiology of many neonatal pulmonary hypertensive disorders, including bronchopulmonary dysplasia, persistent pulmonary hypertension of the newborn, chronic lung disease, and congenital heart disease [25,40–64].

The Postnatal Pulmonary Circulation

The successful transition from the fetal to the postnatal pulmonary circulation is marked by the maintenance of the pulmonary vasculature in a dilated, low-resistance state [65]. Recent evidence suggests that basal NO release, and the subsequent increase in smooth muscle cell cyclic guanosine monophosphate (cGMP) concentrations, in part mediate the low resting pulmonary vascular resistance of the newborn [66]. Other vasoactive substances, including histamine, 5-hydroxytryptamine, bradykinin, and metabolites of arachidonic acid by the cyclooxygenase and lipoxygenase pathways, have also been implicated in mediating postnatal pulmonary vascular tone; however, their roles are not well elucidated. Two of the most important factors affecting pulmonary vascular resistance in the postnatal period are oxygen concentration and pH. Decreasing oxygen tension and decreases in pH elicit pulmonary vasoconstriction [67]. Alveolar hypoxia constricts pulmonary arterioles, diverting blood flow away from hypoxic lung segments, toward well-oxygenated segments, thus enhancing ventilation–perfusion matching [68]. This response to hypoxia, unique to the pulmonary vasculature, is greater in the younger animal than in the adult [69]. Indeed, in most vascular beds (e.g., cerebral vasculature), hypoxia is a potent vasodilator. The exact mechanism of hypoxic pulmonary vasoconstriction remains incompletely under-

stood but likely involves changes in the local concentration of reactive oxygen species that in turn regulate voltage-gated potassium channels and calcium channels [66,70]. Acidosis potentiates hypoxic pulmonary vasoconstriction, whereas alkalosis reduces it [71]. The exact mechanism of pH-mediated pulmonary vascular reactivity also remains incompletely understood but appears to be independent of $PaCO_2$ [72]. Recent data suggest that potassium channels play an important role in mediating these responses as well [73]. Manipulating alveolar oxygen tension and systemic arterial pH are fundamental approaches to changing pulmonary vascular tone in the critical care setting. Alveolar hyperoxia and alkalosis are often used to decrease pulmonary vascular tone because they generally relieve pulmonary vasoconstriction with little effect on the systemic circulation as a whole. However, severe alkalosis is generally avoided because of the detrimental effects of severe hypocarbia or alkalosis on cerebral and myocardial blood flow (see General Treatment Approach, later) [6,8].

Despite extensive innervation of the lung, neural input is not a major determinant of basal pulmonary vascular tone. However, pulmonary neurohumoral receptors are sensitive to α-adrenergic, β-adrenergic, and dopaminergic agonists [74,75]. Therefore, vasoactive agents that stimulate these receptors will affect the vascular tone of both the pulmonary and systemic circulations. Alterations in vascular tone, in response to a given agent, are dependent on the relative tone of the vascular bed at a given time. Therefore, the response of these agents is difficult to predict in an individual critically ill patient.

Determinants of Pulmonary Vascular Resistance

Pulmonary vascular resistance changes throughout gestation and after birth. The resistance of the pulmonary circulation at any one time is related to several factors and can be estimated by applying the resistance equation and the Poiseuille-Hagen relationship [76]. The resistance equation (the hydraulic equivalent of Ohm's law) states that the resistance to flow between two points along a tube equals the decrease in pressure between the two points divided by the flow [77,78]. For the pulmonary vascular bed, where Rp is pulmonary vascular resistance and Qp is pulmonary blood flow, the decrease in mean pressure is from the pulmonary artery (Ppa) to the pulmonary vein (Ppv) or left atrium, where la is mean left atrial pressure:

$$Rp = [Ppa - Ppv \text{ or } la \text{ (mean)}]/Qp$$

Therefore, the calculated pulmonary vascular resistance increases when pulmonary arterial pressure increases or when pulmonary blood flow decreases. Changes in pulmonary venous pressure or mean left atrial pressure are somewhat more complicated. In isolation, increases in pulmonary venous pressure and left atrial pressure would decrease the calculated pulmonary vascular resistance. However, increases in pulmonary venous pressure are generally accompanied by a greater increase in pulmonary arterial pressure (which maintains driving pressure), resulting in an increase in the calculated resistance across the pulmonary vascular bed. Furthermore, changes in left atrial pressure, which occur independent of alterations in pulmonary vascular resistance, must be considered. For example, large intracardiac shunts (e.g., ventricular septal defect) may result in congestive heart failure with an elevation in left atrial pressure. Closure of the ventricular septal defect may acutely decrease left atrial pressure, resulting in an elevation in the calculated pulmonary vascular resistance (provided that pulmonary arterial pressure does not decrease to the same extent), when in fact no change in pulmonary vascular tone has occurred [79].

Other factors that affect pulmonary vascular resistance can be defined by applying a modification of the Poiseuille-Hagen relationship, which describes the resistance (R) to flow of a Newtonian fluid through a system of round, straight glass tubes of constant cross sectional area:

$$Rp = 8 \cdot l \cdot \eta/n\pi r^4$$

where l is length of the system of vessels, n is vessel number, r is the internal radius of the system of vessels, and η is the viscosity of the fluid. According to this relationship, increasing the viscosity of blood perfusing the lungs or decreasing the radius or cross-sectional area (πr^4) of the pulmonary vascular bed increases pulmonary vascular resistance. Because the above equations describe steady, laminar flow of a Newtonian fluid in rigid, glass tubes, differences between physical and biologic systems should be considered. First, blood is not a Newtonian fluid. However, this is probably of little importance at normal hematocrit levels [80]. The viscosity of blood is related to red cell number, fibrinogen concentration, and red cell deformability. An increased hematocrit (secondary to fetal hypoxemia, twin-to-twin transfusion, maternal-to-fetal transfusion, or delayed clamping of the umbilical cord) will increase viscosity [80,81] as pulmonary vascular resistance increases logarithmically when the hematocrit increases. Second, pulmonary vessels are not rigid tubes. Their walls are deformable, and their size and shape are influenced by transmural pressure. For example, as pulmonary blood flow or left atrial pressure increases, vessel diameter may change, and/or the recruitment of additional pulmonary vessels may occur. Therefore, the fall in calculated pulmonary vascular resistance with increases in pulmonary blood flow is nonlinear [65,82,83]. Third, blood flow through the pulmonary circulation is pulsatile, not laminar, and the small pulmonary arteries are branched, curved, and tapered, not smooth [76]. In addition, the small pulmonary arteries are in parallel, and the radii of these arteries may differ in different lung zones.

Despite these differences from physical models, the general effects of changes in physical factors, such as viscosity and radius, do apply [76–78]. In fact, a change in luminal radius is the major factor responsible for maintaining a high pulmonary vascular resistance in the fetus. Consideration of these factors, particularly viscosity and cross-sectional area of the vascular bed, is important in evaluating the pathophysiology of pulmonary hypertensive disorders.

Finally, it is important to note the overall relationship between lung volume and pulmonary vascular resistance, which has been described by several investigators [84,85]. These studies have shown that this relationship to be U-shaped (Figure 20.1) with minimal pulmonary vascular resistance noted at functional residual capacity. Using an open-chest model, pulmonary vascular resistance decreased as lungs were inflated from a collapsed state and then progressively increased at higher lung volumes, which was thought to be related to inflation pressure on the alveolar vessels. These observations support the concept that lung inflation may have a variable effect on the distribution of pulmonary blood flow.

When pressure is expressed in mm of Hg and flow in L/min, units of resistance are derived as mm of Hg/L/min (Wood unit, U). However, comparisons among patients of differing weight and age

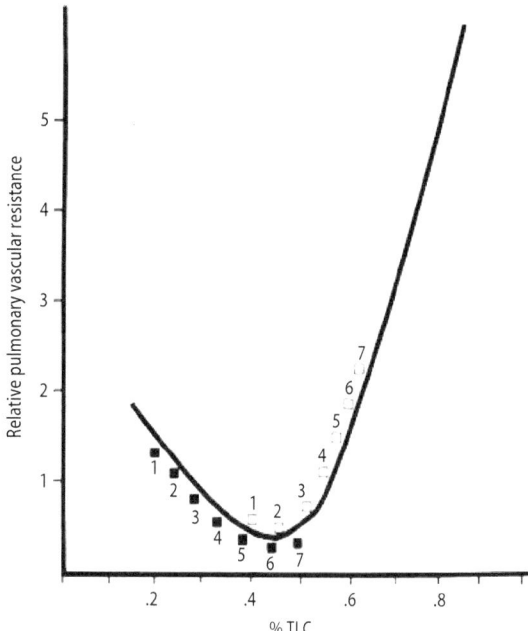

FIGURE 20.1. Diagrammatic plot to illustrate the U-shaped relationship between relative pulmonary vascular resistance (PVR) and relative lung volume (% total lung capacity [TLC]). Regions of the lung are numbered from top (region 7) to bottom (region 1) of the lung for both low (closed squares) and high (open squares) overall lung volumes. (From Baile et al. [84]. Copyright 1982 from American Physiological Socity. Reprinted with perrmission.)

are problematic. Therefore, resistance is more commonly expressed in relation to body surface area, as $U \cdot m^2$. Multiplying U by 80 converts to dynes/sec/cm^{-5}, a common form utilized to express resistance in other settings. Pulmonary vascular resistance may be as high as 8–10 U·m^2 immediately after birth and then, under normal conditions, falls as previously described to adult levels of 1–3 U·m^2 by 6 to 8 weeks of life [27,31].

Pulmonary Hypertensive Disorders

Pulmonary hypertensive disorders are a significant source of morbidity and mortality in the pediatric population. Pulmonary hypertension is defined as a mean pulmonary artery pressure of greater than 25 mm of Hg at rest or greater than 30 mm of Hg during exercise. In addition, a calculated pulmonary vascular resistance of greater than 3 U is generally considered abnormal. In neonates, the most common etiology results from a failure to undergo the normal fall in pulmonary vascular resistance at birth termed *persistent pulmonary hypertension of the newborn* (PPHN) that has an incidence of ~1 per 1,000 live births. However, other pulmonary abnormalities, such as congenital diaphragmatic hernia, respiratory distress syndrome, and bronchopulmonary dysplasia, may also result in neonatal pulmonary hypertension. Beyond the neonatal period, the majority of pediatric pulmonary hypertensive disorders are associated with congenital heart defects. Other, less common causes of pediatric pulmonary vascular disease include primary (idiopathic) pulmonary hypertension, hypoxia-induced pulmonary vascular disease, rheumatologic disorders, sickle cell disease, portal hypertension, chronic thromboembolic disease, human immunodeficiency virus disease, and drug-toxin induced disease. A number of clinical classification systems for

TABLE 20.1. Clinical classification of pulmonary hypertension.

Pulmonary arterial hypertension (PAH)
  Idiopathic (IPAH)
  Familial (FPAH)
  Related to risk factors or associated conditions (APAH)
    Collagen vascular disease
    Congenital systemic-to-pulmonary shunts
    Portal hypertension
    Human immunodeficiency virus infection
    Drugs and toxins
    Other: thyroid disorders, glycogen storage disease, Gaucher disease, hereditary
      hemorrhagic telangiectasia, hemoglobinopathies, myeloproliferative disorders,
      splenectomy
  Associated with venous or capillary involvement
    Pulmonary veno-occlusive disease
    Pulmonary capillary hemangiomatosis
  Persistent pulmonary hypertension of the newborn
Pulmonary hypertension with left heart disease
  Left-sided atrial or ventricular heart disease
  Left-sided valvular heart disease
Pulmonary hypertension associated with lung disease and/or hypoxemia
  Chronic obstructive pulmonary disease
  Interstitial lung disease
  Sleep-disordered breathing
  Alveolar hypoventilation disorders
  Chronic exposure to high altitude
  Developmental abnormalities
Pulmonary hypertension due to chronic thrombotic and/or embolic disease
  Proximal pulmonary arteries
  Distal pulmonary arteries
  Nonthrombotic embolism (tumor, parasites, foreign material)
Miscellaneous
  Sarcoidosis, histiocytosis X, lymphangiomatosis, compression of pulmonary vessels

Source: Adapted from Simonneau et al. [227].

pulmonary hypertension have been proposed, most recently at the 2003 Third World Symposium on Pulmonary Arterial Hypertension (Table 20.1).

Pathobiology of the Pulmonary Vasculature

Vascular endothelial cells are capable of producing a variety of vasoactive substances that participate in the regulation of normal vascular tone. A schematic of some of these endothelial factors is shown in Figure 20.2. These substances, such as NO, ET-1, and prostacyclin are capable of producing vascular relaxation and/or constriction, modulating the propensity of the blood to clot, and inducing and/or inhibiting smooth muscle cell migration and replication [6–20].

Nitric oxide is a labile humoral factor produced by nitric oxide synthase (NOS) from L-arginine in the vascular endothelial cell [86–88]. Nitric oxide diffuses into the smooth muscle cell and produces vascular relaxation by increasing concentrations of guanosine 3′5′-monophosphate (cGMP) via the activation of soluble guanylate cyclase [89,90]. Nitric oxide is released in response to a variety of factors, including shear stress (flow) and the binding of certain endothelium-dependent vasodilators (such as acetylcholine, adenosine triphosphate [ATP], and bradykinin) to receptors on the endothelial cell [4,91]. Basal NO release is an important mediator of both resting pulmonary and systemic vascular tone in the fetus, newborn, and adult, as well as a mediator of the normal fall in pulmonary vascular resistance that occurs

immediately after birth 32,87,92]. In addition, aberrant NO–cGMP signaling is integral to the pathophysiology of pulmonary hypertension, as well as a number of other biologic vascular disorders [10,11,23,25,44,45,48,52].

Endothelin-1 is a 21 amino acid polypeptide also produced by vascular endothelial cells [2]. The vasoactive properties of ET-1 are complex, and studies have shown varying hemodynamic effects on different vascular beds [16–20]. However, its most striking property is its sustained hypertensive action. In fact, ET-1 is the most potent vasoconstricting agent discovered, with a potency 10 times that of angiotensin II. The hemodynamic effects of ET-1 are mediated by at least two distinct receptor populations, ET_A and ET_B [93,94]. The ET_A receptors are located on vascular smooth muscle cells and mediate vasoconstriction, whereas the ET_B receptors are located on endothelial cells and smooth muscle cells and thus may mediate both vasodilation and vasoconstriction, respectively. Individual endothelins occur in low levels in the plasma, generally below their vasoactive thresholds. This suggests that they are primarily effective at the local site of release. Even at these levels, they may potentiate the effects of other vasoconstrictors, such as norepinephrine and serotonin [95]. The role of endogenous ET-1 in the regulation of normal vascular tone is unclear at present [96]. Nevertheless, alterations in ET-1 have been implicated in the pathophysiology of a number of disease states, including pulmonary hypertensive disorders, and has been implicated in the so-called rebound effect of inhaled NO [24,25,54,60,97].

Endothelial-derived hyperpolarizing factor (EDHF), a diffusible substance that causes vascular relaxation by hyperpolarizing the smooth muscle cell, is another important endothelial factor.

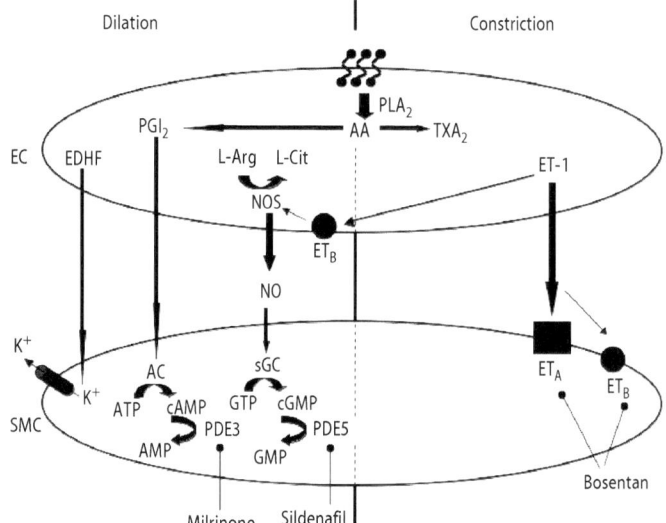

FIGURE 20.2. Schematic of some endothelial-derived factors. EC, pulmonary vascular endothelial cell; SMC, pulmonary vascular smooth muscle cell; EDHF, endothelial-derived hyperpolarizing factor; PGI_2, prostaglandin I_2; PLA_2, phospholipase A_2; AA, arachidonic acid; TXA_2, thromboxane A_2; L-Arg, L-arginine; L-Cit, L-citrulline; NOS, nitric oxide synthase; ET-1, endothelin-1; ET_A, endothelin A receptor; ET_B, endothelin B receptor; NO, nitric oxide; sGC, soluble guanylate cyclase; GTP, guanosine-5′-triphosphate; cGMP, guanosine-3′-5′-cyclic monophosphate; GMP, guanosine monophosphate; AC, adenylate cyclase; ATP, adenosine-5′-triphosphate; cAMP, adenosine-3′-5′-monophosphate; AMP, adenosine monophosphate; PDE, phosphodiesterase (types 3 and 5 shown); K^+, potassium channels. Also shown are sites of action of milrinone (phosphodiesterase 3 inhibitor), sildenafil (phosphodiesterase 5 inhibitor), and bosentan (ET_A and ET_B antagonists).

Endothelial-derived hyperpolarizing factor has not yet been identified, but current evidence suggests that its action is dependent on K+ channels [97]. Activation of potassium channels in the vascular smooth muscle results in cell membrane hyperpolarization, closure of voltage-dependent calcium channels, and ultimately vasodilation. Potassium channels are also present in endothelial cells. Activation within the endothelium results in changes in calcium flux and may be important in the release of NO, prostacyclin, and EDHF. Potassium channel subtypes include ATP-sensitive K+ channels, Ca^{2+}-dependent K+ channels, voltage-dependent K+ channels, and inward-rectifier K+ channels [97].

The breakdown of phospholipids within vascular endothelial cells results in the production of the important byproducts of arachidonic acid, including prostacyclin (PGI_2) and thromboxane (TXA_2). Prostacyclin activates adenylate cyclase, resulting in increased cAMP production and subsequent vasodilation, whereas TXA_2 results in vasoconstriction via phospholipase C signaling. Other prostaglandins and leukotrienes also have potent vasoactive properties. Increasing evidence suggests that endothelial injury and the resulting alteration in the balance of these and other vasoactive substances has a significant role in the development of pulmonary hypertension and increased vascular reactivity [22,98,99]. Support for this hypothesis is strengthened by observations that endothelial injury precedes pulmonary hypertension and its associated vascular remodeling in several animal models of pulmonary hypertension [61,100]. In humans, endothelial dysfunction, including histologic abnormalities of the endothelium, impairment of endothelium-dependent pulmonary vasodilation, and increased plasma ET-1 concentrations have been described in children with congenital heart defects and pulmonary hypertension before the development of significant vascular remodeling [22,98,101]. In addition, neonates with PPHN and adults with advanced pulmonary vascular disease have evidence of endothelial dysfunction, impairment of endothelium-dependent pulmonary vasodilation, increased plasma ET-1 concentrations, and decreased prostacyclin production [23,24,62,99]. The mechanism of injury to the vascular endothelium is unclear but is likely multifactorial and in part dependent on the etiology of the pulmonary hypertension. For example, in children with congenital heart disease and increased pulmonary blood flow, the initiating endothelial injury is likely mediated by increased shear stress. However, once pulmonary arterial pressure is elevated, shear stress-mediated endothelial injury appears to promote the progression of the disease, independent of the underlying etiology. Finally, a genetic disposition appears to be important in some subtypes of pulmonary vascular disease and remains an area of active research. For example, up to 60% of patients with familial idiopathic pulmonary hypertension have mutations resulting in the loss of function of bone morphogenetic protein receptor II [102–105].

Following an initial endothelial injury, smooth muscle proliferation and progressive structural remodeling occurs. The progression of anatomic changes is best characterized in congenital heart disease (see later discussion) [106–109]. However, regardless of the etiology, advanced disease is characterized by medial hypertrophy, intimal hyperplasia, angiomatoid formation, in situ thrombi, and eventual vascular obliteration. If the underlying stress remains untreated (e.g., delayed repair of cardiac shunt), these structural changes can progress to the point of becoming functionally "fixed" or irreversible. An important goal of therapy is to halt this progression and reverse the early vascular remodeling if possible.

General Treatment Approach

Regardless of the underlying etiology, the general treatment approach is similar and can be subdivided into four major goals: (1) prevent and acutely treat active pulmonary vasoconstriction, (2) support the failing right ventricle, (3) treat the underlying etiology, and (4) chronically promote, if possible, the regression of pulmonary vascular remodeling.

Prevent and Acutely Treat Active Pulmonary Vasoconstriction

In the intensive care setting, the prevention and treatment of active pulmonary vasoconstriction is a primary focus for the care of patients with underlying pulmonary vascular disease. It is well appreciated that these patients have augmented pulmonary vasoconstriction in response to such stimuli as hypoxia, acidosis, the catecholamine-mediated α_1-adrenergic stimulation associated with pain and agitation, and increases in intrathoracic pressure [110–112]. In fact, acute increases in pulmonary vascular resistance can lead to significant cardiopulmonary compromise (i.e., a pulmonary hypertensive crisis). The pathophysiology of such a crisis in outlined in Figure 20.3. Following an acute increase in pulmonary arterial pressure, there is an acute increase in right ventricular afterload, producing right ventricular ischemia and, ultimately, failure [113,114]. The resulting increase in right ventricular end diastolic volume shifts the intraventricular septum to the left, decreasing left ventricular volume and cardiac output. Decreased cardiac output results in decreased systemic perfusion and metabolic acidosis. Increased pulmonary vascular resistance and right ventricular failure also decrease pulmonary blood flow, increasing dead space ventilation. Distention of the pulmonary arteries and perivascular edema produce large and small airways obstruction, respectively, which impairs ventilation–perfusion matching and decreases lung compliance. In fact, the decrease in lung compliance can be so dramatic that chest wall movement is impaired, even with manual ventilation. The ensuing hypoxemia, hypercapnia, and acidosis (metabolic and/or respiratory) further increase pulmonary vascular resistance and perpetuate this cascade.

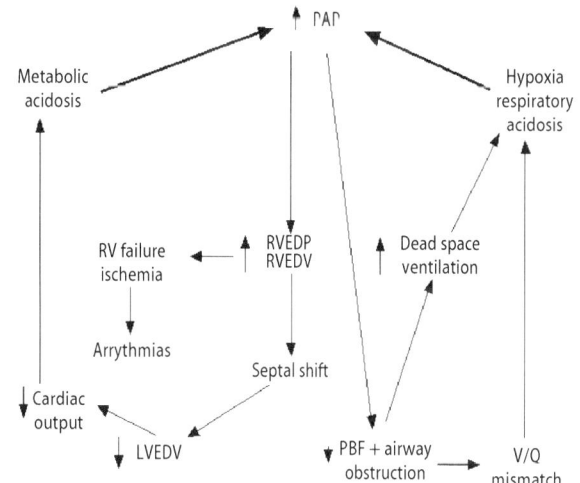

FIGURE 20.3. The cardiopulmonary effects of acute pulmonary hypertension. CO, cardiac output; LVEDV, left ventricular end diastolic volume; PAP, pulmonary arterial pressure; RV, right ventricle; RVEDP, right ventricular end diastolic pressure; RVEDV, right ventricular end diastolic volume; V/Q, ventilation/perfusion.

Prevention of pulmonary hypertensive crises may be accomplished by avoiding stimuli known to increase pulmonary vascular resistance, including hypoxia, acidosis, agitation, pulmonary overdistention, and polycythemia [112]. Various regimens have been utilized for this purpose, including the judicious use of supplemental oxygen, analgesics, sedatives, and muscle relaxants (especially before noxious stimuli, such as suctioning); the maintenance of an alkalotic pH with the use of controlled ventilation and buffer; aggressive evacuation of pneumothoraces and pleural effusions; the utilization of low lung volume ventilator strategies; the minimization of positive end-expiratory pressures; and the maintenance of the hematocrit below 55% [85,115]. In addition, data suggest that the use of pulmonary vasodilator therapy may decrease the incidence of pulmonary hypertensive crises [116–128].

Treatment of active pulmonary vasoconstriction is accomplished with the use of pulmonary vasodilator therapy. The mainstay of acute pulmonary vasodilator therapy remains supplemental oxygen and moderate alkalosis, as these therapies have minimal effects on the systemic vasculature. Interestingly, the dose-dependent response of the pulmonary vasculature to these agents has not been well established. Studies in newborn lambs demonstrate dose-dependent pulmonary vasodilation in response to increasing pH from 7.30 to 7.60, and a dose-dependent response to increasing inspired oxygen concentrations from 0.21 to 0.5, with minimal effects at higher concentrations [129]. Several intravenous agents have been utilized to promote pulmonary vasodilation, including tolazoline, sodium nitroprusside, nitroglycerin, prostacyclin, prostaglandin E$_1$, nifedipine, and α-adrenergic antagonists, such as phenoxybenzamine [130–137]. The efficacies of these agents are variable, at least in part because of their effects on the systemic vasculature. Systemic afterload reduction can be advantageous in the setting of left ventricular dysfunction; however, significant reductions in pulmonary arterial pressure without unacceptable systemic hypotension are often not possible [138–140]. In addition, intravenous vasodilators can override intrinsic hypoxic pulmonary vasoconstriction, resulting in an increase in dead space ventilation, which may not be tolerated in some critically ill patients [141–145].

More recent treatment modalities, most notably inhaled NO, deliver short-acting vasodilators to the pulmonary vasculature via an inhalational route [116–128]. When administered to the lung in its natural gaseous form, NO diffuses through the alveolar wall to reach small pulmonary arteries. It then enters vascular smooth muscle cells, initiating a cascade that results in pulmonary vasodilation via increases in cGMP. After entering the blood vessel lumen, NO is rapidly inactivated by hemoglobin, which confines its effects to the pulmonary vasculature. Because of these properties, inhaled NO has several advantages over other vasodilators, including (1) selective pulmonary vasodilation caused by rapid inactivation by hemoglobin, (2) rapid onset and elimination, and (3) an improvement in ventilation–perfusion matching because of the limitation of delivery to well-ventilated lung regions. Accordingly, inhaled NO has become a mainstay of treatment for acute pulmonary hypertensive disorders and the assessment of pulmonary vascular reactivity. Inhaled prostacyclin has similar pulmonary selectivity, secondary to rapid inactivation by hemoglobin. Its vasodilating effects are secondary to increasing cAMP concentrations. Currently, studies on the use of inhaled prostacyclin for pediatric pulmonary hypertension are sparse, and comparison studies between inhaled NO and inhaled prostacyclin are lacking [146–156].

Inhibitors of phosphodiesterases (PDEs), a family of enzymes that hydrolyze the cyclic nucleotides cAMP and cGMP, are a relatively new class of agents that have potent vasodilating and inotropic effects [157]. Milrinone is a PDE 3 inhibitor that increases cAMP concentrations. Animal and human data demonstrate pulmonary vasodilation in response to milrinone that can be in excess of its systemic effects if the pulmonary vasculature is constricted [158–161]. In addition, a large, randomized study demonstrates that its use decreases the incidence of low cardiac output syndrome following surgery for congenital heart disease [162]. Given these properties, milrinone is increasingly utilized in the postoperative management of patients with congenital heart disease and pulmonary hypertension.

Sildenafil, a PDE5 inhibitor, which increases cGMP concentrations, also has potent pulmonary vasodilating effects [163]. The oral formulation is currently being investigated for chronic pulmonary hypertensive therapy, and recent short-term studies demonstrate beneficial effects in children with advanced pulmonary vascular disease [164]. The intravenous formulation is currently being investigated for acute pediatric pulmonary hypertensive disorders (PPHN and perioperative pulmonary hypertension) [165,166].

Increasing data implicate alterations in ET-1 in the pathophysiology of pulmonary hypertension (see earlier) and suggest that ET-receptor antagonism may be a useful therapeutic strategy [24,25,54,60,97]. In fact, bosentan, an oral combined ET$_A$ and ET$_B$ receptor antagonist, has demonstrated efficacy as a chronic therapy for advanced pulmonary vascular disease [167,168]. To date, there have been no large studies on the use of ET receptor antagonists for acute pulmonary hypertensive disorders. In addition, the use of selective ET receptor antagonism is under investigation but has not yet reached clinical trials.

Support the Failing Right Ventricle

A significant component of the pathophysiology of both acute and chronic pulmonary hypertension is the development of right ventricular dysfunction, which often requires pharmacologic support. Maintenance of adequate preload is necessary to optimize cardiac output in patients with pulmonary hypertension. Continuous central venous pressure monitoring may be helpful to guide volume therapy, keeping in mind that patients with a poorly compliant right ventricle or increased right ventricular afterload may require elevated central venous pressures to maintain an adequate cardiac output. Frequent clinical assessment of liver size can be helpful, particularly in infants.

Despite adequate preload, cardiac output may be compromised secondary to elevated right ventricular afterload and/or biventricular myocardial dysfunction after cardiac surgery and cardiopulmonary bypass, necessitating the use of inotropic agents [111,169]. These agents increase stroke volume at a given preload and afterload by stimulating ß$_1$-adrenergic receptors [170,171]. However, some of these agents also stimulate ß$_2$- or α_1-adrenergic receptors, which are found on the smooth muscle cells of both the pulmonary and systemic arteries. Agents that stimulate ß$_2$-adrenergic receptors decrease both pulmonary and systemic vascular resistance and improve right and left ventricular function [172,173]. Agents that stimulate α_1-adrenergic receptors may increase both systemic and pulmonary vascular resistance. Therefore, a rational approach to using inotropic agents in the setting of pulmonary hypertension is to utilize agents with ß$_2$-receptor selectivity and minimal α_1-

adrenergic stimulation (i.e., dobutamine). Although animal studies have shown that high doses of dopamine increase pulmonary vascular resistance, human studies have shown increased cardiac output with minimal effects on pulmonary vascular resistance [130,174]. Milrinone is also a useful therapy for patients with pulmonary hypertension and myocardial dysfunction, given its vasodilatory and inotropic properties [162].

In the setting of pulmonary hypertension secondary to congenital heart defects, an atrial communication can be beneficial in that it allows the failing right ventricle to decompress when right atrial pressure rises [175]. Accordingly, atrial septal defects can be left unclosed (i.e., patent foramen ovale) or created at the time of surgery. The existence of an atrial level communication decreases the risk of right ventricular failure and maintains left-sided cardiac output. The resulting right-to-left shunt is generally well tolerated, particularly if high hemoglobin concentrations are maintained. As right ventricular function improves, right-to-left shunting decreases and oxygenation improves. Atrial septostomy as a part of management for chronic pulmonary hypertension (e.g., primary pulmonary hypertension) has been advocated but must be considered carefully on an individual basis [176–180].

In patients with refractory pulmonary hypertension, short-term postoperative extracorporeal support has been useful during the postoperative period of extreme vasoreactivity. However, its use should be limited to support those patients in which the underlying pulmonary vascular disease is deemed reversible.

Treat the Underlying Etiology

Whenever possible, treatment of the underlying disorder must coincide with symptomatic treatment for pulmonary hypertension if attenuation and/ reversal of the disease are to be successful. For example, in neonates, this may involve correction of underlying metabolic disturbances, antibiotics for infectious etiologies, and exchange transfusions for polycythemia. For patients with congenital heart disease, repair of the underlying defect, after determining that the pulmonary vascular disease is reversible (see later), is mandatory. For hypoxia-induced disease, tonsillectomy and adenoidectomy may be required for sleep apnea, and a descent to sea level may be needed for high-altitude–related disease. Finally, for rheumatologic disease, immunosuppression may be required.

Chronically Promote, if Possible, the Regression of Pulmonary Vascular Remodeling

The mainstay of chronic therapy has been aimed at decreasing pulmonary vascular resistance, thereby assisting right ventricular function and perhaps attenuating the progression of vascular remodeling by decreasing the pressure to which the vasculature is exposed. The continuous infusion of prostacyclin (epoprostin) has been the most successful therapy to date in this regard [181–185]. In fact, several studies in humans with advanced pulmonary vascular disease demonstrate improved 5-year survival and improved exercise tolerance. Interestingly, even those patients without an initial vasodilating response to the infusion show significant long-term benefit, suggesting that effects beyond vasodilation, such as antiplatelet effects, cAMP-mediated inhibition of smooth muscle cell growth, or other unknown mechanisms may be responsible for the treatment effect [186]. Despite the impressive results, several factors limit its utilization, including the need for chronic intravascular assess with the associated infectious and thrombotic risks, and many other untoward effects, including headache, flushing,

and acute cardiopulmonary compromise with disruption of the infusion [187].

With the increasing appreciation for the role of ET-1 in the pathophysiology of pulmonary vascular disease, ET receptor antagonists have been developed as a potential treatment modality. To date, bosentan, a combined ET_A and ET_B receptor antagonist, is the most widely studied agent and is the only receptor antagonist approved for the treatment of pulmonary hypertension [167,168]. Recent studies in adults with primary pulmonary hypertension demonstrate similar improvements in survival and exercise tolerance as those demonstrated with epoprostenol [188]. The use of ET receptor antagonists for pediatric pulmonary hypertensive disorders is currently under investigation.

Deficiencies in the NO–cGMP cascade in pulmonary vascular disease are well documented. In addition, the vasodilating effects, antiplatelet effects, and antiproliferative effects of augmenting this cascade are well appreciated. Therefore, new chronic therapies that augment NO–cGMP signaling, which include chronic inhaled NO delivered by nasal cannula and sildenafil, are currently under investigation [187]. In fact, the short-term benefit of sildenafil in children with advanced pulmonary hypertension has recently been reported [164].

Data indicate that several of these new oral therapies, such as bosentan and sildenafil, may offer additional benefit by virtue of their ability to inhibit vascular smooth muscle growth and fibrosis [187]. A number of other treatment strategies, including combination drug therapies, are currently under investigation. To date they have been used predominantly in advanced pulmonary vascular disease, but, due to these favorable characteristics, several potential applications warrant investigation. This includes their use in lung hypoplastic syndromes, in hypoxia-associated disease, and in congenital heart disease in order to improve the operability of patients with modest vascular changes [189].

Persistent Pulmonary Hypertension of the Newborn

In a number of clinical conditions, pulmonary vascular resistance does not decrease normally at birth. As a result, pulmonary blood flow remains reduced and pulmonary arterial pressure remains high. The pathophysiologic effects are hypoxemia, myocardial dysfunction, and a resulting reduction in systemic oxygen delivery. The hypoxemia is most often secondary to extrapulmonary right-to-left shunting of blood at the atrial and/or ductal levels but may also be secondary to intrapulmonary right-to-left shunting of blood when associated with parenchymal lung disease. The pathophysiologic mechanisms preventing the normal pulmonary vasodilatation at birth remain unclear and are most likely multifactorial in etiology.

Within this definition of PPHN, three major subgroups are often characterized: those with underdevelopment of the lung, those with maladaptation of the lung, and those with maldevelopment of the lung [58]. These subgroups represent a spectrum of etiologies and pathophysiology. For example, underdevelopment of the lung represents disorders of vascular hypoplasia, which are usually associated with varying degrees of lung hypoplasia. Within this subgroup, patients with congenital diaphragmatic hernia have been most thoroughly investigated. Although the structural abnormalities are greatest on the side of the hernia, both of the lungs of these patients are smaller and have fewer alveoli than do lungs from a normal control population [190–192]. Their lungs also have fewer vessels per unit of lung [192]. Thus, the total cross-sectional area of the vascular bed is markedly decreased. Furthermore, the existing pulmonary arteries have increased muscle mass with medial hypertrophy in normally muscularized arteries and an abnormal extension of muscle into the intra-acinar arteries. The increased muscularization may explain the labile, right-to-left extrapulmonary shunting of blood seen in such patients [193,194]. The response to therapy and long-term outcome is dictated by the degree of hypoplasia of the underlying vasculature. Following acute therapies, which often include surgical repair, mechanical ventilation with inhaled NO, and extracorporeal support, subacute and chronic pulmonary hypertension has been increasingly recognized as a major outcome variable in these patients. Because ultimately lung and vascular growth are necessary to reverse the disease process, aggressive long-term support with agents that inhibit vascular remodeling (i.e., ET receptor antagonists and PDE inhibitors) is an emerging treatment approach to support these infants as they grow.

Maladaptation of the lung represents a stress event at the time of delivery that does not allow the normal dilating stimuli, such as increases in systemic arterial pH and oxygen tension, to occur. This may occur in the setting of apnea, pneumonia, sepsis, and aspiration of meconium or amniotic fluid [195–197]. The underlying pulmonary vasculature is often normal, and, thus, these neonates are likely to respond to vasodilator therapy and the correction of contributory metabolic abnormalities.

Maldevelopment of the lung represents a group of conditions in which the vasculature is thickened and abnormally distributed. For example, some newborns who die from persistent pulmonary hypertension have abnormally muscular pulmonary vascular beds, even when they die on the first day of life. In particular, they have thickened muscular coats in the normally muscular preacinar arteries, and extension of muscle into the normally nonmuscular intra-acinar arteries [56,57]. Because vascular remodeling takes time to develop, it has been hypothesized that this increased muscularization is caused by a chronic intrauterine stress. In animal models, this pathophysiology can be mimicked by chronic placental insufficiency, fetal hypoxemia, chronic constriction of the ductus arteriosus, and chronic NO inhibition [40,55,198–203]. Interestingly, PPHN has been associated with maternal indomethacin use, which causes constriction of the ductus arteriosus [204,205]. The response to therapy in neonates with maldevelopment of the lung is variable and may be related to the extent and type of underlying structural vascular pathology.

The primary therapeutic approach is to decrease pulmonary vascular resistance and support myocardial function. The specific treatment modality depends on the underlying etiology. If the cause is perinatal asphyxia, correcting alveolar hypoxia, hypercarbia, and metabolic acidosis by ventilation with 100% oxygen, and by administration of buffer, should decrease pulmonary vascular tone toward normal levels. If parenchymal disease (i.e., respiratory distress syndrome, meconium aspiration, or pneumonia) is causing pulmonary vasospasm due to alveolar hypoxia and hypercarbia, then inflation of the alveoli with positive end-expiratory pressure, surfactant administration, and mechanical ventilation may reverse the pulmonary hypertension [206–208]. The near-term child can exert substantial intrathoracic pressure opposing mechanical ventilation; thus, sedation and occasionally muscle paralysis may be necessary to obtain stable mechanical ventilation [209].

When treatment of the underlying pulmonary parenchymal, infectious, or inflammatory disease is ineffective, or if there is no such underlying disease, therapy is directed at reversing abnormal pulmonary vasoconstriction. This is generally accomplished with sedation, mechanical ventilation with 100% oxygen, and alkalinization. When further pulmonary vasodilation is needed, inhaled NO is utilized with or without high-frequency ventilation. In fact, several multicentered, randomized trials have demonstrated that inhaled NO improves oxygenation and decreases the need for extracorporeal life support in newborns with persistent pulmonary hypertension [117,121,126], although no differences in mortality were noted. The use of extracorporeal membrane oxygenation has substantially decreased overall mortality for most subsets of PPHN. However, overall mortality rates remain substantial at 5%–15% [210–213].

Pulmonary Hypertension Associated with Congenital Heart Disease

The development of pulmonary hypertension and increased pulmonary vascular reactivity is associated with two major types of congenital heart disease: (1) those with increased pulmonary blood flow and pulmonary arterial pressure and (2) those with increased pulmonary venous pressure [110–112,169]. After birth, large communications at the level of the ventricles or great vessels result in increased pulmonary blood flow and pulmonary arterial pressure, which produces progressive structural and functional abnormalities of the pulmonary vasculature [59,106–110,214–217]. Similarly, elevated pulmonary venous pressure results in progressive increases in pulmonary venous and arterial pressure, which produces structural abnormalities of the pulmonary vasculature. Heath and Edwards first described the progression of these pulmonary vascular changes in 1958 [217]. In their classification, changes progress from medial hypertrophy (grade I) to intimal hyperplasia (grade II), lumen occlusion (grade III), arterial dilatation (grade IV), angiomatoid formation (grade V) and fibrinoid necrosis (grade VI). In addition, morphometric analysis shows progression of disturbed arterial growth and remodeling of the pulmonary vascular bed, which correlates with the aberrant hemodynamic state of the pulmonary circulation [108,109,214–216]. These changes are characterized by (1) abnormal extension of vascular smooth muscle into small peripheral pulmonary arteries and mild medial hypertrophy of normally muscular arteries (grade A), (2) severe medial hypertrophy of normally muscular arteries (grade B), and (3) decreased pulmonary arterial number (grade C). Uncorrected, these vascular changes result in decreased cross-sectional area and obliteration of the pulmonary vascular bed and death secondary to severe cyanosis or myocardial failure.

Different congenital heart defects vary considerably in the frequency and severity of pulmonary hypertension. The risks and frequencies of developing advanced pulmonary vascular disease (PVD) for particular heart defects are summarized in Table 20.2. Importantly, children with trisomy 21 and congenital heart defects often have an accelerated development of advanced pulmonary vascular disease [218]. This may be secondary to confounding factors such as airway obstruction or another unidentified predisposition. After surgical correction, early vascular changes (grades I–III, grades A, B) are reversible; however, more severe changes are irreversible and progressive. Therefore, the pathophysiologic state of the pulmonary circulation is the main determinant of the clinical course and the success of surgical treatment, and it explains the trend toward early repair of congenital heart defects [169].

Although early surgical repair of congenital heart defects has decreased the incidence of irreversible pulmonary vascular disease,

TABLE 20.2. Risks and frequencies of developing advanced pulmonary vascular disease (PVD) in the presence of a heart defect.

Defect	Risk of PVD	Age
Increased pulmonary blood flow		
Truncus arteriosus	~100%	<2 years
Atrioventricular canal	~100%	~2 years
Ventricular septal defect (VSD)	~15%–20%	>2 years
Patent ductus arteriosus	~15%–20%	>2 years
Transposition of the great arteries with VSD	~70%–100%	1–2 years
Atrial septal defect	~20%	>20 years
Increased pulmonary venous pressure		
Obstructed TAPVR (total anomalous pulmonary venous return)	Variable	Variable
Cor triatriatum	Variable	Variable
Mitral stenosis	Variable	Variable

even those children with reversible vascular changes suffer morbidity and mortality in the perioperative period secondary to chronic and/or acute elevations in pulmonary vascular resistance [10–112,219]. Chronic elevations are related to the structural changes that decrease the cross-sectional area of the pulmonary vascular bed. These alterations may take several months to normalize following surgical repair. Acute elevations in pulmonary vascular resistance are often seen immediately following surgery with cardiopulmonary bypass, when there is often a period of enhanced pulmonary vascular reactivity [8,22,98]. This period may last up to 5–7 days and is most likely a manifestation of preexisting aberrant endothelial cell–smooth muscle cell interactions that are exacerbated at the time of surgery. During cardiopulmonary bypass, several factors including the disruption of pulmonary blood flow, complement activation, and neutrophil activation induce pulmonary vascular endothelial dysfunction. This results in an increase in the production and/or release of endothelial factors that promote vasoconstriction, such ET-1 and TXA_2, and a decrease in endothelial relaxing factors, most importantly NO [220]. This period of extreme reactivity may produce severe hypoxemia, acidosis, low cardiac output, and death if not treated immediately.

Classically, a preoperative determination of pulmonary vascular reactivity is made in the cardiac catheterization laboratory in order to assess the operability of a given patient, that is, the degree to which the pulmonary vascular disease is reversible, as well as the postoperative risk. This testing involves measuring pulmonary arterial pressure and calculating pulmonary vascular resistance under varying conditions. The vascular resistance following acute maximal vasodilator therapy (e.g., oxygen and NO) represents the degree of structural pulmonary vascular disease that is present. Despite the frequent utilization of such testing, there is no absolute pulmonary vascular resistance that is universally considered inoperable. In general, a larger reduction in resistance in response to vasodilator therapy correlates with an increased chance of reversibility and a lower risk of perioperative morbidity from pulmonary hypertension. Recent studies suggest that the combination of 100% oxygen and inhaled NO produces maximal pulmonary vasodilation and has some perioperative predictive value [221,222]. In fact, a 20% decrease in the ratio of the pulmonary-to-systemic vascular resistance with vasodilator therapy, and a nadir in this ratio of less than 33%, was 97% sensitive and 90% accurate in predicting a good surgical outcome. Therefore, the combination of oxygen and inhaled NO is now most commonly used for pulmonary vascular reactivity

testing. Reactivity testing may also be helpful in the intensive care unit in the setting of a persistent postoperative elevation of pulmonary arterial pressure in order to differentiate between residual anatomic defects and prolonged periods of increased tone [118].

The optimal treatment for perioperative pulmonary hypertensive morbidity is prevention with early surgical repair. It is increasingly clear that the longer the pulmonary vasculature is exposed to the abnormal forces associated with increased blood flow and/or pressure, the greater the risk of perioperative pulmonary vascular reactivity. Following surgery, the goal of perioperative management is to minimize active pulmonary vasoconstriction during the period of exaggerated reactivity and support the right ventricle. To this end, avoidance of those stimuli that increase pulmonary vascular resistance (hypoxia, acidosis, pain, agitation, increased intrathoracic pressure) is critical. Continuous pulmonary arterial and right atrial pressure monitoring is often helpful by allowing prompt recognition of pulmonary hypertensive crises and evaluation of the response to therapeutic maneuvers. Monitoring systemic arterial pressure and systemic arterial oxygen saturation is essential in that it allows changes in pulmonary arterial pressure to be interpreted in the context of the total cardiopulmonary response. For example, if systemic and pulmonary arterial pressures increase in response to pain and agitation, but right atrial pressure does not increase, and systemic perfusion and oxygen saturation remain adequate, then specific treatment directed at the pulmonary vasculature is not necessary. Conversely, increases in pulmonary arterial pressure that are associated with increased right atrial pressure, decreased systemic pressure, and/or decreased systemic saturation might herald imminent collapse.

The objective of vasodilator therapy is to decrease right ventricular afterload and prevent acute increases in pulmonary arterial pressure. Inhaled NO, in combination with oxygen, has been increasingly utilized because of its potent vasodilating effects, pulmonary selectivity, and rapid onset and elimination (see earlier). Several studies demonstrate its potent vasodilating effects in this population [223–226]; however, large, randomized trails are lacking. One randomized trial did demonstrate that inhaled NO decreased postoperative pulmonary vascular resistance, the incidence of pulmonary hypertensive crises, and the days of mechanical ventilation compared with placebo [226]. In patients with a history of pulmonary venous hypertension (total anomalous pulmonary venous return, mitral valve disease), aggressive diuresis may be helpful because interstitial pulmonary edema may contribute significantly to elevations in pulmonary vascular resistance.

Therapies that maintain an adequate cardiac output in this patient population are not dissimilar to therapies utilized in other patient populations, with the exception of the particular emphasis placed on right ventricular afterload reduction and support. It is noteworthy that patients with a poorly compliant right ventricle or with increased right ventricular afterload may require elevated central venous pressures to maintain an adequate preload. In addition, the use of inotropic agents with significant α_1-adrenergic effect should be minimized to avoid the associated pulmonary vasoconstriction. Agents such as dobutamine, milrinone, and dopamine are routinely utilized.

The use of high levels of positive end-expiratory pressure (PEEP) is somewhat controversial. Mechanical hyperventilation with high PEEP increases intrathoracic pressure and pulmonary vascular resistance [85,115]. This therapy should be avoided if adequate systemic arterial saturation can be achieved by other means. However, at low lung volumes, the use of PEEP may increase lung volume toward functional residual capacity and, thus, improve gas exchange and may lower pulmonary vascular resistance. Mechanical ventilation without PEEP (especially in patients after partial and total caval-pulmonary shunts) predisposes patients to atelectasis, worsens ventilation–perfusion matching, results in systemic arterial hypoxemia, and increases pulmonary vascular resistance [85]. Thus, low levels of PEEP (3–4 cm H_2O), which have minimal effects on pulmonary vascular resistance, should be used to prevent atelectasis in this patient population.

Primary Pulmonary Hypertension

Until very recently, pulmonary arterial hypertension of unknown etiology was termed *primary pulmonary hypertension*. However, recent evidence indicates a genetic disposition in a subset of patients with primary pulmonary hypertension, and a number of diseases that lead to pulmonary arterial hypertension with similar histological and pathophysiologic features have been uncovered [102–105]. Thus, at the 2003 Third World Symposium on Pulmonary Arterial Hypertension, a new classification was proposed to further classify primary pulmonary hypertension into the following subgroups: (1) idiopathic pulmonary arterial hypertension (IPAH), (2) familial pulmonary arterial hypertension (FPAH), and (3) pulmonary arterial hypertension related to risk factors or associated conditions (APAH) [227].

Unfortunately, mortality from primary pulmonary hypertension remains high and may be higher for children than adults. In fact, the Primary Pulmonary Hypertension National Institutes of Health Registry reports a median survival of only 10 months for pediatric patients [228]. However, recent data suggest that pediatric patients may respond differently than adults to new therapies and that these differences may portend a better outcome in younger patients [229,230]. The frequency of primary pulmonary hypertension in pediatric patients is not known, but it appears that the number of confirmed cases is increasing. The incidence is slightly increased in females [231]. The most common causes of death in children with primary pulmonary hypertension are right ventricular failure and sudden death, which may be related to malignant cardiac arrhythmias, pulmonary emboli, or acute right ventricular ischemia [228]. Physicians caring for children in an intensive care unit setting must be cognizant of this disorder, albeit rare, because relatively benign disease processes, such as pneumonia, can be life threatening for children with primary pulmonary hypertension, which may not have been previously identified.

As opposed to adults with primary pulmonary hypertension, who often have severe plexiform lesions resulting in relatively fixed vascular changes, children display greater medial hypertrophy with less intimal fibrosis and fewer plexiform lesions [187,229]. In addition, pediatric patients have a decreased pulmonary arterial number and increased pulmonary vascular reactivity compared with adult patients. The molecular mechanisms underlying primary pulmonary hypertension remain speculative; however, studies suggest an integral role for endothelial dysfunction, resulting in an increase in factors that favor both vasoconstriction and mitogenesis, such as ET-1 and TXA_2, and a decrease in factors that promote vasodilation and smooth muscle antiproliferation, such as NO and prostacyclin [23,101,187,232–235]. Other mechanisms have been investigated including, altered gene expression, coagulation abnormalities (resulting in intravascular thrombosis), and defects of pulmonary vascular smooth muscle cell potassium channels [236–238].

Recent advances in the understanding of pulmonary hypertension have established an association with a number of disease processes and toxins. Thus, it is now known that pulmonary hypertension can be related to collagen vascular disease, portal hypertension, human immunodeficiency virus infection, chronic obstructive pulmonary disease, interstitial lung disease, sleep-disordered breathing, alveolar hypoventilation disorders, chronic exposure to high altitudes, thromboembolic disease, sickle cell disease, *Schistosomiasis*, sarcoidosis, thyroid disorders, glycogen storage disease, Gaucher disease, hereditary hemorrhagic telangiectasia, myeloproliferative disorders, and pulmonary capillary hemangiomatosis. In addition, drugs or toxins, most notably anorexigens, have been associated with the development of pulmonary hypertension [187,227]. In general the diagnostic work-up includes history and physical examination, electrocardiography, chest radiography, echocardiography, and cardiac catheterization. Serologic evaluation in order to exclude secondary causes is required, and V/Q scanning to evaluate for pulmonary emboli may be necessary.

Treatment strategies for pediatric pulmonary arterial hypertension are evolving. When the disease is associated with a known disorder, treatment must include specific therapy aimed at the underlying condition. However, general treatments include the approach reviewed above, with oxygen, calcium channel blockers, anticoagulation, ET receptor antagonists, prostacyclin analogues, acute and chronic inhaled NO, PDE type 5 inhibitors, atrial septostomy, and lung or heart–lung transplant considerations as indicated [187].

Patients with pulmonary arterial hypertension have histologic evidence of in situ pulmonary vascular thrombosis, which is the rationale for anticoagulation therapy. Although several adult studies have demonstrated its efficacy, pediatric studies are lacking [239,240]. Currently, warfarin is the treatment of choice for adult patients and in large pediatric centers with significant experience with pediatric pulmonary arterial hypertension. Low-molecular-weight heparin is another alternative [241]; aspirin does not have any demonstrated efficacy.

Chronic calcium channel blockade is efficacious for a subset of adults and children with pulmonary arterial hypertension. In fact, whereas less than 25% of adults respond to calcium channel blockers, up to 40% of children are positive responders [186,242]. It is worth noting that calcium channel blockers are not utilized in the management of other common causes of pediatric pulmonary hypertension, such as PPHN and congenital heart disease. Indeed, calcium channel blockade should be avoided in neonates and after congenital heart surgery. However, studies indicate that long-acting calcium channel blockers, such as nifedipine and amlodipine, are well tolerated in children with primary pulmonary hypertension. An important caveat is that a positive response to calcium channel blockers (i.e., an acute reduction in pulmonary arterial pressure) must be demonstrated as a part of acute vasodilator reactivity testing. Children without a positive acute response do not benefit from chronic treatment.

Prostaglandins are a mainstay of therapy for patients with pulmonary arterial hypertension. In general, prostacyclin (epoprostenol) is administered as a continuous infusion, necessitating a permanent indwelling central catheter, with its associated risks [181–185]. However, various other formulations including oral, inhaled, and subcutaneous prostacyclin analogues have been developed and are in various stages of clinical investigation [243–246].

Supplemental oxygen, cardiac glycosides, antiarrhythmic therapy, and inotropic agents are also variably utilized in certain patients [187,247]. Diuretic therapy is also often beneficial, keeping in mind that these patients may require elevated right ventricular preload. Based on an expanding understanding of the disease process, future therapies might include elastase inhibitors and gene therapy [248,249]. As noted previously, atrial septostomy may have a role in the management of a select group of patients [250]. However, atrial septostomy in the setting of an acute exacerbation of chronic pulmonary hypertension may lead to unacceptable hypoxemia because of excess right-to-left atrial shunting. Finally, heart–lung, single-lung, or bilateral lung transplantation has been successful in pediatric patients with terminal pulmonary hypertension [251,252]. The International Society for Heart and Lung Transplantation reports survival of approximately 50% at 5 years in pediatric patients [253]. Consensus is lacking as to the best type of transplant.

Other

Hypoxia

Increases in pulmonary arterial pressure in response to hypoxia are well described. Clinical and experimental evidence suggests that prolonged exposure or chronic intermittent exposure to hypoxia can result in functional and structural derangements of the pulmonary vasculature, leading to pulmonary hypertension [254–256]. Fortunately, elevations in pulmonary arterial pressure that occur in response to acute hypoxia (such as an acute ascent in altitude) are rapidly reversible. Interestingly, there is great clinical variability in the response to hypoxia. For example, increased susceptibility to high-altitude pulmonary edema, which is associated with increased pulmonary arterial pressure, has been linked to certain major histocompatibility complexes [257,258]. The mechanisms of hypoxia-induced pulmonary hypertension continue to be an area of intense investigation. To date the precise mechanisms remain unclear, but it is known that a number of endothelial derived factors, such as NO, ET-1, leukotrienes, and potassium channels, participate [10,259–262]. Furthermore, additional genetic polymorphisms are also under investigation. Pediatricians must consider this physiology in patients with conditions such as upper airway obstruction, central hypoventilation, and neuromuscular disorders that affect ventilation. In fact, many of these patients do develop evidence of pulmonary hypertension, with right ventricular enlargement. In most cases, addressing the underlying pathology is curative, but it can take some time to fully reverse the structural changes that have occurred.

Acute Lung Injury

The pathophysiology of acute lung injury involves damage to both the alveolar epithelium and pulmonary vascular endothelium. Vascular endothelial injury accounts for key features of acute lung injury, including intravascular thrombosis and capillary permeability that increases alveolar fluid [263]. In fact, pulmonary vascular injury, in the setting of acute lung injury, can lead to pulmonary arterial hypertension, resulting in increased intrapulmonary shunting, hypoxia, pulmonary edema, and right ventricular dysfunction [264–267]. In children with acute lung injury, persistently elevated pulmonary arterial pressures have been associated with worse outcomes [268]; therefore, vasodilators have been utilized in the management of these patients. However, intravenous vasodila-

tors that dilate both the systemic and pulmonary vasculature have significant problems, including systemic hypotension, right ventricular ischemia, increased intrapulmonary shunting (i.e., increased V/Q mismatch), and increased hypoxemia [141–145]. Consequently, selective pulmonary vasodilation with inhaled NO has been utilized, as it improves V/Q matching and oxygenation without untoward systemic effects [269,270]. Unfortunately, improvements in oxygenation associated with inhaled NO are transient, and large randomized trials have failed to demonstrate an improvement in mortality with its use [120,271,272]. The routine use of inhaled NO in patients with acute lung injury, therefore, cannot be justified; however, it may be indicated in individual patients, particularly those with an acute hemodynamic compromise and refractory hypoxemia caused by elevated pulmonary arterial pressures. Clearly, physicians caring for pediatric patients with acute lung injury must include an awareness of the pulmonary vascular aberrations associated with the disease in their management considerations.

Conclusion

Historically, diseases of the pulmonary vasculature, although not uncommon, have been underrecognized. This was caused, in part, by the paucity of effective treatments as well as an incomplete understanding of the vascular biologic mechanisms. In fact, over the past decade, the therapeutic gold standard has been the continuous infusion of prostacyclin. Although certainly extending and improving the lives of many patients, intravenous prostacyclin administration has been predominantly limited to patients with irreversible disease, given the inconvenience and morbidity associated with its delivery. Fortunately, an expanded understanding of the vascular endothelium, vascular smooth muscle cells, and the role of their interactions in the pathophysiology of pulmonary vascular disease have resulted in new effective treatments, with additional potential therapies evolving rapidly. Oral agents such as bosentan and sildenafil are two examples with great promise. In addition, accumulated experience and focused research have uncovered a multitude of disease processes that contribute directly or indirectly to the development of pulmonary hypertension. Physicians caring for critically ill children must be aware of these illnesses, the pathophysiology of pulmonary hypertension, and the available treatment options in order to translate these advances into improved outcomes for patients.

References

1. McIntyre TM, Zimmerman GA, Satoh K, Prescott SM. Cultured endothelial cells synthesize both platelet-activating factor and prostacyclin in response to histamine, bradykinin, and adenosine triphosphate. J Clin Invest 1985;76(1):271–280.
2. Yanagisawa M, Kurihara H, Kimura S, Tomobe Y, Kobayashi M, Mitsui Y, et al. A novel potent vasoconstrictor peptide produced by vascular endothelial cells. Nature 1988;332(6163):411–415.
3. Palmer RM, Ashton DS, Moncada S. Vascular endothelial cells synthesize nitric oxide from L-arginine. Nature 1988;333(6174):664–666.
4. Rubanyi GM, Romero JC, Vanhoutte PM. Flow-induced release of endothelium-derived relaxing factor. Am J Physiol 1986;250(6 Pt 2):H1145–H1149.
5. Fiscus RR. Molecular mechanisms of endothelium-mediated vasodilation. Semin Thromb Haemost 1988;14(Suppl):12–22.

6. Moncada S, Higgs A. The L-arginine-nitric oxide pathway. N Engl J Med 1993;329(27):2002–2012.

7. Fineman JR, Heymann MA, Soifer SJ. N omega-nitro-L-arginine attenuates endothelium-dependent pulmonary vasodilation in lambs. Am J Physiol 1991;260(4 Pt 2):H1299–H1306.

8. Dinh-Xuan AT. Endothelial modulation of pulmonary vascular tone. Eur Respir J 1992;5(6):757–762.

9. Garg UC, Hassid A. Nitric oxide-generating vasodilators and 8-bromo-cyclic guanosine monophosphate inhibit mitogenesis and proliferation of cultured rat vascular smooth muscle cells. J Clin Invest 1989;83(5):1774–1777.

10. Fineman JR, Chang R, Soifer SJ. EDRF inhibition augments pulmonary hypertension in intact newborn lambs. Am J Physiol 1992;262(5 Pt 2):H1365–H1371.

11. Fineman JR, Crowley MR, Heymann MA, Soifer SJ. In vivo attenuation of endothelium-dependent pulmonary vasodilation by methylene blue. J Appl Physiol 1991;71(2):735–741.

12. Braner DA, Fineman JR, Chang R, Soifer SJ. M&B 22948, a cGMP phosphodiesterase inhibitor, is a pulmonary vasodilator in lambs. Am J Physiol 1993;264(1 Pt 2):H252–H258.

13. Kourembanas S, McQuillan LP, Leung GK, Faller DV. Nitric oxide regulates the expression of vasoconstrictors and growth factors by vascular endothelium under both normoxia and hypoxia. J Clin Invest 1993;92(1):99–104.

14. Budhiraja R, Tuder RM, Hassoun PM. Endothelial dysfunction in pulmonary hypertension. Circulation 2004;109(2):159–165.

15. Matsuura A, Kawashima S, Yamochi W, Hirata K, Yamaguchi T, Emoto N, et al. Vascular endothelial growth factor increases endothelin-converting enzyme expression in vascular endothelial cells. Biochem Biophys Res Commun 1997;235(3):713–716.

16. Cassin S, Kristova V, Davis T, Kadowitz P, Gause G. Tone-dependent responses to endothelin in the isolated perfused fetal sheep pulmonary circulation in situ. J Appl Physiol 1991;70(3):1228–1234.

17. Wong J, Vanderford PA, Fineman JR, Chang R, Soifer SJ. Endothelin-1 produces pulmonary vasodilation in the intact newborn lamb. Am J Physiol 1993;265(4 Pt 2):H1318–H1325.

18. Wong J, Vanderford PA, Fineman JR, Soifer SJ. Developmental effects of endothelin-1 on the pulmonary circulation in sheep. Pediatr Res 1994;36(3):394–401.

19. Bradley LM, Czaja JF, Goldstein RE. Circulatory effects of endothelin in newborn piglets. Am J Physiol 1990;259(5 Pt 2):H1613–H1617.

20. Perreault T, De Marte J. Maturational changes in endothelium-derived relaxations in newborn piglet pulmonary circulation. Am J Physiol 1993;264(2 Pt 2):H302–H309.

21. Rudolph AM, Heymann MA. Circulatory changes during growth in the fetal lamb. Circ Res 1970;26(3):289–299.

22. Celermajer DS, Cullen S, Deanfield JE. Impairment of endothelium-dependent pulmonary artery relaxation in children with congenital heart disease and abnormal pulmonary hemodynamics. Circulation 1993;87(2):440–446.

23. Giaid A, Saleh D. Reduced expression of endothelial nitric oxide synthase in the lungs of patients with pulmonary hypertension. N Engl J Med 1995;333(4):214–221.

24. Giaid A, Yanagisawa M, Langleben D, Michel RP, Levy R, Shennib H, et al. Expression of endothelin-1 in the lungs of patients with pulmonary hypertension. N Engl J Med 1993;328(24):1732–1739.

25. Reddy VM, Wong J, Liddicoat JR, Johengen M, Chang R, Fineman JR. Altered endothelium-dependent responses in lambs with pulmonary hypertension and increased pulmonary blood flow. Am J Physiol 1996;271(2 Pt 2):H562–H570.

26. Levin DL, Rudolph AM, Heymann MA, Phibbs RH. Morphological development of the pulmonary vascular bed in fetal lambs. Circulation 1976;53(1):144–151.

27. Iwamoto HS, Teitel D, Rudolph AM. Effects of birth-related events on blood flow distribution. Pediatr Res 1987;22(6):634–640.

28. Rudolph AM. Fetal and neonatal pulmonary circulation. Annu Rev Physiol 1979;41:383–395.

29. Dawes GS, Mott JC, Widdicombe JG, Wyatt DG. Changes in the lungs of the new-born lamb. J Physiol 1953;121(1):141–162.

30. Heyman MA, Soifer S. Control of the fetal and neonatal pulmonary circulation. In: Weir EK, Reeves JT, eds. Pulmonary Vascular Physiology and Pathophysiology. New York: Dekker; 1989.

31. Rudolph AM. Distribution and regulation of blood flow in the fetal and neonatal lamb. Circ Res 1985;57(6):811–821.

32. Fineman JR, Soifer SJ, Heymann MA. Regulation of pulmonary vascular tone in the perinatal period. Annu Rev Physiol 1995;57:115–134.

33. Enhorning G, Adams FH, Norman A. Effect of lung expansion on the fetal lamb circulation. Acta Paediatr Scand 1966;55(5):441–451.

34. Leffler CW, Hessler JR, Green RS. The onset of breathing at birth stimulates pulmonary vascular prostacyclin synthesis. Pediatr Res 1984;18(10):938–942.

35. Tiktinsky MH, Morin FC, 3rd. Increasing oxygen tension dilates fetal pulmonary circulation via endothelium-derived relaxing factor. Am J Physiol 1993;265(1 Pt 2):H376–H3780.

36. Shaul PW, Farrar MA, Zellers TM. Oxygen modulates endothelium-derived relaxing factor production in fetal pulmonary arteries. Am J Physiol 1992;262(2 Pt 2):H355–H364.

37. Shaul PW, Farrar MA, Magness RR. Pulmonary endothelial nitric oxide production is developmentally regulated in the fetus and newborn. Am J Physiol 1993;265(4 Pt 2):H1056–H1063.

38. Cornfield DN, Chatfield BA, McQueston JA, McMurtry IF, Abman SH. Effects of birth-related stimuli on L-arginine-dependent pulmonary vasodilation in ovine fetus. Am J Physiol 1992;262(5 Pt 2):H1474–H1481.

39. Black SM, Johengen MJ, Ma ZD, Bristow J, Soifer SJ. Ventilation and oxygenation induce endothelial nitric oxide synthase gene expression in the lungs of fetal lambs. J Clin Invest 1997;100(6):1448–1458.

40. Fineman JR, Wong J, Morin FC, 3rd, Wild LM, Soifer SJ. Chronic nitric oxide inhibition in utero produces persistent pulmonary hypertension in newborn lambs. J Clin Invest 1994;93(6):2675–2683.

41. Beghetti M, Black SM, Fineman JR. Endothelin-1 in congenital heart disease. Pediatr Res 2005;57(5 Pt 2):16R–20R.

42. Black S, Fineman J, Johengen M, Bristow J, Soifer S. Increased pulmonary blood flow alters the molecular regulation of vascular reactivity in the lamb. Chest 1998;114(1 Suppl):39S.

43. Black SM, Bekker JM, Johengen MJ, Parry AJ, Soifer SJ, Fineman JR. Altered regulation of the ET-1 cascade in lambs with increased pulmonary blood flow and pulmonary hypertension. Pediatr Res 2000;47(1):97–106.

44. Black SM, Bekker JM, McMullan DM, Parry AJ, Ovadia B, Reinhartz O, et al. Alterations in nitric oxide production in 8-week-old lambs with increased pulmonary blood flow. Pediatr Res 2002;52(2):233–244.

45. Black SM, Fineman JR, Steinhorn RH, Bristow J, Soifer SJ. Increased endothelial NOS in lambs with increased pulmonary blood flow and pulmonary hypertension. Am J Physiol 1998;275(5 Pt 2):H1643–H1651.

46. Black SM, Mata-Greenwood E, Dettman RW, Ovadia B, Fitzgerald RK, Reinhartz O, et al. Emergence of smooth muscle cell endothelin B-mediated vasoconstriction in lambs with experimental congenital heart disease and increased pulmonary blood flow. Circulation 2003;108(13):1646–1654.

47. Black SM, Sanchez LS, Mata-Greenwood E, Bekker JM, Steinhorn RH, Fineman JR. sGC and PDE5 are elevated in lambs with increased pulmonary blood flow and pulmonary hypertension. Am J Physiol Lung Cell Mol Physiol 2001;281(5):L1051–L1057.

48. Fineman JR, Wong J, Mikhailov T, Vanderford PA, Jerome HE, Soifer SJ. Altered endothelial function in lambs with pulmonary hypertension and acute lung injury. Pediatr Pulmonol 1999;27(3):147–156.

49. Mata-Greenwood E, Meyrick B, Steinhorn RH, Fineman JR, Black SM. Alterations in TGF-beta1 expression in lambs with increased pulmonary blood flow and pulmonary hypertension. Am J Physiol Lung Cell Mol Physiol 2003;285(1):L209–L221.

50. Ovadia B, Reinhartz O, Fitzgerald R, Bekker JM, Johengen MJ, Azakie A, et al. Alterations in ET-1, not nitric oxide, in 1-week-old lambs with increased pulmonary blood flow. Am J Physiol Heart Circ Physiol 2003;284(2):H480–H490.

51. Reddy VM, Meyrick B, Wong J, Khoor A, Liddicoat JR, Hanley FL, et al. In utero placement of aortopulmonary shunts. A model of postnatal pulmonary hypertension with increased pulmonary blood flow in lambs. Circulation 1995;92(3):606–613.

52. Steinhorn RH, Fineman JR. The pathophysiology of pulmonary hypertension in congenital heart disease. Artif Organs 1999;23(11):970–974.

53. Steinhorn RH, Russell JA, Lakshminrusimha S, Gugino SF, Black SM, Fineman JR. Altered endothelium-dependent relaxations in lambs with high pulmonary blood flow and pulmonary hypertension. Am J Physiol Heart Circ Physiol 2001;280(1):H311–H317.

54. Wong J, Reddy VM, Hendricks-Munoz K, Liddicoat JR, Gerrets R, Fineman JR. Endothelin-1 vasoactive responses in lambs with pulmonary hypertension and increased pulmonary blood flow. Am J Physiol 1995;269(6 Pt 2):H1965–H1972.

55. Abman SH, Shanley PF, Accurso FJ. Failure of postnatal adaptation of the pulmonary circulation after chronic intrauterine pulmonary hypertension in fetal lambs. J Clin Invest 1989;83(6):1849–1858.

56. Haworth SG, Reid L. Persistent fetal circulation: newly recognized structural features. J Pediatr 1976;88(4 Pt 1):614–620.

57. Murphy JD, Rabinovitch M, Goldstein JD, Reid LM. The structural basis of persistent pulmonary hypertension of the newborn infant. J Pediatr 1981;98(6):962–967.

58. Oishi P, Fineman JR. Pharmacologic therapy for persistent pulmonary hypertension of the newborn: as "poly" as the disease itself. Pediatr Crit Care Med 2004;5(1):94–96.

59. Reid LM. Structure and function in pulmonary hypertension. New perceptions. Chest 1986;89(2):279–288.

60. Rosenberg AA, Kennaugh J, Koppenhafer SL, Loomis M, Chatfield BA, Abman SH. Elevated immunoreactive endothelin-1 levels in newborn infants with persistent pulmonary hypertension. J Pediatr 1993;123(1):109–114.

61. Adnot S, Raffestin B, Eddahibi S, Braquet P, Chabrier PE. Loss of endothelium-dependent relaxant activity in the pulmonary circulation of rats exposed to chronic hypoxia. J Clin Invest 1991;87(1):155–162.

62. Christman BW, McPherson CD, Newman JH, King GA, Bernard GR, Groves BM, et al. An imbalance between the excretion of thromboxane and prostacyclin metabolites in pulmonary hypertension. N Engl J Med 1992;327(2):70–75.

63. Jernigan NL, Walker BR, Resta TC. Pulmonary PKG-1 is upregulated following chronic hypoxia. Am J Physiol Lung Cell Mol Physiol 2003;285(3):L634–L642.

64. Steinhorn RH, Morin FC, 3rd, Fineman JR. Models of persistent pulmonary hypertension of the newborn (PPHN) and the role of cyclic guanosine monophosphate (GMP) in pulmonary vasorelaxation. Semin Perinatol 1997;21(5):393–408.

65. Rudolph AM, Auld PA. Physical factors affecting normal and serotonin-constricted pulmonary vessels. Am J Physiol 1960;198:864–872.

66. Rudolph AM, Yuan S. Response of the pulmonary vasculature to hypoxia and H+ ion concentration changes. J Clin Invest 1966;45(3):399–411.

67. Marshall C, Marshall B. Site and sensitivity for stimulation of hypoxic pulmonary vasoconstriction. J Appl Physiol 1983;55(3):711–716.

68. Custer JR, Hales CA. Influence of alveolar oxygen on pulmonary vasoconstriction in newborn lambs versus sheep. Am Rev Respir Dis 1985;132(2):326–331.

69. Cutaia M, Rounds S. Hypoxic pulmonary vasoconstriction. Physiologic significance, mechanism, and clinical relevance. Chest 1990;97(3):706–718.

70. Moudgil R, Michelakis ED, Archer SL. Hypoxic pulmonary vasoconstriction. J Appl Physiol 2005;98(1):390–403.

71. Schreiber MD, Heymann MA, Soifer SJ. Increased arterial pH, not decreased PaCO$_2$, attenuates hypoxia-induced pulmonary vasoconstriction in newborn lambs. Pediatr Res 1986;20(2):113–117.

72. Cartwright D, Gregory GA, Lou H, Heyman MA. The effect of hypocarbia on the cardiovascular system of puppies. Pediatr Res 1984;18(8):685–690.

73. Cornfield DN, Resnik ER, Herron JM, Reinhartz O, Fineman JR. Pulmonary vascular K+ channel expression and vasoreactivity in a model of congenital heart disease. Am J Physiol Lung Cell Mol Physiol 2002;283(6):L1210–L1219.

74. Colebatch HJ, Dawes GS, Goodwin JW, Nadeau RA. The nervous control of the circulation in the foetal and newly expanded lungs of the lamb. J Physiol 1965;178(3):544–562.

75. Rudolph AM, Heyman MA, Lewis AB. Physiology and pharmacology of the pulmonary circulation in the fetus and newborn. In: Hodson WA, ed. Lung Biology and Disease. Development of the Lung. New York: Dekker.

76. Roos A. Poiseuille's law and its limitations in vascular systems. Med Thorac 1962;19:224–238.

77. Caro CG. Mechanics of the pulmonary circulation. In: Caro CG, ed. Advances in Pulmonary Physiology. London: Edwin Arnold; 1966.

78. Prandtl L, Tietjens OG. Applied Hydro- and Aeromechanics. New York: Dover; 1957.

79. Rudolph AM. Congenital Diseases of the Heart: Clinical-Physiological Considerations, 2nd ed. Armonk, NY: Futura; 2001.

80. Agarwal JB, Paltoo R, Palmer WH. Relative viscosity of blood at varying hematocrits in pulmonary circulation. J Appl Physiol 1970;29(6):866–871.

81. Benis AM, Usami S, Chien S. Effect of hematocrit and inertial losses on pressure-flow relations in the isolated hindpaw o the dog. Circ Res 1970;27(6):1047–1068.

82. Culver BH, Butler J. Mechanical influences on the pulmonary microcirculation. Annu Rev Physiol 1980;42:187–198.

83. Permutt S, Caldini P, Maseri A. Recruitment vs. distensibility in the pulmonary vascular bed. In: Fishman AP, Hecht HH, eds. The Pulmonary Circulation and Interstitial Space. Chicago: University of Chicago Press; 1969.

84. Baile EM, Pare PD, Brooks LA, Hogg JC. Relationship between regional lung volume and regional pulmonary vascular resistance. J Appl Physiol 1982;52(4):914–920.

85. Whittenberger JL, Mc GM, Berglund E, Borst HG. Influence of state of inflation of the lung on pulmonary vascular resistance. J Appl Physiol 1960;15:878–882.

86. Bush PA, Gonzalez NE, Ignarro LJ. Biosynthesis of nitric oxide and citrulline from L-arginine by constitutive nitric oxide synthase present in rabbit corpus cavernosum. Biochem Biophys Res Commun 1992;186(1):308–314.

87. Ignarro LJ, Byrns RE, Buga GM, Wood KS. Endothelium-derived relaxing factor from pulmonary artery and vein possesses pharmacologic and chemical properties identical to those of nitric oxide radical. Circ Res 1987;61(6):866–879.

88. Ignarro LJ, Ross G, Tillisch J. Pharmacology of endothelium-derived nitric oxide and nitrovasodilators. West J Med 1991;154(1):51–62.

89. Ignarro LJ, Harbison RG, Wood KS, Kadowitz PJ. Activation of purified soluble guanylate cyclase by endothelium-derived relaxing factor from intrapulmonary artery and vein: stimulation by acetylcholine, bradykinin and arachidonic acid. J Pharmacol Exp Ther 1986;237(3):893–900.

90. Murad F. Cyclic guanosine monophosphate as a mediator of vasodilation. J Clin Invest 1986;78(1):1–5.

91. Mulsch A, Bassenge E, Busse R. Nitric oxide synthesis in endothelial cytosol: evidence for a calcium-dependent and a calcium-independent mechanism. Naunyn Schmiedebergs Arch Pharmacol 1989;340(6 Pt 2):767–770.

92. Brashers VL, Peach MJ, Rose CE, Jr. Augmentation of hypoxic pulmonary vasoconstriction in the isolated perfused rat lung by in vitro

antagonists of endothelium-dependent relaxation. J Clin Invest 1988;82(5):1495–1502.

93. Arai H, Hori S, Aramori I, Ohkubo H, Nakanishi S. Cloning and expression of a cDNA encoding an endothelin receptor. Nature 1990;348(6303):730–732.

94. Sakurai T, Yanagisawa M, Takuwa Y, Miyazaki H, Kimura S, Goto K, et al. Cloning of a cDNA encoding a non-isopeptide-selective subtype of the endothelin receptor. Nature 1990;348(6303):732–735.

95. Rubanyi GM, ed. Endothelin. New York: Oxford University Press for the American Physiological Society; 1992.

96. Vane JR, Anggard EE, Botting RM. Regulatory functions of the vascular endothelium. N Engl J Med 1990;323(1):27–36.

97. Faraci FM, Heistad DD. Regulation of the cerebral circulation: role of endothelium and potassium channels. Physiol Rev 1998;78(1):53–97.

98. Rabinovitch M, Bothwell T, Hayakawa BN, Williams WG, Trusler GA, Rowe RD, et al. Pulmonary artery endothelial abnormalities in patients with congenital heart defects and pulmonary hypertension. A correlation of light with scanning electron microscopy and transmission electron microscopy. Lab Invest 1986;55(6):632–653.

99. Dinh Xuan AT, Higenbottam TW, Clelland C, Pepke-Zaba J, Cremona G, Wallwork J. Impairment of pulmonary endothelium-dependent relaxation in patients with Eisenmenger's syndrome. Br J Pharmacol 1990;99(1):9–10.

100. Meyrick B, Gamble W, Reid L. Development of Crotalaria pulmonary hypertension: hemodynamic and structural study. Am J Physiol 1980;239(5):H692–H702.

101. Yoshibayashi M, Nishioka K, Nakao K, Saito Y, Matsumura M, Ueda T, et al. Plasma endothelin concentrations in patients with pulmonary hypertension associated with congenital heart defects. Evidence for increased production of endothelin in pulmonary circulation. Circulation 1991;84(6):2280–2285.

102. Lane KB, Machado RD, Pauciulo MW, Thomson JR, Phillips JA, 3rd, Loyd JE, et al. Heterozygous germline mutations in BMPR2, encoding a TGF-beta receptor, cause familial primary pulmonary hypertension. The International PPH Consortium. Nat Genet 2000; 26(1):81–84.

103. Thomson JR, Machado RD, Pauciulo MW, Morgan NV, Humbert M, Elliott GC, et al. Sporadic primary pulmonary hypertension is associated with germline mutations of the gene encoding BMPR-II, a receptor member of the TGF-beta family. J Med Genet 2000;37(10): 741–745.

104. Newman JH, Wheeler L, Lane KB, Loyd E, Gaddipati R, Phillips JA, 3rd, et al. Mutation in the gene for bone morphogenetic protein receptor II as a cause of primary pulmonary hypertension in a large kindred. N Engl J Med 2001;345(5):319–324.

105. Humbert M, Deng Z, Simonneau G, Barst RJ, Sitbon O, Wolf M, et al. BMPR2 germline mutations in pulmonary hypertension associated with fenfluramine derivatives. Eur Respir J 2002;20(3):518–523.

106. Rabinovitch M, Haworth SG, Castaneda AR, Nadas AS, Reid LM. Lung biopsy in congenital heart disease: a morphometric approach to pulmonary vascular disease. Circulation 1978;58(6):1107–1122.

107. Meyrick B, Reid L. Ultrastructural findings in lung biopsy material from children with congenital heart defects. Am J Pathol 1980;101(3): 527–542.

108. Hislop A, Haworth SG, Shinebourne EA, Reid L. Quantitative structural analysis of pulmonary vessels in isolated ventricular septal defect in infancy. Br Heart J 1975;37(10):1014–1021.

109. Haworth SG. Pulmonary vascular disease in different types of congenital heart disease. Implications for interpretation of lung biopsy findings in early childhood. Br Heart J 1984;52(5):557–571.

110. Hoffman JI, Rudolph AM, Heymann MA. Pulmonary vascular disease with congenital heart lesions: pathologic features and causes. Circulation 1981;64(5):873–877.

111. Burrows FA, Klinck JR, Rabinovitch M, Bohn DJ. Pulmonary hypertension in children: perioperative management. Can Anaesth Soc J 1986;33(5):606–628.

112. Wheller J, George BL, Mulder DG, Jarmakani JM. Diagnosis and management of postoperative pulmonary hypertensive crisis. Circulation 1979;60(7):1640–1644.

113. Rowe RD, Hoffman T. Transient myocardial ischemia of the newborn infant: a form of severe cardiorespiratory distress in full-term infants. J Pediatr 1972;81(2):243–250.

114. Turner-Gomes SO, Izukawa T, Rowe RD. Persistence of atrioventricular valve regurgitation and electrocardiographic abnormalities following transient myocardial ischemia of the newborn. Pediatr Cardiol 1989;10(4):191–194.

115. Bancalari E, Jesse MJ, Gelband H, Garcia O. Lung mechanics in congenital heart disease with increased and decreased pulmonary blood flow. J Pediatr 1977;90(2):192–195.

116. Day RW, Allen EM, Witte MK. A randomized, controlled study of the 1-hour and 24-hour effects of inhaled nitric oxide therapy in children with acute hypoxemic respiratory failure. Chest 1997;112(5):1324–1331.

117. Inhaled nitric oxide in full-term and nearly full-term infants with hypoxic respiratory failure. The Neonatal Inhaled Nitric Oxide Study Group. N Engl J Med 1997;336(9):597–604.

118. Atz AM, Wessel DL. Inhaled nitric oxide in the neonate with cardiac disease. Semin Perinatol 1997;21(5):441–155.

119. Clark RH, Kueser TJ, Walker MW, Southgate WM, Huckaby JL, Perez JA, et al. Low-dose nitric oxide therapy for persistent pulmonary hypertension of the newborn. Clinical Inhaled Nitric Oxide Research Group. N Engl J Med 2000;342(7):469–474.

120. Dellinger RP, Zimmerman JL, Taylor RW, Straube RC, Hauser DL, Criner GJ, et al. Effects of inhaled nitric oxide in patients with acute respiratory distress syndrome: results of a randomized phase II trial. Inhaled Nitric Oxide in ARDS Study Group. Crit Care Med 1998;26(1): 15–23.

121. Dobyns EL, Cornfield DN, Anas NG, Fortenberry JD, Tasker RC, Lynch A, et al. Multicenter randomized controlled trial of the effects of inhaled nitric oxide therapy on gas exchange in children with acute hypoxemic respiratory failure. J Pediatr 1999;134(4):406–412.

122. Fineman JR, Zwass MS. Inhaled nitric oxide therapy for persistent pulmonary hypertension of the newborn. Acta Paediatr Jpn 1995; 37(4):425–430.

123. Karamanoukian HL, Glick PL, Zayek M, Steinhorn RH, Zwass MS, Fineman JR, et al. Inhaled nitric oxide in congenital hypoplasia of the lungs due to diaphragmatic hernia or oligohydramnios. Pediatrics 1994;94(5):715–718.

124. Kinsella JP, Truog WE, Walsh WF, Goldberg RN, Bancalari E, Mayock DE, et al. Randomized, multicenter trial of inhaled nitric oxide and high-frequency oscillatory ventilation in severe, persistent pulmonary hypertension of the newborn. J Pediatr 1997;131(1 Pt 1):55–62.

125. Lunn RJ. Inhaled nitric oxide therapy. Mayo Clin Proc 1995;70(3):247–255.

126. Roberts JD, Jr., Fineman JR, Morin FC, 3rd, Shaul PW, Rimar S, Schreiber MD, et al. Inhaled nitric oxide and persistent pulmonary hypertension of the newborn. The Inhaled Nitric Oxide Study Group. N Engl J Med 1997;336(9):605–610.

127. Russell IA, Zwass MS, Fineman JR, Balea M, Rouine-Rapp K, Brook M, et al. The effects of inhaled nitric oxide on postoperative pulmonary hypertension in infants and children undergoing surgical repair of congenital heart disease. Anesth Analg 1998;87(1):46–51.

128. Schreiber MD, Gin-Mestan K, Marks JD, Huo D, Lee G, Srisuparp P. Inhaled nitric oxide in premature infants with the respiratory distress syndrome. N Engl J Med 2003;349(22):2099–2107.

129. Heidersbach RS, Johengen MJ, Bekker JM, Fineman JR. Inhaled nitric oxide, oxygen, and alkalosis: dose-response interactions in a lamb model of pulmonary hypertension. Pediatr Pulmonol 1999;28(1): 3–11.

130. Stephenson LW, Edmunds LH, Jr., Raphaely R, Morrison DF, Hoffman WS, Rubis LJ. Effects of nitroprusside and dopamine on pulmonary arterial vasculature in children after cardiac surgery. Circulation 1979;60(2 Pt 2):104–110.

131. Rubis LJ, Stephenson LW, Johnston MR, Nagaraj S, Edmunds LH, Jr. Comparison of effects of prostaglandin E1 and nitroprusside on pulmonary vascular resistance in children after open-heart surgery. Ann Thorac Surg 1981;32(6):563–570.

132. Wimmer M, Schlemmer M, Ebner F. Hemodynamic effects of nifedipine and oxygen in children with pulmonary hypertension. Cardiovasc Drugs Ther 1988;2(5):661–668.

133. Bush A, Busst C, Booth K, Knight WB, Shinebourne EA. Does prostacyclin enhance the selective pulmonary vasodilator effect of oxygen in children with congenital heart disease? Circulation 1986;74(1):135–144.

134. Uglov FG, Davydenko VV, Orlovskii PI, Grigor'ev EE, Bushmarin ON. [Intravascular hemolysis in patients with artificial heart valves]. Vestn Khir Im I I Grek 1986;136(4):135–141.

135. Weesner KM. Hemodynamic effects of prostaglandin E1 in patients with congenital heart disease and pulmonary hypertension. Cathet Cardiovasc Diagn 1991;24(1):10–15.

136. Kermode J, Butt W, Shann F. Comparison between prostaglandin E1 and epoprostenol (prostacyclin) in infants after heart surgery. Br Heart J 1991;66(2):175–178.

137. Brook MM, Fineman JR, Bolinger AM, Wong AF, Heymann MA, Soifer SJ. Use of ATP-MgCl2 in the evaluation and treatment of children with pulmonary hypertension secondary to congenital heart defects. Circulation 1994;90(3):1287–1293.

138. Stevenson DK, Kasting DS, Darnall RA, Jr., Ariagno RL, Johnson JD, Malachowski N, et al. Refractory hypoxemia associated with neonatal pulmonary disease: the use and limitations of tolazoline. J Pediatr 1979;95(4):595–599.

139. Tripp ME, Drummond WH, Heymann MA, Rudolph AM. Hemodynamic effects of pulmonary arterial infusion of vasodilators in newborn lambs. Pediatr Res 1980;14(12):1311–1315.

140. Starling MB, Neutze JM, Elliott RL, Elliott RB. Comparative studies on the hemodynamic effects of prostaglandin E1 prostacyclin, and tolazoline upon elevated pulmonary vascular resistance in neonatal swine. Prostaglandins Med 1981;7(5):349–361.

141. Radermacher P, Huet Y, Pluskwa F, Herigault R, Mal H, Teisseire B, et al. Comparison of ketanserin and sodium nitroprusside in patients with severe ARDS. Anesthesiology 1988;68(1):152–157.

142. Radermacher P, Santak B, Becker H, Falke KJ. Prostaglandin E1 and nitroglycerin reduce pulmonary capillary pressure but worsen ventilation-perfusion distributions in patients with adult respiratory distress syndrome. Anesthesiology 1989;70(4):601–606.

143. Vlahakes GJ, Turley K, Hoffman JI. The pathophysiology of failure in acute right ventricular hypertension: hemodynamic and biochemical correlations. Circulation 1981;63(1):87–95.

144. Melot C, Lejeune P, Leeman M, Moraine JJ, Naeije R. Prostaglandin E1 in the adult respiratory distress syndrome. Benefit for pulmonary hypertension and cost for pulmonary gas exchange. Am Rev Respir Dis 1989;139(1):106–110.

145. Radermacher P, Santak B, Wust HJ, Tarnow J, Falke KJ. Prostacyclin for the treatment of pulmonary hypertension in the adult respiratory distress syndrome: effects on pulmonary capillary pressure and ventilation-perfusion distributions. Anesthesiology 1990;72(2):238–244.

146. De Wet CJ, Affleck DG, Jacobsohn E, Avidan MS, Tymkew H, Hill LL, et al. Inhaled prostacyclin is safe, effective, and affordable in patients with pulmonary hypertension, right heart dysfunction, and refractory hypoxemia after cardiothoracic surgery. J Thorac Cardiovasc Surg 2004;127(4):1058–1067.

147. Hache M, Denault A, Belisle S, Robitaille D, Couture P, Sheridan P, et al. Inhaled epoprostenol (prostacyclin) and pulmonary hypertension before cardiac surgery. J Thorac Cardiovasc Surg 2003;125(3):642–649.

148. Kelly LK, Porta NF, Goodman DM, Carroll CL, Steinhorn RH. Inhaled prostacyclin for term infants with persistent pulmonary hypertension refractory to inhaled nitric oxide. J Pediatr 2002;141(6):830–832.

149. Weston MW, Isaac BF, Crain C. The use of inhaled prostacyclin in nitroprusside-resistant pulmonary artery hypertension. J Heart Lung Transplant 2001;20(12):1340–1344.

150. Hache M, Denault AY, Belisle S, Couture P, Babin D, Tetrault F, et al. Inhaled prostacyclin (PGI2) is an effective addition to the treatment of pulmonary hypertension and hypoxia in the operating room and intensive care unit. Can J Anaesth 2001;48(9):924–929.

151. Fiser SM, Cope JT, Kron IL, Kaza AK, Long SM, Kern JA, et al. Aerosolized prostacyclin (epoprostenol) as an alternative to inhaled nitric oxide for patients with reperfusion injury after lung transplantation. J Thorac Cardiovasc Surg 2001;121(5):981–982.

152. Della Rocca G, Coccia C, Costa MG, Pompei L, Di Marco P, Vizza CD, et al. Inhaled aerosolized prostacyclin and pulmonary hypertension during anesthesia for lung transplantation. Transplant Proc 2001;33(1–2):1634–1636.

153. Abe Y, Tatsumi K, Sugito K, Ikeda Y, Kimura H, Kuriyama T. Effects of inhaled prostacyclin analogue on chronic hypoxic pulmonary hypertension. J Cardiovasc Pharmacol 2001;37(3):239–251.

154. van Heerden PV, Barden A, Michalopoulos N, Bulsara MK, Roberts BL. Dose-response to inhaled aerosolized prostacyclin for hypoxemia due to ARDS. Chest 2000;117(3):819–827.

155. Max M, Rossaint R. Inhaled prostacyclin in the treatment of pulmonary hypertension. Eur J Pediatr 1999;158 Suppl 1:S23–S26.

156. Olschewski H, Ghofrani HA, Walmrath D, Schermuly R, Temmesfeld-Wollbruck B, Grimminger F, et al. Inhaled prostacyclin and iloprost in severe pulmonary hypertension secondary to lung fibrosis. Am J Respir Crit Care Med 1999;160(2):600–607.

157. Beavo JA. Cyclic nucleotide phosphodiesterases: functional implications of multiple isoforms. Physiol Rev 1995;75(4):725–748.

158. Kato R, Sato J, Nishino T. Milrinone decreases both pulmonary arterial and venous resistances in the hypoxic dog. Br J Anaesth 1998;81(6):920–924.

159. Chen EP, Bittner HB, Davis RD, Jr., Van Trigt P 3rd. Milrinone improves pulmonary hemodynamics and right ventricular function in chronic pulmonary hypertension. Ann Thorac Surg 1997;63(3):814–821.

160. Chen EP, Bittner HB, Davis RD, Van Trigt P. Hemodynamic and inotropic effects of milrinone after heart transplantation in the setting of recipient pulmonary hypertension. J Heart Lung Transplant 1998;17(7):669–678.

161. Chang AC, Atz AM, Wernovsky G, Burke RP, Wessel DL. Milrinone: systemic and pulmonary hemodynamic effects in neonates after cardiac surgery. Crit Care Med 1995;23(11):1907–1914.

162. Hoffman TM, Wernovsky G, Atz AM, Kulik TJ, Nelson DP, Chang AC, et al. Efficacy and safety of milrinone in preventing low cardiac output syndrome in infants and children after corrective surgery for congenital heart disease. Circulation 2003;107(7):996–1002.

163. Watanabe H, Ohashi K, Takeuchi K, Yamashita K, Yokoyama T, Tran QK, et al. Sildenafil for primary and secondary pulmonary hypertension. Clin Pharmacol Ther 2002;71(5):398–402.

164. Humpl T, Reyes JT, Holtby H, Stephens D, Adatia I. Beneficial effect of oral sildenafil therapy on childhood pulmonary arterial hypertension: twelve-month clinical trial of a single-drug, open-label, pilot study. Circulation 2005;111(24):3274–3280.

165. Shekerdemian LS, Ravn HB, Penny DJ. Interaction between inhaled nitric oxide and intravenous sildenafil in a porcine model of meconium aspiration syndrome. Pediatr Res 2004;55(3):413–418.

166. Stocker C, Penny DJ, Brizard CP, Cochrane AD, Soto R, Shekerdemian LS. Intravenous sildenafil and inhaled nitric oxide: a randomised trial in infants after cardiac surgery. Intensive Care Med 2003;29(11):1996–2003.

167. Channick RN, Simonneau G, Sitbon O, Robbins IM, Frost A, Tapson VF, et al. Effects of the dual endothelin-receptor antagonist bosentan in patients with pulmonary hypertension: a randomised placebo-controlled study. Lancet 2001;358(9288):1119–1123.

168. Rubin LJ, Badesch DB, Barst RJ, Galie N, Black CM, Keogh A, et al. Bosentan therapy for pulmonary arterial hypertension. N Engl J Med 2002;346(12):896–903.

169. Kouchoukos NT, Blackstone EH, Kirklin JW. Surgical implications of pulmonary hypertension in congenital heart disease. Adv Cardiol 1978(22):225–231.

170. Mentzer RM, Alegre CA, Nolan SP. The effects of dopamine and isoproterenol on the pulmonary circulation. J Thorac Cardiovasc Surg 1976;71(6):807–814.

171. Holloway EL, Polumbo RA, Harrison DC. Acute circulatory effects of dopamine in patients with pulmonary hypertension. Br Heart J 1975;37(5):482–485.

172. Martinez AM, Padbury JF, Thio S. Dobutamine pharmacokinetics and cardiovascular responses in critically ill neonates. Pediatrics 1992;89(1):47–51.

173. Perkin RM, Levin DL, Webb R, Aquino A, Reedy J. Dobutamine: a hemodynamic evaluation in children with shock. J Pediatr 1982;100(6):977–983.

174. Crowley MR, Fineman JR, Soifer SJ. Effects of vasoactive drugs on thromboxane A2 mimetic-induced pulmonary hypertension in newborn lambs. Pediatr Res 1991;29(2):167–172.

175. Rozkovec A, Montanes P, Oakley CM. Factors that influence the outcome of primary pulmonary hypertension. Br Heart J 1986;55(5):449–458.

176. Rich S, Lam W. Atrial septostomy as palliative therapy for refractory primary pulmonary hypertension. Am J Cardiol 1983;51(9):1560–1561.

177. Mullins CE, Nihill MR, Vick GW, 3rd, Ludomirsky A, O'Laughlin MP, Bricker JT, et al. Double balloon technique for dilation of valvular or vessel stenosis in congenital and acquired heart disease. J Am Coll Cardiol 1987;10(1):107–114.

178. Hausknecht MJ, Sims RE, Nihill MR, Cashion WR. Successful palliation of primary pulmonary hypertension by atrial septostomy. Am J Cardiol 1990;65(15):1045–1046.

179. Kerstein D, Levy PS, Hsu DT, Hordof AJ, Gersony WM, Barst RJ. Blade balloon atrial septostomy in patients with severe primary pulmonary hypertension. Circulation 1995;91(7):2028–2035.

180. Sandoval J, Gaspar J, Pulido T, Bautista E, Martinez-Guerra ML, Zeballos M, et al. Graded balloon dilation atrial septostomy in severe primary pulmonary hypertension. A therapeutic alternative for patients nonresponsive to vasodilator treatment. J Am Coll Cardiol 1998;32(2):297–304.

181. Higenbottam T, Wheeldon D, Wells F, Wallwork J. Long-term treatment of primary pulmonary hypertension with continuous intravenous epoprostenol (prostacyclin). Lancet 1984;1(8385):1046–1047.

182. Barst RJ, Rubin LJ, McGoon MD, Caldwell EJ, Long WA, Levy PS. Survival in primary pulmonary hypertension with long-term continuous intravenous prostacyclin. Ann Intern Med 1994;121(6):409–415.

183. Barst RJ, Rubin LJ, Long WA, McGoon MD, Rich S, Badesch DB, et al. A comparison of continuous intravenous epoprostenol (prostacyclin) with conventional therapy for primary pulmonary hypertension. The Primary Pulmonary Hypertension Study Group. N Engl J Med 1996;334(5):296–302.

184. Shapiro SM, Oudiz RJ, Cao T, Romano MA, Beckmann XJ, Georgiou D, et al. Primary pulmonary hypertension: improved long-term effects and survival with continuous intravenous epoprostenol infusion. J Am Coll Cardiol 1997;30(2):343–349.

185. McLaughlin VV, Genthner DE, Panella MM, Rich S. Reduction in pulmonary vascular resistance with long-term epoprostenol (prostacyclin) therapy in primary pulmonary hypertension. N Engl J Med 1998;338(5):273–277.

186. Barst RJ, Maislin G, Fishman AP. Vasodilator therapy for primary pulmonary hypertension in children. Circulation 1999;99(9):1197–1208.

187. Widlitz A, Barst RJ. Pulmonary arterial hypertension in children. Eur Respir J 2003;21(1):155–176.

188. McLaughlin VV, Sitbon O, Badesch DB, Barst RJ, Black C, Galie N, et al. Survival with first-line bosentan in patients with primary pulmonary hypertension. Eur Respir J 2005;25(2):244–249.

189. Keller RL, Hamrick SE, Kitterman JA, Fineman JR, Hawgood S. Treatment of rebound and chronic pulmonary hypertension with oral sildenafil in an infant with congenital diaphragmatic hernia. Pediatr Crit Care Med 2004;5(2):184–187.

190. Bohn D, Tamura M, Perrin D, Barker G, Rabinovitch M. Ventilatory predictors of pulmonary hypoplasia in congenital diaphragmatic hernia, confirmed by morphologic assessment. J Pediatr 1987;111(3):423–431.

191. Naeye RL, Shochat SJ, Whitman V, Maisels MJ. Unsuspected pulmonary vascular abnormalities associated with diaphragmatic hernia. Pediatrics 1976;58(6):902–906.

192. Levin DL. Morphologic analysis of the pulmonary vascular bed in congenital left-sided diaphragmatic hernia. J Pediatr 1978;92(5):805–809.

193. Dibbins AW, Wiener ES. Mortality from neonatal diaphragmatic hernia. J Pediatr Surg 1974;9(5):653–662.

194. Bloss RS, Aranda JV, Beardmore HE. Vasodilator response and prediction of survival in congenital diaphragmatic hernia. J Pediatr Surg 1981;16(2):118–121.

195. Fox WW, Gewitz MH, Dinwiddie R, Drummond WH, Peckham GJ. Pulmonary hypertension in the perinatal aspiration syndromes. Pediatrics 1977;59(2):205–211.

196. Shankaran S, Farooki ZQ, Desai R. beta-hemolytic streptococcal infection appearing as persistent fetal circulation. Am J Dis Child 1982;136(8):725–727.

197. Reece EA, Moya F, Yazigi R, Holford T, Duncan C, Ehrenkranz RA. Persistent pulmonary hypertension: assessment of perinatal risk factors. Obstet Gynecol 1987;70(5):696–700.

198. Soifer SJ, Kaslow D, Roman C, Heymann MA. Umbilical cord compression produces pulmonary hypertension in newborn lambs: a model to study the pathophysiology of persistent pulmonary hypertension in the newborn. J Dev Physiol 1987;9(3):239–252.

199. Levin DL, Mills LJ, Weinberg AG. Hemodynamic, pulmonary vascular, and myocardial abnormalities secondary to pharmacologic constriction of the fetal ductus arteriosus. A possible mechanism for persistent pulmonary hypertension and transient tricuspid insufficiency in the newborn infant. Circulation 1979;60(2):360–364.

200. Morin FC, 3rd. Ligating the ductus arteriosus before birth causes persistent pulmonary hypertension in the newborn lamb. Pediatr Res 1989;25(3):245–250.

201. Wild LM, Nickerson PA, Morin FC, 3rd. Ligating the ductus arteriosus before birth remodels the pulmonary vasculature of the lamb. Pediatr Res 1989;25(3):251–257.

202. McQueston JA, Kinsella JP, Ivy DD, McMurtry IF, Abman SH. Chronic pulmonary hypertension in utero impairs endothelium-dependent vasodilation. Am J Physiol 1995;268(1 Pt 2):H288–H294.

203. Shaul PW, Yuhanna IS, German Z, Chen Z, Steinhorn RH, Morin FC, 3rd. Pulmonary endothelial NO synthase gene expression is decreased in fetal lambs with pulmonary hypertension. Am J Physiol 1997;272(5 Pt 1):L1005–L1012.

204. Manchester D, Margolis HS, Sheldon RE. Possible association between maternal indomethacin therapy and primary pulmonary hypertension of the newborn. Am J Obstet Gynecol 1976;126(4):467–469.

205. Levin DL, Fixler DE, Morriss FC, Tyson J. Morphologic analysis of the pulmonary vascular bed in infants exposed in utero to prostaglandin synthetase inhibitors. J Pediatr 1978;92(3):478–483.

206. Fox WW, Berman LS, Downes JJ, Jr., Peckham GJ. The therapeutic application of end-expiratory pressure in the meconium aspiration syndrome. Pediatrics 1975;56(2):214–217.

207. Truog WE, Lyrene RK, Standaert TA, Murphy J, Woodrum DE. Effects of PEEP and tolazoline infusion on respiratory and inert gas exchange in experimental meconium aspiration. J Pediatr 1982;100(2):284–290.

208. Auten RL, Notter RH, Kendig JW, Davis JM, Shapiro DL. Surfactant treatment of full-term newborns with respiratory failure. Pediatrics 1991;87(1):101–107.

209. Henry GW, Stevens DC, Schreiner RL, Grosfeld JL, Ballantine TV. Respiratory paralysis to improve oxygenation and mortality in large newborn infants with respiratory distress. J Pediatr Surg 1979; 14(6):761–767.

210. Toomasian JM, Snedecor SM, Cornell RG, Cilley RE, Bartlett RH. National experience with extracorporeal membrane oxygenation for newborn respiratory failure. Data from 715 cases. ASAIO Trans 1988;34(2):140–147.

211. O'Rourke PP, Crone RK, Vacanti JP, Ware JH, Lillehei CW, Parad RB, et al. Extracorporeal membrane oxygenation and conventional medical therapy in neonates with persistent pulmonary hypertension of the newborn: a prospective randomized study. Pediatrics 1989;84(6): 957–963.

212. Meinert CL. Extracorporeal membrane oxygenation trials. Pediatrics 1990;85(3):365–366.

213. Bahrami KR, Van Meurs KP. ECMO for neonatal respiratory failure. Semin Perinatol 2005;29(1):15–23.

214. Reid LM. The pulmonary circulation: remodeling in growth and disease. The 1978 J. Burns Amberson lecture. Am Rev Respir Dis 1979;119(4):531–546.

215. Rabinovitch M, Keane JF, Norwood WI, Castaneda AR, Reid L. Vascular structure in lung tissue obtained at biopsy correlated with pulmonary hemodynamic findings after repair of congenital heart defects. Circulation 1984;69(4):655–667.

216. Haworth SG, Reid L. Quantitative structural study of pulmonary circulation in the newborn with aortic atresia, stenosis, or coarctation. Thorax 1977;32(2):121–128.

217. Heath D, Edwards JE. The pathology of hypertensive pulmonary vascular disease; a description of six grades of structural changes in the pulmonary arteries with special reference to congenital cardiac septal defects. Circulation 1958;18(4 Part 1):533–547.

218. Clapp S, Perry BL, Farooki ZQ, Jackson WL, Karpawich PP, Hakimi M, et al. Down's syndrome, complete atrioventricular canal, and pulmonary vascular obstructive disease. J Thorac Cardiovasc Surg 1990;100(1):115–121.

219. Hallidie-Smith KA, Hollman A, Cleland WP, Bentall HH, Goodwin JF. Effects of surgical closure of ventricular septal defects upon pulmonary vascular disease. Br Heart J 1969;31(2):246–260.

220. Wessel DL, Adatia I, Giglia TM, Thompson JE, Kulik TJ. Use of inhaled nitric oxide and acetylcholine in the evaluation of pulmonary hypertension and endothelial function after cardiopulmonary bypass. Circulation 1993;88(5 Pt 1):2128–2138.

221. Atz AM, Adatia I, Lock JE, Wessel DL. Combined effects of nitric oxide and oxygen during acute pulmonary vasodilator testing. J Am Coll Cardiol 1999;33(3):813–819.

222. Balzer DT, Kort HW, Day RW, Corneli HM, Kovalchin JP, Cannon BC, et al. Inhaled Nitric Oxide as a Preoperative Test (INOP Test I): the INOP Test Study Group. Circulation 2002;106(12 Suppl 1):I76–I81.

223. Beghetti M, Adatia I. Inhaled nitric oxide and congenital cardiac disease. Cardiol Young 2001;11(2):142–152.

224. Yoshimura N, Yamaguchi M, Oka S, Yoshida M, Murakami H, Kagawa T, et al. Inhaled nitric oxide therapy after Fontan-type operations. Surg Today 2005;35(1):31–35.

225. Kawakami H, Ichinose F. Inhaled nitric oxide in pediatric cardiac surgery. Int Anesthesiol Clin 2004;42(4):93–100.

226. Miller OI, Tang SF, Keech A, Pigott NB, Beller E, Celermajer DS. Inhaled nitric oxide and prevention of pulmonary hypertension after congenital heart surgery: a randomised double-blind study. Lancet 2000;356(9240):1464–1469.

227. Simonneau G, Galie N, Rubin LJ, Langleben D, Seeger W, Domenighetti G, et al. Clinical classification of pulmonary hypertension. J Am Coll Cardiol 2004;43(12 Suppl S):5S–12S.

228. D'Alonzo GE, Barst RJ, Ayres SM, Bergofsky EH, Brundage BH, Detre KM, et al. Survival in patients with primary pulmonary hypertension. Results from a national prospective registry. Ann Intern Med 1991;115(5):343–349.

229. Yamaki S, Wagenvoort CA. Comparison of primary plexogenic arteriopathy in adults and children. A morphometric study in 40 patients. Br Heart J 1985;54(4):428–434.

230. Sandoval J, Bauerle O, Gomez A, Palomar A, Martinez Guerra ML, Furuya ME. Primary pulmonary hypertension in children: clinical characterization and survival. J Am Coll Cardiol 1995;25(2):466–474.

231. Rich S, Dantzker DR, Ayres SM, Bergofsky EH, Brundage BH, Detre KM, et al. Primary pulmonary hypertension. A national prospective study. Ann Intern Med 1987;107(2):216–223.

232. Barst RJ, Stalcup SA, Steeg CN, Hall JC, Frosolono MF, Cato AE, et al. Relation of arachidonate metabolites to abnormal control of the pulmonary circulation in a child. Am Rev Respir Dis 1985;131(1):171–177.

233. Newman CW, Jacobson GP, Hug GA, Weinstein BE, Malinoff RL. Practical method for quantifying hearing aid benefit in older adults. J Am Acad Audiol 1991;2(2):70–75.

234. Stewart DJ, Levy RD, Cernacek P, Langleben D. Increased plasma endothelin-1 in pulmonary hypertension: marker or mediator of disease? Ann Intern Med 1991;114(6):464–469.

235. Giaid A. Nitric oxide and endothelin-1 in pulmonary hypertension. Chest 1998;114(3 Suppl):208S–212S.

236. Yuan JX, Aldinger AM, Juhaszova M, Wang J, Conte JV, Jr., Gaine SP, et al. Dysfunctional voltage-gated K+ channels in pulmonary artery smooth muscle cells of patients with primary pulmonary hypertension. Circulation 1998;98(14):1400–1406.

237. Rabinovitch M, Andrew M, Thom H, Trusler GA, Williams WG, Rowe RD, et al. Abnormal endothelial factor VIII associated with pulmonary hypertension and congenital heart defects. Circulation 1987;76(5): 1043–1052.

238. Geggel RL, Carvalho AC, Hoyer LW, Reid LM. von Willebrand factor abnormalities in primary pulmonary hypertension. Am Rev Respir Dis 1987;135(2):294–299.

239. Fuster V, Steele PM, Edwards WD, Gersh BJ, McGoon MD, Frye RL. Primary pulmonary hypertension: natural history and the importance of thrombosis. Circulation 1984;70(4):580–587.

240. Frank H, Mlczoch J, Huber K, Schuster E, Gurtner HP, Kneussl M. The effect of anticoagulant therapy in primary and anorectic drug-induced pulmonary hypertension. Chest 1997;112(3):714–721.

241. Thompson BT, Spence CR, Janssens SP, Joseph PM, Hales CA. Inhibition of hypoxic pulmonary hypertension by heparins of differing in vitro antiproliferative potency. Am J Respir Crit Care Med 1994;149(6): 1512–1517.

242. Rich S, Kaufmann E, Levy PS. The effect of high doses of calcium-channel blockers on survival in primary pulmonary hypertension. N Engl J Med 1992;327(2):76–81.

243. Saji T, Ozawa Y, Ishikita T, Matsuura H, Matsuo N. Short-term hemodynamic effect of a new oral PGI2 analogue, beraprost, in primary and secondary pulmonary hypertension. Am J Cardiol 1996;78(2):244–247.

244. Nagaya N, Uematsu M, Okano Y, Satoh T, Kyotani S, Sakamaki F, et al. Effect of orally active prostacyclin analogue on survival of outpatients with primary pulmonary hypertension. J Am Coll Cardiol 1999;34(4):1188–1192.

245. Hoeper MM, Schwarze M, Ehlerding S, Adler-Schuermeyer A, Spiekerkoetter E, Niedermeyer J, et al. Long-term treatment of primary pulmonary hypertension with aerosolized iloprost, a prostacyclin analogue. N Engl J Med 2000;342(25):1866–1870.

246. Higenbottam TW, Butt AY, Dinh-Xaun AT, Takao M, Cremona G, Akamine S. Treatment of pulmonary hypertension with the continuous infusion of a prostacyclin analogue, iloprost. Heart 1998;79(2): 175–179.

247. Rich S, Seidlitz M, Dodin E, Osimani D, Judd D, Genthner D, et al. The short-term effects of digoxin in patients with right ventricular dysfunction from pulmonary hypertension. Chest 1998;114(3):787–792.

248. Cowan KN, Jones PL, Rabinovitch M. Elastase and matrix metalloproteinase inhibitors induce regression, and tenascin-C antisense prevents progression, of vascular disease. J Clin Invest 2000;105(1):21–34.

249. Cowan KN, Heilbut A, Humpl T, Lam C, Ito S, Rabinovitch M. Complete reversal of fatal pulmonary hypertension in rats by a serine elastase inhibitor. Nat Med 2000;6(6):698–702.

250. Barst RJ. Role of atrial septostomy in the treatment of pulmonary vascular disease. Thorax 2000;55(2):95–96.

251. Mallory GB, Spray TL. Paediatric lung transplantation. Eur Respir J 2004;24(5):839–845.

252. Mendeloff EN, Meyers BF, Sundt TM, Guthrie TJ, Sweet SC, de la Morena M, et al. Lung transplantation for pulmonary vascular disease. Ann Thorac Surg 2002;73(1):209–219.

253. Boucek MM, Edwards LB, Keck BM, Trulock EP, Taylor DO, Hertz MI. Registry for the International Society for Heart and Lung Transplantation: seventh official pediatric report—2004. J Heart Lung Transplant 2004;23(8):933–947.

254. Grover RF, Vogel JH, Voigt GC, Blount SG Jr. Reversal of high altitude pulmonary hypertension. Am J Cardiol 1966;18(6):928–932.

255. Tucker A, McMurtry IF, Reeves JT, Alexander AF, Will DH, Grover RF. Lung vascular smooth muscle as a determinant of pulmonary hypertension at high altitude. Am J Physiol 1975;228(3):762–767.

256. Meyrick B, Reid L. Endothelial and subintimal changes in rat hilar pulmonary artery during recovery from hypoxia. A quantitative ultrastructural study. Lab Invest 1980;42(6):603–615.

257. Hultgren HN, Grover RF, Hartley LH. Abnormal circulatory responses to high altitude in subjects with a previous history of high-altitude pulmonary edema. Circulation 1971;44(5):759–770.

258. Hanaoka M, Kubo K, Yamazaki Y, Miyahara T, Matsuzawa Y, Kobayashi T, et al. Association of high-altitude pulmonary edema with the major histocompatibility complex. Circulation 1998;97(12):1124–1128.

259. Cornfield DN, Reeve HL, Tolarova S, Weir EK, Archer S. Oxygen causes fetal pulmonary vasodilation through activation of a calcium-dependent potassium channel. Proc Natl Acad Sci USA 1996;93(15):8089–8094.

260. Wang Y, Coceani F. Isolated pulmonary resistance vessels from fetal lambs. Contractile behavior and responses to indomethacin and endothelin-1. Circ Res 1992;71(2):320–330.

261. Ivy DD, Parker TA, Kinsella JP, Abman SH. Endothelin A receptor blockade decreases pulmonary vascular resistance in premature lambs with hyaline membrane disease. Pediatr Res 1998;44(2):175–180.

262. Chang JK, Moore P, Fineman JR, Soifer SJ, Heymann MA. K+ channel pulmonary vasodilation in fetal lambs: role of endothelium-derived nitric oxide. J Appl Physiol 1992;73(1):188–194.

263. Ware LB, Matthay MA. The acute respiratory distress syndrome. N Engl J Med 2000;342(18):1334–1349.

264. Zapol WM, Snider MT. Pulmonary hypertension in severe acute respiratory failure. N Engl J Med 1977;296(9):476–480.

265. Tomashefski JF Jr, Davies P, Boggis C, Greene R, Zapol WM, Reid LM. The pulmonary vascular lesions of the adult respiratory distress syndrome. Am J Pathol 1983;112(1):112–126.

266. Erdmann AJ, 3rd, Vaughan TR, Jr., Brigham KL, Woolverton WC, Staub NC. Effect of increased vascular pressure on lung fluid balance in unanesthetized sheep. Circ Res 1975;37(3):271–284.

267. Sibbald WJ, Driedger AA, Myers ML, Short AI, Wells GA. Biventricular function in the adult respiratory distress syndrome. Chest 1983;84(2):126–134.

268. Katz R, Pollack M, Spady D. Cardiopulmonary abnormalities in severe acute respiratory failure. J Pediatr 1984;104(3):357–364.

269. Rossaint R, Falke KJ, Lopez F, Slama K, Pison U, Zapol WM. Inhaled nitric oxide for the adult respiratory distress syndrome. N Engl J Med 1993;328(6):399–405.

270. Fioretto JR, de Moraes MA, Bonatto RC, Ricchetti SM, Carpi MF. Acute and sustained effects of early administration of inhaled nitric oxide to children with acute respiratory distress syndrome. Pediatr Crit Care Med 2004;5(5):469–474.

271. Taylor RW, Zimmerman JL, Dellinger RP, Straube RC, Criner GJ, Davis K Jr, et al. Low-dose inhaled nitric oxide in patients with acute lung injury: a randomized controlled trial. JAMA 2004;291(13):1603–1609.

272. Lundin S, Mang H, Smithies M, Stenqvist O, Frostell C. Inhalation of nitric oxide in acute lung injury: results of a European multicentre study. The European Study Group of Inhaled Nitric Oxide. Intensive Care Med 1999;25(9):911–919.

Index